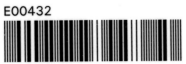

EPILEPSY
IN
CHILDREN

EPILEPSY IN CHILDREN

Edited by

Sheila Wallace

*Department of Child Health,
University Hospital of Wales,
Cardiff, UK*

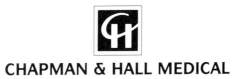

CHAPMAN & HALL MEDICAL

London · Glasgow · Weinheim · New York · Tokyo · Melbourne · Madras

Published by Chapman & Hall, 2–6 Boundary Row, London SE1 8HN, UK

Chapman & Hall, 2–6 Boundary Row, London SE1 8HN, UK

Blackie Academic & Professional, Wester Cleddens Road, Bishopbriggs, Glasgow G64 2NZ, UK

Chapman & Hall GmbH, Pappelallee 3, 69469 Weinheim, Germany

Chapman & Hall USA, 115 Fifth Avenue, New York NY 10003, USA

Chapman & Hall Japan, ITP-Japan, Kyowa Building, 3F, 2-2-1 Hirakawacho, Chiyoda-ku, Tokyo 102, Japan

Chapman & Hall Australia, 102 Dodds Street, South Melbourne, Victoria 3205, Australia

Chapman & Hall India, R. Seshadri, 32 Second Main Road, CIT East, Madras 600 035, India

First edition 1996

© 1996 Chapman & Hall

Typeset in 10/12pt Palatino by Photoprint, 9–11 Alexandra Lane, Torquay
Printed in Great Britain at the University Press, Cambridge

ISBN 0 412 56860 8

In memory of William

CONTENTS

CONTRIBUTORS

JEAN AICARDI
The Neurosciences Unit
The Wolfson Centre
Mecklenburgh Square
London WC1N 2AP
UK

PETER G. BARTH
University of Amsterdam Hospital
Department of Pediatric Neurology
Amsterdam
NL 1105 AZ
Netherlands

FRANK M.C. BESAG
St Piers Lingfield
Lingfield
Surrey
UK

PAULO ROGÉRIO M. DE BITTENCOURT
Unidade de Neurologia Clinica
Hospital Nossa Senhora das Graças
Rua Alcides Munhoz, 433, 80810
Curitiba
Brazil

BLAISE F.D. BOURGEOIS
Dept of Neurology, Washington University
Box 8111 660 S. Euclid Avenue
St Louis, MO 63110
USA

MICHELLE BUREAU
Centre Saint-Paul
300 Boulevard Sainte-Marguerite
13009 Marseille
France

DAVID CHADWICK
Department of Neurological Science
Walton Hospital
Rice Lane
Liverpool L9 1AE
UK

HARRY T. CHUGANI
Division of Pediatric Neurology
Children's Hospital of Michigan,
3901 Beaubien Blvd.,
Detroit, MI 48201
USA

PAOLO CURATOLO
Institute of Child Neuropsychiatry
University of Rome
Via Dei Sabelli 108
00185 Rome
Italy

THIERRY DEONNA
Unité de Neuropédiatrie
Centre Hospitalier Universitaire Vaudois
1011 Lausanne, le
Switzerland

CHARLOTTE DRAVET
Centre Saint-Paul
300 Boulevard Sainte-Marguerite
13009 Marseille
France

OLIVIER DULAC
Hôpital Saint Vincent-de-Paul
75674 Paris Cedex 14
France

NATALIO FEJERMAN
Department of Neurology
Hospital de Pediatria
Prof. Juan. P. Garrahan Hospital
Combate de los Pozos
1881 Buenos Aires
1245 Argentina

LARS FORSGREN
Umeå University
Department of Neurology
SE-901 85 Umeå
Sweden

R. MARK GARDINER
Department of Paediatrics
University College London Medical School,
    Rayne Institute
University Street
London WC1E 6JJ
UK

PIERRE GENTON
Centre Saint-Paul
300 Boulevard Sainte-Marguerite
13009 Marseille
France

F.M. GIBBON
Department of Child Health
University Hospital of Wales
Heath Park
Cardiff CF4 4XW
UK

OLAF HENRIKESEN
Statens Center for Epilepsi
Postboks 900
1301 Sandvika
Norway

JOHN G.R. JEFFERYS
Department of Physiology and Biophysics
St Mary's Hospital Medical School
Norfolk Place
London W2 1PG
UK

currently at:
Department of Physiology
University of Birmingham
Edgbaston
Birmingham B15 2TT
UK

DOROTHÉE G.A. KASTELEIJN-NOLST
    TRENITÉ
Instituut voor Epilepsiebestrijding
'Meer en Bosch'
'De Cruquiushoeve'
Heemstede
Netherlands

JOHN LIVINGSTON
Room 140B Clarendon Wing
The Infirmary at Leeds
Belmont Grove
Leeds LS2 9NS
UK

ROBERTO MICHELUCCI
Ospedale Bellaria
Cattedra di Clinica Neurologica
Universita di Bologna
40139 Bologna – via Altura 3
Italy

ELI M. MIZRAHI
The Methodist Hospital
Baylor College of Medicine
Epilepsy Research Center
1 Baylor Plaza
6565 Fannin, Houston
Texas 77030
USA

MAURICIO COELHO NETO
Unidade de Neurologia Clinica
Hospital Nossa Senhora das Graças
Rua Alcides Munhoz, 433, 80810
Curitiba
Brazil

SHUNSUKE OHTAHARA
Department of Child Neurology
Okayama University Medical School
5–1 Shikatachio – 2 Chome
Okayama
Japan

YOKO OHTSUKA
Department of Child Neurology
Okayama University Medical School
5–1 Shikatachio – 2 Chome
Okayama
Japan

C.P. PANAYIOTOPOULOS
Consultant in Clinical Neurophysiology &
  Epilepsy
St Thomas' Hospital, Lambeth Palace Road
London SE1 7EH
UK

CHARLES E. POLKEY
The Neurosurgical Unit
The Maudsley Hospital
De Crespigny Park
London SE5 8AZ
UK

C. RAMESH
Department of Child Health
University Hospital of Wales
Heath Park
Cardiff CF4 4XW
UK

DAVID RAVINE
Institute of Medical Genetics
University Hospital of Wales
Heath Park
Cardiff CF4 4XW
UK

ALAN RICHENS
Department of Clinical Pharmacology &
  Therapeutics
University of Wales College of Medicine
Heath Park
Cardiff CF4 4XN
UK

RAILI RIIKONEN
Department of Child Neurology
University of Helsinki
Lastenlinnantie 2
00250 Helsinki
Finland

JOSEPH ROGER
Centre Saint-Paul
300 Boulevard Sainte-Marguerite
13009 Marseille
France

GUIDO RUBBOLI
Ospedale Bellaria
Cattedra di Clinica Neurologica
Universita di Bologna
40139 Bologna – via Altura 3
Italy

MATTI SILLANPÄÄ
Lastenneurologian Yksikkö TYKS
20520 Turku
Finland

JOHN B.P. STEPHENSON
Fraser of Allander Unit
Royal Hospital for Sick Children
Glasgow G3 8SJ
UK

DAVID C. TAYLOR
Pentre Grange
Llanover
Near Abergavenny
Gwent
UK

CARLO ALBERTO TASSINARI
Ospedale Bellaria
Cattedra di Clinica Neurologica
Universita di Bologna
40139 Bologna – via Altura 3
Italy

ROGER D. TRAUB
IBM Research Division
T.J. Watson Research Centre
PO Box 218
Yorktown Heights
NY 10598
USA

and
Department of Neurology
Columbia University
New York
NY 10032
USA

HARRY V. VINTERS
Department of Pathology and Lab Medicine
  (Neuropathology)
UCLA School of Medicine
Los Angeles
CA 90024–1732
USA

SHEILA J. WALLACE
Department of Child Health
University Hospital of Wales
Heath Park
Cardiff CF4 4XW
UK

CLAUDE G. WASTERLAIN
Department of Neurology
Reid Neurological Research Center
UCLA School of Medicine
710 Westwood Plaza
Los Angeles
CA 90024–1769
USA

KAZUYOSHI WATANABE
Department of Pediatrics
Nagoya University School of Medicine
65 Tsuruma-cho
Showa-ku
Nagoya 466
Japan

FOREWORD

When I first agreed to write the Foreword to this book, I was expecting it to be yet another volume on epilepsy complete with the usual approaches. It was with great delight that I read the manuscript and realized that this text is quite different and an excellent addition to the literature. Dr Wallace has made a distinct contribution by breaking some of the usual molds that have, in the past, hampered multi-authored texts on epilepsy.

First, Dr Wallace has assembled a truly international list of contributors. Although she has leaned heavily on her European colleagues, she has also drawn on experts from North and South America as well as the Far East to complement her own expertise and extensive experience. By masterful advance planning, she has gathered contributors to her volume who are the best clinical investigators in the field of childhood epilepsy and who have the most to say about the disorder.

Second, the text is unequivocally and unabashedly about epileptic syndromes. Those of us who spent most of our productive scientific years working out the nature of seizures can only be delighted to see that the really meaningful clinical approach to epilepsy – that which seeks the nature of epileptic syndromes – has now arrived at a sufficient state of sophistication that pediatric epileptologists now converse in this language.

Finally, this book is comprehensive without being overpowering. It brings the best of the basic science to the reader in a manner that is approachable but not superficial. Yet the book is primarily a clinical volume; it carefully leads the clinician from a discourse on febrile seizures to a sophisticated analysis of the differential diagnosis of Aicardi's syndrome to the psychiatric aspects of childhood seizures.

Every doctor who treats seizures in childhood will benefit from having this book not only for the knowlede it brings – and I have learned much – but for the extraordinary reference it will provide when one is confronted with a child with epilepsy.

Roger J. Porter MD
Adjunct Professor Neurology
University of Pennsylvania
Philadelphia
USA

PREFACE

Epilepsy is the commonest neurologic disorder of childhood. Both those whose physical and cognitive states are otherwise normal, and those in whom seizures may be but one facet of a severe debilitating generalized brain disease, can present with epileptic seizures. An understanding of the nature of epilepsy requires knowledge of brain development, extending from genetic coding to the relative stability of mid-to-late childhood. The underlying metabolic factors which govern neurotransmission and the appropriate development of cerebral microconnections are clearly of critical importance. Acquired problems, particularly trauma and infection, must also be considered. Epidemiologic studies help to define populations most at risk. The many clinical and electroencephalographic manifestations of different types of epilepsy are diverse in underlying pathology, responses to treatment, and prognosis. Cognitive, psychiatric, and social factors impinge on the overall lifestyles of affected children.

This book on epilepsy aims to provide an up-to-date text for the specialist reader. It starts with an overview of definitions. An extensive review examines nonepileptic seizures, so that due clarification of the presentation of alternative disorders can be emphasized. An assessment of the incidence and prevalence, overall, and under specific circumstances, is provided. Structural anomalies, chromosomal abnormalities, disorders of metabolism and infections are considered as etiologic factors. Both pathologic and pathophysiologic aspects are presented. Overviews of the classifications of both epileptic seizures and syndromes are given. The difficult subject of genetics receives due attention. Details of seizures in the neonate and of those occurring in febrile children are followed by information on specific syndromes. These are reviewed as they present, in order of age of onset. Special consideration is given to epilepsies symptomatic of structural lesions, and to those occurring in the mentally retarded. There is a review of the problems of status epilepticus. Appropriate neurophysiologic, imaging, hematologic, biochemical, and microbiologic investigations are presented. After consideration of the pharmacology of antiepileptic drugs, their uses are detailed; also, there is information on diets, behavioral and social therapy, and surgery. Cognitive and psychiatric problems which present in association with the etiologic aspects, following the development of epilepsy, or related to therapeutic interventions, are considered. A brief statement on special centers for epilepsy reviews such facilities. Information on epilepsy persisting into adulthood concludes the volume.

ABBREVIATIONS

ACh	acetylcholine
ACTH	adrenocorticotrophic hormone
AD	afterdischarge
AEA	acquired epileptic aphasia
AED	antiepileptic drug
AHP	afterhyperpolarization
AL	argininosuccinate lyase
AMPA	α-amino-3-hydroxy-5-methyl-4-isoxazole propionic acid
4AP	4-aminopyridine
AS	absence seizures
BAEP	brainstem auditory evoked potentials
BCECT	benign childhood epilepsy with centrotemporal spikes
BCEOP	benign partial epilepsy with occipital paroxysms
BFIC	benign familial infantile convulsions
BFNC	benign familial neonatal convulsions
BH_4	tetrahydrobiopterin
BMEI	benign myoclonic epilepsy in childhood
BPEAS	benign partial epilepsy with affective symptomatology
BRE	benign rolandic epilepsy
CA	conceptional age
CAE	childhood absence epilepsy
CAl, CA3	subregions of the hippocampus proper
CD	cortical dysplasia
CCK	cholecystokinin
CFM/CFAM	cerebral function monitors
CMV	cytomegalovirus
CNS	central nervous system
CP	cerebral palsy
CPS	complex partial seizures
CPSE	complex partial status epilepticus
CRH	corticotrophin releasing hormone
CSF	cerebrospinal fluid
CSWSS	continuous spike-waves of slow sleep
CT	computed tomography
CVST	computerized visual search task
DCSWS	dementia with continuing spike-waves during slow wave sleep

DG	dentate gyrus
DHAP-AT	dihydroxyacetonephosphate acyltransferase
DHCA	dihydroxycholestanoic acid
DNET	dysembryoplastic neuroepithelial tumors
DR	delayed rectifier
DRPLA	dentato-rubral-pallido-laysian atrophy
ECMO	extracorporeal membrane oxygenation
EEG	electroencephalograph
EBV	Epstein–Barr virus
ECoG	electrocorticography
EGTCSA	epilepsy with generalized tonic-clonic seizures on awakening
EOG	electro-oculogram
EPC	epilepsia partialis continua
EP	evoked potential
EPSC	excitatory postsynaptic current
EPSP	excitatory postsynaptic potential
ERG	electroretinogram
ESR	erythrocyte sedimentation rate
FFA	free fatty acid
FDG	2-deoxy-2[^{18}F]fluoro-D-glucose
FOS	fixation-off sensitivity
FS	febrile seizure
GAD	glutamic acid decarboxylase
GABA	γ-amino-butyric acid
GABA-T	GABA-transaminase
GAERS	Genetic Absence Epilepsy Rats from Strasbourg
g_{Ca}	Ca conductance
GAP	GTPase activating protein
GD	Gaucher's disease
GFAP	glial fibrillary acidic protein
GTCS	generalized tonic-clonic seizures
HD	Huntington's disease
HME	hemimegalencephaly
HMPAO	technetium-99m hexamethyl propyleneamine oxime
HPA	hypophyseal-adrenal axis
HS	horn sclerosis
HSV	herpes simplex virus
5-HTP	5-hydroxytryptamine
IGE	idiopathic generalized epilepsy
IH	infantile hydrocephalus
ILAE	International League Against Epilepsy
IPS	intermittent photic stimulation

IPSP	inhibitory postsynaptic potential
IS	infantile spasms
JAE	juvenile absence epilepsy
JME	juvenile myoclonic epilepsy
KS	Kojewnikow's syndrome
LD	Lafora's disease
LGS	Lennox–Gastaut syndrome
MA	myoclonic absences
MAE	myoclonic astatic epilepsy
MAS	myoclonic astatic seizures
ME	myoclonic epilepsies
MEG	magnetoencephalography
MELAS syndrome	Mitochondrial Encephalopathy Lactic Acidosis Stroke-like episodes
MERRF syndrome	Myoclonus Epilepsy and Ragged-Red Fibers
MR	mental retardation
MRI	magnetic resonance imaging
MRS	magnetic resonance spectroscopy
MS	myoclonic seizures
MST	multiple subpial transection
MTS	mesial temporal sclerosis
mtDNA	mitochondrial DNA
NCL	neuronal ceroid lipofuscinosis
NCPP	National Collaborative Perinatal Project
NCS	neurocutaneous syndromes
NCSE	nonconvulsive status epilepticus
NF-1	neurofibromatosis type 1
NKH	nonketotic hyperglycinemia
NMD	neuronal migration disorders
NMDA	N-methyl-D-aspartate
NRT	nucleus reticularis thalami
OCT	ornithine transcarbamylase
PCR	photoconvulsive responses
PDHC	pyruvate dehydrogenase complex
PE	photosensitive epilepsy
PEHO syndrome	Progressive Encephalopathy with edema, Hypsarrhythmia and Optic atrophy
PEMA	phenylethylmalonamide
PET	positron emission tomography
PGS	primary generalized seizures
PKU	phenylketonuria

PLP	pyridoxal-5′-phosphate
PME	progressive myoclonic epilepsy
PMG	polymicrogyria
PSW	polyspike-waves
RAKIT	Revised Amsterdamse Kinder Intelligentie Test
RE	reading epilepsy
REM	rapid eye movement
SBS	secondary bilateral synchrony
S-B	suppression burst
SE	status epilepticus
SMEI	severe myoclonic epilepsy in infancy
SPECT	single photon emission computed tomography
SQUID	superconducting quantum interference device
SSCP	single strand conformation polymorphism
SSE	stimulus-sensitive epilepsy
SSPE	subacute sclerosing panencephalitis
SSW	slow spike-wave
SW	spike-wave
TA	typical absences
TCI	transitory cognitive impairment
TCR	thalamocortical relay
THCA	trihydroxycholestanoic acid
TLE	temporal lobe epilepsy
TS	tuberous sclerosis
TSC	tuberous sclerosis complex
ULD	Unverricht–Lündborg disease
VAPSE	Variation Affecting Protein Structure or Expression
VEP	visually evoked potential
VGS	video-game-induced seizure
VIP	videointerface processor
VPA	valproic acid
WHO	World Health Organization
WISC	Wechsler Intelligience Scales for Children
WISC-R	revised WISC
ZCA	zone of cortical abnormality

DEFINITIONS

Sheila J. Wallace

In terms prepared for a nonmedical readership, epilepsy is defined as 'a chronic nervous disorder that involves changes in the state of consciousness and of motion and that is due either to an inborn defect which produces convulsions of greater or lesser severity with clouding of consciousness or to an organic lesion of the brain produced by tumour, injury, toxic agents or glandular disturbances' (*Webster's Third New International Dictionary*, 1981). The emphases on the motor component and the disturbance of awareness are sufficiently restrictive to give this definition a somewhat archaic ring. However, there are real difficulties in defining epilepsy sufficiently precisely so that all types of the epilepsies can be accommodated and all seizures which are not epileptic are excluded.

The word 'epilepsy' is derived from the Greek *epi*, upon, and *lambanein*, to seize. Thus the suddenness of the attacks is emphasized by the Greek, but somewhat lost in the English description, unless the definition of seizures is itself examined. This allows a rather less precise interpretation: a sudden fit or attack of illness. The recent North American use of the verb to seize, meaning the actual physical act of having a seizure, is at variance with the usual dictionary interpretation which suggests that an outside agent is responsible for seizing the victim. This latter view leads to a better understanding of epileptic seizures, since there must always be a precipitating event.

It is useful to look at the definitions suggested throughout history and to examine their refinement as anatomic and physiologic aspects have become more sophisticated.

HISTORIC PERSPECTIVES

The growth of the understanding of epilepsy in childhood has been reviewed in a publication on the evolution of developmental medicine (Wallace, 1986). In keeping with the sudden, unexpected nature of the attacks, Hippocrates considered epilepsy to be a sacred disease; by noting that seizures might be partial, as well as generalized, he sowed the early seeds of a classification system. The Arabians, writing in the ninth and tenth centuries AD, were beginning to separate the more benign seizure disorders, such as those precipitated by febrile illness, from those which were chronic and lifelong. For the next few centuries, afflictions of the brain were considered in a predominantly philosophical manner. References to epilepsy in the German literature in the fifteenth century emphasize the frequency in childhood by calling it 'infants' disease'. Meanwhile, the use of the term 'the falling sickness' underlined the common association with sudden loss of posture. On the other hand, signs related to raised intracranial pressure, meningitis or strychnine poisoning were also considered convulsions. This tendency was summarized in a medical dictionary produced in the eighteenth century by Quincy, when he commented that 'a great many

Epilepsy in Children. Edited by Sheila Wallace. Published in 1996 by Chapman & Hall, London. ISBN 0 412 56860 8

disorders are included under this term'. Quincy also stated that epilepsy 'is a convulsion' and 'differs only in this, that in an Epilepsy, sensation suddenly ceases, with an immediate prostration of the body'. By the beginning of the nineteenth century, epileptic convulsions were recognized as secondary rather than primary conditions. Even so, Charles West, writing in 1842, considered them due to 'the predominance of the spinal over the cerebral system early in life'. Poupart has recently been credited with the first delineation, in 1705, of absence epilepsy. A definite major milestone in the recognition of a specific seizure type came with the description of infantile spasms by W.J. West in 1841.

Since the early part of the twentieth century, the expansion of knowledge in the basic sciences and pathology has made it increasingly possible to develop definitions which take into account features additional to those which are purely clinical, in particular, the electroencephalograph (EEG).

MODERN DEFINITIONS

The first major attempt to define the vocabulary of epilepsy was published just over 20 years ago. It was the result of the deliberations of a Working Group of the World Health Organization (WHO) (Gastant, 1973). Seizures are therein defined as sudden and transitory abnormal phenomena of a motor, sensory, autonomic or psychic nature, resulting from transient dysfunction of part or all of the brain. Epileptic seizures were further characterized as due to excessive discharges of hyperexcitable populations of neurons. Detailed descriptions of over 100 events which can be epileptic seizures were provided. In later years these definitions have been examined critically and an internationally accepted classification of seizures agreed (Commission on Classification and Terminology of the International League Against Epilepsy, 1981). However, even in 1973, a large number of terms, including

'grand mal', were deemed obsolete. On the other hand, petit mal seizures were precisely defined, with the particular aims of emphasizing their specificity to a type of primary generalized epilepsy, and, of exclusion of the use of this term for epileptic drop attacks and for those seizures which are not associated with bilateral, synchronous, symmetric discharges of rhythmic 2.5–3.5 Hz spike-wave complexes. Seizure was considered a more appropriate term for an epileptic attack than convulsion, since the latter implies body movement.

In a later chapter in this book (Chapter 6), the pathophysiologic criteria for an epileptic event are given as: a paroxysm in which there is quick emergence from and quick return to normal brain function, with resultant disruption of normal brain function, during which there is an increased firing rate in all or most neurons in a defined brain region. At a neurochemical level, it is recognized that an imbalance between excitatory and inhibitory mechanisms exists, resulting in excessive synchronization of abnormal numbers of potentials in a neuronal aggregate.

Epileptic seizures have been further characterized as partial, generalized and secondary generalized. Complete confidence in making these distinctions is easiest for seizures which are obviously partial; some apparently generalized episodes can be shown by EEG, etiology or even therapeutic response to be secondary, rather than primary generalized, so that other parameters may need to be considered. Nevertheless, the starting point is inevitably clinical.

Partial seizures are considered simple if consciousness is not lost and complex if loss of awareness occurs. However, the difficulties with defining consciousness and responsiveness are highlighted by Porter (1993). The problems are greatest with young children and in patients who have aphasia without loss of awareness as the major component. Porter (1993) emphasizes that amnesia for the event does not necessarily mean that consciousness is lost or altered during it, and points out that a lay person may have a different idea of responsiveness or consciousness from a professional worker.

Seizures, and epilepsies, are further defined as: (1) idiopathic – a disease not occasioned by another .... primary; (2) cryptogenic – hidden .... of obscure or unknown etiology (but considered secondary to an anatomic or pathologic change); (3) symptomatic .... the underlying anatomic/pathologic substrate is defined. Clearly where seizures are partial, knowledge of the clinical and EEG manifestations helps to localize the underlying lesion.

All definitions of epilepsy emphasize the recurring nature of the seizures. The WHO Working Group (Gastaut, 1973) defined epilepsy as a chronic brain disorder of various etiologies characterized by recurrent seizures, due to excessive discharge of cerebral neurons, associated with a variety of clinical and laboratory manifestations. Primary generalized epilepsies are defined as those in which seizures are generalized from the outset. These can be tonic-clonic, typical absence or bilateral massive myoclonus. Furthermore, in primary generalized epilepsies, there are no neurologic or psychologic deficits between seizures; no clear etiologic factors; and, bilateral synchronous and symmetrical discharges are found on EEG. All other epilepsies are either partial or secondary generalized. The possibility that more than one seizure type may occur in an epilepsy, and the associations between certain clinical, EEG and etiologic factors and, patterns of response to treatment, were noted in 1973, with the resultant development of internationally accepted definitions of epileptic syndromes, i.e. groups of symptoms and signs usually occurring together (Commission on Classification and Terminology of the International League Against Epilepsy, 1989). An overview of the classifications of seizures and epilepsies and more detailed individual

accounts of syndromes are given later in this book (Chapters 7, 11–15).

The problems with defining status epilepticus are at least as great as those in other areas. Most of the publications reviewed by Hauser (1983) used duration as the main criterion, with 30 minutes the most usual time span. However, Shorvon (1994) has highlighted the particular difficulties related to nonconvulsive status, where clinical abnormalities are often minimal and the duration may be very long and difficult to define. After due deliberation about the uses of 'unvarying' and 'recurrent' and 'prolonged', Shorvon (1994) suggests that status epilepticus 'is a condition in which epileptic activity persists for 30 minutes or more, causing a wide spectrum of clinical symptoms, and with a highly variable pathophysiological, anatomical and aetiological basis' (Chapter 18).

CONCLUSIONS

Definitions in epilepsy continue to be refined. In brief, seizures are episodes of sudden disruption in brain function associated with abnormally high firing rates and synchronization of discharges in neurons in defined regions of the brain; epilepsy is the recurrence of such seizures.

REFERENCES

Commission on Classification and Terminology of the International League Against Epilepsy (1981) Proposal for revised clinical and electroencephalographic classification of epileptic seizures. *Epilepsia*, **22**, 489–501.

Commission on Classification and Terminology of the International League Against Epilepsy (1989) Proposal for revised classification of epilepsies and epileptic syndromes. *Epilepsia*, **30**, 389–99.

Gastant, H. (1973) *Dictionary of Epilepsy. Part I: Definitions*. World Health Organization, Geneva.

Hauser, W.A. (1983) Status epilepticus: frequency, etiology and neurological sequelae, in *Advances in Neurology*, vol 34; *Status Epilepticus*. (eds

A.V. Delgado-Escueta, C.G. Wasterlain, D.M. Treiman and R.J. Porter), Raven Press, New York, pp. 3–14.

Porter, R.J. (1993) Classification of epileptic seizures and epileptic syndromes, in *A Textbook of Epilepsy*, 4th edn, (eds J. Laidlaw, A. Richens, and D. Chadwick), Churchill Livingstone, Edinburgh, pp. 1–22.

Shorvon, S. (1994) Definition, classification and frequency of status epilepticus, in *Status Epilepticus*, (ed. S. Shorvon), Cambridge University Press, Cambridge, pp. 21–30.

Wallace, S.J. (1986) The evolution of developmental medicine, in *Child Care Through the Ages*, (eds J. Cule and T. Turner), STS Publishing, Cardiff, pp. 80–107.

Webster's Third New International Dictionary (1981) Encyclopaedia Britannica Inc., Chicago.

John B.P. Stephenson

This chapter justifies its place in a book on epilepsy in order to emphasize three points. The first and most important is to underline some aspects of the large differential diagnosis of epilepsy and to pay particular attention to those seizures which are not epileptic in origin. Secondly, attention is drawn to a poorly recognized situation where true epileptic seizures are preceded by syncopes to produce a combinatory episode, the anoxic-epileptic seizure; this is not normally associated with epilepsy, as the term is usually understood. Thirdly, a few examples of the other side of the coin are cited, in which there are not only true epileptic seizures but true epilepsy, albeit unrecognized, because the episodes resemble nonepileptic events. Questions of therapy are discussed only briefly: this chapter concentrates on diagnosis, that most difficult, lonely and clinical process.

NONEPILEPTIC SEIZURES

The enormous diversity of epileptic seizures is well known and described elsewhere. The diversity of nonepileptic events may not be so great but is certainly considerable and all such variations have certainly not yet been described. Some of these nonepileptic events fully justify the term seizure (Stephenson, 1990; Aicardi, 1992). The most common type

of nonepileptic seizure is the anoxic seizure, or syncopal convulsion. Those who dislike using the term seizure for such fainting fits are nonetheless more ready to use it when speaking of episodes with apparent psychological mechanism, the so-called pseudo-epileptic seizures. It is a general habit or practice to use the term seizure when one does not know the mechanism of the episode. For example, all convulsive and non-convulsive episodes associated with high fever in young children may be called febrile seizures, even though it is not established that every one of these events has an epileptic mechanism.

What follows is an imperfect and temporary classification, dividing nonepileptic events into syncopes, psychologic disorders, derangements of the sleep process, and miscellaneous neurologic events.

SYNCOPES AND ANOXIC SEIZURES

An anoxic seizure is a consequence of a syncope which is an abrupt cutting off of the energy substrates to the cerebral cortex, usually through a sudden decrease in cerebral perfusion by oxygenated blood either from a reduction in cerebral blood flow itself, or from a drop in the oxygen content, or a

Epilepsy in Children. Edited by Sheila Wallace. Published in 1996 by Chapman & Hall, London. ISBN 0 412 56860 8

combination of these (Stephenson, 1990). The term 'anoxic seizure' is shorthand for the clinical or electroclinical event that occurs as a result of the cessation of nutrition to the most metabolically active neurons. Less complete, or less rapidly evolving syncope will have less dramatic consequences. For ease of reference the syncopes have been subdivided, but it must be recognized that overlaps occur and present knowledge is inevitably incomplete.

Reflex anoxic seizures

Gastaut (1968) used the term reflex anoxic cerebral seizures to describe all the various syncopes, sobbing spasms and breath-holding spells, which followed noxious stimuli in young children. Since 1978, reflex anoxic seizure has been used more specifically to describe a particular type of nonepileptic convulsive event, most commonly induced in young children by an unexpected bump to the head (Stephenson, 1978). Although other terminology, such as pallid breath-holding and pallid infantile syncope, have been applied to such episodes (Lombroso and Lerman, 1967), the term reflex anoxic seizure is now widely recognized (Roddy, Ashwal and Schrieider, 1983; Appleton, 1993).

The clinical picture has been extensively documented (Stephenson, 1990), but evidence as to precisely what happens is hard to find. Almost all the available information comes from the description of parents who have witnessed their child's attack, or from observations of episodes reproduced by ocular compression, more recently with split-screen video-EEG/ECG control. Reproduced should perhaps be described as supposedly reproduced, because one relies on a parent stating that what happens when the heart stops following ocular compression is exactly the same as the episode which has occurred at home when the young child fell and bumped his head. Many of the descriptions are absolutely convincing, but there is as yet no

known home movie, or domiciliary videotape, of a natural reflex anoxic seizure. Such recordings would certainly be of interest, particularly as from parental reports the natural syncopes may be much worse than those induced by ocular compression in the EEG laboratory: one parent indeed describes unconsciousness with pallor (after the motor event) lasting 1 hour and 11 minutes! The closest to a videorecord of a 'natural' attack was obtained personally at the end of 1993 when filming a 4-year-old girl having capillary blood taken. The accompanying convulsive syncope was more severe than that previously recorded in the same child after ocular compression. The duration of postictal stupor was also longer, but other mothers who watched the videotape were surprised at how quickly the child recovered! Direct evidence with respect to the pathophysiology is also very limited. A single child had two episodes while connected to EEG and ECG recorders (Stephenson, 1983), and pure cardiac asystole appeared to account precisely for the resultant electroclinical anoxic seizure (Stephenson, 1990). Since then only three further recordings have been obtained. A 4-year-old girl (the same child who was videotaped having the blood sample) collapsed and twitched when a balloon burst unexpectedly in a supermarket. The cardiac monitor ('King of Hearts') recorded 20 seconds asystole. Another girl, aged 2 years, had a typical reflex anoxic seizure when she knocked herself in a Citizens' Advice Bureau and the attached cassette recorder demonstrated cardiac asystole of 30 seconds with slow escape rhythm of the ECG at the conclusion. The same child had approximately 25 seconds asystole 6 months later (also when wearing a 'King of Hearts' cardiac monitor). Observations on the anoxic seizure induced by ocular compression in this child are of considerable interest and may to some extent explain the confusion which often obtains regarding the distinction between reflex anoxic seizures and breath-holding spells. When this particular girl had ocular compression no heart-beat systole was apparent from the moment the thumbs began the ocular pressure (the usual finding in such cases). At the same time, in the first few seconds of this asystolic period, there were rapid expiratory grunts at about three grunts per second. The parents recognized these grunts as similar to those noticed in the natural events, but the anoxic seizure in this case was entirely accounted for by the cardiac asystole and the expiratory grunting was apparently an epiphenomenon. In true breath-holding attacks (see 'Breath-holding attacks' below), the amount and duration of expiratory grunting may be greater and longer and undoubtedly the latency between the stimulus and the motor seizure is greater.

Extracts from a recent letter from a consultant neurologist may give the reader some idea of the diagnostic difficulties still experienced:

Thank you for asking me to see this seven year old young man

he wrote

As a toddler he began to have attacks of loss of awareness, rigidity and eye rolling which would be induced by minor knocks. This has continued and recently an episode occurred in which he had an undoubted tonic/clonic seizure with incontinence of urine. Curiously, as far as I can tell from mother's account, every attack has been triggered by a minor bump on the head and he has never had an attack out of the blue. He had difficulties at birth. The family history is clear except for a convulsion in the mother when she was tiny, about which there is no further information. It seems to me that this boy is having a form of reflex epileptic seizure and my inclination would have been to start treatment with sodium valproate. In fact mother told me that he is attending the paediatric department at . . . and that he was started on Epilim just a couple of weeks ago. Even though two EEGs have been normal I do not doubt that he has an epileptic tendency and I am sure that he should be on treatment for at least a couple of years free from attacks.

When I saw this boy he was beginning to become an 'epileptic', his school knew about his 'epilepsy', his mother was in touch with an epilepsy association, and invalidity benefit had been applied for on the basis of epilepsy. Presumably the difficulty here was that neither the pediatrician nor the neurologist knew that this was precisely the story of nonepileptic reflex anoxic seizures of vagal-mediated cardioinhibitory type. It is probable that the diagnosis of breath-holding spells had been entertained earlier, but quite rightly discarded, if only because the boy was by now over the age of 7 years. The alternative 'reflex' cardiac syncope such as is seen in the long QT syndrome (see 'Long QT disorders' below) was not considered, again quite rightly, because such syncopes have not been described as *solely* as a sequel to minor bumps to the head.

As children grow older reflex anoxic seizures may cease altogether or change to more obvious convulsive or nonconvulsive vasovagal syncope in childhood and adolescence. It is possible, although proper long-term studies have not been done, that syncopes may reappear in old age. Beyond the toddler stage, children may report sensory disturbances along with the syncopes. These include out-of-body experiences with a dream-like quality which may include the child feeling as if he or she has floated up to the ceiling and is watching his or her body lying on the floor in a seizure. Night terrors (see 'Pavor Nocturnus' below) as a sequel to such episodes have also been reported by parents.

It is often said that breath-holding spells (see 'Breath-holding attacks' below) may also occur in children who have reflex anoxic seizures. It is certainly true that in some children some episodes may be more blue or cyanotic and some more pale and blanched looking, but there are no good recordings which confirm this proposition. It is best to try to make a precise diagnosis whether a convulsive syncope in a young child is cardiogenic or respiratory in origin. If it is cardiogenic, then the main differential diagnosis is reflex anoxic seizures versus long QT syndrome or other cardiac syncope. If it appears to be a respiratory syncope, then the differential diagnosis is breath-holding spells (prolonged expiratory apnea) or suffocation (Meadow's syndrome, see 'Suffocation' below).

Vasovagal syncope

If reflex anoxic seizures represent a fairly pure 'vagal' attack, vasovagal syncope involves a vasodepressor component with variable vagal accompaniment. Episodes may begin in infancy (then well described as pallid infantile syncope) and thereafter are seen at all ages, becoming most dramatic perhaps in old age (Fitzpatrick and Sutton, 1989). Tables in medical textbooks or works of epileptology tend to perpetuate gross errors with respect to the distinction between vasovagal syncope and comparable epileptic seizures. This may be in part because many authors equate syncope with some sort of limp pallid swooning in the Victorian manner. Here, for example, are the features previously said to distinguish between syncope and seizures – posture: upright; pallor and sweating: invariable; onset: gradual; injury: rare; convulsive jerks: rare; incontinence: rare; unconsciousness: seconds; recovery: rapid; postictal confusion: rare; frequency: infrequent; precipitating factors: crowded places, lack of food and unpleasant circumstances. In reality the situation is different. Vasovagal syncope may well occur supine, particularly in the case of venepuncture fits; though some (e.g. Roddy, Ashwal and Schneider, 1983) would call these reflex anoxic seizures insofar as the mechanism is strongly cardioinhibitory, but there is probably a vasodepressor element in

addition. Pallor and sweating are certainly not invariable, nor need onset be gradual. There is no difference between the liability to injury in convulsive syncope as opposed to a comparable epileptic seizure. Convulsive jerks are certainly not rare but occur in perhaps 50% of vasovagal syncopes (Ziegler, Lin and Bayer, 1978). Incontinence is common (urinary incontinence occurred in 10% of cases in one experimental study – Stephenson, 1990). Unconsciousness may be much more than seconds and recovery, although it is usually rapid to a degree, is not necessarily complete early on. It is true that postictal confusion, proper, is rare but it can occur. The frequency of vasovagal syncope may be very great, up to more than once a day. Stimuli may be very subtle, but it is true that some sort of stimulus should be detected for at least some attacks.

The setting and stimulus are indeed the most important factors in allowing the presumptive diagnosis of vasovagal syncope, together with elicitation of the warning symptoms or aura. A seizure which occurs after a bath while the child is having her hair blow dried, or brushed, is – without need for further investigation – a vasovagal nonepileptic convulsive syncope. Premonitory symptoms are usually present in older children even if the duration is only a second or two, but sometimes these are forgotten and only recalled when syncope is reproduced as in head-up tilt. All physicians are aware of the usual symptoms of cerebral ischemia, such as dizziness and greying out of vision and tinnitus, but an important additional symptom is abdominal pain. It may be difficult to tell whether abdominal pain is a symptom or trigger of a vasovagal syncope or an actual intestinal symptom of a strong vagal discharge. The latter is quite common (Stephenson, 1990), and sometimes leads to confusion with the so-called epigastric aura which may precede the complex partial component of the temporal lobe epileptic seizure.

Almost all children with vasovagal syncope

have a first-degree relative, commonly a parent, affected (Camfield and Camfield, 1990). It is unfortunately common (histories are included in Stephenson, 1990) to find that the parent who now seems convincingly to have vasovagal convulsive syncope has become irredeemably 'epileptic' and too habituated (or too frightened of losing a precious driving licence) to discontinue years of useless antiepileptic medicine.

Such considerations have led to the use of head-up tilt testing, not only as a diagnostic aid but as a diagnostic reinforcer. If for example a child, a family doctor and a pediatrician have all been convinced that the child has had 'grand mal epilepsy' since the age of 3, then some dramatic theatre may be necessary at the age of 12–14 years to make the switch from epilepsy to the nicer diagnosis of vasovagal syncope. There are no good data on this point, but there is an impression that if the diagnosis is not properly instilled by this age, it may be too late to prevent a life of being 'epileptic'. Head-up tilt testing of children has now been reported by a number of authors (Samoil *et al.*, 1993). I have used a technique of 60 degrees head-up tilt with foot-plate support, recording simultaneous EEG and ECG on cassette tape (Medilog 9200 system) linked to a videocamera through a videointerface processor (VIP). At the same time beat to beat blood pressure is measured noninvasively using the Finapres method. A witness to natural events, normally a parent, is always present during this tilt test to confirm that what is reproduced is identical to natural episodes. The child is also able to say whether premonitory symptoms are the same as those experienced 'in the field'. At the time of writing we have reproduced **convulsive** syncope in nine children aged 8–13 years, in all of whom there has been marked cardioinhibition (in contrast to the adult situation, Grossi *et al.*, 1990), asystole varying from 4 to 30 seconds. Of particular interest was the high incidence of behaviors resembling syncope, but without the cardiovascular or cerebral effects expected in true syncope. We have called these 'psychic' or psychologic or psychogenic syncopes or pseudo-syncopes. Similar episodes have been described in adults (Linzer *et al.*, 1992) and are discussed under 'Pseudo-syncope' below. It is common for individuals to have both vasovagal syncope and some quite similar psychologic event. Such interactions deserve much further exploration.

A case history illustrates the transition from reflex anoxic seizure in infancy through short latency pain-induced vasovagal syncope to blood-illness-injury phobia (Connolly, Hallam and Marks, 1976) in adolescence: the history was given by the mother when her affected daughter was aged 13 years. A consultation was requested immediately the mother had seen on television the recording of the finger-prick-induced reflex anoxic seizure referred to under 'Reflex anoxic seizures' above. The previous diagnoses had included epilepsy, hypoglycemia and hysterical behavior.

The first episode occurred at the age of 10 months after a very slight bump to the infant's head. The appearance of the attacks has been similar from then to now, except that severity has varied and tended to increase. Typically there is latency of 10–20 seconds during which she may say 'oh mum I've hurt myself'. By this time the blood has drained from her face, she goes limp and falls as if dead, going totally rigid making a noise like a cackle or gurgle, with her hands and feet turned in and her back sometimes forming the shape of an arc. Sometimes her arms and legs jerk, but not violently, as though pedaling her bicycle, but on occasion thrashing wildly like a full seizure (as her mother describes it). Again she looks like death and then wakes up as if coming out of a very deep sleep. She is then very disorientated, does not know what has happened or where she is, but within a couple of minutes she has come to herself and may then want to lie down again and have a proper sleep. Since about the age of 7 or 8 years she has described an aura. *She hears a noise like a high-pitched screaming and sometimes hears a voice but cannot describe the voice precisely. Sometimes she sees red, a colour she does not like. More recently she has had strange hallucinations during the warning period, such as seeing a train rushing towards her. The stimuli have modified over the years after the first head bump. All episodes in earlier years followed small pains like a finger being bent back. Then she developed the same reaction to seeing a minor injury such as a scab which had come off a wound, and then inevitable syncope at the sight of blood. Most recently merely the thought of self-injury was sufficient.*

On the evening before the intended consultation she was told (wrongly) that her eyeballs would be pressed down and within 2 minutes she was stiff and snorting. Although the mother's sister had had some type of genuine epilepsy, a family history of syncope of any kind was denied. Actually the mother later admitted to several faints in adolescence and in pregnancy, but did not mention them because she did not have a **fit**.

Vagovagal syncope

In contrast to vasovagal syncope, vagovagal syncope is rare. The reflex is usually triggered by swallowing or vomiting and cardiac standstill results, with a motor anoxic seizure if the asystole is sufficiently prolonged. This is probably not a life-threatening disorder, but the symptoms can be troublesome, particularly if the patient also has migraine with associated vomiting. Pacemaker therapy can be used successfully in this situation (Stephenson, 1990).

Orthostasis

Syncope due to orthostatic hypotension secondary to autonomic failure is rare in childhood. Dopamine β-decarboxylase deficiency (Mathias *et al.*, 1990) is a possibility in such a clinical situation. Clues may be tiredness and excessive dislike of exercise. The simplest way of detecting orthostatic incompetence is to stand the child on a foam mat (to avoid injury when falling) for 10 minutes with continuous blood pressure measurements, which is best done using Finapres recording from a finger with the hand secured at heart level. This method may also be used to provoke vasovagal syncope (see 'Vasovagal syncope' above) in young children, including those too young to tilt (Oslizlok *et al.*, 1992).

Long QT disorders

The long QT syndromes are associated with genuinely life-threatening syncopes which may be simple or convulsive. The mechanism of the syncopes is a ventricular tachyarrhythmia, normally torsades de pointes. As a rule, there is no great difficulty in the diagnosis of the syndrome of Jervell and Lange-Nielsen (1957), in which congenital deafness is associated with an autosomal recessive inheritance. Much more difficult is the Ward–Romano syndrome (Ward, 1964), which is dominantly inherited but with incomplete penetrance. It has been suggested (Singh *et al.*, 1993) that the diagnosis may fairly easily be made by asking the right question, in particular asking whether the child lost consciousness and remained completely still 'like a dead body' for several seconds before having 'tonic/clonic seizures'. Actually what these authors describe is a cardiogenic syncope, not fundamentally different from the reflex anoxic seizure or a convulsive vasovagal syncope in which the vagal component predominates. The observation that the child lies like a dead body is not necessarily made, and of course the seizure is normally not a tonic/clonic seizure but an anoxic seizure with a combination of spasms and jerks and stiffening. There is a degree of overlap between the stimuli which induce reflex anoxic seizures and vasovagal syncopes and those which trigger the ventricular tachyarrhythmias of the long QT syndrome, but the most important hint in favor of a long QT disorder is the story of convulsions triggered by fear or fright and particularly in two situations:

1. **during exercise**, especially when that exercise is emotionally charged;
2. during **sleep**.

A personal example illustrates diagnostic difficulties. A 5-year-old girl presented with a history of convulsive syncope since the age of 2. At the first consultation the parents said that when she fell, not necessarily hurting herself and not necessarily falling on any particular part of her, she went gray or gray/purple around the mouth, looked faintish as if dead, went very very rigid as her eyes rolled and her head flopped, she moaned and 'she was dead in my arms'. One of the episodes was said to have occurred as a splinter was being taken out of her finger by her mother. There was a positive family history in that the father had fainted on cutting his finger and the mother had faints in pregnancy. A 24-hour cassette ECG on the child had been reported as normal. A diagnosis of reflex anoxic seizures was made and it was decided that it would not be necessary to do ocular compression as a confirmatory test. Three years later the consultant pediatrician wrote again:

> 'She had approximately one year without any episodes but has had two close episodes in the last few weeks both of which occurred during physical exertion during play. At least one of these episodes seemed to be associated with an olfactory aura, the child describing strange smells before the event. In both situations she was found unconscious, stiff and mottled grey but recovered fairly promptly. I guess this is still a vagally-mediated event but the parents would value further assessment and reassurance.'

Review of the history revealed that although two of the episodes had originally been associated with falling when playing with a ball, other episodes had occurred when chasing a dog, trying to catch the waves at the edge of the sea, playing being chased on her bicycle and **during** a hopping race. The new historical details prompted immediate measurement of her QT interval, the corrected value of which (QTc) was 479 milliseconds (normal value less than 440 milliseconds). A review of the original 24-hour ECG from 3 years previously showed that the QTc was prolonged then also at 470 milliseconds. Her mother had a marginally prolonged QTc of 449 milliseconds, whereas her father and sister had normal QTc measurements of 387 and 390 milliseconds respectively.

Long QT disorders are much less common than reflex anoxic seizures, but this diagnosis should be sought when the precipitants of a cardiac syncope are not of the typical benign reflex anoxic seizure type (that is to say unexpected bumps to the head) and particularly when exercise or sleep are triggers. This diagnostic consideration is another reason for trying to separate by history cardiac and respiratory syncopes.

Other cardiac syncopes

Diagnostic difficulties do not usually arise with respect to endogenous cardiac syncopes other than those of the long QT syndromes. However it is up to the clinician to obtain a sufficiently clear history to determine whether a seizure or convulsion is an epileptic seizure or is a nonepileptic convulsive syncope. Sometimes ventricular tachyarrhythmias occur with normal QT intervals (Shaw, 1981; Brown and Godman, 1991; Yabek, 1991; Leenhardt *et al.*, 1995), and there are occasions in obvious congenital heart disease when, for example, paroxysmal pulmonary hypertension may have to be inferred by the precise description, indicating an anoxic seizure precipitated by exercise (Stephenson, 1990).

Breath-holding attacks

Breath-holding spells have been described for centuries (Culpepper, 1737), but controversy as to what they are remains (Gordon, 1987). The term 'breath-holding' is not at all satisfactory (DiMario, 1992). It tends to give offence to parents of affected children. It seems to imply temper tantrums and bad behavior. One imagines that many pediatricians actually do believe that breath-holding spells are a manifestation of a behavior disorder and, in some pediatric textbooks breath-holding attacks are to be found in the section on psychiatric or psychologic disorders. However, recent studies have shown that however one defines breath-holding spells, behavioral disorders in those afflicted do not differ from those in control children (DiMario and Burleson, 1993).

Breath-holding seems to imply some sort of voluntary 'I'll hold my breath until I get what I want' behavior, whereas none of the behaviors so described seems to involve this mechanism. There is no difficulty nowadays in recognizing that what used to be called white or pallid breath-holding (Lombroso and Lerman, 1967) has a cardiac rather than a respiratory mechanism, as discussed earlier in the section on reflex anoxic seizures (p. 6). The term prolonged expiratory apnea (Southall, Samuels and Talbert, 1985) is certainly helpful in discussing those episodes in which the mechanism is predominantly respiratory, even though the pathophysiologic details may be in dispute.

A difficulty is, as with so many paroxysmal disorders, that precise detailed documentation of what happens is in short supply. Cinematographic registration has been described (Gauk, Kidd and Prichard, 1963). Videorecordings – predominantly of several episodes in a single child – have been obtained (Stephenson, 1990, 1991a); Southall, Samuels and Talbert (1990) have polygraphic recordings of a few children, but the total information compared to the frequency of occurrence of natural episodes is very small. There appears to be a pure respiratory 'breath-holding' spell, without any change in cardiac rate or rhythm (albeit information on cardiac output is not available), such attacks being clearly cyanotic or 'blue' breath-holding. There are also episodes which may be described as 'mixed' breath-holding in so far as not only is there expiratory apnea but also a degree of bradycardia or cardiac asystole (Stephenson, 1990, 1991a). At the present time there does not seem any particular reason to distinguish pure respiratory or expiratory breath-holding from 'mixed' breath-holding. In both situations there is, perhaps associated with a series of expiratory grunts, a rapid development of cyanosis or arterial desaturation, with decerebration and an anoxic seizure in the more severe cases. Differentiation from reflex anoxic seizures (see 'Reflex anoxic seizures' above) is mainly in the latency, which, although quite short, is not at all as brief as the 10 seconds which it takes between cardiac standstill and the onset of the symptoms of syncope.

There is an argument about the prognosis of these cyanotic breath-holding spells or prolonged expiratory apneas (Samuels, Talbert and Southall, 1991; Stephenson, 1991). Part of the explanation for the published disagreements may be that various subpopulations of children experience what appear to be similar attacks. For example, infants with tracheal anomalies may have similar episodes (Gauk, Kidd and Prichard, 1966; Filler, Rossello and Lebowitz, 1976). Also, severe cyanotic breath-holding spells which resemble prolonged expiratory apnea may be seen in infants with structural malformations of the posterior fossa. I have seen such attacks in a variety of Joubert's syndrome, with some evidence that these episodes may be fatal. However, management of neurodevelopmentally intact children does depend on the general assumption that cyanotic breath-holding is benign (Gordon, 1987).

Compulsive Valsalva

Children with aberrant development including those with autistic disorders may have their atonic or more dramatic syncopal attacks compulsively self-induced by something akin to a Valsalva or Weber maneuver (Gastaut, Broughton and De Leo, 1982). Such episodes may be very severe and, indeed, have a fatal outcome (Genton and Busserre, 1993). The child seems able to obstruct the cerebral circulation completely, so that an anoxic seizure results. Perhaps, because of the cerebral abnormality already present, this is one situation in which anoxic-epileptic seizures (see 'Anoxic-epileptic seizures' below) may result (Aicardi, Gastaut and Mises, 1988; Battaglia, Guerrini and Gastaut, 1989; Li, Lombroso and Stephenson 1989). If the episodes are very frequent, as is often the case, detailed analysis by videorecording and polygraphic registration (Genton and Busserre, 1993) may allow precise elucidation of the diagnosis. Clues include the video-picture of 'breath-holding', reduction of the amplitude of the QRS complexes on ECG, and then a burst of high-voltage slow waves on EEG.

Gastroesophageal reflux

Much has been written about gastroesophageal reflux in infants, but cinematographic or videorecording or full polygraphic registration of a reflux-associated episode which might be described as a seizure has not been reported, though a true reflux associated with an epileptic seizure has been described (Navelet *et al.*, 1989). Nonetheless, there is a persuasively recognizable condition – the 'awake apnea syndrome' (Spitzer *et al.*, 1984). Having been fed within the previous hour, often following imposed change of posture, the infant gasps, is apneic, stiffens, changes colour and may then look startled. A personal case is described in Stephenson (1990).

Suffocation

An important, unusual but difficult, diagnosis relates to serial suffocation of a baby (usually) by the mother (Meadow, 1990). This can be termed the active form of Munchausen syndrome by proxy, or Meadow syndrome, or the fictitious epilepsy type (Meadow, 1984). In this situation the parent repeatedly suffocates the baby by either pressing a hand or some other material over the baby's mouth or else the mother presses the baby's face against her bosom (Stephenson, 1990) with a resultant anoxic seizure. The evolution here is much longer than in the usual endogenous cyanotic breath-holding attack, with a latency of something of the order of 2 minutes. Diagnosis may be exceedingly difficult, but depends on such factors as recognizing that the episodes only **begin in the presence of the mother**, even when various other people, such as relatives or nursing or medical staff, observe the conclusion of the episodes. There is a particular sequence of abnormalities of the EEG/ECG and movement and muscle potentials when such an episode is recorded on cassette (Stephenson, 1990, 1994), and a suggestive appearance on polygraphic recordings including measurements of hypoxemia (Poets *et al.*, 1993). Definitive diagnosis may require covert video recording (Samuels *et al.*, 1992). Transmission of the diagnosis to the family presents great difficulties. I have found it helpful to involve a psychiatrist before discussion with the family of the mechanism of induction of these anoxic seizures (Stephenson, 1990).

Hyperekplexia

Hyperekplexia is a rare disorder (or group of disorders) which may include dramatic neonatal onset (Pascotto and Coppola, 1952) with nonepileptic convulsive syncopes which may prove fatal. Insofar as effective treatment is possible (Vigevano *et al.*, 1989), diagnostic awareness should be high. An early major paper on this topic (Suhren, Bruyn and Tuynman, 1966) described a dominantly inherited disorder in which there were stiff hypertonic neonates with later pathologic startle. Some confusion has been engendered by the title of this first paper which referred to hyperexplexia, whereas the proper Greek term is hyperekplexia (Gastaut and Villeneuve, 1967). The consistent specific diagnostic sign of hyperekplexia is elicited by tapping the infant's nose (Kurczynski, 1983). In a normal infant nose-tapping produces a minimal response, whereas in affected children there is an obvious and reproducible startle response including head retraction. This startle may be induced over and over again. The diagnosis in sporadic cases in which the baby is stiff and tends to startle is not too difficult. More difficult is the situation in which the baby is not stiff but does have neonatal onset convulsions with severe syncope (Stephenson, 1992). These dramatic nonepileptic seizures may be induced by bathing but the nose-tap test is clearly positive. Also of diagnostic value is the EEG recording during a seizure (Fig. 2.1). A series of what superficially may appear to be spikes appears on the EEG, but these are actually rapidly recurring muscle potentials from scalp muscle (synchronous potentials also are seen on the ECG channel) whose fire rate decreases *pari passu* with slowing of both EEG and ECG in the resultant severe syncope. It is now suggested that the gene for the usual dominantly inherited variety of hyperekplexia is on chromosome 5q related to a defect in the strychnine-sensitive alpha$_1$ subunit of the glycine receptor (Shiang *et al.*, 1993), but it is not known whether the sporadic normal tone type of hyperekplexia has the same origin. Whatever the variety, clonazepam remains the treatment of choice.

Other syncopes and pre-syncopes

All varieties of syncope and pre-syncope have certainly not yet been described. The most common variety of apparently life-threatening event (a syncope for sure) consists of initial hypoxemia of entirely unexplained mechanism (Poets *et al.*, 1993).

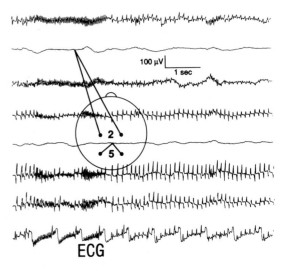

Fig. 2.1 10 second segment of cassette EEG/ECG (Medilog 9200) during a severe nonepileptic convulsive syncope in neonatally manifesting sporadic hyperekplexia. Note that 'spikes', whether very rapidly recurring ('tonic') or at around 8 per second ('clonic'), are confined to scalp areas overlying muscle and so are absent at the vertex (channels 2 and 5, arrowed); similar activity is seen on the ECG channel. These 'spikes' represent repetitive muscle action potentials, whereas the EEG is virtually isoelectric. The underlying ECG also demonstrates severe (hypoxic-ischaemic) bradycardia (see 'Hyperekplexia', p. 13).

Spontaneous hyperventilation (see also 'Hyperventilation' below) may lead to apparent absences (North, Ouvrier and Nugent, 1990), but it should be remembered that a possibly difficult-to-diagnose absence-like seizure may be of frontal lobe origin (Swartz, 1992).

'PSYCHIC' SEIZURES

The disorders listed in this section may not be fundamentally different from some of the other disorders here described, particularly in the section on 'Syncopes and anoxic seizures' above, but what are often called psychological mechanisms seem of more obvious importance (Chapter 25).

Daydreams

There is general awareness of episodes referred to as Daydreams which may be mistaken for epileptic or anoxic (syncopal) absences. There may not be a fundamental difference from that described in the next subsection as gratification, but the subsequent conditions are more likely to lead to diagnostic difficulties.

Gratification

More or less pleasurable appearing masturbatory behaviour may be seen from infancy onwards, perhaps more in girls. Rhythmic hip flexion and adduction may be accompanied by a distant expression and perhaps somnolence thereafter.

Sometimes more difficult may be the phenomenon in slightly older children, of the 'television in the sky'. Affected children may appear to stare into space or have unvocalized speech with imaginary individuals and perhaps seem to twitch or move one or more limbs for several minutes at a time. They may also have disorders of sleep (see 'Parasomnias' below). If continuous EEG recordings are undertaken, no abnormality will be demonstrated.

Out-of-body experiences

There are several situations in which children may describe experiences in which they appear to lose immediate contact with their bodies and perhaps see themselves from above. Such hallucinations have been described in epileptic seizures, anoxic seizures, migraine and as a 'normal' phenomenon. Some of these perceptual disorders may be described as the 'Alice in Wonderland phenomenon'. Dissociated states have been well described by Mahowald and Schenck (1992).

Panic/anxiety

Panic attacks are well recognized in adults and criteria for their presence in children have been described and recently well reviewed (Ollendick, Mattis and King, 1994). However, it is important to recognize that panic attacks may actually be manifestations of epileptic seizures (Laidlaw and Zaw, 1993, McNamara, 1993). In many cases hyperventilation may be involved.

Hyperventilation

Hyperventilation in any human induces various 'organic' symptoms which may in certain individuals stimulate further hyperventilation and exacerbation of the original symptoms. A degree of panic may be so engendered. Asking the child to hyperventilate (whether by getting the child to repeatedly blow out a candle or to blow a tissue or to directly hyperventilate) may induce symptoms similar to those of which the child complains. Continuation of hyperventilation once the directed hyperventilation has been stopped may be of additional diagnostic value.

Hysteria

Whether the term hysteria should be used is debated but self-induced nonepileptic nonsyncopal seizures are not rare. Such episodes are called various names, such as pseudoepileptic seizures, or nonepileptic seizures or nonepileptic attack disorder; none of these terms are satisfactory. The sort of episodes described crudely mimic epileptic seizures and have some resemblance to certain frontal lobe epileptic seizures but often have prominent sexual and aggressive components. They are usually recognized readily by observation and particularly by videotape observation and do not include alteration in background EEG. In some cases incest may be the etiology (Goodwin, Simms and Bergman, 1979; Alper *et al.*, 1993); whether or not this can be determined, psychiatric management tends to lead to resolution.

Depression

In adults depression may be an explanation of 'psychic' syncopes (Linzer *et al.*, 1992). Whether this is a feature of childhood depression has not yet been determined.

Schizophrenia

Alterations of behavior related to hallucinations in childhood, such as in schizophrenia, may resemble certain types of epileptic seizure. Detailed psychiatric evaluation may be necessary to clarify the diagnosis.

Invention

In some families seizures, syncopes or whatever are not induced but are invented (Meadow, 1984). This can be termed the passive form of Meadow's syndrome. In a personal case the affected child was supposed to be having daily seizures which were no longer observed after admission to the ward in a children's hospital. However, when the mother was, at the same time, interviewed by adult psychiatrists she affirmed that the seizures were continuing with the same frequency as previously.

Pseudo-syncope

Insofar as a swoon, or fall, or atonic collapse with apparent loss of consciousness is some physicians' conception of syncope, 'pseudo-syncope' may be a suitable description when true syncope is not present. What has been called a 'psychosomatic' syncope has been described in adults who collapse on head-up tilt with normal vital signs (Linzer *et al.*, 1992). This sort of response can be seen quite frequently in head-up tilt testing in children. One such child had been expelled from school because of frequent 'fainting'. Collapse occurred on head-up tilt without change in heart rate, blood pressure (continuously recorded by Finapres) or EEG. Simple psychotherapy was followed by prompt recovery.

PARASOMNIAS

While it is certain that all the 'funny turns' which may occur in the day time have not yet been properly described in the literature, it is even more likely that the disorders of the organization of sleep, the parasomnias, are by no means fully described. There are great intrinsic difficulties in readily determining what happens during sleep. Even ordinary visual observation may be difficult, whereas videorecording and even more so, polygraphic recording, may only be possible in exceptional cases where episodes are very frequent. It is important to recognize that all parasomnias have not yet been described and to question carefully the origin of any episode which occurs only during sleep.

Benign neonatal sleep myoclonus

The major importance of benign neonatal sleep myoclonus is that it may be misdiagnosed as epilepsy and even treated with such heavy doses of antiepileptic medication that the neonate ends up in the intensive care unit on a ventilator (Stephenson, 1990). Recognition is easy for someone who has seen a videotape of the condition in which the baby has repetitive, usually rhythmic but possibly arrhythmic, jerks of one or more limbs only during sleep. In some instances there is a report of the occasional jerk in the waking state but sometimes in very young infants it is difficult to tell whether the sleep state is actually present. If there are difficulties in the diagnosis, an EEG has to be obtained during a period of jerking but it is imperative to ensure that artifacts which result from the perhaps quite violent jerking are not misinterpreted as epileptic spike discharges. While it is important for pediatricians or pediatric neurologists to have, if possible, seen a videotape of as many of the various paroxysmal phenomena described in this chapter, it is absolutely essential that they have seen the appearance of benign neonatal sleep myoclonus so that misdiagnosis of epilepsy may be avoided.

Jactatio capitis nocturna

There are various repetitive movement disorders of sleep, of which the most common may be jactatio capitis. In this situation the individual repeatedly bangs his or her head on the pillow perhaps for hours at a time, a behavior which may persist for years.

Pavor nocturnus

Most pediatricians are aware of the parasomnia normally called night terrors. Usually occuring only once a night, the child sits up looking very frightened and perhaps quivering and behaving to some extent as if awake, but with no knowledge thereafter of what has transpired. It is important to differentiate this from a true epileptic seizure of frontal origin in which sitting up, frightened-looking behavior may occur several times nightly; dominant inheritance has now been found in several families (Scheffer et al., 1994).

New parasomnias

Other parasomnias are becoming recognized (Tuxhorn and Hoppe, 1993). It is important to note the emergent possibility of these and to refer for specialist polygraphic recording children who might otherwise be diagnosed as having epilepsy (and also of course to recognize the contrary possibility of epileptic seizures masquerading as parasomnias).

Paroxysmal nocturnal dystonia

It is not at the moment clear whether dystonic episodes in sleep are really parasomnias. Some instances of what has previously been described as paroxysmal dystonia (Lugaresi and Cirignotta, 1981) seem likely to be true epileptic seizures, probably of frontal lobe origin (Tinuper *et al.*, 1990; Meierkord *et al.*, 1992). Video recording of episodes may

clarify the situation, and multiple episodes nightly will suggest an epileptic origin. Whether or not one accepts an epileptic origin of such episodes of paroxysmal nocturnal dystonia, this is one situation in which a trial of therapy (slow-release carbamazepine at bedtime) seems eminently justified. Excessive daytime somnolence as a presenting feature of such episodes has been described in adults (Maccario and Lustman, 1990) and might be expected in childhood.

NEUROLOGIC MISCELLANEA

There are many neurologic disorders or episodic phenomena which can be described as of neurologic origin and which may be mistaken for epileptic seizures. Some more or less well-recognized examples are briefly described. It is not possible to give a complete picture – many types of fit, attack, turn, spell, or whatever have surely yet to be described.

Tics

Tics, whether simple or complex or as part of Tourette syndrome, do not usually pose diagnostic difficulty, but if tics are frequent, as they usually are, the alternative diagnosis of an epileptic origin of, for example, the vocalization, may be determined by recording an EEG **during** the tic, preferably with simultaneous videorecording.

Myoclonus

Nonepileptic myoclonus occurs in many situations. If there is difficulty in diagnostic distinction, EEG will determine whether the myoclonus is epileptic or not. The EEG (preferably with videorecording simultaneously) will show obvious spike discharges during epileptic myoclonus.

Cataplexy (narcolepsy)

Although narcolepsy which consists of irresistible onset of daytime sleep, cataplexy and hypnagogic hallucinations may infrequently begin in childhood, its recognition and diagnosis is rare. Cataplexy, or something akin to cataplexy with atonia on emotional stimulation, is more commonly noted in the rare disorder of ophthalmoplegia and neurovisceral storage (Niemann–Pick type 2S) in which a history of neonatal jaundice followed much later by difficulty with vertical eye movements will give a clue. Something akin to cataplexy may also be noted in the Prader–Willi syndrome (Stephenson, 1990).

Craniocervical junction disorders

Disorders of the craniocervical junction, particularly congenital disorders such as type 1 Chiari malformation, may be responsible for syncopes which are distinctive in not being associated with EEG or ECG change. Diagnostic clues may include syncope on sudden increase in intracranial pressure. The fullness of the brain filling the foramen magnum may be missed on superficial examination of the brain by CT scanning, but sagittal magnetic resonance imaging of the craniocervical junction should prove diagnostic and may allow therapeutic occipital decompression.

Tetany

Apart from metabolic derangements in which the diagnosis is obvious, tetany is most often seen in the hyperventilation syndrome with, or without, panic attacks (see 'Psychic seizures' above). In hypoparathyroidism it is more usual to have some form of epileptic seizure rather than tetany.

Sandifer's syndrome

Intermittent contortions of the neck with marked lateral flexion are occasionally seen with serious gastroesophageal reflux, either in normal or in neurologically impaired children (Werlin *et al.*, 1980). Sometimes it is very difficult to tell whether such contortions are a manifestation of a separate dystonia which might be dopa-sensitive.

Benign paroxysmal torticollis

Benign paroxysmal torticollis in infancy (Deonna and Martin, 1981) lasts for hours to days and is not associated with spasm or pain in the muscles. A possible relationship to migraine remains speculative.

Paroxysmal vertigo and episodic ataxia

Preschool children with benign paroxysmal vertigo of childhood are commonly referred as possible epilepsy, but the characteristic story of recurrent arrest of motion with a frightened expression but without impairment of consciousness gives the diagnosis.

Dominantly inherited episodic ataxias are rare but potentially treatable. Presentation may be as early as infancy. The family history needs careful evaluation since affected members tend to acquire a number of different false diagnoses. Effort is justified since these ion channel disorders respond to acetazolamide (Griggs and Nutt, 1995).

Complicated migraine

In some series, for example that of Gibbs and Appleton (1992), migraine equalled reflex anoxic seizure or vasovagal syncope in being one of the three most common conditions misdiagnosed as epilepsy in childhood. Not surprisingly such migraine was most commonly of the complicated variety. Confusional migraine and migraine complicated by convulsive syncope are perhaps most likely to be confused with epilepsy, hemiplegic migraine having a more clear-cut identifiable course.

Alternating hemiplegia

The paroxysmal features and neurology of alternating hemiplegia of childhood are remarkable and fascinating. In their original report, Verret and Steele (1971) presented eight cases from the Hospital for Sick Children, Toronto; they regarded the condition as an infantile-onset complicated migraine. Casaer (1987) only managed to include 12 cases in a multicentre European therapeutic trial. Recently 10 patients were reported from Montreal (Silver and Andermann, 1993) and a further 22 cases from Aicardi's group in Paris (Bourgeois, Aicardi and Goutières, 1993). These and other figures suggest that the condition is both underdiagnosed and underreported.

The general features are well known to all pediatric neurologists, with attacks of flaccid hemiplegia on one or other, or both sides, beginning in the first 18 months of life associated with autonomic phenomena and the gradual appearance of developmental delay and a degree of choreoathetosis. Actually, paroxysmal hemiplegia is not the first symptom at all, and usually the first attack is not noticed until after the age of 6 months. The **initial** manifestations begin before the age of 6 months, often much earlier. These consist of predominently brief and perhaps clustered tonic attacks which may be regarded as nonepileptic tonic seizures. These stiffenings are commonly unilateral with some resemblence to the asymmetric tonic neck reflex, that may also be bilateral, with a degree of opisthotonus and up-deviation of the eyes. Pallor and crying or screaming and general misery tend to accompany these attacks. Eye movement abnormalities, in particular strabismus or nystagmus which may be unilateral, commonly accompany these early tonic episodes.

Once hemiplegic episodes begin they may affect one or both sides (or even one upper limb and a contralateral lower limb as in case 3 of Casaer, 1987).

Some sort of trigger precedes attacks in almost all affected children. Emotional factors – excitement, bright lights and bathing including hot baths – are reported. The frequency of bathing (in the bathroom, not in the sea) is probably underreported – in one family (case 3, Casaer, 1987) this regular trigger was not recognized until the child was 15 years old.

The relationship to migraine is difficult, at present, to determine and the symptoms of migraine may not be elicited in the older affected child if cognitive impairment is severe. However, the later development of absolutely typical migraine symptoms has been recorded (case 3, Casaer, 1987; Silver and Andermann, 1993).

Paroxysmal dyskinesias

An increasing number of familial and non-familial paroxysmal dyskinesias are reported (e.g. see Nardocci *et al.*, 1989). **Paroxysmal kinesigenic choreoathetosis** is most commonly seen. The 'wobblies' whenever the young child stands up or makes other definitive movements, may respond to antiepileptic medication, although it is not established that the mechanism is an epileptic one.

Benign paroxysmal tonic up-gaze of childhood (Ouvrier and Billson, 1988; Deonna, Roulet and Meyer, 1990)

This is, as it is titled, sometimes associated with forward bending of the head, or downbeat nystagmus. Two reported patients had some sort of collapse which might have been a syncope (possibly a breath-holding spell), but sufficient patients with this combination have not yet been reported to make any conclusion. It is conceivable that this disorder resembles the better-known dopa-sensitive dystonia.

Functional blinking (Vrabec, Levin and Nelson, 1989)

Functional blinking should perhaps be in the psychogenic section: it is a differential diagnosis of the epileptic syndrome of absences with eyelid myoclonus.

Nonepileptic head-drops (Brunquell, McKeever and Russman, 1990)

These have been characterized by there being no difference in the speed of the initial flexion of the neck and the subsequent extension. Brunquell, McKeever and Russman also found that repetitive head-nods, which they described as 'bobs' (in which the velocity of recovery matched that of descent) and in which the episodes were repeated (bobbing), were a consistent feature of nonepileptic head-drops. Defining head-nods as those accompanied by 'epileptic' scalp EEG discharges, they found that head-bobbing did not occur as an epileptic phenomenon.

Shuddering

Shuddering may begin in infancy (Holmes and Russman, 1986); this does not usually precede essential tremor. If urination accompanies shuddering, confusion with epilepsy may be engendered.

Benign nonepileptic infantile spasms

This is the preferred term of Dravet *et al.* (1986) for the condition first described by Lombroso and Fejerman (1977). Serial jerks or spasms (actually each component of the salvo may be a combination of a mild clonic jerk lasting a few milliseconds and a spasm component lasting perhaps 1 second) resemble those serial spasms seen in West's syndrome and other static encephalopathies in which spasms have an epileptic or 'subepileptic' mechanism (Stephenson, 1991b).

Toxic attacks and seizures

The explanation of drug-induced oculogyric crisis is usually obvious, but sometimes there is a contrary mistake in which an absence with ocular revulsion is not recognized as epileptic. Repeated nonepileptic tonic seizures may be a feature of acute carbamazepine poisoning, and misinterpretation may occur if there has been covert ingestion of carbamazepine in a family where others have been taking this drug for genuine epilepsy (e.g. see Stephenson 1990, case 5.1).

Pyogenic meningitis

Pyogenic meningitis has to be mentioned here because the tonic or vibratory nonepileptic seizures which accompany brain swelling in *Hemophilus influenzae* meningitis were often misdiagnosed as epilepsy and treated with repeated injections of diazepam with disastrous results (e.g. Stephenson, 1990, case 15.46). Although immunization may now prevent serious hemophilus infections, the situation of brain swelling and herniation is by no means confined to this disorder.

Subacute sclerosing panencephalitis (SSPE)

The periodic transient blanks or sags subtly explaining decline in school performance might perhaps be regarded as true epileptic seizures, but, whatever one's definition, it is important to recognize that an antiepileptic drug, such as carbamazepine, may at least temporarily halt the cognitive decline in this chronic measles virus disease.

ANOXIC-EPILEPTIC SEIZURES

It is only in the past 40 years that those who have paid close attention to the mechanisms of seizures have recognized that the common motor seizure which is a manifestation of severe convulsive syncope is a nonepileptic seizure, the so-called anoxic seizure (see 'Nonepileptic seizures' above). It is true that there are many comments in the literature suggesting that it is 'common knowledge' that severe anoxia produces epileptic convulsions or even specifically tonic-clonic epileptic seizures, but, in fact, such remarks have until recently been based on a misinterpretation of the data. Indeed, there is no published, well-documented instance of a generalized tonic-clonic epileptic seizure, as currently defined, ever having been an immediate sequel of acute anoxia either asphyxial or ischemic. Nonetheless, true epileptic seizures as an immediate consequence of syncope have now been properly described and recorded, and it is this particular syncope/seizure combination which is defined as the anoxic-epileptic seizure.

It has long been known that hypoxia (as from experimental nitrogen inhalation) or oligemia (secondary to the hypocapnia of hyperventilation) may activate the spike-wave discharges of absence epilepsy (Gastaut *et al.*, 1961). With this in mind, and on the basis of a detailed study of a large number of children with febrile seizures (Stephenson and Ounsted, 1982, summarized in Stephenson, 1990), it was hypothesized that the anoxic-epileptic seizure mechanism might 'explain' some febrile seizures. Difficulties in recording brief febrile seizures – even with only videotape, far less with polygraphy – have prevented any confirmation or contradiction of this proposal. However, since the first published documentation of an afebrile anoxic-epileptic seizure (Stephenson, 1983), several further cases have been reported (Aicardi, Gastaut and Mises *et al.* 1988, Battaglia, Guerrini and Gastaut, 1989; Emery, 1990; Stephenson 1990). Anecdotal evidence suggests that these anoxic-epileptic seizures are distinctly more common than the few published cases suggest. So far no instances in adolescence or adulthood are on record.

CLINICAL DESCRIPTIONS

Details of the best documented cases are shown in Table 2.1. Most were infants or young children who also had a history of reflex syncopes without an epileptic component. These syncopes were reflex anoxic seizures, cyanotic breath-holding spells, or syncopes which from the description might have been 'mixed' breath-holding or of an indeterminate cardiorespiratory mechanism. In two of the publications (Battaglia, Guerrini and Gastaut, 1989; Emery, 1990), the term **tonic-clonic** is used, but true tonic-clonic epileptic seizures, in the currently accepted sense, were never a sequel to syncopes. What was seen in most cases was a **clonic** epileptic seizure often long enough to be classed as clonic status epilepticus. Confusion may arise in a short episode if the trigger or provoking stimulus is not recognized because the tonic component of the anoxic seizure followed by the clonic epileptic component superficially resembles a tonic-clonic epileptic seizure.

Table 2.1 Anoxic-epileptic seizures: published cases

Reference* and case no.	Sex	Age (yr)	Trigger	Syncope	Epileptic component (duration: min)
(a) EEG/polygraphic recording					
1;4 [11.1]	M	1.4	Bump/OC	RAS (asystole 22 s)	Clonic (9.5)
2;3 [3]	F	11	?(Autistic)	Valsalva	Absence (0.2)†
3 [1]	F	2.6	Falls/frustration	BBH	Clonic (1)†
3 [2]	F	2.6	Anger/OC	RAS (asystole 33 s)	Absence status (2.4)
4 [11.2]	M	0.9	Hurt/OC	RAS (asystole 25 s)	Clonic (0.4)
(b) Witnessed by a physician					
4 [4.8]	F	1	Bump	RAS	Clonic (15)
4 [11.4]	F	1.3	Hurt	BBH ('mixed')	Clonic (4)
4 [11.5]	F	4	Hurt	RAS	Clonic (25)
5 [1]	F	1	Bump	?BBH ?RAS	Clonic (45 – twice)
5 [2]	M	1	Frustration	BBH	Clonic (?60)

s = seconds, OC = ocular compression, BBH = blue breath holding, RAS = reflex anoxic seizure (vagal asystole).
*1, Stephenson, 1983; 2, Aicardi, Gastaut and Mises, 1988; 3, Battaglia, Guerrini and Gastaut, 1989; 4, Stephenson, 1990; 5, Emery, 1990.
†Also evidence of epilepsy.

Prolonged absence amounting to absence status has been reported in one child (Battaglia *et al.*, 1989). As is also emphasized by Guerrini, Battaglia and Gastaut (1991), this is a situation in which confirmation of the diagnosis requires experimental provocation under polygraphic recording. If a child has repeated episodes of trauma-triggered pallor and stiffening and prolonged unconsciousness, it may be impossible on clinical grounds to distinguish between a pure reflex anoxic seizure and an anoxic-epileptic absence. In this situation ocular compression is justifiable and necessary.

Compulsive Valsalva manoeuvre as a mechanism of syncopes and anoxic seizures has been alluded to earlier (see 'Compulsive Valsalva' above). Again, the distinction between pure syncopes and anoxic-epileptic seizures may be difficult without polygraphy (Aicardi, Gastaut and Mises, 1988; Battaglia *et al.*, 1989). An example of this diagnostic difficulty has been reported in abstract (Li, Lombroso and Stephenson, 1989) and as case 8.4 in Stephenson (1990). An 8-year-old autistic boy had frequent syncopes from compulsive Valsalvas since the age of 2½ years, often followed by prolonged tonic and vibratory seizures with postictal stupor. On polygraphic recording it was not possible to be certain that the motor seizure was epileptic rather than anoxic but from the video-recordings an epileptic mechanism was highly likely and his later development of spontaneous complex partial epileptic seizures with a tonic component supports this interpretation.

DRUG THERAPY

In most families studied personally, parents have preferred not to give either atropine (if the syncopal component was a reflex anoxic seizure) or antiepileptic medication. However, eliminating the epileptic component while the tendency to syncopes continues may be helpful and improve the quality of life. In all three children reported by Battaglia, Guerrini

and Gastaut (1989), sodium valproate was effective. In their case 1 it is possible that phenobarbitone was also effective, but clobazam was ineffective. Emery (1990) reported that phenobarbitone and carbamazepine seemed to be effective but polygraphic recordings were not used to confirm this.

Rectal or intravenous diazepam was used to terminate all the clonic seizures listed in Table 2.1, in which the reported duration was 15 minutes or more, apparently with good effect.

Therapeutic considerations are illustrated by the following case report:

A boy began to have reflex syncopes ('mixed' breath-holding) at the age of 13 months. Provocations included annoyance or frustration or head bumps. About half of the syncopes were followed by a clonic epileptic seizure. Clonic status epilepticus followed syncope induced by a minor bump to the head at the age of 16 months. Rectal diazepam to a total of 10 mg was given and shortly afterwards he had a respiratory arrest (a blood level of diazepam was reported as negligible at this time). Respiration returned after 2–3 minutes and he recovered consciousness in half an hour. Sodium valproate at 200 mg daily eliminated the epileptic component of his anoxic epileptic seizures until the age of 26 months when hurt induced syncope and then 40 minutes' clonic twitching. This slowed and ceased spontaneously (parents in attendance were afraid to give further diazepam). Consciousness was not regained for 3 hours. Sodium valproate was discontinued at the age of 3 years and subsequent breath-holding spells were not followed by epileptic seizures beyond the age of 4 years. Unprovoked epileptic seizures (epilepsy) did not develop, as with most reported cases, but subsequently his younger sister suffered a 2-hour clonic convulsion, when febrile, aged 10 months.

EPILEPTIC-ANOXIC SEIZURES

It is as important to recognize seizures which are not epileptic or epileptic seizures which do not signify epilepsy, as is the reverse error of failing to recognize epileptic seizures which masquerade as nonepileptic, the 'pseudo-epileptic seizures'. This small section briefly highlights a particular subgroup which I have called the **epileptic-anoxic seizure** (Stephenson, 1990). This is a seizure in which the syncopal component is dominant and the epileptic component subtle or difficult to recognize. In this context epileptic-anoxic seizures may be classified under the headings 'Epileptic apnea without bradycardia', 'Epileptic apnea with bradycardia' and 'Epileptic asystole' (Stephenson, 1990). Anoxic seizures secondary to epileptic asystole are well described in adults (for references see Stephenson, 1990), but in young children the most important area of difficulty lies with epileptic apnea.

EPILEPTIC APNEA

Epileptic apnea has been described for over a century. References up to 1990 are included in Stephenson (1990). Since then important publications have included Helmers, Weiss and Holmes (1991), Singh, Al Shawan and Al Deeb (1993) and Hewertson *et al.* (1994). Probably the most common situation is of repeated unexplained apneas beyond the neonatal period, such as described in case 6.1 in Stephenson (1990). Videorecording may be helpful in confirming a history of an initial stare before oxygen desaturation and cyanosis, and ictal EEG recording by cassette or otherwise will show discharges, whether repetitive spikes or monomorphous theta activity arising in one or other temporal region. Remarkably, discharges may begin in the same child in either the right or the left temporal region in different apneas (Singh, Al Shawan and Al Deeb, 1993). This particular phenomenon of origin of epileptic apnea from right or left temporal lobe in the same child can occur in both apparently 'normal' infants and in a child with 18q− chromosomal constitution.

CONCLUDING DIAGNOSTIC REMARKS

It is fortunate for innovative practitioners of the future that much of epileptic, nonepileptic and composite seizures has yet to be adequately described. The precise, detailed, consecutive, all-embracing history remains paramount (Stephenson 1990), but the use of home videorecording increasingly supplants or expands the spoken or mimed history. Constraints on the physician's time must be a factor in allowing misdiagnoses and unnecessary EEGs and brain images when the full story with, or without, video evidence would make all clear. During the week in which I write these lines I have had the privilege of taking a 90-minute history which conclusively showed that a particular child's 'epilepsy' was nothing of the kind. This may seem luxury medicine but to that family the time was worthwhile.

The most useful addition to those history-gathering processes (including home videotaping) which have been described in Stephenson (1990) has been the method of showing videorecordings of different epileptic and nonepileptic seizure examples to parents to discover which, if any, resemble their own child's attacks – the 'that's it!' phenomenon. But, since every paroxysmal disorder is not yet on film, far less described at all, the ancient art of history taking must be paramount. And the historian is you.

REFERENCES

Aicardi, J. (1992) *Diseases of the Nervous System in Childhood*, MacKeith Press and Cambridge University Press, Cambridge and New York.
Aicardi, J., Gastaut, H. and Mises, J. (1988) Syncopal attacks compulsively self-induced by Valsalva's manoeuvre associated with typical absence seizures. *Archives of Neurology* **45**, 923–5.
Alper K., Devinski O., Perrine K. *et al.* (1993) Non epileptic seizures and childhood sexual and physical abuse. *Neurology*, **43**, 1950–3.
Appleton, R. E. (1993) Reflex anoxic seizures. *British Medical Journal*, **307**, 214–5.
Battaglia, A., Guerrini, R. and Gastaut, H. (1989)

Epileptic seizures induced by syncopal attacks. *Journal of Epilepsy*, **2**, 137–46.

Bourgeois, M., Aicardi, J. and Goutières, F. (1993) Alternating hemiplegia of childhood. *Journal of Pediatrics*, **122**, 673–9.

Brown, D.C. and Godman, M.J. (1991) Life threatening 'epilepsy'. *Archives of Disease in Childhood*, **66**, 986–7.

Brunquell, P., McKeever, M. and Russman, B.S. (1990) Differentiation of epileptic from non-epileptic head drops in children. *Epilepsia*, **31**, 401–5.

Camfield, P.R. and Camfield, C.S. (1990) Syncope in childhood: a case control clinical study of the familial tendency to faint.' *Canadian Journal of Neurological Science*, **17**, 306–8.

Casaer, P. (1987) Flunarizine in alternating hemiplegia in childhood. An international study in 12 children. *Neuropediatrics*, **18**, 191–5.

Connolly, J., Hallam, R.S. and Marks, I.M. (1976) Selective association of fainting with blood-injury-illness fear. *Behaviour Therapy*, **7**, 8–13.

Culpeper, N. (1737) *A Directory for Midwives; or a Guide for Women in their Conception, Bearing (etc.)*, Bettersworth & Hitch, London.

Deonna, T.W. and Martin, D. (1981) Benign paroxysmal torticollis in infancy. *Archives of Disease in Childhood*, **56**, 956–9.

Deonna, Th., Roulet, E. and Meyer H.V. (1990) Benign paroxysmal tonic upgaze of childhood – a new syndrome. *Neuropediatrics*, **21**, 213–4.

DiMario, F.J. (1992) Breath-holding spells in childhood. *American Journal of Diseases of Childhood*, **146**, 125–31.

DiMario, F.J. and Burleson, J.A. (1993) Behaviour profile of children with severe breath-holding spells. *Journal of Pediatrics*, **122**, 488–91.

Dravet, C., Giraud, N., Bureau, M. *et al.*, (1986) Benign myoclonus of early infancy or benign non-epileptic infantile spasms. *Neuropediatrics*, **17**, 33–8.

Emery, E.S. (1990) Status epilepticus secondary to breath-holding and pallid syncopal spells. *Neurology*, **40**, 859.

Filler R.M., Rossello, P.J. and Lebowitz, R.L. (1976) Life-threatening anoxic spells caused by tracheal compression after repair of esophageal atresia: correction by surgery. *Journal of Pediatric Surgery*, **11**, 739–48.

Fitzpatrick, A. and Sutton, R. (1989) Tilting towards a diagnosis in recurrent unexplained syncope. *Lancet*, **i**, 658–60.

Gastaut, H. (1968) A physiopathogenic study of reflex anoxic cerebral seizures in children (syncopes, sobbing spasms and breath-holding spells), *Clinical Electroencephalography of Children*, (eds P. Kellaway and I. Petersen), Almquist & Wiksell, Stockholm.

Gastaut, H., Bostem, F., Fernandez-Guardiola, A. et al., (1961) Hypoxic activation of the EEG by nitrogen inhalation, *Cerebral Anoxia and the Electroencephalogram*, (eds H. Gastaut and J.S. Meyer), Charles C. Thomas, Springfield, IL.

Gastaut, H., Broughton, R. and De Leo, G. (1982) Syncopal attacks compulsively self-induced by the Valsalva manoeuvre in children with mental retardation. *Electroencephalography and Clinical Neurophysiology*, **35** (Suppl.), 323–9.

Gastaut, H. and Villeneuve, A. (1967) The startle disease or hyperekplexia: pathological surprise reaction. *Journal of Neurological Science*, **5**, 523–42.

Gauk, E.W., Kidd, L. and Prichard, J.S. (1963) Mechanism of seizures associated with breath-holding spells. *New England Journal of Medicine*, **268**, 1436–41.

Gauk, E.W., Kidd, L. and Prichard, J.S. (1966) Aglottic breath-holding spells. *New England Journal of Medicine*, **275**, 1361–2.

Genton, P. and Busserre, A. (1993) Pseudo-absences atoniques par syncopes auto-provoquees (manoeuvre de Valsalva). *Epilepsies*, **5**, 223–7.

Gibbs, J. and Appleton, R.E. (1992) False diagnosis of epilepsy in children. *Seizure*, **1**, 15–18.

Goodwin, D.S., Simms, M., Bergman R. (1979) Hysterical seizures: a sequel to incest. *American Journal of Orthopsychiatry*, **49**, 698–703.

Gordon, N. (1987) Breath-holding spells. *Developmental Medicine and Child Neurology*, **29**, 810–4.

Griggs, R.C. and Nutt, J.G. (1995) Episodic ataxias as channelopathies. *Annals of Neurology*, **37**, 285–6.

Grossi, D., Buonomo, C., Mirizzi, F. *et al.* (1990) Electroencephalographic and electrocardiographic features of vasovagal syncope induced by head-up tilt. *Functional Neurology*, **5**, 257–60.

Guerrini, R., Battaglia, A. and Gastaut, H. (1991) Absence status triggered by pallid syncopal spells. *Neurology*, **41**, 1528–9.

Helmers, S.L., Weiss, M.J. and Holmes, G.L. (1991) Apneic seizures with bradycardia in a newborn. *Journal of Epilepsy*, **4**, 173–80.

Hewertson, J., Poets, C.F., Samuels, M.P. *et al.* 1994) Epileptic seizure-induced hypoxaemia in infants presenting with apparent life-threatening events. *Pediatrics*, **94**, 148–56.

Holmes, G.L. and Russman, B.S. (1986) Shuddering attacks. *American Journal of Diseases of Children*, **140**, 72–4.

Jervell, A. and Lange-Nielsen, F. (1957) Congenital deaf-mutism, functional heart disease with prolongation of the Q–T interval and sudden death. *American Heart Journal*, **54**, 59–67.

Kurczynski, T.W. (1983) Hyperekplexia. *Archives of Neurology*, **40**, 246–8.

Laidlaw, J.D.D. and Zaw, K.M. (1993) Epilepsy mistaken for panic attacks in an adolescent girl. *British Medical Journal*, **306**, 709–10.

Leenhardt, A., Lucet, V., Denjoy, I. *et al.* (1995) Catecholaminergic polymorphic ventricular tachycardia in children. A 7-year follow-up of 21 patients. *Circulation*, **91**, 1512–19.

Li, W.W., Lombroso, C.T. and Stephenson, J.B.P. (1989) Eradication of incapacitating self-induced ischaemic seizures by opioid receptor blockade. *Epilepsia*, **30**, 679 (abstr).

Linzer, M., Varia, I., Pontinen, M. *et al.* (1992) Medically unexplained syncope: relationship to psychiatric illness. *American Journal of Medicine*, **92**, (Suppl. 1A), 18S–25S.

Lombroso, C.T. and Fejerman, N. (1977) Benign myoclonus of early infancy. *Annals of Neurology*, **1**, 138–43.

Lombroso, C.T. and Lerman, P. (1967) Breath-holding spells (cyanotic and pallid infantile syncope). *Pediatrics*, **39**, 563–81.

Lugaresi, E. and Cirignotta, F. (1981) Hypogenic paroxysmal dystonia: epileptic seizure or a new syndrome? *Sleep*, **4**, 129–38.

McNamara, M.E. (1993) Absence seizure associated with panic attacks initially misdiagnosed as temporal lobe epilepsy: the importance of prolonged EEG monitoring in diagnosis. *Journal of Psychiatry and Neuroscience*, **18**, 46–8.

Maccario, M. and Lustman, L.I. (1990) Paroxysmal nocturnal dystonia presenting as excessive daytime somnolence. *Archives of Neurology*, **47**, 291–94.

Mahowald, M.W. and Schenck, C.H. (1992) Dissociated states of wakefulness and sleep. *Neurology*, **42**(suppl.6), 44–52.

Mathias, C.J., Bannister, R., Cortelli, P. *et al.* (1990) Clinical autonomic and therapeutic observations in two siblings with postural hypotension and sympathetic failure due to an inability to synthesize noradrenaline from dopamine because of a deficiency of dopamine betahydroxylase. *Quarterly Journal of Medicine*, **75**, 617–33.

Meadow, R. (1984) Fictitious epilepsy. *Lancet*, **ii**, 25–8.

Meadow, R. (1990) Suffocation, recurrent apnea, and sudden infant death. *Journal of Pediatrics*, **117**, 351–7.

Meierkord, H., Fish, D.R., Smith, S.J.M. *et al.* (1992) Is nocturnal paroxysmal dystonia a form of frontal lobe epilepsy? *Movement Disorders*, **7**, 38–42.

Nardocci, N., Lamperti, E., Rumi, V. and Angelini, L. (1989) Typical and atypical forms of paroxysmal choreoathetosis. *Developmental Medicine and Child Neurology*, **31**, 670–4.

Navelet, Y., Wood, C., Robieux, C. and Tardieu, M. (1989) Seizures presenting as apnoea. *Archives of Disease in Childhood*, **64**, 357–9.

North, K.N., Ouvrier, R.A. and Nugent, M. (1990) Pseudoseizures caused by hyperventilation resembling absence epilepsy. *Journal of Child Neurology*, **5**, 288–94.

Ollendick, T.H., Mattis, S.G. and King, N.J. (1994) Panic in children and adolescents: a review. *Journal of Child Psychology and Psychiatry*, **35**, 113–34.

Oslizlok, P., Allen, M., Griffin, M. and Gillette, P. (1992) Clinical features and management of young patients with cardioinhibitory response during orthostatic testing. *American Journal of Cardiology*, **69**, 1363–5.

Ouvrier, R.A. and Billson, M.D. (1988) Benign paroxysmal tonic upgaze of childhood. *Journal of Child Neurology*, **3**, 177–80.

Pascotto, A. and Coppola, G. (1992) Neonatal hyperekplexia: a case report. *Epilepsia*, **33**, 817–20.

Poets, C.F., Samuels, M.P., Noyes, J.P. *et al.*, (1993) Home event recordings of oxygenation, breathing movements, and heart rate and rhythm in infants with recurrent life-threatening events. *Journal of Pediatrics*, **123**, 693–701.

Roddy, S.M., Ashwal, S. and Schneider, S. (1983) Venepuncture fits: a form of reflex anoxic seizure. *Pediatrics*, **72**, 715–8.

Samoil, D., Grubb, B.P., Kip, K. and Kosinski, D.J. (1993) Head-upright tilt table testing in children with unexplained syncope. *Pediatrics*, **92**, 426–30.

Samuels, M.P., Talbert, D.G. and Southall, D.P. (1991) Cyanotic 'breath-holding' and sudden death. *Archives of Disease in Childhood*, **66**, 257–8.

Samuels, M.P., McClaughlin, W., Jacobson, R.R. *et al.* (1992) Fourteen cases of imposed upper airway obstruction. *Archives of Disease of Child-hood*, **67**, 162–70.

Scheffer, I.E., Bhatia, K.P., Lopes-Cendes, I. *et al.* (1994) Autosomal dominant frontal lobe epilepsy misdiagnosed as sleep disorder. *Lancet*, **343**, 515–7.

Shaw, T.R.D. (1981) Recurrent ventricular fibrillation associated with normal QT intervals. *Quarterly Journal of Medicine*, **200**, 451–62.

Shiang, R., Ryan, S.G., Zhu, Y. Z. *et al.* (1993) Mutations in the α_1 subset of the inhibitory glycine receptor cause the dominant neurologic disorder, hyperekplexia. *Nature Genetics*, **5**, 351–7.

Silver, K. and Andermann, F. (1993) Alternating hemiplegia of childhood: a study of 10 patients and results of flunarizine treatment. *Neurology*, **43**, 36–41.

Singh, B., Al Shawan, S.A. and Al Deeb, S.M. (1993) Partial seizures presenting as life-threatening apnea. *Epilepsia*, **34**, 901–3.

Singh, B., Al Shahwan, S.A., Habbab, M.A. *et al.* (1993) Idiopathic long QT syndrome: asking the right question. *Lancet*, **341**, 741–2.

Southall, D.P., Johnson, P., Morley, C.J. *et al.* (1985) Prolonged expiratory apnoea: a disorder resulting in episodes of severe arterial hypoxaemia in infants and young children. *Lancet*, **ii**, 571–7.

Southall, D.P., Samuels, M.P. and Talbert, D.G. (1990) Recurrent cyanotic episodes with severe arterial hypoxaemia and intrapulmonary shunting: a mechanism for sudden death. *Archives of Disease in Childhood*, **65**, 953–61.

Spitzer, A.R., Boyle, J.T., Tuchman, D.N. and Fox, W.W. (1984) Awake apnea associated with gastroesophageal reflux: a specific clinical syndrome. *Journal of Pediatrics*, **104**, 200–5.

Stephenson, J.B.P. (1978) Reflex anoxic seizures ('white breathholding'): nonepileptic vagal attacks. *Archives of Disease in Childhood*, **53**, 193–200.

Stephenson, J.B.P. (1983) Febrile convulsions and reflex anoxic seizures, in *Research progress in Epilepsy* (ed. F.C. Rose), Pitman, London.

Stephenson, J.B.P. (1990) *Fits and Faints*, MacKeith Press and Cambridge University Press, Cambridge and New York.

Stephenson, J.B.P. (1991a) Blue breath-holding is benign. *Archives of Disease in Childhood*, **66**, 255–7.

Stephenson, J.B.P. (1991b) Epilepsy. *Current Opinion in Neurology and Neurosurgery*, **4**, 406–9.

Stephenson, J.B.P. (1992) Vigabatrin for startle disease with altered cerebrospinal-fluid free gamma-aminobutyric acid. *Lancet*, **340**, 430–1.

Stephenson, J.B.P. (1994) Video surveillance in diagnosis of intentional suffocation. *Lancet*, **344**, 414–5.

Stephenson, J.B.P. and Ounsted, C. (1982) Febrile convulsions, in *Handbook of Experimental Pharmacology*, (ed. A. S. Milton), Springer-Verlag, Berlin.

Suhren, O., Bruyn, G.W. and Tuynman, J.A. (1966) Hyperexplexia: a hereditary startle syndrome. *Journal of the Neurological Sciences*, **31**, 577–605.

Swartz, B.E. (1992) Pseudo-absence seizures: a frontal lobe phenomenon. *Journal of Epilepsy*, **5**, 80–93.

Tinuper, P., Cerullo, A., Cirignotta, F. *et al.* (1990) Nocturnal paroxysmal dystonia with short-lasting attacks: three cases with evidence for an epileptic frontal lobe origin of seizures. *Epilepsia*, **31**, 549–56.

Tuxhorn, I. and Hoppe, M. (1993) Parasomnia with rhythmic movements manifesting as nocturnal tongue biting. *Neuropediatrics*, **24**, 167–8.

Verret, S. and Steele, J.C. (1971) Alternating hemiplegia in childhood: a report of eight patients with complicated migraine beginning in infancy. *Pediatrics*, **47**, 675–80.

Vigevano, F., DiCapua, M. and Dalla Bernardina, B. (1989) Startle disease: an avoidable cause of sudden infant death. *Lancet*, **i**, 216.

Vrabec, T.R., Levin, A.V. and Nelson, L.B. (1989) Functional blinking in childhood. *Pediatrics*, **83**, 967–70.

Ward, O.C. (1964) A new familial cardiac syndrome in children. *Journal of the Irish Medical Association*, **54**, 103–6.

Werlin, S.L., D'Souza, B.J., Hogan, W.J. *et al.* (1980) Sandifer syndrome: an unappreciated clinical entity. *Developmental Medicine and Child Neurology*, **22**, 374–8.

Yabek, S.M. (1991) Ventricular arrhythmias in children with an apparently normal heart. *Journal of Pediatrics*, **119**, 1–11.

Ziegler, D.K., Lin, J. and Bayer, W.L. (1978) Convulsive syncope: its relationship to cerebral ischemia. *Transactions of the American Neurological Association*, **103**, 150–4.

EPIDEMIOLOGY: INCIDENCE AND PREVALENCE

Lars Forsgren

DEFINITIONS

Incidence is defined as the number of new persons with a disease that occur in a specified population during a given period. The incidence of epilepsy is usually calculated for a period of 1 year, so-called annual incidence rates, and expressed per 100 000 inhabitants.

Prevalence (point prevalence) is defined as the number of persons with a given disease at a particular time, the prevalence day, in a specified population. The prevalence of epilepsy is usually expressed per 1000 inhabitants.

A number of factors have to be taken into consideration when results of epidemiological studies are compared. Such factors are definition of the studied disorder, the sources for identification of the study population and the composition of the study population. Usually only children with active epilepsy are included. Active epilepsy refers to children who had their most recent seizure during the last 5-year period preceding the prevalence date (some investigators limit the period to the last 1, 2, or 3 years) or are receiving treatment with antiepileptic drugs because of epilepsy on the prevalence day, regardless of when the last seizure occurred. Although not fulfilling the definition of epilepsy, children with single seizures, febrile convulsions or seizures due to other acute disorders are sometimes included in incidence and prevalence rates of epilepsy.

The general relevance of studies depends on the identification of the study population. Studies of children identified only from hospital clinics with a special interest in epilepsy underestimate incidence and prevalence, since it is unlikely that all children with epilepsy are referred to these clinics. Furthermore, the proportion of children with severe epilepsy and bad prognoses is overestimated, as they are more likely to be referred to special clinics than other children with epilepsy. In general, the more sources of information used in identifying children with epilepsy, the more correctly do the epidemiological findings represent the true situation. However, despite extensive searches, there will always be a proportion of unknown size, of children with unidentified epilepsy. Finally, incidence and prevalence vary in different subgroups of children with epilepsy. By using rates specified by age, sex and other variables, a more detailed picture emerges allowing a better base for evaluation of differences between studies. The rates presented below were either directly quoted from the cited papers or calculated by the author from information on the denominator and nominator given in the papers. Previously unpublished data on seizure frequency are also presented.

Epilepsy in Children. Edited by Sheila Wallace. Published in 1996 by Chapman & Hall, London. ISBN 0 412 56860 8

Table 3.1   Crude annual incidence (I)/100 000 of epilepsy/seizures in children

Country reference and year	Age group (yr)	I	Population
England and Wales Crombie *et al.*, 1960	0–14	152	Febrile convulsions and SS included
USA Shamansky and Glaser, 1979	0–14	73	Symptomatic seizures and SS included
Denmark Juul-Jensen and Foldspang, 1983	0–14	73	Febrile convulsions excluded. SS included
Sweden Heijbel *et al.*, 1975	0–15	134	Febrile convulsions excluded. SS included
Sweden Sidenvall *et al.*, 1993	0–15	73	Febrile convulsions excluded. SS included
Norway de Graaf, 1974	0–14	66	Febrile convulsions with abnormal EEG included ≥2 seizures
Poland Zielinski, 1974	0–10	45 (32)	SS included. (≥2 unprovoked seizures)
Sweden Blom *et al.*, 1978	0–15	82	≥2 unprovoked seizures
Sweden Brorson and Wranne, 1987	0–19	50	≥2 unprovoked seizures
Faroe Islands Joensen, 1986	0–19	71	≥2 unprovoked seizures
England Brewis *et al.*, 1966	0–14	53	≥2 unprovoked seizures
United Kingdom Verity *et al.*, 1992	0–10	43	≥2 unprovoked seizures
Chile Lavados *et al.*, 1992	0–14	124	≥2 unprovoked seizures
USA Hauser and Kurland, 1975	0–19	56–81	≥2 unprovoked seizures

SS = single seizures.
*Incidence for four different intervals 1935–67.

INCIDENCE

CRUDE INCIDENCE

The crude annual incidence ranges from 43 to 152 per 100 000 children (Table 3.1). Neonatal seizures were not included in most studies. The more than threefold variance largely depends on differences in methodology and definitions in different studies. Studies including febrile convulsions and single unprovoked seizures in general show higher incidence rates than studies only including recurrent unprovoked seizures. The median annual incidence rate of epilepsy, excluding neonatal seizures, is about 60/100 000 children at risk. If single unprovoked seizures are included the incidence rises to approximately 80–100/100 000. In adults the incidence is lower, about 30–50/100 000 than in children. The incidence rises in old age to rates similar to those found in children.

AGE-SPECIFIC INCIDENCE

The highest incidence was found during the first year of life in almost all studies (Fig. 3.1). The rates decline with increasing age during

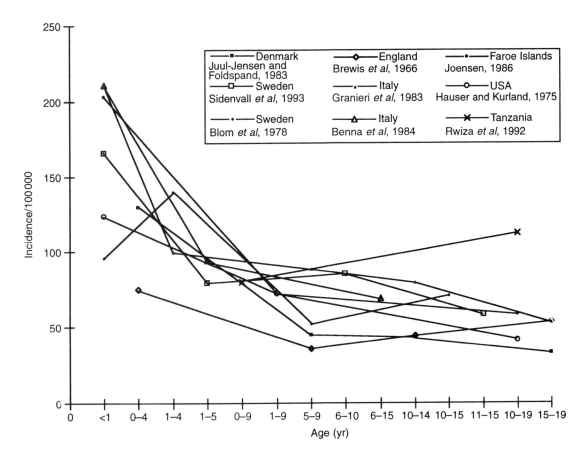

Fig. 3.1 Age-specific incidence of epilepsy in children. Danish and Swedish study from 1993 includes single seizures. The median incidence for four different intervals 1935–67 is shown for the American study.

childhood. The mean age-specific incidences /100 000 from the studies in Fig. 3.1 are: 169 (≤1 year, neonatal seizures excluded; six studies), 103 (1 to 4 or 5 years; four studies), 61 (5 or 6 to 9 or 10 years; five studies), 59 (10 or 11 to 14 or 15 years; five studies), 46 (15 to 19 years; three studies). Very high rates were reported from Equador with incidences of 174 and 268/100 000 in age groups 0–9 and 10–19 years respectively (Placencia *et al.*, 1992). In part they depend on inclusion of single and acute symptomatic afebrile seizures. An incidence of 82/100 000 was reported in Italian 5–14-year-old schoolchildren (Cavazutti, 1980).

Neonatal seizures are often excluded in epidemiologic studies of epilepsy, mainly due to diagnostic uncertainty whether various subtle attack phenomena are of epileptic or nonepileptic nature. Furthermore, in epidemiologic studies of epilepsy, seizures are unprovoked while many neonatal seizures are symptomatic due to various acute events. The neonatal seizure incidence ranges from 150/100 000 of live term births (Eriksson and Zetterström, 1979) to 20 200/100 000 in preterm infants (Seay and Bray, 1977). When both term and preterm infants are included, rates of 500/100 000 (Holden, Mellits and

Freeman, 1982) and 3200/100 000 have been reported (Sidenvall *et al.*, 1993). (See also chapter 9.)

SEX-SPECIFIC INCIDENCE

Most studies report a slightly higher incidence in boys than in girls (Crombie *et al.*, 1960; Zielinski, 1974; Hauser and Kurland, 1975; Shamansky and Glaser, 1979; Granieri *et al.*, 1983; Juul-Jensen and Foldspang, 1983; Lavados *et al.*, 1992). However, Sidenvall *et al.* (1993) reported a higher incidence in girls and in the majority of studies reporting a higher incidence in boys than girls, the reverse was found during specific childhood ages. Thus, Granieri *et al.* (1983) found a higher incidence in girls aged 1–4 years, Crombie *et al.* (1960) in girls aged 5–9 years, Juul-Jensen and Foldspang (1983) in girls aged 10–14 years, Hauser and Kurland (1975) in girls aged 10–19 years and Shamansky and Glaser (1979) in almost half of each individual year of age investigated. In conclusion, there is no consistent difference in incidence between boys and girls.

CUMULATIVE INCIDENCE

The cumulative incidence of epilepsy is the estimated proportion of a population which develops epilepsy over a specified time interval. A cumulative incidence rate can be calculated from known age-specific incidence rates and increases with advancing age. Up to age 14 years, 1.1–1.7% of children have had at least one afebrile seizure (Shamansky and Glaser, 1979; von Wendt *et al.*, 1985; Tsuboi, 1988) and 0.8% repeated afebrile seizures, i.e. epilepsy (Tsuboi, 1988). In British cohort studies epilepsy occurred in 0.4% of children <10 years (Verity, Ross and Golding, 1992) and <11 years (Ross *et al.*, 1980). At least one afebrile seizure occurred in 0.6% in the study of Verity, Ross and Golding (1992). Birth weight <2500 g is associated with increased cumulative inci-

dence (van den Berg and Yerushalmy, 1969; von Wendt *et al.*, 1985).

PREVALENCE

CRUDE PREVALENCE

There are many studies on the prevalence of epilepsy. The rates presented here refer to active epilepsy (see 'Definitions' above) unless otherwise specified. The prevalence rates reported from 15 studies are shown in Table 3.2. Despite great variations in the studies regarding the period of investigation, resources and methodology, most studies (febrile convulsions excluded) find a prevalence between 3 and 6/1000 children. The prevalence rates are similar on different continents with the exception of South America and small African isolates, where higher rates have been reported (Jilek-Aall, Jilek and Miller, 1979; Lavados *et al.*, 1992; Goudsmit, van der Waals and Gajdusek, 1983; Placencia *et al.*, 1992). The cause of these high rates may be genetic or due to various infections, particularly cysticercosis. However, there is no consistent observation of the high rates being due to particular etiologies in the African and South American studies (Lavados *et al.*, 1992; Senanayake and Roman, 1993).

AGE-SPECIFIC PREVALENCE

The prevalence of epilepsy increases with increasing age during childhood. The age-specific prevalences of 17 studies are summarized in Fig. 3.2 (Crombie *et al.*, 1960; Brewis *et al.*, 1966; Gudmundsson, 1966; Stanhope, Brody and Brink, 1972; Zielinski, 1974; Granieri *et al.*, 1983; Haerer, Anderson and Schoenberg, 1986; Joensen, 1986; Osuntokun *et al.*, 1987; Bharucha *et al.* 1988; Cowan *et al.* 1989; Tekle-Haimanot *et al.*, 1990; Hauser, Annegers and Kurland, 1991; Maremmani *et al.*, 1991; Guiliani *et al.*, 1992; Placencia *et al.*, 1992; Rwiza *et al.*, 1992). The mean prevalence was 3.8 in children aged 0–4

Table 3.2 Crude prevalence of childhood epilepsy

Country reference and year	Prevalence/1000	Comments
England Pond *et al.*, 1960	9.6	Includes single seizures and febrile convulsions. 0–19 yr
England and Wales Crombie *et al.*, 1960	3.7	Includes repeated febrile convulsions. 0–14 yr
Iceland Gudmundsson, 1966	3.2	Includes single unprovoked seizures. 0–19 yr
England Brewis *et al.*, 1966	4.7	0–19 yr
Guam Stanhope *et al.*, 1972	4.5	0–19 yr
Finland Sillanpää, 1973	3.2	0–15 yr
Norway de Graaf, 1974	4.4	Includes repeated febrile convulsions with abnormal EEG. 0–19 yr
China Li *et al.*, 1985	4.2	0–19 yr
Faroe Islands Joensen, 1986	6.5	0–19 yr
USA Haerer *et al.*, 1986	6.0	0–19 yr. Includes 22% with 'possible epilepsy'
Nigeria Osuntokun *et al.*, 1987	6.0	0–19 yr
India Bharucha *et al.*, 1988	3.6	0–19 yr
USA Cowan *et al.*, 1989	4.7	0–19 yr
USA* Hauser *et al.*, 1991	2.7 3.6 2.8 3.5 3.9	0–14 yr
Tanzania Rwiza *et al.*, 1992	6.6	0–19 yr
Chile Lavados *et al.*, 1992	17.0	0–14 yr

*Prevalence years 1940, 1950, 1960, 1970, 1980.

or 0–9 years, 4.2 in children aged 5–9 years, 5.3 in children 10–14 years old and 7.8 in children 10–19 years old.

Some studies have reported on the prevalence in school age children. A prevalence of 3.0 was found in Italian children aged 6–14 years (Pazzaglia and Frank–Pazzaglia, 1976), of 5.7–9.3/1000 in American children aged 6–15 years (Baumann, Marx and Leonidakis, 1977, 1978), of 3.4 in Japanese children aged 9–14 years (Tsuboi, 1988), and 5.7 in Spanish children aged 6–14 years (Sangrador

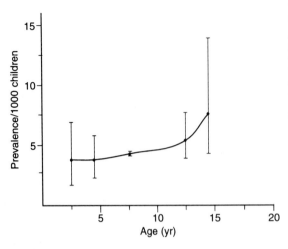

Fig. 3.2 The mean age-specific prevalence of epilepsy in children based on 17 studies. Scale bars indicate the range.

and Luaces, 1991). The prevalence of epilepsy in school age children, all studies combined, is about 5–6/1000.

SEX-SPECIFIC PREVALENCE

The reports on sex-specific prevalence are similar to reports on sex-specific incidence, i.e. the majority of studies report a slightly higher prevalence in boys than girls (Wajsbort, Haral and Alhandury, 1967; Stanhope, Brady and Brink, 1972; Granieri *et al.*, 1983; Joensen, 1986; Bharucha *et al.*, 1988; Koul, Razdan and Motta, 1988; Cowan *et al.*, 1989; Maremmani *et al.*, 1991; Guiliani *et al.*, 1992; Lavados *et al.*, 1992; Rwiza *et al.*, 1992). Several studies report a higher prevalence of girls in some specific childhood ages (Crombie *et al.*, 1960; Pond, Bidwell and Stein, 1960; Gudmundsson, 1966; de Graaf, 1974; Haerer, Anderson and Schoenberg, 1986; Tekle-Haimanot *et al.*, 1990; Hauser, Annegers and Kurland, 1991). Higher crude prevalences in girls than boys have also been found (Goudsmit *et al.*, 1983; Osuntokun *et al.*, 1987). In conclusion, as for incidence, there is no consistent difference in prevalence between boys and girls.

LIFETIME PREVALENCE

The lifetime prevalence of epilepsy is the proportion of a population who have ever had epilepsy up to a specified age or during the entire lifetime. Lifetime prevalence rate is partly based upon persons who had seizures many years ago, and thus includes persons with both active and inactive epilepsy.

The lifetime prevalence in schoolchildren of 8–9 years old varies widely despite the use of similar methodology. Prevalences of 7.8 (Meighan, Queener and Westman, 1976) and 14.1 (Rose *et al.*, 1973) were reported from the USA, 21.1 from Chile (Chiofalo *et al.*, 1979) and 18.3 from Mexico (Garcia-Pedroza *et al.*, 1983). All these studies included single seizures and complex febrile seizures. There were no analyses of risk factors, which may explain the rate differences. Lower lifetime prevalences, 4.4–4.8, were found in children <14 years when only children with epilepsy were included (Benna *et al.*, 1984; Doerfer and Wässer, 1987). Since these rates are lower than rates of active epilepsy (see 'Age-specific prevalence' above), there was probably an underascertainment of cases.

TIME TRENDS

The prevalence of active epilepsy in children aged 0–14 years increased moderately over a 40-year period, from 2.7/1000 in 1940 to 3.9 in 1980 (Hauser, Annegers and Kurland, 1991). No increase during this period was seen in 0–9-year-old children, while there was an increase in prevalence for each successive decade investigated in children aged 10–14 years. The increase in prevalence may be due to improvement in ascertainment of cases and by the retention of identified cases in the numerator over time (Hauser and Hesdorffer, 1990).

Incidence rates increase from the first to second period of investigation (Hauser and Kurland, 1975; Doose and Sitepu, 1983; Doerfer and Wässer, 1987). Rates decrease in the final period of investigation (Hauser and

Kurland, 1975; Doerfer and Wässer, 1987). No statistically significant difference in incidence was found by Shamansky and Glaser (1979) during an 11-year period, by Cavazutti (1980) during a 6-year period and by Lavados *et al.* (1992) during a 5-year period. In conclusion, there is no certain change in incidence of epilepsy and single seizures over time.

SEIZURE TYPES

The incidence of primary generalized seizure disorders is higher than that of partial seizures, 39–44 vs 21–32/100 000 (Blom, Heijbel and Bergfors, 1978; Sidenvall *et al.*, 1993). Primary generalized seizures were also more common than partial seizures in the study of Verity, Ross and Golding (1992). Hauser and Kurland (1975) found a primary generalized seizure to be more common as the initial seizure in children aged 0–9 years, while in children aged 10–19 years primary generalized and partial seizures were almost equally common.

In contrast to adults where prevalence rates show a predominance of partial seizures (Zielinski, 1974; Hauser and Kurland, 1975; Forsgren, 1992), either primary generalized (Cowan *et al.*, 1989; Lavados *et al.*, 1992) or partial seizures (Cavazutti, 1980) are predominant in children or these major seizure types are equally common (Hauser, Annegers and Kurland, 1991).

The incidence/prevalence of specific epileptic syndromes are sometimes specified. For benign childhood epilepsy with centrotemporal spikes (BECT), there is a wide difference. BECT is not mentioned at all in some studies, while other studies found incidences of 11–21/100 000 (Blom, Heijbel and Bergfors, 1978; Sidenvall *et al.*, 1993). BECT accounted for every fourth child with epilepsy in the studies of Blom, Heijbel and Bergfors (1978) and Cavazutti (1980). The incidence of absence epilepsy was 7/100 000 in two recent studies (Olsson, 1988; Sidenvall

et al., 1993), which is comparable to the incidence of juvenile myoclonic epilepsy, 6–8/100 000 (Blom *et al.* 1978; Sidenvall *et al.*, 1993). The studies of Blom, Heijbel and Bergfors (1978), Olsson (1988) and Sidenvall *et al.* (1993) are all from a single country, Sweden. Since the above-mentioned epileptic syndromes have a strong genetic influence, the rates presented may differ substantially in other populations.

SEIZURE FREQUENCY

Published prevalence studies seldom report the seizure frequency in the population studied, and when doing so both children and adults are lumped together. Unpublished results from northern Sweden by the present author and colleagues found that of children with active epilepsy, 49% were free from seizures, 22% had a seizure less than once per fortnight and 24% had at least one seizure every fortnight, in the year preceding the investigation date.

EPILEPSY IN OTHER DISORDERS

MENTAL RETARDATION

The most common disorder associated with epilepsy is mental retardation (MR) (see Chapter 17). Epilepsy occurred in 21–36% of children with severe MR (Corbett, Harris and Robinson, 1975; Gustavson *et al.*, 1977) and in 12–18% with mild MR (Blomquist *et al.*, 1981; Hagberg *et al.*, 1981). The prevalence in children aged 0–19 years with both epilepsy and MR has been reported as 1.4/1000 (Forsgren *et al.*, 1990).

CEREBRAL PALSY

Epilepsy was reported in 15% (prevalence 0.32/1000 live births; similar rates in term and preterm children) of children with cerebral palsy (CP) who were followed up to age 4–8 years (Hagberg *et al.*, 1989) and CP in 23% of children with epilepsy (Brorson, 1970); see

Chapter 16). In children with hemiplegic CP, a history of epilepsy was recorded in 34%, more often in postnatal cases (78%) than in congenital cases (28%). Active epilepsy occurred in 23% (Uvebrant, 1988). In an epidemiologic study of children with spastic tetraplegic CP, all cases were found to have severe mental retardation and 94% had epilepsy (Edebol-Tysk, 1989).

INFANTILE HYDROCEPHALUS

Epilepsy occurred at 2–6 years of age in 33% of children with infantile hydrocephalus (IH) (Fernell, Hagberg and Hagberg, 1990). The proportion with epilepsy was higher in children with a gestational age of <32 full weeks (56%) than in children born at term (31%) During a mean follow-up period of 9 years, 48% had a history of epilepsy (Saukkonen, Serlo and von Wendt, 1990). In 22% the initial seizure occurred before shunting and in 26% after shunting, in the majority >2 years after the shunting (Saukkonen, Serlo and von Wendt, 1990). Children with IH and autistic symptoms were reported to have epilepsy in 50%, 7/8 with partial seizures and secondary generalization, compared with 9% in children with IH and no autistic symptoms (Fernell, Gillberg and von Wendt, 1991).

NEUROCUTANEOUS SYNDROMES

In a hospital-based study, 98% of children with tuberous sclerosis (TS) also had epilepsy and 69% of children had infantile spasms (IS) during the first 2 years of life (Pampiglione and Moynahan, 1976). In population-based studies 50–93% had a history of epilepsy (Nevin and Pearce, 1968; Wiederholt, Gomez and Kurland, 1985; Umapathy and Johnston, 1989). Mild cases with TS were included in the study of Webb, Fryer and Osborne (1991), who besides clinical findings also used radiology in the investigation of relatives of known cases with TS. A history of epilepsy was found in 62%. Of 40 children with TS and

Table 3.3 Estimated number of children aged 0–14 years with new* and established† active epilepsy worldwide

Region	New cases annually	Established epilepsy
Europe	58 000	580 000
Former Soviet Union	46 000	460 000
North America	36 000	360 000
Latin America and the Caribbean	98 000	980 000
Sub-Saharan Africa	153 000	1 530 000
Near East and North Africa	63 000	630 000
Asia	593 000	5 930 000
Oceania	4 000	42 000
World	1 051 000	10 512 000

*Assuming an annual incidence of 60/100 000 and a prevalence of 0.6%†.

epilepsy, about 70% developed complex partial seizures and this occurred as often in children who had prior IS as in those without IS (Yamamoto *et al.*, 1987). Sturge–Weber syndrome is the other major neurocutaneous syndrome where epilepsy is common, being reported in 75–90% (Gilly *et al.*, 1977; Gomez and Bebin, 1987; Chapter 16).

GLOBAL PERSPECTIVE

Table 3.3 is based on the worldwide childhood population (Jamison, 1991) and assumes an annual incidence of childhood epilepsy of 60/100 000 and a prevalence of active epilepsy of 0.6%. High incidence and prevalence rates reported from Latin America (Placencia *et al.*, 1992) indicate that the figures for Latin America are too low. The vast majority of children are found in the developing world, where at present it is expected that about 900 000 new children develop epilepsy every year and 9000 000 children have epilepsy. The majority of these children probably do not receive antiepileptic treatment! The corresponding figures in the developed world are about 150 000 new children with epilepsy yearly and 1500 000 with an established epilepsy.

REFERENCES

Baumann, R.J., Marx, M.B., Leonidakis, M.G. (1977) An estimate of the prevalence of epilepsy in a rural Appalachian population. *American Journal of Epidemiology*, **106**, 42–52.

Baumann, R.J., Marx, M.B. and Leonidakis, M.G. (1978) Epilepsy in rural Kentucky: prevalence in a population of school age children. *Epilepsia*, **19**, 75–80.

Benna, P., Ferrero, P., Bianco, C. *et al.* (1984) Epidemiologic aspects of epilepsy in the children of a Piedmontese district (Alba-Bra). *Panminerva Medica*, **26**, 113–8.

Bharucha, N.E., Bharucha, E.P., Bharucha, A.E. *et al.* (1988) Prevalence of epilepsy in the Parsi community of Bombay. *Epilepsia*, **29**, 111–5.

Blom, S., Heijbel, J. and Bergfors, P.G. (1978) Incidence of epilepsy in children: a follow-up study three years after the first seizure. *Epilepsia*, **19**, 343–50.

Blomquist, H.K., Gustavson, K-H. and Holmgren, G. (1981) Mild mental retardation in children in a northern Swedish county. *Journal of Mental Deficiency Research*, **25**, 169–86.

Brewis, M., Poskanzer, D., Rolland, C. and Miller, H. (1966) Neurological disease in an English city. *Acta Neurologica Scandinavica*, **42** (suppl 24), 1–89.

Brorson, L.-O. (1970) *Epilepsi hos barn och ungdom. En klinisk, psykometrisk och social undersökning inom Uppsala län. I.* Socialstyrelsen redovisar: Epileptiker vården, Stockholm.

Brorson, L.-O. and Wranne, L. (1987) Long-term prognosis in childhood epilepsy: survival and seizure prognosis. *Epilepsia*, **28**, 324–30.

Cavazutti, G.B. (1980) Epidemiology of different types of epilepsy in school age children of Modena, Italy. *Epilepsia*, **21**, 57–62.

Chiofalo, N., Kirschbaum, A., Fuentes, A. *et al.* (1979) Prevalence of epilepsy in children of Melipilla, Chile. *Epilepsia*, **20**, 261–8.

Corbett, J.A., Harris, R. and Robinson, R.G. (1975) Epilepsy, in *Mental retardation and developmental disabilities*, vol VII, (ed J. Wortis), Bruner Mazel, New York, pp. 79–111.

Cowan, L.D., Bodensteiner, J.B., Leviton, A. and Doherty, L. (1989) Prevalence of the epilepsies in children and adolescents. *Epilepsia*, **30**, 94–106.

Crombie, D.L., Cross, K.W., Try, J. *et al.* (1960) A survey of the epilepsies in general practice. *British Medical Journal*, **2**, 416–22.

de Graaf, A. S. (1974) Epidemiological aspects of epilepsy in northern Norway. *Epilepsia*, **15**, 291–9.

Doerfer, J. and Wässer, S. (1987) An epidemiologic study of febrile convulsions and epilepsy among children. *Epilepsy Research*, **1**, 149–51.

Doose, H. and Sitepu, B. (1983) Childhood epilepsy in a German city. *Neuropediatrics*, **14**, 220–4.

Edebol-Tysk, K. (1989) Epidemiology of spastic tetraplegic cerebral palsy in Sweden. I. Impairments and disabilities. *Neuropediatrics*, **20**, 41–5.

Eriksson, M. and Zetterström, R. (1979) Neonatal convulsions. *Acta Paediatrica Scandinavica*, **68**, 807–11.

Fernell, E., Hagberg, G. and Hagberg, B. (1990) Infantile hydrocephalus – the impact of enhanced preterm survival. *Acta Paediatrica Scandinavica*, **79**, 1080–6.

Fernell, E., Gillberg, C. and von Wendt, L. (1991) Autistic symptoms in children with infantile hydrocephalus. *Acta Paediatrica Scandinavica*, **80**, 451–7.

Forsgren, L. (1992) Prevalence of epilepsy in adults in northern Sweden. *Epilepsia*, **33**, 450–8.

Forsgren, L., Edvinsson, S-O., Blomquist, H.K. *et al.* (1990) Epilepsy in a population of mentally retarded children and adults. *Epilepsy Research*, **6**, 234–48.

Garcia-Pedroza, E., Rubio-Donnadieu, F., Garcia-Ramos, G. *et al.* (1983) Prevalence of epilepsy in children: Tlalpan, Mexico City, Mexico. *Neuroepidemiology*, **2**, 16–23.

Gilly, R., Lapras, C., Tommasi, M. *et al.* (1977) Maladie de Sturge–Weber–Krabbe. Réflexions a partir de 21 cas. *Pédiatrie*, **32**, 45–64.

Gomez, M.R. and Bebin, E.M. (1987) Sturge–Weber syndrome, in *Neurocutaneous Diseases: A Practical Approach*, (ed. R.M. Gomez), Butterworths, London, pp. 365–7.

Goudsmit, J., van der Waals, F.W. and Gajdusek, D.C. (1983) Epilepsy in the Gbawein and Wroughbarh clan of Grand Bassa county, Liberia: the endemic occurrence of 'See-ee' in the native population. *Neuroepidemiology*, **2**, 24–34.

Granieri, E., Rosati, G., Tola, R. *et al.* (1983) A descriptive study of epilepsy in the district of Copporo, Italy, 1964–1978. *Epilepsia*, **24**, 502–14.

Gudmundsson, G. (1966) Epilepsy in Iceland. *Acta Neurologica Scandinavica*, **43** (suppl 25), 1–124.

Guiliani, G., Terziani, S., Senigaglia, A.R. *et al.* (1992) Epilepsy in an Italian community as assessed by a survey for prescriptions of antiepileptic drugs: epidemiology and patterns of care. *Acta Neurologica Scandinavica*, **85**, 23–31.

Gustavson, K-H., Holmgren, G., Jonsell, R. and Blomquist, H.K. (1977) Severe mental retardation in children in a northern Swedish county. *Journal of Mental Deficiency Research*, **21**, 161–180.

Haerer, A.F., Anderson, D.W. and Schoenberg, B.S. (1986) Prevalence and clinical features of epilepsy in a biracial population. *Epilepsia*, **27**, 66–75.

Hagberg, B., Hagberg, G., Lewerth, A. and Lindberg, U. (1981) Mild mental retardation in Swedish school children, II etiologic and pathogenetic aspects. *Acta Paediatrica Scandinavica*, **70**, 445–52.

Hagberg, B., Hagberg, G., Olow, I. and von Wendt, L. (1989) The changing panorama of cerebral palsy in Sweden. V. The birth year period 1979–1982. *Acta Paediatrica Scandinavica*, **78**, 283–90.

Hauser, W.A. and Hesdorffer, D.C. (1990) *Epilepsy. Frequency, Causes and Consequences*, Demos Publications, New York.

Hauser, W.A. and Kurland, L.T. (1975) The epidemiology of epilepsy in Rochester, Minnesota, 1935 through 1967. *Epilepsia*, **16**, 1–66.

Hauser, W.A., Annegers, J.F. and Kurland L.T. (1991) Prevalence of epilepsy in Rochester, Minnesota: 1940–1980. *Epilepsia*, **32**, 429–45.

Heijbel, J., Blom, S. and Bergfors, P.G. (1975) Benign epilepsy of children with centrotemporal EEG foci. A study of incidence rate in outpatient care. *Epilepsia*, **16**, 657–64.

Holden, K.R., Mellits, E.D. and Freeman, J.M. (1982) Neonatal seizures. 1. Correlation of prenatal and perinatal events with outcomes. *Pediatrics*, **70**, 165–76.

Jamison, E. (1991) *World Population Profile: 1991*, US Department of Commerce.

Jilek-Aall, L., Jilek, W. and Miller, J.R. (1979) Clinical and genetic aspects of seizure disorders prevalent in an isolated African population. *Epilepsia*, **20**, 613–22.

Joensen, P. (1986) Prevalence, incidence, and classification of epilepsy in the Faroes. *Acta Neurologica Scandinavica*, **74**, 150–5.

Juul-Jensen, P. and Foldspang, A. (1983) Natural history of epileptic seizures. *Epilepsia*, **24**, 297–312.

Koul, R., Razdan, S. and Motta, A. (1988) Prevalence and pattern of epilepsy (LathIMirgi/Laran) in rural Kashmir, India. *Epilepsia*, **29**, 116–22.

Lavados, J., Germain, L., Morales, A. *et al.* (1992) A descriptive study of epilepsy in the district of El salvador, Chile, 1984–1988. *Acta Neurologica Scandinavica*, **85**, 249–56.

Li, S., Schoenberg, B.S., Wang, C. *et al.* (1985) Epidemiology of epilepsy in urban areas of the People's Republic of China. *Epilepsia*, **26**, 391–94.

Maremmani, C., Rossi, G., Bonuccelli, U. and Murri, L. (1991) Descriptive epidemiologic study of epilepsy syndromes in a district of northwest Tuscany, Italy. *Epilepsia*, **32**, 294–8.

Meighan, S.S., Queener, L., Weitman, M. (1976) Prevalence of epilepsy in children of Multnomah county, Oregon. *Epilepsia*, **17**, 245–56.

Nevin, N.C. and Pearce, W.G. (1968) Diagnostic and genetical aspects of tuberous sclerosis. *Journal of Medical Genetics*, **5**, 273–80.

Olsson, I. (1988) Epidemiology of absence epilepsy. I. Concept and incidence. *Acta Paediatrica Scandinavica*, **73**, 860–6.

Osuntokun, B.O., Adeuja, A.O.G., Schoenberg, B.S. *et al.* (1987) Prevalence of the epilepsies in Nigerian Africans: a community-based study. *Epilepsia*, **28**, 272–9.

Pampiglione, G. and Moynahan, E.J. (1976) The tuberous sclerosis syndrome: clinical and EEG studies in 100 children. *Journal of Neurology, Neurosurgery and Psychiatry*, **39**, 663–73.

Pazzaglia, P. and Frank-Pazzaglia, L. (1976) Record in grade school of pupils with epilepsy: an epidemiological study. *Epilepsia*, **17**, 361–6.

Placencia, M., Shorvon, S.D., Paredes, V. *et al.* (1992) Epileptic seizures in an Andean region of Equador. Incidence and prevalence and regional variation. *Brain*, **115**, 771–82.

Pond, D.A., Bidwell, B.H. and Stein, L. (1960) A survey of epilepsy in fourteen general practices. I. Demographic and medical data. *Psychiatrica Neurologica Neurochirurgica*, **63**, 217–36.

Rose, S.W., Penry, J.K., Markush, R.E. *et al.* (1973) Prevalence of epilepsy in children. *Epilepsia*, **14**, 113–52.

Ross, E.M., Peckham, C.S., West, P.B. and Butler, N.R. (1980) Epilepsy in childhood: findings from the National Child Development Study. *British Medical Journal*, **280**, 207–10.

Rwiza, H.T., Kilonzo, G.P., Haule, J. *et al.* (1992) Prevalence and incidence of epilepsy in Ulanga, a rural Tanzanian district: a community-based study. *Epilepsia*, **3**, 1051–6.

Sangrador, C.O. and Luaces, R.P. (1991) Study of

the prevalence of epilepsy among schoolchildren in Valladolid, Spain. *Epilepsia*, **32**, 791–7.

Saukkonen, A.-L., Serlo, W. and von Wendt, L. (1990) Epilepsy in hydrocephalic children. *Acta Paediatrica Scandinavica*, **79**, 212–8.

Seay, A.R. and Bray, P.F. (1977) Significance of seizures in infants weighing less than 2500 grams. *Archives of Neurology*, **34**, 381–2.

Senanayake, N. and Roman, G.C. (1993) Epidemiology of epilepsy in developing countries. *Bulletin of the World Health Organization*, **71**, 247–58.

Shamansky, S.L. and Glaser, G.H. (1979) Socio-economic characteristics of childhood seizure disorders in the New Haven area: an epidemiological study. *Epilepsia*, **20**, 457–74.

Sidenvall, R., Forsgren, L., Blomquist, H.K., Heijbel, J. (1993) A community based prospective incidence study of epileptic seizures in children. *Acta Paediatrica*, **82**, 60–5.

Sillanpää, M. (1973) Medico-social prognosis of children with epilepsy. Epidemiological study and analysis of 245 patients. *Acta Paediatrica Scandinavica*, **62** (suppl. 237), 1–104.

Stanhope, J.M., Brody, J.A. and Brink, E. (1972) Convulsions among the Chamorro people of Guam, Mariana Islands. I. Seizure disorders. *American Journal of Epidemiology*, **95**, 292–8.

Tekle-Haimanot, R., Forsgren, L., Abebe, M. *et al.* (1990) Clinical and electroencephalographic characteristics of epilepsy in rural Ethiopia: a community-based study. *Epilepsy Research*, **7**, 230–9.

Tsuboi, T. (1988) Prevalence and incidence of epilepsy in Tokyo. *Epilepsia*, **29**, 103–10.

Umapathy, D. and Johnston, A.W. (1989) Tuberous sclerosis: prevalence in the Grampian Region of Scotland. *Journal of Mental Deficiency Research*, **33**, 349–55.

Uvebrant, P. (1988) Hemiplegic cerebral palsy. Aetiology and outcome. *Acta Paediatrica Scandinavica*, (suppl 345).

van den Berg, B.J. and Yerushalmy, J. (1969) Studies on convulsive disorders in young children. I. Incidence of febrile and and nonfebrile convulsions by age and other factors. *Pediatric Research*, **3**, 298–304.

Verity, C.M., Ross, E.M. and Golding, J. (1992) Epilepsy in the first 10 years of life: findings of the child health and education study. *British Medical Journal*, **305**, 857–61.

von Wendt, L., Rantakallio, P., Saukkonen, A.L. and Mäkinen, H. (1985) Epilepsy and associated handicaps in a 1 year birth cohort in Northern Finland. *European Journal of Pediatrics*, **144**, 149–51.

Wajsbort, J., Haral, N. and Alfandary, I. (1967) A study of chronic epilepsy in northern Israel. *Epilepsia*, **8**, 105–16.

Webb, D.W., Fryer, A.E. and Osborne, J.P. (1991) On the incidence of fits and mental retardation. *Journal of Medical Genetics*, **28**, 395–7.

Wiederholt, W.C., Gomez, M.R. and Kurland, L.T. (1985) Incidence and prevalence of tuberous sclerosis in Rochester, Minnesota, 1950 through 1982. *Neurology*, **35**, 600–3.

Yamamoto, N., Watanabe, K., Negoro, T. *et al.* (1987) Long-term prognosis of tuberous sclerosis with epilepsy in children. *Brain Development*, **9**, 292–5.

Zielinski, J.J. (1974) *Epidemiology and Medicosocial Problems of Epilepsy in Warsaw. Final Report on Research Program no. 19-P-5832-F-01*, Psycho-neurological Institute, Warsaw.

ASPECTS OF ETIOLOGY 4

STRUCTURAL ABNORMALITIES

4a

Sheila J. Wallace

INTRODUCTION

In the past, identification of structural abnormalities relied on the recognition of major changes, visible to the naked eye, or on painstaking and very time-consuming analyses of the histologic appearances of brain obtained after death or at operation, when the changes found were not necessarily precursors of the epilepsy. The advent of sophisticated imaging techniques has allowed identification, early in life, of changes in brain formation which are increasingly recognized as important substrates for the development and persistence of epilepsy. Details of neuroimaging techniques and their applications are given in Chapter 20; of pathologic changes which can be of etiologic importance in Chapter 5; and, of epilepsies symptomatic of structural lesions in Chapter 16. This chapter reviews information on the normal development of the brain and examines how deviations from the normal sequence of events may predispose to epilepsy.

NORMAL DEVELOPMENT (Lou, 1982)

The central nervous system is formed from ectodermal cells. By a process termed gastrulation, mesodermal cells migrate to a position between the ectoderm and the endoderm and induce the formation, from the ectoderm, of the neural plate, at about 2–3 weeks' gestation. In the next 2–3 weeks, neurulation, with the formation of a closed cylinder of cells, the neural tube, from the neural plate,

acts as a basis for later growth and differentiation. During neurulation, there is rapid neuronal multiplication. Following this, the neurons migrate to their permanent positions. Migration occurs maximally between the first and sixth months of gestation. It is followed by differentiation of the neurons. Differentiation is particularly active up to 6 months postnatally, after which the rate slows down considerably, but some differentiation probably continues throughout life. There is concomitant development in the supporting and guiding cells. Dendritic and axonal development, columnar organization and synaptogenesis all proceed in an orderly fashion. There is an initial overproduction of neurons, dendritic spines and cellular contacts, with later pruning and remodelling, which leads to greater specificity and sophistication in cerebral activity.

Of the stages of cerebral development, neuronal migration seems the most relevant to later epilepsy, and an understanding of this process is useful (Caviness, 1989; Bayer and Altman, 1991; Evrard *et al.*, 1992; Palmini *et al.*, 1993).

NEURONAL MIGRATION

Neurons going to the dorsal cortex migrate in combination with radial glial fibers. The latter stretch the entire length of the cerebral wall and act as neuronal guides. Neuroblasts form in the periventricular germinal matrix and are closely, but dynamically, attached to glial

Epilepsy in Children. Edited by Sheila Wallace. Published in 1996 by Chapman & Hall, London. ISBN 0 412 56860 8

fibers through the actions of cell adhesion molecules (Palmini *et al.*, 1993). Earlier studies suggested that the final positions of neurons were always determined by simple radial migration. However, more recent work has shown that neurons which settle in the ventrolateral and lateral parts of the anterior cortex migrate laterally, and arrive at these situations later than simultaneously generated neocortical neurons which go to the dorsal part of the cortical plate (Bayer and Altman, 1991). Those neurons which migrate laterally in what is termed the lateral cortical stream, leave this stream at specific points and go to predetermined loci in the cortical plate. It is believed that thalamocortical fibers may determine the location and timing of the departure of particular neurons from the lateral cortical stream. A fundamental aspect of the radial migration pattern is that the neurons which are produced earliest in the periventricular region settle deep in the cortex, adjacent to the white matter, whereas later produced neurons settle progressively more superficially, in an 'inside-out' fashion. Considering that these younger neurons must migrate past the older, already established, cells and that lateral migration also takes place, it is not surprising that migration may at times be aberrant and that neurons might settle in areas where their contacts with other cells could cause abnormal direction of intracerebral messages, and thus predispose to epilepsy.

In most instances, once migration has been completed, there is considerable enlargement of the neuronal soma and neurite outgrowth; also, progressive elaboration of the dendritic surfaces and axonal systems takes place. However, in large-projection neurons of neocortical layers V and VI and cerebellar granular cells, some axonal elaboration may take place concurrently with migration. Both axonal and dendritic outgrowth is directed by the growth cone. Many classes of receptors are contained on the membranous surface of the growth cone, which seems to release

transmitter substances as it moves (Caviness, 1989). Axons which synthesize and contain noradrenergic and GABAergic transmitters, ramify early in plexuses of the molecular and subplate layers of the neocortex. Axons of long projection tend to grow together in common fascicles which defasciculate only when they direct their terminal arborizations to selected synaptic targets, though collaterals may arise from the fascicule along its length. The final targeting of axons is not yet fully understood, and specification of neuronal function, originally thought to have been determined before migration, is now believed to take place at a later stage.

The formation of synapses is a relatively late event (Caviness, 1989). Type I asymmetric synapses appear first and predominate; they are mainly on dendritic spines and on smaller, relatively distal segments of the dendritic arbors. Type II symmetric synapses are fewer and appear later; they are found principally on the soma and proximal dendritic trunks of target neurons. In a given projection, synapses are selective in relation to the target cell class, and their morphology can be highly characteristic in specific circumstances. Modifications which are uncharacteristic may occur if conditions of development are not normal.

Regressive events are as important in the final development of the neocortex as the arrival of the migrating cells, their organization, and the formation of synapses. Such regressive events consist of cell death, axonal pruning, and elimination of synapses. It is considered that the resultant change in the functioning of the neuronal network can be substantial (Caviness, 1989). In particular, neurons appear to be eliminated from the superficial cortical layer in a programmed manner. Even without death of the cell of origin, pruning of axons seems to be a vigorous phenomenon. The early overprovision of synapses can amount to as much as 30–40%. Synaptic numbers reach their peak in the first 6–12 months of postnatal life and remain high for about 1–2 years. Adult numbers of synapses are found from 5–10 years onwards. Such plasticity in the establishment of neuronal contacts is important in the context of epilepsy. Reinforcement of aberrant and unwanted synaptic connections may be potentiated by seizure discharges, and the development of more desirable pathways inhibited.

ABERRANT DEVELOPMENT

In children in whom disorders of neuronal proliferation result in microcephaly, epilepsy is unusual. However, when macrocephaly results, as may occur in tuberous sclerosis, seizures are often of early onset and persistent. As causes of seizures, disorders of neuronal organization are less readily defined than those of migration, but Huttenlocher (1974) demonstrated defective dendritic development in children with severe mental retardation, infantile myoclonic seizures, and hypsarrhythmia on EEG. Seizures tend to occur late in the evolution of conditions in which defective myelination or demyelination are the predominant features.

Abnormalities in neuronal migratory patterns are increasingly recognized as the underlying causes in many patients with epilepsy. They may be generalized and/or diffuse; or, focal, lateralized, or localized.

GENERALIZED OR DIFFUSE MIGRATORY ABNORMALITIES

Lissencephaly

If migration of the neurons is arrested at 12–15 weeks' gestation, there is failure of development of the gyri; or, only a few abnormally broad, gyri are formed, so that the brain has an unusually smooth appearance. The resulting cortex is very thick and consists of a molecular layer and an incompletely formed true cortex (layers I and II), which are separated from a wide field of heterotopic neurons (layer IV) by a thin zone which has a few cells in it (layer III) (Caviness, 1989). In the subcortical heterotopia, the neurons are well differentiated and are indistinguishable from those normally found in the neocortex; they survive and differentiate normally and are, therefore, capable of forming synapses and transmitting impulses. Children with lissencephaly present early with intractable epilepsy and severe mental retardation. The seizure types are varied, and often include tonic and atonic attacks. Lissencephaly usually presents as an isolated phenomenon, but can also be a component of the Miller–Dieker syndrome, when facial and somatic anomalies coexist and there is a deletion of part of the short arm of chromosome 17. The lissencephaly (type II) found in the Walker–Warburg syndrome is pathologically different, with complete disruption of the cortical architecture. Unlayered, poorly orientated cells are separated by trabeculae of gliomesenchymal tissue which is in continuity with massively proliferated meningeal mesenchyme. Although severe neurologic disability is present in the Walker–Warburg syndrome, seizures are not prominent.

Pachygyria

This exists when cerebral gyri are reduced in number, but are not completely absent. All the affected patients reported by Guerrini *et al.* (1993) were mentally retarded and had epilepsy, which was largely resistant to drug treatment.

Abnormalities of gyral formation

These may be found in a number of metabolic disorders, including nonketotic hyperglycinemia, Zellweger's syndrome, neonatal adrenoleucodystrophy, Menkes' disease, Leigh's syndrome, glutaric aciduria type II, and in the fetal alcohol syndrome (Aicardi, 1992). However, not all these disorders are as diffuse or generalized as in typical lissencephaly. In particular, multiple verrucose collections of heterotopic neurons are found throughout the cortex in glutaric aciduria type II.

Band heterotopia/double cortex
(Palmini *et al.*, 1993)

In this condition, a substantial number of neurons reach their normal positions in the cortex, but others remain in a distinct heterotopic layer which may be subcortical or periventricular. There is always a clear-cut white matter layer between the cortex and the heterotopia. The gyral pattern may or may not be normal. These abnormalities are demonstrable by MRI, and can be missed if reliance is on CT scanning only. The spectrum of disability associated with double cortex/band heterotopias is very wide. Some children have only mild mental retardation and seizures, usually secondary generalized or partial, which respond readily to drug therapy; others are severely disabled by very resistant epilepsy and significant mental retardation.

Aicardi's syndrome

This syndrome is characterized by its occurrence in females, agenesis of the corpus callosum, choroidoretinal lacunae, and infantile spasms. The cortex is thin and unlayered; there is diffuse polymicrogyria with fused molecular layers, and nodular heterotopias are found in the periventricular region and in the centrum ovale. Although the seizures resemble infantile spasms, hypsarrhythmia is not found, but asymmetric and asynchronous abnormalities, with or without suppression-burst, are recorded on the EEG in both waking and sleeping states.

FOCAL, LATERALIZED OR LOCALIZED MIGRATORY ABNORMALITIES

Hemimegalencephaly

In hemimegalencephaly, a variety of abnormalities of the cortical architecture are found. They include areas of pachygyria and polymicrogyria, in addition to subcortical neuronal heterotopias. The affected hemisphere and the ipsilateral ventricle are enlarged. The seizures which develop are partial, with or without secondary generalization, and are likely to be resistant to medical treatment.

Focal cortical dysplasia, focal pachygyria, and focal polymicrogyria

These can all present with therapy-resistant partial seizures.

Nodular gray matter heterotopias

These heterotopias are probably the commonest form of neuronal migration disorder. They are not always associated with recognizable seizure disorders and, when small, are possibly a feature of brain development which is not necessarily abnormal. Although if seizures present in association with heterotopias recognizable on imaging, they are usually partial, microscopic areas of dysgenesis have been identified at postmortem in the brains of patients who have had epilepsies considered to be primary generalized (Meencke and Janz, 1984).

The congenital bilateral perisylvian syndrome

This syndrome is characterized clinically by a combination of congenital facio-pharyngo-masticatory diplegia, epilepsy, and mental retardation (Kuzniecky, Anderman and the CBPS Multicenter Collaborative Study Group, 1993). Bilateral, symmetric perisylvian structural abnormalities are found on imaging. Only two brains have become available for examination pathologically: in one, there was asymmetric opercularization; in the other, bilateral opercular hypoplasia with exposure of the insula was found. Four-layered polymicrogyria was observed in the insular and opercular region, extending to the inferior frontal and parietal regions. The polymicrogyric cortex intermixed abruptly with normal cortex. The seizures in this condition include atypical absences and tonic, atonic, and generalized tonic-clonic attacks.

CONCLUSIONS

Although cerebral development as a whole is clearly important in any condition giving rise to neurologic handicap, disorders of neuronal migration, particularly those in which neurons behave normally, but are misplaced, are very important substrates on which epilepsy may develop. In children with persisting therapy-resistant seizures of partial onset, current imaging techniques should be used to the greatest possible extent, so that heterotopias, which might be amenable to surgery, can be identified.

REFERENCES

Aicardi, J. (1992) Malformations of the CNS, in *Diseases of the Nervous System in Childhood* (ed. J. Aicardi), MacKeith Press, London, pp. 108–202.

Bayer, S.A. and Altman, J. (1991) *Neocortical Development*, Raven Press, New York.

Caviness, V.S. (1989) Normal development of the cerebral neocortex, in *Developmental Neurobiology* (eds P. Evrard and A. Minkowski), Raven Press, New York, pp. 1–10.

Evrard, P., Miladi, N., Bonnier, C. and Gressens, P. (1992) Normal and abnormal development of the brain, in *Handbook of Neuropsychology*, Vol 6: *Child Neuropsychology* (eds I. Rapin and S.J. Segalowitz), Elsevier, Amsterdam.

Guerrini, R., Robain, O., Dravet, Ch. *et al.* (1993) Clinical, electrographic and pathological findings in the malformations of the cerebral cortex, in *New Trends in Pediatric Neurology* (eds N. Fejerman and N.A. Chamoles), Elsevier, Amsterdam, pp. 101–7.

Huttenlocher, P.R. (1974) Dendritic development in neocortex of children with mental defect and infantile spasms. *Neurology*, **24**, 203–10.

Kuzniecky, R., Andermann, F. and the CBPS Multicenter Collaborative Study Group (1993) The congenital bilateral perisylvian syndrome: a study of 31 patients, in *New Trends in Pediatric Neurology* (eds N. Fejerman and N.A. Chamoles), Elsevier, Amsterdam, pp. 95–100.

Lou, H.C. (1982) *Developmental Neurology*, Raven Press, New York.

Meencke, H.-J. and Janz, D. (1984) Neuropathological findings in primary generalized epilepsy. A study of eight cases. *Epilepsia*, **25**, 8–21.

Palmini, A., da Costa, J.C., Andermann, F. and Neto, P.R. (1993) Neuronal migration disorders and seizures in children: neurobiology, epileptic syndromes, neuroimaging and surgical treatment, in *New Trends in Pediatric Neurology* (eds N. Fejerman and N.A. Chamoles), Elsevier, Amsterdam, pp. 87–94.

ASSOCIATIONS WITH CHROMOSOMAL ABNORMALITIES

4b

David Ravine

The past decade has witnessed both a convergence of molecular genetics and cytogenetics and ongoing technical improvements in cytogenetics, particularly in high-resolution banding. These advances are responsible for a revolution in the understanding of the etiology of a number of conditions which were previously the domain of clinicians skilled in syndromic pattern recognition. An ever-increasing number of syndromes, some with epilepsy as part of their clinical spectra, are now known to have an underlying chromosomal abnormality with an associated molecular counterpart. Epilepsies associated with mental retardation are further considered in Chapter 17.

Small chromosomal deletions, duplications, or variations in copy number of repeated sequences cause loss, imbalance, or disruption of a gene or a number of contiguous genes with a resultant clinical phenotype. The size of a deletion can vary from loss of microscopically visible chromosomal segments through to submicroscopic molecular deletions involving only the 'critical region' responsible for the development of the phenotype. Phenotypic expression may not only be determined by the presence of a deletion, but also by the sex of the transmitting parent. This modification of gene expression by parental origin of the gene is termed genomic imprinting, and is now known to be an important factor in the Angelman and Prader–Willi syndrome phenotypes. Another recently recognized genetic mechanism is gene disruption due to variation in copy number of repeated DNA sequences. These variable repeated sequences, some of which may be detected cytogenetically, are now known to be responsible for several inherited human diseases, including the fragile X syndrome.

In addition to the syndromes that have epilepsy and an underlying cytogenetic abnormality, there are a large number of other apparently nonspecific chromosomal deletions and duplications in which epilepsy is a prominent feature. This section focuses on the more frequent or distinctive syndromes with an underlying chromosomal abnormality which have epilepsy as a prominent feature. A more comprehensive review of neurologic disorders, including epilepsy, associated with chromosomal anomalies has been previously published (Kunze, 1980). Although lacking the additional information now available from more recent clinical and molecular advances, the scope of Kunze's review ensures that it will remain a valuable reference.

FRAGILE X SYNDROME

The fragile X syndrome, with an estimated prevalence of 0.4–8 per 1000 males, is the most common human chromosomal anomaly associated with heritable mental retardation.

Epilepsy in Children. Edited by Sheila Wallace. Published in 1996 by Chapman & Hall, London. ISBN 0 412 56860 8

It is also the first condition identified in a class of genetic disorders now known to be due to dynamic mutation in heritable unstable DNA (Richards and Sutherland 1992). Both males and females can be affected phenotypically although, in keeping with X-linked inheritance, the phenotype is much more severe in males. The DNA instability is due to variation in the copy number of a trinucleotide repeat p(CCG)n, within the region of the FMR-1 (Fragile X Mental Retardation-1) gene located at Xq27.3. Prior to the discovery of the molecular abnormality, the syndrome was identified through cytogenetic recognition of a fragile site at the Xq27.3 locus when folate deficient culture media was used. In addition to mental retardation, hypotonia is common, as is a degree of incoordination. Affected individuals frequently have a distinctive long, narrow facies with prominent ears. Macro-orchidism is common, as are orthopedic problems including scoliosis, joint laxity, and pes planus. While focal neurologic signs are absent, seizures, either generalized or complex partial in nature, occur with some frequency (Wisniewski *et al.* 1991). An EEG pattern of medium- to high-voltage unilateral or bilateral spikes in the temporal area is common and can be identified in affected males with and without seizures. The temporal or central spikes are sometimes multifocal, with two or more independent, occasionally alternating, foci that occur primarily during sleep (Musumeci *et al.* 1988). A behavioral phenotype is also recognized, and while many have an interest in relating socially, affected people are frequently anxious, easily overstimulated and subsequently avoidant, with autistic-like features including hyperactivity, perseverative speech, hand-biting, hand-flapping, and poor eye contact (Hagerman *et al.*, 1986).

ANGELMAN'S SYNDROME

Seizures are common in Angelman's syndrome, which is characterized by a specific facial appearance, severe mental retardation, virtually absent language, laughter, and ataxic movements. The condition results from absence of a maternally contributed segment of chromosome 15 (15q11–13). Convulsions, which often fluctuate in an episodic pattern, generally commence between 18 and 24 months of age and become less frequent in later childhood (Clayton-Smith and Pembrey, 1992). They can be of any type and control is often difficult, particularly during periods of exacerbation. A number of characteristic EEG changes have been described. The most consistent finding is posterior slow wave activity with discharges, facilitated by or seen only on passive eye closure (Boyd *et al.*, 1988). Repeated EEGs may be necessary before the typical appearances are demonstrated. A gene encoding a receptor subunit for the inhibitory neuropeptide GABA (GABARB3) has been localized to the 15q11–13 region (Wagstaff *et al.*, 1991). However, while deletions in Angelman's syndrome have included this gene, the gene is also deleted in Prader–Willi syndrome, a condition where seizures are uncommon. Thus, while GABARB3 involvement may have some role in predisposing those with Angelman's syndrome to epilepsy, it is not the only factor involved.

PRADER–WILLI SYNDROME

Clinical manifestations include reduced fetal movements, infantile hypotonia and feeding problems, mental retardation, childhood hyperphagia and obesity, short stature, small hands and feet, hypogonadism, and a distinctive facial appearance. Epilepsy is uncommon. In one survey of 63 affected adults, only two had a history of seizures (Clarke *et al.*, 1989). In contrast to Angelman's syndrome, the cause of Prader–Willi syndrome appears to be the absence of a paternal contribution of 15q11–q13, whether by a paternally derived deletion or maternal uniparental disomy.

CYTOGENETIC AND MOLECULAR STUDIES IN THE ANGELMAN AND PRADER–WILLI SYNDROMES

The majority of patients with Angelman's syndrome and Prader–Willi syndrome have a deletion of chromosome 15q11–13, the primary difference being in the parental origin of the deletion. The clinical differences and the apparent cytogenetic similarity of Angelman's syndrome and Prader–Willi syndrome raise many intriguing questions and have provoked a number of intensive investigations. Gene(s) in 15q11–13 appear to be maternally or paternally imprinted during gametogenesis, so that copies from each parent are required for normal development (Knoll *et al.*, 1993). Deletions from parents of the opposite sex manifest clinically distinct syndromes, and additional copies of genes from one parent do not balance missing genes from the other parent. Angelman's syndrome results from a lack of maternal contribution from chromosome 15q11–13. Loss of the maternal copy occurs either by maternal deletion of 15q11–13, or, more rarely, by paternal uniparental disomy involving chromosome 15. In contrast, the cause of Prader–Willi syndrome appears to be the absence of a paternal contribution of 15q11–13, whether by a paternally derived deletion or maternal uniparental disomy. The segment of 15q11–13 considered to contain the critical region(s) for the two syndromes is currently being narrowed down.

MILLER–DIEKER SYNDROME

Miller–Dieker syndrome is characterized by severe disturbance of neuronal migration (type 1 lissencephaly) and a distinctive facies, including prominent forehead, bitemporal hollowing, and a short nose with upturned nares. (See Chapter 4a) Crying often brings out prominent vertical forehead furrowing. Apneic or tonic seizures usually begin between 3 and 6 months, and life expectancy is about 2 years. Cytogenetically visible 17p13.3 deletions, both maternally and paternally derived, have been observed in some patients, while in others, molecular studies have established the existence of submicroscopic deletions (Dobyns *et al.*, 1991).

SMITH–MAGENIS SYNDROME

Seizures, psychomotor retardation, and pathologic evidence of a neuronal migration defect occur in the Smith–Magenis syndrome, which is also associated with small deletions of the short arm of chromosome 17 (Smith *et al.*, 1986). Although on the same arm of chromosome 17, the Smith–Magenis deletion at 17p11.2 is proximal to the deletion responsible for the Miller–Dieker syndrome, and while seizures, congenital heart disease and microcephaly occur in both conditions, they have little else in common. Smith–Magenis syndrome has a distinctive facies, including midfacial hypoplasia and brachycephaly, and other distinctive features, including short, broad hands, pronounced speech delay and mental retardation ranging from mild to severe. Approximately 60% have seizures, while 70% exhibit selfmutilatory behavior. The ages at which patients have been described range from the neonatal period to 62 years.

WOLF–HIRSCHHORN SYNDROME

Small deletions involving distal 4p are responsible for the Wolf–Hirschhorn syndrome, another clinically recognizable, multiple-anomaly syndrome. The phenotype is striking, featuring growth and mental retardation, seizures, microcephaly, hypertelorism, colobomas, prominent glabella, cleft lip or palate, and cardiac defects. The majority of 4p deletions are de novo and paternally derived (Quarrell *et al.*, 1991). A submicroscopic deletion, detectable only by molecular probes, has been reported (Alherr *et al.*, 1991).

PALLISTER–KILLIAN SYNDROME

This syndrome of severe mental retardation, distinctive facies with bitemporal alopecia, forehead prominence, ptosis and short anteverted nostrils has an underlying tissue-limited chromosomal mosaicism involving tetrasomy of the short arm of chromosome 12. A small marker chromosome, isochromosome 12p(i(12p)), is found in fibroblasts. At birth the i(12p) is to be found in metaphases from direct bone marrow preparations, and often in mosaic form in peripheral lymphocytes, although the abnormal population rapidly disappears from the circulation. Culture of skin fibroblasts prior to cytogenetic studies may also result in loss of the abnormal cell line. The majority of patients will develop a seizure disorder, mostly starting in early infancy, although onset in young adult life has been documented. In adulthood, features include a coarse face, enlarged tongue, profound mental handicap, and epilepsy (Quarrell, Hamill and Hughes, 1988).

TRISOMY 12p

The phenotype of the 12p trisomy syndrome is well defined and characterized by turricephaly, flat occiput, and characteristic facies which bears strong similarities to the features of the Pallister–Killian syndrome (Schinzel, 1983). Neurologic features include early hypotonia, severe mental retardation, and seizures. EEG findings of 3 Hz generalized spike and wave discharges have been reported in some cases (Guerrini *et al.*, 1990).

RING CHROMOSOME 14

Common to all cases are seizures that appear in early infancy and which are often difficult to control (Schinzel, 1983). Growth retardation is prominent and characteristic dysmorphic signs include dolichocephaly with biparietal narrowing, epicanthic folds, flat nasal bridge, anteverted nostrils, and abnormal

pigmentation of skin and retina. Microcephaly and moderate to severe psychomotor retardation are frequent, as are variable neurologic abnormalities, including tremor, athetoid movements, hypotonia, and hypertonia (Schmidt *et al.*, 1981).

TRISOMY 21 (DOWN'S SYNDROME)

In a large retrospective study of adults with Down's syndrome, 6.4% had seizures, of whom 62% had an identifiable etiology, usually related to a common medical complication of Down's syndrome such as neonatal hypoxia-ischemia, hypoxia from congenital heart disease, or infection (Strafstrom *et al.*, 1991). In contrast to those with an identifiable etiology, half of those with seizures of unknown etiology had no diagnostic work-up beyond an EEG. While there is some evidence that brains from individuals with Down's syndrome have a unique pathophysiology that would tend to shift the balance in favour of net cortical excitation (Wisniewski *et al.*, 1986), it appears that the majority with seizures have had an acute medical illness that has precipitated seizures in brains already predisposed to hyperexcitability. It is recommended that all Down's syndrome children with seizures undergo investigations to determine the likely etiology (Stafstrom *et al.*, 1991).

TRISOMY 13 (PATAU'S SYNDROME)

Major structural defects are a common occurrence, and include brain defects such as holoprosencephaly and cerebellar hypoplasia. Seizures and apneic episodes occur, and the mean life expectancy is 130 days. While approximately half die during the first month, 15% survive the first year. Survival beyond 3 years is exceptional.

TRISOMY 18 (EDWARD'S SYNDROME)

The median life expectancy for liveborn infants with trisomy 18 is less than 1 week, with a range from 1 hour to 18 months.

Mental deficiency is severe and, like trisomy 13, major structural brain defects are common, as are seizures and apneic episodes.

SEX CHROMOSOME ANEUPLOIDY

Sex chromosome abnormalities, including Turner's syndrome (45,X), Kleinfelter's syndrome (47,XXY) and the various X-aneuploidies are not generally associated with an increased susceptibility to seizures. An exception to this is the sometimes severe phenotype associated with ring (X) and ring (Y) chromosomes (van Dyke *et al.*, 1992). It is now recognized that there is a syndrome of growth deficiency, mental retardation, seizures, facial dysmorphism, in some cases streaky hypo- or hyperpigmentation of the skin, and occasional limb defects, usually associated with mosaicism for small ring (X) chromosomes but sometimes with ring (Y) and occasionally with 45,X/46,XY mosaicism (Dennis *et al.*, 1993). It is apparent that this syndrome accounts for some cases categorized as hypomelanosis of Ito.

HYPOMELANOSIS OF ITO

This condition has hypopigmented lesions, distributed in a swirling or streaked pattern over the body according to the lines of Blaschko (Happle, 1993). Three-quarters of reported cases also have one or more abnormalities of the CNS, eyes, hair, teeth, or musculoskeletal system. CNS manifestations include seizures, mental retardation of varying degrees, and autistic symptoms. Chromosomal mosaicism of autosomes or sex chromosomes is frequently detected, and the mosaic cytogenetic defect is considered responsible for the pigmentary patterns as well as the other features present. Usually, the chromosomal mosaicism is detectable in fibroblasts and/or peripheral blood lymphocytes, although occasionally it is detectable only in epidermal keratinocytes.

REFERENCES

Alherr, M.R., Bengtsson, U., Elder, F.F.B. *et al.* (1991) Molecular confirmation of Wolf–Hirshhorn syndrome with a subtle translocation of chromosome 4. *American Journal of Medical Genetics*, **49**, 1235–42.

Boyd, S.G., Harden, A. and Patton, M.A. (1988) The EEG in early diagnosis of the Angelman (Happy Puppet) syndrome. *European Journal of Pediatrics*, **147**, 508–13.

Clarke, D.J., Waters, J. and Corbett, J.A. (1989) Adults with Prader–Willi syndrome: abnormalities of sleep and behaviour. *Journal of the Royal Society of Medicine*, **82**, 21–4.

Clayton-Smith, J. and Pembrey, M.E. (1992) Angelman syndrome. *Journal of Medical Genetics*, **29**, 412–5.

Dennis, N.R., Collins, A.L., Crolla, J.A. *et al.* (1993) Three patients with ring (X) chromosomes and a severe phenotype. *Journal of Medical Genetics*, **30**, 482–6.

Dobyns, W.B., Curry, C.J.R., Hoyme, E.H. *et al.* (1991) Clinical and molecular diagnosis of Miller–Dieker syndrome. *American Journal of Human Genetics*, **48**, 584–94.

Guerrini, R., Bureau, M., Mattei, M.-G. *et al.* (1990) Trisomy 12p syndrome: a chromosomal disorder associated with generalized 3-Hz spike and wave discharges. *Epilepsia*, **31**, 557–66.

Hagerman, R.J., Jackson, A.W., Levitas, A. *et al.* (1986) An analysis of autism in 50 males with fragile X syndrome. *American Journal of Medical Genetics*, **23**, 359–74.

Happle, R. (1993) An early drawing of Blaschko's lines. *British Journal of Dermatology*, **128**, 464.

Knoll, J.H.M., Wagstaff, J. and Lalande, M. (1993) Cytogenetic and molecular studies in the Prader–Willi and Angelman syndromes: an overview. *American Journal of Medical Genetics*, **46**, 2–6.

Kunze, J. (1980) Neurological disorders in patients with chromosomal anomalies. *Neuropediatrics*, **11**, 203–49.

Musumeci, D.A., Ferri, R., Colognola, R.M. *et al.* (1988) Prevalence of a novel epileptogenic EEG pattern in the Martin–Bell syndrome. *American Journal of Medical Genetics*, **30**, 207–12.

Quarrell, O.W.J., Hamill, M.A. and Hughes H.E. (1988) Pallister–Killian mosaic syndrome with emphasis on the adult phenotype. *American Journal of Medical Genetics*, **31**, 841–4.

Quarrell, O.W.J., Snell, R.G., Curtis, M.A. *et al.* (1991) Paternal origin of the chromosomal deletion resulting in Wolf–Hirschhorn syndrome. *Journal of Medical Genetics*, **28**, 256–9.

Richards, R.I. and Sutherland, G.R. (1992) Heritable unstable DNA sequences. *Nature Genetics*, **1**, 7–9.

Schmidt, R., Eviatar, L., Nitowsky, H.M. *et al.* (1981) Ring chromosome 14: a distinct clinical entity. *Journal of Medical Genetics*, **18**, 304–7.

Schinzel, A. (1983) *Catalogue of Unbalanced Chromosome Aberrations in Man*, de Gruyter, New York.

Smith, A.C.M., McGavran, L., Robinson, J. *et al.* (1986) Interstitial deletion of (17)(p11.2p11.2) in nine patients. *American Journal of Medical Genetics*, **24**, 393–414.

Stafstrom, C.E., Patxot, O.F., Gilmore, H.E. and Wisniewski, K.E. (1991) Seizures in children with Down syndrome: etiology, characteristics and outcome. *Developmental Medicine and Child Neurology*, **33**, 191–200.

van Dyke, D.L., Wiktor, A., Palmer, C.G. *et al.* (1992) Ullrich–Turner syndrome with a small ring X chromosome and presence of mental retardation. *American Journal of Medical Genetics*, **43**, 996–1005.

Wagstaff, J., Knoll, J.H.M., Fleming, J. *et al.* (1991) Localization of the gene encoding the $GABA_A$ receptor B3 subunit to the Angelman/Prader–Willi region of human chromosome 15. *American Journal of Medical Genetics*, **49**, 330–7.

Wisniewski, K.E., Laure-Kamionowska, M., Connell, F. and Wen, G.Y. (1986) Neuronal density and synaptogenesis in the postnatal stages of brain maturation in Down syndrome, in *The Neurobiology of Down Syndrome* (ed. C. Epstein), Raven Press, New York

Wisniewski, K.E., Segan, S.M., Miezejeski, C.M. *et al.* (1991) The fra(x) syndrome: neurological, electrophysiologic, and neuropathological abnormalities. *American Journal of Medical Genetics*, **38**, 476–80.

Peter G. Barth

INTRODUCTION

Epileptic seizures as components of inherited disorders of metabolism are dealt with here. The part played by epileptic seizures in such disorders is variable. For example, in the mucopolysaccharidoses, the propensity to seizures is low, manifesting only in the terminal stage, and even then the impact on the general status of the patient may be limited and easy to manage. By contrast, in other disorders, such as Alpers' disease, epilepsy is an early sign or even the first symptom, and difficult to manage. Epilepsy may be nonspecific, or take such a typical course that its clinical pattern or its EEG features, or both, may aid significantly in early diagnosis. Such is the case in the ceroid-lipofuscinoses. Not all inherited metabolic disorders that may cause seizures at some time in some patients are included. A selection had to be made, in order to present the most important disorders in detail. Inclusion in this chapter was prompted by those disorders where:

1. Epilepsy is seen early in the course of the disease and plays a significant role in the diagnostic process, or
2. Typical epileptic syndromes such as myoclonus, infantile spasms, or neonatal seizures are present, or
3. Management of seizures causes special problems.

Epilepsy plays a role in some well-defined inherited neurodegenerative disorders which still await the identification of the biochemical defects involved. It was decided to include these disorders.

In the field of inherited neurometabolic disorders one and the same genetic defect may present at all ages, even in adulthood, dependent on: the amount of residual activity of the deficient enzyme; the effects of modifying genes, or, external factors. This expression of the same gene defect across different age groups would provide a good argument for disregarding age in the plan of this chapter part. However, considerations of clinical diagnosis and of treatment make it necessary to take into account the age at onset. This applies especially to the neonatal period with its peculiar and unique metabolic demands during adaptation from intrauterine to extrauterine life. Hence the neonatal period has been singled out for special attention. More detailed classification, based on age, may be appropriate in some disorders, but will not enhance understanding in others. Therefore a further subclassification based on age has been deliberately omitted. A summary of investigations which can be appropriate is given in Chapter 21.

DISORDERS WITH NEONATAL ONSET

Inborn errors of metabolism may cause neonatal seizures first, followed by other symptoms or, alternatively, may have alarming symptoms such as progressive drowsiness and 'irritability' before convulsions appear,

Epilepsy in Children. Edited by Sheila Wallace. Published in 1996 by Chapman & Hall, London. ISBN 0 412 56860 8

or drowsiness and irritability may start co-incidentally with a series of seizures. The presence of other neurologic symptoms beside seizures depends on whether the nature of the underlying disorder is destructive.

In any newborn presenting with seizures, hypoglycemia or hypocalcemia should be ruled out. Routine transfontanellar ultrasonography will exclude major brain malformations or intraparenchymal hemorrhage responsible for seizures.

Cerebrospinal fluid must be taken to rule out infectious disease. Metabolic causes of neonatal seizures will have to be considered if these more frequent causes have been ruled out.

Antepartum fetal hypoxia/ischemia may cause meconium-stained amniotic fluid and low Apgar scores. However, a bad start may also be an early symptom in some inborn errors. Therefore such symptoms should not be taken to exclude inborn errors if further deterioration takes place. Nonoptimal adaptation to the birth process may be the first symptom of an inborn error. Seizures in the neonate are further considered in Chapter 9.

The inherited metabolic disorders detailed below should be considered and probed by diagnostic procedures in the neonate with unexpected seizures.

AMINO ACID DISORDERS INCLUDING DISORDERS OF GABA METABOLISM

Neonatal seizures due to vitamin B_6 dependency

Vitamin B_6 is present in various dietary products such as pyridoxal, pyridoxamine, and pyridoxine. The phosphorylated active compound, pyridoxal-5'-phosphate (PLP), is a cofactor to enzymes catalyzing decarboxylation and transamination of amino acids. Consequently the deficiency of pyridoxine may be expected to cause widely different clinical symptoms. These include hypochromic an-

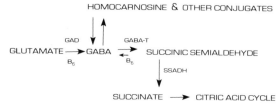

Fig. 4c.1 Disorders of GABA metabolism. GAD = glutamic acid decarboxylase; GABA = gamma-amino-butyric acid; SSADH = succinic-semi-aldehyde dehydrogenase.

emia, mucous membrane and skin lesions, polyneuropathy, and epileptic seizures. Seizures due to dietary B_6 deficiency are related to diminished activity of glutamic acid decarboxylase (GAD). The enzyme catalyzes the formation of GABA (γ-amino-butyric acid), the most important inhibitory neurotransmitter of the brain, from glutamate. This enzyme also requires PLP as cofactor (Fig. 4c.1). Dietary B_6 deficiency impairs activity of GAD by causing deficiency of PLP.

In neonatal seizures due to vitamin B_6 dependency, no dietary deficiency has been found. It is an inherited disorder. The first report by Hunt *et al.* (1954) followed the observation of a neonate whose convulsions started at 3 hours of age and were refractory to phenobarbitone, but disappeared after a multivitamin injection. The active ingredient finally turned out to be pyridoxine given in a dosage of 6 mg daily. Pyridoxine at 2 mg given daily orally was effective in preventing recurrence of seizures. In 1967, Bejsovec, Kulenda and Ponca were able to review 16 previous reports and added the first family history with intrauterine seizures.

In the typical case, seizures occur in a newborn within hours after birth, are difficult to control by conventional antiepileptic therapy, and respond promptly to administration of a high dose of pyridoxine intramuscularly or intravenously. Mothers may sense these seizures prenatally as hiccup-like movements of the fetus. The history may be compounded by fetal distress and meconium-stained amniotic fluid (Bankier, Turner and Hopkins, 1983). Continuation of vitamin B_6 in high oral doses is required to keep the baby seizure free.

Studies on the biochemical background of the disorder have excluded abnormal uptake of B_6, or deficient synthesis of PLP (Heeley *et al.*, 1978). A genetic mutation is thought to affect the binding site of the apo-enzyme to its co-enzyme PLP (Fig. 4c.1). Vitamin B_6 dependency responds to pharmacologic doses of parenteral pyridoxine by expanding the co-enzyme pool and thus off-setting adverse kinetics (Minns, 1980). The activity of GAD in biopsied kidney tissue of a patient with B_6 dependency was deficient (Yoshida, Tada and Ara Rawa, 1971), but the significance of the finding has been questioned because GAD proteins in kidney and brain are not identical. Deficient activity in autopsied brain from a patient was found by Lot *et al.* (1978). One more practical approach to clinical biochemical diagnosis is measurement of GABA in CSF. GABA is present in CSF in two forms: as the free amino acid and in its peptide bound forms, such as in the tripeptide homocarnosine (Jaeken *et al.*, 1990). GABA in the CSF reflects production in the brain, rather than peripheral production. Sensitive methods are available for GABA measurement in the CSF. However, concentration gradients both for free and total GABA and for homocarnosine should be taken into account, with the lowest concentrations being present in the lowest part (the first fraction obtained at lumbar puncture), and higher concentrations at higher levels (Grove *et al.*, 1982). Comparison between samples is possible only when they are drawn from corresponding fractions. CSF samples for GABA measurement should be deeply frozen immediately after lumbar puncture, because enzymatic peptide degradation may cause an artefactual increase (Jaeken *et al.*, 1990). GABA was found to be deficient in the CSF in B_6 dependent seizures (Kurlemann *et al.*, 1987), but more observations on free and

bound GABA in this disease will be needed. Finally, although its existence in man has yet to be proved, the existence of a B_6 resistant GAD deficiency should be kept in mind.

Diagnosis and treatment

In any baby or infant who presents with refractory seizures or has seizures known to be familial, pyridoxine should be tried as therapy. The amount of pyridoxine required to control the seizures may vary, but 100 mg intravenously or intramuscularly may be required. The effect, monitored by EEG before and after administration, should be quick. Continuation of oral therapy should be with the lowest daily dose required to prevent seizures from recurring. A CSF sample for determination of GABA and GABA-containing peptides should ideally be taken before the start of treatment. Facilities for resuscitation should be kept at hand, because of a danger of respiratory depression following the first large dose of pyridoxine (Kroll, 1985).

GABA transaminase (GABA-T) deficiency (Fig. 4c.1)

This is the only other disorder in the metabolic routes of GABA which leads to neonatal seizures. Only one family has been described (Jaeken *et al.*, 1984). Furthermore the deficiency leads to increased somatic growth, megalencephaly, and spongiform degeneration of myelin. Increased levels of GABA and β-alanine in urine and increased levels of GABA, homocarnosine and β-alanine were found in the CSF. GABA-T activity was diminished in a liver biopsy.

Disorders of the urea cycle (hyperammonemias)

Inherited deficiency of an urea cycle enzyme may result in a severe neonatal encephalopathy, with coma and epileptic seizures. The most frequently affected enzymes in the neonate are carbamyl phosphate synthetase (CPS), argininosuccinic acid synthetase (AS), argininosuccinate lyase (AL), and ornithine transcarbamylase (OCT). Disorders of the first three are inherited in an autosomal recessive mode. OCT deficiency is X-linked, and although female carriers may be clinically affected, usually, only males suffer the severe neonatal form.

Prematurely born neonates may suffer from a transient hyperammonemia which is not genetic and may be caused by micro-thrombi in the portal system (Van Geet *et al.*, 1991).

Diagnosis and treatment

Patients with neonatal hyperammonemia behave perfectly normally at birth. Until birth, clearance of their ammonia overload is through their mother's liver. After birth ammonia starts to accumulate, and will lead to seizures and drowsiness, usually after the first 24 hours. Ammonia levels of 100–150 μM/l cause lethargy, poor feeding and vomiting, hyperventilation, and grunting respiration. Focal or generalized seizures may occur, together with abnormal posturing and diaphoresis. Levels above 400 μM/l result in coma, and above 500 μM/l in brain swelling and irreversible brain damage (Breningstall, 1986). Prompt diagnosis and treatment may prevent lethal brain damage. Treatment includes hemodialysis, and intravenously administered ligands such as benzoate which binds glycine and prevents excess ammonia formation from amino acid breakdown. Administration of arginine enhances disposal of NH_3 in cases of AS and AL deficiency.

Sulfite oxidase deficiency and molybdenum cofactor deficiency

Sulfite oxidase, a mitochondrial enzyme, catalyzes the oxidation of inorganic sulfite ($SO_3^=$) to sulfate ($SO_4^=$). The oxidation takes place in the space between the outer and inner mitochondrial membranes. A major source of sulfite in the body is the S atom of cysteine. Sulfite oxidase contains molybdenum complexed to a pterin as cofactor. The molybdenum cofactor is present in two other oxidases, xanthine dehydrogenase, an enzyme involved in the tandem oxidations of hypoxanthine to xanthine and xanthine to uric acid, and, also aldehyde oxidase. Sulfite oxidase deficiency occurs in two forms: as an isolated enzyme defect and as part of a general deficiency of the molybdenum cofactor-containing enzymes.

Sulfite oxidase deficiency and molybdenum cofactor deficiency both lead to the accumulation of sulfite, and share the same clinical symptomatology.

The accumulation of hypoxanthine in molybdenum cofactor deficiency does not cause cerebral symptoms. Sulfite oxidase deficiency was first reported in 1967 by Irreverre *et al.*, and molybdenum cofactor deficiency in 1978 by Duran *et al.*

The deficiency of sulfite oxidase, either as single deficiency or as part of general deficiency of the molybdenum cofactor, leads to severe and irreversible cerebral damage which starts to develop immediately after birth. In fact, this is one of the most destructive and unmanageable inborn errors of metabolism that affects the neonatal brain. Both deficiencies have autosomal recessive inheritance.

Patients with either defect are born normally, and may not display dysmorphic features, but abnormal facial features, especially enophthalmy, microcephaly, and, in one case, palatoschisis have been described (Wadman *et al.*, 1983). Patients usually develop convulsions as early as the first week of life. Their CT scan or ultrasonography will display early and severe signs of brain damage, which may be very similar to the effects of brain damage due to perinatal asphyxia. CT scans show universal hypo-

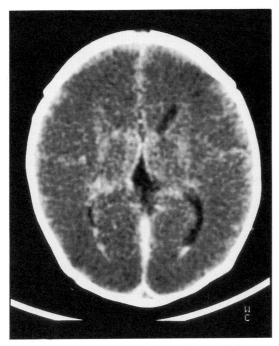

Fig. 4c.2 CT scan of newborn with molybdenum co-factor deficiency (contrast enhanced). Loss of distinction between neocortex and central white matter suggests cytotoxic edema. Hypodensity of neocortex and thalamus. Minor hemorrhage in the posterior horns. The picture is similar to severe hypoxic/ischemic damage.

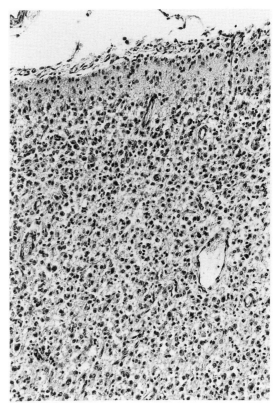

Fig. 4c.3 Neocortex of 9-day-old newborn with molybdenum co-factor deficiency displays severe destruction. Loss of normal distinction between cortical layers is caused by severe loss of neurons and dense infiltration with macrophages. (HE stain).

density and loss of distinction between cortex and central and subcortical white matter (Fig. 4c.2) Later CT scanning may reveal generalized shrinkage and cortical and thalamic calcification (Endres *et al.*, 1988; Brown *et al.*, 1989; Slot *et al.*, 1993). Even the later pictures may suggest perinatal asphyxia as the cause of the damage. Severe neonatal encephalopathy may lead to early central hypoventilation and ventilator dependency (Brown *et al.*, 1989; Slot *et al.*, 1993). Patients may die in the neonatal period or later. Later symptoms of severe damage include spastic quadriplegia and severe cognitive impairment. Lens dislocation has been found in older cases, but this symptom, though highly characteristic, is not present in all cases. Neuropathologic

descriptions (Rosenblum, 1968; Barth *et al.*, 1985; Roth *et al.*, 1985; Brown *et al.*, 1989) point to a severe destructive process operating both on the cerebral cortex and on the subcortical and deep white matter, with subsequent atrophy and patchy mineralization. In the newborn cases spongiosis of the cerebral cortex and subcortical and deep white matter is striking. Microcavitation is found in the white matter. The loss of neurons, especially in the cerebral cortex, is extreme, and is more severe than is usually encountered in perinatal hypoxic-ischemic encephalopathy (Fig. 4c.3).

Diagnosis and treatment

Sulfite oxidase deficiency should be suspected in any neonate with unexpected encephalopathy and seizures following normal birth, and in any neonate with progressive encephalopathy. Fresh urine specimens should be screened for the presence of sulfite, because sulfite in the sample will be oxidized to sulfate on standing. General screening should include amino acid and purine analysis. Typical metabolic findings in the urine in both disorders include increased levels of sulfite, S-sulphocysteine, thiosulfate, taurine, and decreased cystine. In molybdenum cofactor deficiency, in addition, elevated levels of xanthine and hypoxanthine are found. No effective rational treatment is available.

Nonketotic hyperglycinemia (NKH)

Glycine is a nonessential amino acid. It is formed endogenously from serine or from ethanolamine by way of glyoxylate. Hyperglycinemia is found in a number of inborn errors of fatty acid catabolism, associated with often life-threatening acidosis, and collectively known as ketotic hyperglycinemia. The latter name was given before gas chromatography identified the fatty acid abnormalities in the disorders now known as propionic acidemia and methylmalonic acidemia. NKH, on the other hand, causes no acidosis and no fatty acid abnormality is found on gas chromatography. NKH is an autosomal recessive disorder which causes an excess of glycine in CSF, blood, and urine, due to an impairment in the glycine cleavage system (Hayasaka *et al.*, 1987). Glycine is an inhibitory neurotransmitter mediating postsynaptic inhibition to motor neurons in the spinal cord. More recently the focus has been on the relationship of glycine to the NMDA (*N*-methyl-D-aspartate) receptor, the main receptor for excitatory amino acids in the brain, as it was found that application of glycine allosterically increases the number of synaptic potentials in the receptor (Thomson, Walker and Flynn, 1989; Huettner, 1991). Overstimulation of the NMDA receptor for any reason causes cell death, especially in the immature brain. Affected babies usually are asymptomatic at normal term birth but become obtunded within hours to some days after birth, with failure to suck, feed or cry, shallow breathing, apneic spells which progress to coma, and respiratory failure. Latency of symptoms after birth has been given as between 7 hours and 8 days (Gitzelmann and Steinmann, 1982). Neurologic symptoms include brisk tendon reflexes and depressed Moro response. Myoclonus, i.e. very brief focal or generalized contractions, often stimulus evoked, as well as generalized seizures have been observed. Seizures may become difficult to manage by routine anticonvulsants. The EEG in NKH in the neonatal period is highly characteristic, with brief high-voltage paroxysms, predominantly over the vertex in a burst-suppression pattern. This burst-suppression pattern has been described in 11 of 12 neonates with NKH, before the ninth day of life (Mises *et al.*, 1978). The EEG pattern is not pathognomonic. It may be seen in other metabolic encephalopathies with neonatal onset, and in the acute phase of severe hypoxic-ischemic encephalopathy, but its finding in an initially normal neonate together with a rapidly progressive encephalopathy should always arouse the suspicion of NKH.

Babies with NKH may die in the neonatal period or may spontaneously improve in vital function and survive with severe brain damage. Their epilepsy may proceed to hypsarrhythmia and infantile spasms.

In NKH glycine is relatively more elevated in CSF than in plasma (Carson, 1982). CSF concentration has been correlated with outcome, the highest CSF/plasma ratios belonging to a group with the poorest outcome (Hayasaka *et al.*, 1987). The mechanism of brain damage in NKH is unknown. Neuropathologic studies have shown spongiosis of myelinated white matter with myelin splitting at the intraperiod line (Agamanolis *et al.*, 1982), both in the cerebral hemispheres and in the brainstem. Prenatal onset of the cerebral damage is indicated by the occasional finding of dysgenesis of the corpus callosum (Scher *et al.*, 1986; Dobyns, 1989). No therapy has proved effective yet. A promising clinical and EEG response to treatment with the NMDA-receptor antagonist dextrometorphan has been described (Schmitt *et al.*, 1993). Because of the destructive nature of the disorder, early diagnosis and treatment should be achieved. Routine antiepileptic medication may be provided in the case of NKH, except for valproic acid which should be avoided because it tends to increase glycine levels (Jaeken *et al.*, 1977).

PEROXISOMAL DISORDERS

Biochemistry (Fig. 4c.4)

Peroxisomes are cell organelles present in all cell types except erythrocytes. Enzymes contained in peroxisomes subserve different metabolic pathways. Enzymes contained in

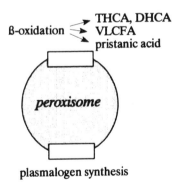

Fig. 4c.4 β-Oxidation and plasmalogen synthesis represent different enzyme systems, each within the peroxisomal membrane. Impairment of both systems results from a peroxisomal assembly disorder (generalized peroxisomal disorder). THCA = trihydroxycholestanoic acid; DHCA = dihydroxycholestanoic acid; VLCFA = very long chain fatty acid.

the peroxisomal membrane are topographically linked to act in tandem as metabolic pathways. The most important pathway is the β-oxidation system with its high affinity for very long straight chain (> 22C) fatty acids, dicarboxylic acids, bile acids precursors, and very long branched chain fatty acids such as phytanic acid and its α-oxidation product pristanic acid (Wanders *et al.*, 1990a; Clayton, 1991). This system is different in structure and function from the fatty acid chain shortening system in mitochondria. The mitochondrial system is mainly involved in chain shortening of long chain (< 22C), medium chain, and short chain fatty acids by β-oxidation. Enzyme proteins in peroxisomes and mitochondria are structurally different. Functional differences between the β-oxidation in peroxisomes and in mitochondria have been extensively reviewed. (Wanders *et al.*, 1990a; Schulz, 1991). Very long chain polyenoic fatty acids constitute an important part of complex lipids, such as phosphatidyl choline, in the central nervous system (Poulos *et al.*, 1988). Regular turnover of these lipids is mandatory for the maintenance of myelin and requires intact peroxisomes. Other peroxisomal metabolic pathways include part of the synthetic machinery for plasmalogens (ether phospholipids) that constitute a quantitatively important part of complex lipids in the brain. Impairment of these pathways can be discovered by investigation of plasma (serum), erythrocytes, and cultured skin fibroblasts. Peroxisomes proliferate by budding from preexisting peroxisomes, but peroxisomal enzymes are synthesized in the endoplasmic reticulum to become imported into peroxisomes by targeting systems that require address-labels in the form of specific amino acid-targeting sequences (Van den Bosch *et al.*, 1992). Biosynthesis of peroxisomes requires the presence of a number of membrane proteins. The absence of a family member of these peroxisomal membrane proteins leads to 'leaky' peroxisomes that do not import enzymes and fail to show up on routine electronmicroscopy, but can be made visible by immunochemical staining as 'peroxisomal ghosts' (Santos *et al.*, 1988; Brul *et al.*, 1989; Santos *et al.*, 1992). Generalized peroxisomal disorders are therefore peroxisomal assembly disorders. At least nine complementation groups exist, proving that at least an equal number of genes are involved in peroxisomal assembly (Shimozawa *et al.*, 1993).

Peroxisomal phenotypes

Only those peroxisomal disorders that express abnormalities in the oxidation of very long chain fatty acids have been reported to give rise to neonatal seizures. These include generalized peroxisomal disorders (disorders of peroxisomal assembly) and isolated deficiencies of one peroxisomal β-oxidation enzyme with intact peroxisomes. Rhizomelic chondrodysplasia, a disorder with multiple peroxisomal dysfunctions, has not been extensively studied with respect to its neurologic status in the neonatal period.

GENERALIZED PEROXISOMAL DISORDERS

Three clinical phenotypes are recognized in the generalized peroxisomal disorders. The most lethal form, Zellweger's syndrome, presents with severe hypotonia and paresis, dystrophy, swallowing disorder, and early death (Bowen *et al.*, 1964; Opitz *et al.*, 1969). A moderate expression is the infantile phytanic acid storage or infantile Refsum's disease (Scotto *et al.*, 1982; Poll-Thé *et al.*, 1987) and neonatal adrenoleukodystrophy (Aubourg *et al.*, 1986; Kelley *et al.*, 1986) lies in between these two. All three are inherited as autosomal recessive disorders. The name of a fourth phenotype, hyperpipecolic acidemia (Gatfield *et al.*, 1968), seems to have gone into oblivion because of its overlap with other phenotypes. (Historically this may be considered odd: the original publication must be

recognized as the first in which a peroxisomal disorder was decorated with a biochemical label!)

Zellweger's syndrome and neonatal adrenoleukodystrophy cause neonatal seizures and will be briefly discussed here. Zellweger's syndrome was the first of these phenotypes to become known by its clinical features, although it was a decade before its association with apparent absence of peroxisomes was recognized (Goldfischer *et al.*, 1973). Its external features (very large fontanelle, abnormal earlobes with hypoplastic lobule, hypoplastic supraorbital ridges, etc.) are well known in literature and displayed by many textbooks. The most impressive clinical findings are severe hypotonia and paresis, club feet which result from intrauterine moulding, swallowing disorder, and sometimes respiratory insufficiency. The cerebral malformations are probably mainly responsible for epileptic phenomena. Common to all patients is neocortical dysplasia and clusters of neuronal heterotopia stemming from a neuronal migration disorder (Volpe and Adams, 1972; Evrard *et al.*, 1978), originating early in gestation (Powers *et al.*, 1985).

Radiological procedures may help the clinician to support a presumptive diagnosis of Zellweger's syndrome. A radiologic survey of the skeleton may reveal periarticular calcifications. Structural abnormalities of the brain are present, such as various types of disturbed neuronal migration, some of which show up on MRI. Heterotopic subcortical clusters may be seen (Van der Knaap and Valk, 1991), but are often of minute size and below the threshold of resolution. Polymicrogyria is a regular feature of large parts of the neocortex. The most characteristic, although not pathognomonic, sign in Zellweger's can be seen on MRI and is also discernible on CT, as a steep parietal cleft which joins the Sylvian fissure to the superior part of the cerebral hemisphere. Also present are pachymicrogyria, patches of apparently thickened cortex, especially around the Sylvian fissure,

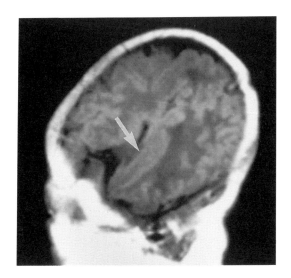

Fig. 4c.5 Neocortical dysplasia in a newborn with Zellweger's syndrome. Lateral sagittal T1-weighted magnetic resonance image shows patch of thickened cortex adjacent to Sylvian fissure (arrow). In Zellweger's syndrome this abnormal image represents crowded microgyri, rather than true pachygyria.

and its abnormal extension (Fig. 4c.5). Other features, such as the periventricular germinolytic cysts (Sarnat, Trevenen and Darwish, 1993) are likely to be seen on transfontanellar ultrasonography. Other malformations, outside the CNS, are renal cortical cysts and the dysmorphic external appearance (Opitz *et al.*, 1969) which is due to interference with embryonic shaping processes. Degenerative tissue changes are a major aspect of Zellweger's syndrome. Examples are the periarticular calcification, especially visible around the knees, pigmentary retinopathy, hepatic fibrosis or cirrhosis (Opitz *et al.*, 1969), and fatty changes in astrocytes (Aubourg *et al.*, 1985). A variety of epileptic seizures may be present in the first days of a patient with Zellweger's syndrome. While status epilepticus is unusual, seizures may be difficult to treat and present as apneic spells, blinking spells, generalized and partial clonic seizures. Effective treatment may be difficult.

The neurophysiologic features of Zellweger's syndrome, including the EEG features, have been described (Govaerts *et al.*, 1985).

Neonatal adrenoleukodystrophy (Ulrich *et al.*, 1978; Aubourg *et al.*, 1986; Kelley *et al.*, 1986) has many similarities to Zellweger's syndrome, but the facial dysmorphia is less typical than in the latter. No renal cortical cysts and no periarticular calcifications are found in neonatal adrenoleukodystrophy. Malformations in the brain are limited to polymicrogyric patches of neocortex. Degenerative changes are progressive myelin breakdown with perivascular cuffing, not unlike the histopathology seen in X-linked adrenoleukodystrophy. Some features, such as pigmentary retinopathy, sensory deafness, and liver pathology (fibrosis, cirrhosis), are shared by all generalized peroxisomal disorders: Zellweger's syndrome, neonatal adrenoleukodystrophy, infantile Refsum disease.

SINGLE DEFECTS OF PEROXISOMAL β-OXIDATION

Phenocopies of Zellweger's syndrome and neonatal adrenoleukodystrophy exist in the form of isolated peroxisomal β-oxidation defects with intact peroxisomes. The β-oxidation cycle requires an activating enzyme, peroxisomal acyl-CoA synthetase, and three enzymes for the repeating cycle which cleaves off 2 carbon units per cycle each time until the 8-carbon unit octanoic acid is reached which is further oxidized in the mitochondria (Wanders *et al.*, 1990a). Deficiency of the first enzyme, peroxisomal acyl-CoA synthetase, leads to X-linked adrenoleukodystrophy/adrenomyeloneuropathy in childhood or adulthood. Deficiency of one of the other three: acyl-CoA oxidase (Poll-Thé *et al.*, 1988), bifunctional protein (Watkins *et al.*, 1989; Wanders *et al.*, 1990b, 1992), and thiolase (Schram *et al.*, 1987) will cause neurologic symptoms, including seizures in the neonatal period. In some reports dealing with isolated β-oxidation defects no enzyme deficiency could be pinpointed (Naidu *et al.*, 1988; Barth *et al.*, 1990; Kyllerman *et al.*, 1990; Mandel *et al.*, 1992; Van Maldergem *et al.*, 1992).

DIAGNOSIS AND TREATMENT IN PEROXISOMAL DISORDERS

A peroxisomal disorder should be suspected in any neonate with seizures and severe generalized hypotonia that cannot be otherwise explained. Clinical and radiologic signs and symptoms may aid in presumptive diagnosis. As cultured skin fibroblasts take a long time to grow before determinations can be done and decisions on treatment have to be taken in a neonate who is often critically ill, rapid diagnosis should rest on determinations in plasma/serum and erythrocytes.

Determination of very long chain fatty acids in plasma or serum should be the first step. Definite elevation of C26 (hexacosanoic acid) is proof of a disorder of peroxisomal β-oxidation. Measurement of the activity of the first peroxisomal enzyme in the plasmalogen synthesis route – dihydroxyacetonephosphate acyltransferase (DHAP-AT) – which can be done in thrombocytes (Wanders *et al.*, 1985), or measurement of the concentration of plasmalogens in erythrocytes (Heymans *et al.*, 1984), is the next diagnostic step. A deficiency of plasmalogen synthesis means that one other enzyme system attached to the peroxisomal membrane, not dependent on the first, is absent. This gives evidence of a generalized peroxisomal disorder, i.e. either Zellweger's syndrome or neonatal adrenoleukodystrophy (Wanders *et al.*, 1993). If plasmalogen synthesis is normal, an isolated β-oxidation defect is likely. Determination of bile acids in plasma (Clayton *et al.*, 1988; Clayton, 1991) should determine whether abnormal bile acid precursors (dihydroxy- and trihydroxycholestanoic acids; DHCA, THCA) are present. Oxidation of these bile

acid precursors requires bifunctional protein and thiolase, both of which are also involved in oxidation of very long chain fatty acids. The presence of these abnormal bile acids, in the case of a single β-oxidation defect, points to either bifunctional protein or thiolase as the site of the deficiency. With the first enzyme, acyl-CoA oxidase, the situation is different. Bile acid precursors are not dependent on this enzyme, because they have a different peroxisomal oxidase (THCA-CoA oxidase) as first step in their β-oxidation route. Absence of abnormal bile acids together with an isolated defect in β-oxidation therefore suggests acyl-CoA oxidase as the site of the defect. This simplified flow scheme is useful in the search for peroxisomal deficiencies in neonates with seizures, but does not exclude all peroxisomal disorders. When the plasmalogen step in diagnosis is omitted, elevation of very long chain fatty acids and bile acids suggests the neonate has a generalized peroxisomal disorder, but does not rule out isolated deficiencies. Fibroblasts should be taken in any case of very long chain fatty acid elevation for final studies and as a reference for future prenatal diagnosis. A note should be made on a single instance of isolated accumulation of di- and trihydroxycholestanoic acid without elevation of C26 in hypotonic sibs with seizures at 3 months (Wanders *et al.*, 1991). They probably suffered from an isolated abnormality of peroxisomal bile acid metabolism.

There is no specific treatment for seizures, thus standard medication should be tried. There are no objections to giving standard antiepileptic medication to children with peroxisomal disorders. Where there is hepatic disease, caution should be exerted, and the dosage of drugs that are metabolized and excreted by the liver adjusted according to plasma levels. Renal excretion is usually unimpaired, even in the presence of renal cortical cysts.

INFANTS AND CHILDREN

AMINO ACID AND ORGANIC ACID DISORDERS

Glutaric acidemia type 1

Glutaric acidemia type 1 is due to an autosomal recessive deficiency of the enzyme glutaryl CoA dehydrogenase. It leads to accumulation of glutaric acid and 3-hydroxyglutaric acid and causes secondary impairment of the mitochondrial β-oxidation route with overflow of dicarboxylic acids, especially adipic acid. Because of the binding of glutaric acid to circulating free carnitine as the conjugate glutarylcarnitine, a decreased level of free carnitine results.

Infants and children with glutaric acidemia have megalencephaly with a characteristic wide gap between the frontal and parietal opercula on CT or MRI without initial signs of a destructive process. This peculiar finding can be observed before the onset of symptoms. In most cases symptoms start acutely between 6 and 18 months, often provoked by mild infection. Initial symptoms are decreased consciousness, hypotonia, and often seizures. Recovery is most often incomplete and severe incapacitating dystonia is usual (Kyllerman and Steen, 1977; Hoffmann *et al.*, 1991; Morton *et al.*, 1991). The disease has a predilection for the caudate nucleus which shows destructive changes at autopsy, explaining the severe dystonia (Leibel *et al.*, 1980). Spongiform changes in the cerebral white matter may also be found. In the first infant of an affected family, the peculiar presentation often leads to a false diagnosis of infectious encephalitis, despite the fact that the CSF shows no signs of inflammation. Children who are diagnosed in the presymptomatic phase should be put on dietary protein restriction to keep glutaric acid production as low as possible. Specific restriction of lysine and tryptophan, precursors of glutaric acid, may be needed. Other therapies, consisting of riboflavin as cofactor to the deficient enzyme, and a GABA analog and *l*-carnitine have been advocated (Brandt *et al.*, 1979; Seccombe, James and Booth, 1986). This treatment has been offered to symptomatic children, but no improvement has been reported in children who have reached this stage.

Disorders of the urea cycle with late onset

Inherited urea cycle disorders may present after the neonatal period with symptoms of intermittent hyperammonemia. These can be checked by restriction of protein intake. Acute episodes are rarely accompanied by seizures. The most important exception to this rule is arginase deficiency, which has a different course (Terheggen *et al.*, 1969; Mizutani *et al.*, 1983). In this disorder a progressive spastic paraparesis may develop, together with epileptic seizures, even when hyperammonemia is well controlled. Toxicity may be due to arginine itself or to its guanidino metabolites (Lambert *et al.*, 1991), and regular control of arginine is of great importance in the prevention of deterioration.

Biotinidase deficiency

Biotin is a water soluble vitamin which, after ingestion, becomes part, through enzymic action, of four carboxylases in a covalent binding. These enzymes are 3-methylcrotonyl-CoA carboxylase, acetyl-CoA carboxylase, pyruvate carboxylase, and propionyl-CoA carboxylase. They are involved in leucine catabolism, fatty acid synthesis through malonyl-CoA, gluconeogenesis and catabolism of odd-chain fatty acids and a number of amino acids. Common to the carboxylases is the incorporation and recycling of their biotin component by two other enzymes: holocarboxylase synthetase and biotinidase. Deficiency of one of these enzymes leads to functional deficiency of all the carboxylases. The holocarboxylase synthetase deficiency is mainly seen to manifest before 3 months of age and the biotinidase at later ages. Deficiency causes profound metabolic effects. The early-onset synthetase-deficient patients have seizures in a small proportion, but a majority of the late-onset biotinidase-deficient patients have seizures both as initial manifestation and as a major neurologic problem. Recognition may be delayed since the characteristic skin rash and alopecia only develop in a minority and the metabolic acidosis, hyperammonemia, and ketosis are not seen initially (Wolf and Heard, 1989). Seizures in unrecognized biotinidase deficiency are difficult to control by conventional anticonvulsants. In the large series of Salbert, Pellock and Wolf (1993) biotin therapy stopped the seizures within 24 hours in 12 of 16 (75%) of those whose seizures were uncontrolled by anticonvulsants. A daily schedule of 5–10 mg biotin orally is usually effective. Multivitamin preparations, given in the absence of a specific diagnosis, may contain enough biotin to suppress the symptoms of the disease (Diamantopoulos *et al.*, 1986).

Outside periods of crisis abnormal metabolic abnormalities in the urine may be minimal. Sometimes only small amounts of the leucine metabolite 3-hydroxy-isovaleric acid are found on gas chromatography of the urine. CSF to plasma ratios for lactate and 3-hydroxy-isovaleric acid may be elevated (Duran *et al.*, 1993). Biotinidase can be determined in plasma, obviating the necessity to subject the patient to loading or fasting studies that are not without danger. Early recognition of this disorder is important, because of its excellent response to treatment. The pathology of the disease is similar to and as destructive as Leigh's syndrome (Honavar *et al.*, 1992).

Postneonatal vitamin B$_6$ dependency

The initial impression that vitamin B$_6$ dependency is limited to neonatal seizures had to be modified following several reports on postneonatal onset. These included onset of therapy-refractory epilepsy with generalized, focal, myoclonic, partial motor, or partial complex types (Goutières and Aicardi, 1985; Bankier, Turner and Hopkins, 1983; Krishnamoorthy, 1983; Coker, 1992). Goutières and Aicardi (1985) recommend that a trial of pyridoxine should be performed in all seizure disorders with onset before 18 months of age, regardless of type. Circulatory collapse following the first large dose of pyridoxine has been reported in postneonatal pyridoxine-dependency seizures (Tanaka *et al.*, 1992). Therefore proper facilities for resuscitation should be kept at hand.

DISORDERS OF AMINE METABOLISM

Disorders of tetrahydrobiopterin metabolism ('malignant phenylketonuria')

Since neonatal screening for phenylketonuria (PKU) became a routine procedure in many countries, classic PKU (phenylalanine hydroxylase deficiency) has become rare. However, the regulation of the enzyme requires the presence of tetrahydrobiopterin (BH$_4$) which is oxidized to qBH$_2$, or quinonoid dihydrobiopterin as a source of hydrogen for the hydroxylation reaction. The replenishment of BH$_4$ from qBH$_2$ requires the integrity of a number of other enzymes. At least three enzyme deficiencies lead to disordered BH$_4$ homeostasis. The importance of this system derives from the fact that two other hydroxylases besides phenylalanine hydroxylase are dependent on an adequate supply of BH$_4$. These are tryptophan hydroxylase and tyrosine hydroxylase in the pathways for the synthesis of the neurotransmitters serotonin and dopamine respectively. Typically the patient with a disorder of tetrahydrobiopterin homeostasis suffers from neurologic deterioration despite excellent dietary control of his hyperphenylalaninemia. The deterioration may include seizures, although the main symptoms are probably extrapyramidal (Dhondt, 1987; Hyland, 1993).

Aromatic amino acid decarboxylase deficiency

This condition is mentioned for completeness. Only one family has been described with this disorder in which serotonin and dopamine are depleted, because the common decarboxylase which acts on L-DOPA and on 5-hydroxytryptophan (5-HTP) is deficient (Hyland, 1993). Contrary to the situation in BH$_4$ deficiencies, phenylalanine is not elevated. Therefore biogenic amines have to be determined. The patients presented with hypotonia, oculogyric crises, defective temperature regulation, and later hypotension (Fig. 4c.6).

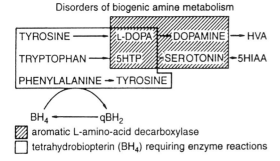

Disorders of biogenic amine metabolism

☒ aromatic L-amino-acid decarboxylase

☐ tetrahydrobiopterin (BH$_4$) requiring enzyme reactions

Fig. 4c.6 Disorders of biogenic amine metabolism. Tetrahydrobiopterin (BH$_4$) deficiency results in the loss of activity of three enzyme activities depicted in the unshaded rectangle. Resulting deficiency of L-DOPA and 5HTP, in turn causes deficiency of the neurotransmitters dopamine and serotonin. Aromatic L-amino acid decarboxylase catalyzes the reactions indicated in the shaded rectangle. Deficiency also results in deficiency of dopamine and serotonin. L-DOPA = L-dihydroxyphenylalanine; 5HTP = 5-hydroxytryptophan; HVA = homovanillic acid; 5HIAA = 5-hydroxyindolic acid; qBH$_2$ = quinonoid form of dihydrobiopterin.

DISORDERS OF PYRIMIDINE METABOLISM: DIHYDROPYRIMIDINE DEHYDROGENASE DEFICIENCY

Combined excretion of thymine and uracil was first described by Berger *et al.* (1984) in patients with dihydropyrimidine dehydrogenase deficiency. The abnormal pyrimidine pattern is due to deficiency of an enzyme which is active in the metabolic pathways of cytosine and 5-methylcytosine. A study by Braakhekke *et al.* (1987) showed that affected persons have mental retardation, microcephaly, and epilepsy. Interestingly some have only epilepsy. Autosomal recessive inheritance is suggested by pedigrees.

GLUCOSE TRANSPORTER DEFICIENCY (De Vivo *et al.*, 1991)

Infants with the disorder had repeated generalized seizures starting within a few months after birth with normal interictal EEG. CSF/blood ratio for glucose was decreased (0.19–0.35; normal 0.65) and CSF lactate was 0.31–1.5 (normal 1–2.8 m mol/l), suggesting that there was diminished availability of blood glucose and its metabolites to the brain. A glucose transporter deficiency in red blood cells has been proven. This transporter is identical to the transporter in endothelial cells of the brain. Both children described improved dramatically with the provision of an alternative energy source to their brains; i.e. a ketogenic diet.

DISORDERS OF THE RESPIRATORY CHAIN AND PYRUVATE DEHYDROGENASE COMPLEX

Seizures in infants and children caused by mitochondrial disorders are mainly related to deficiencies of the respiratory chain and the pyruvate dehydrogenase complex (PDHC). Deficiencies in these pathways may lead to functional and structural impairment of the brain and hence to seizures. Less frequently a deficiency of the citric acid (Krebs) cycle or pyruvate carboxylase may be involved. Biotinidase deficiency has been addressed in a preceding paragraph. Disorders of mitochondrial β-oxidation affect the brain indirectly by causing hypoglycemic episodes. The existence of a mitochondrial genome beside the nuclear genome and the complex interactions between these two has broad implications for clinical expression and inheritance. Point mutations in nuclear or mitochondrial DNA (mtDNA), large deletions in mitochondrial DNA, and variable tissue distribution of mutant mtDNA (heteroplasmy) give rise to a wealth of different disorders. mtDNA depletion or intergenomic signalling defects are recent discoveries (Wallace 1992; De Vivo, 1993). Clinical syndromes such as Leigh's syndrome, Alpers' syndrome, Kearns–Sayre syndrome, MELAS, MERRF, NARP, and Pearson's syndrome are each caused by more than a single defect. The encephalopathies in children caused by respiratory chain deficiency are known by the names Leigh's syndrome, Alpers' syndrome, MELAS, and MERRF. In addition, Leigh's syndrome may be caused by deficiency of PDHC. The use of the names Leigh's and Alpers' disease has been questioned because of overlapping biochemical and even clinical features. However, there is sufficient difference between them to keep these names for the time being as belonging to clinically different entities.

Leigh's syndrome is a neurologic entity defined by its pathologic features. These consist of bilateral, symmetric gray and white matter lesions in the brain and spinal cord, microscopically characterized by loss of axons and dendrites (neuropil), intense capillary proliferation, and sometimes accompanied by cavity formation. The lesions are frequently found in the basal ganglia, especially the putamina, and the brainstem. The neocortex is not preferentially affected. The lesions are reminiscent of Wernicke's disease (Leigh, 1951; Montpetit *et al.*, 1971). Clinically Leigh's syndrome is highly variable, with a remitting course and exacerbations often provoked by intercurrent infections. Major symptoms are hypotonia, vomiting and brainstem and extraocular eye symptoms. Leigh's syndrome has become firmly linked to various sites of the respiratory chain and

PDHC (Miyabayashi *et al.*, 1985; Van Erven *et al.*, 1986; Arts *et al.*, 1987; DiMauro *et al.*, 1987; Van Coster *et al.*, 1991; Sakuta *et al.*, 1992; Shoffner *et al.*, 1992). Lactic acidemia and elevated lactic acid in the CSF are usually but not invariably present (Wijburg *et al.*, 1991). In a review of 173 proven cases (Van Erven *et al.*, 1987), seizures were seen at the onset of the disease in 8%. Therapy-resistant epilepsy and status epilepticus are less frequent. Alpers' disease is a degeneration of gray matter in which severe cortical degeneration and degeneration of basal ganglia and nuclear systems in the brainstem is found. Degeneration of neurons and decay of the intervening structures (spongiosis) with increase and dilatation of capillaries is found (Alpers, 1931; Blackwood *et al.*, 1963; Laurence and Cavanagh, 1968; Janota, 1974; Huttenlocher, Solitaire and Adams, 1976; Jellinger and Seitelberger, 1979). Destruction may lead to extreme cortical atrophy and microscopic devastation of the cortex, so much that cortical layers become indistinct because of the loss of neurons and reactive infiltration with macrophages and astrocytes. This happens especially in the infantile cases. In other cases changes may be macroscopically indistinct. This disease has been variously called 'progressive degeneration of the cerebral cortex in infancy' (Laurence and Cavanagh, 1968), 'spongy glio-neuronal dystrophy' (Jellinger and Seitelberger, 1979), 'spongy degeneration of grey matter' (Janota, 1974), and 'infantile diffuse cerebral degeneration' (Huttenlocher, Solitare and Adams, 1976) After normal early development, convulsions and myoclonus appear during infancy or childhood with coincident arrest in motor development. A special type, which combines with diffuse liver disease, was first mentioned incidentally in two out of a series of five by Blackwood *et al.* (1963). A succinct description of this disorder appears in the report of Boyd *et al.* 1986 on 12 children – 10 autopsy proven and two siblings to proven cases: 'All the children developed fits, often with explosive onset as a major feature of their disease. These seizures frequently consisted of isolated twitching of one or other limb, sometimes for weeks on end.' Electroencephalograms were characterized by focal very high voltage (200–1000 μV) very slow (< 1 Hz) waves, alternating with low voltage superimposed polyspikes usually contralateral to the focal seizures. The electroretinogram is normal, which serves to differentiate this disorder from late-infantile Batten's disease, another degenerative disorder with severe epilepsy. The onset of this disease is mostly before 2 years of age. An association between Alpers' disease, ragged-red muscle fibers and elevation of lactic acid in blood, urine, and CSF was reported by Shapira *et al.* in 1975. Complex I deficiency (Prick *et al.* 1981; Tulinius *et al.*, 1991), Complex IV deficiency (Prick *et al.*, 1983), and a defect in the citric acid cycle between succinyl-CoA and fumarate (Prick *et al.* 1982) have been reported in association with Alpers' disease. There appears, therefore, to be a strong association between Alpers' disease and various disorders of the respiratory chain. One specific risk in the hepatocerebral form of Alpers's disease is related to an apparent specific vulnerability to toxic effects of valproic acid (Bicknese *et al.*, 1992). Thus the mitochondrial route of valproate degradation has to be kept in mind. Valproate is activated to valproyl-CoA, and as such might tie up already impaired mitochondrial fatty acid degradation ('CoA trapping'). Animal experiments stress the possible value of carnitine (to increase excretion of valproic acid) and pantothenic acid (as a precursor of CoA) in the case of valproate toxicity (Thurston and Hauhart, 1992).

MELAS syndrome (Mitochondrial myopathy, Encephalopathy, Lactic acidosis and Stroke-like episodes) was first described in 1984 (Pavlakis *et al.*, 1984). Onset is from the age of 3 to 40 years. Progressive encephalopathy is typically accompanied by migraine-like headache, dementia, seizures, and stroke-like episodes (Montagna *et al.*, 1988). Lactic acidosis is usual and ragged-red fibers are seen in the muscle biopsies. One-third of the patients have basal ganglia calcifications and some have external ophthalmoploplegia. Two point mutations in the mtDNA gene for tRNA[leu(UUR)] have been identified. In accordance with the localization of the defect in the mitochondria, inheritance of the disorder is matrilinear (De Vivo, 1993). Myoclonus epilepsy and ragged-red fibers (MERRF) was first delineated by Fukuhara *et al.*, in 1980 as a disorder with onset in childhood with bursts of myoclonus, seizures, intention tremor, ataxia, mental deterioration, muscular weakness, and pes cavus. Lactic acidemia is usual. Neuropathologic findings in the original two patients (Takeda *et al.*, 1988) showed degeneration of cerebellar cortex, dentate and red nuclei, globus pallidus and subthalamic nucleus. Degeneration in the spinal cord included posterior columns and posterior spinocerebellar tracts. Peripheral nerves were also affected. Like MELAS, MERRF is transmitted by maternal inheritance and a point mutation in the mitochondrial genome has been reported in a number of, but not all, patients in the mtDNA gene for tRNA[lys] by Shoffner *et al.* (1990). Findings were summarized in a review (Pavlakis *et al.*, 1988). This disorder with its prominent myoclonus epilepsy and ataxia has to be kept in mind when considering a diagnosis of Ramsey–Hunt disease.

PEROXISOMAL DISORDERS

The most important peroxisomal disease with onset after birth is X-linked adrenoleukodystrophy. Symptoms begin during childhood. Seizures are the presenting feature in a small minority, and can be secondary to hypoglycemia, associated with the adrenal insufficiency (Aubourg *et al.*, 1982).

LYSOSOMAL DISORDERS

Lysosomal disorders are typically storage disorders with a progressive course. In the majority the storage includes neurons. The propensity to epileptic seizures varies. It is low in the mucopolysaccharidoses, somewhat higher in some oligosaccharidoses, e.g. reported as 34% in fucosidosis (Willems *et al.*, 1991), and prominent in α-*N*-acetylgalactosaminidase deficiency or Schindler's disease (Desnick and Wang, 1990). Sialidosis and galactosialidosis have in common a defect in the catabolism of sialic acid containing glycoconjugates (Cantz and Ulrich-Bott, 1990). Both may present as the so-called cherry-red spot-myoclonus syndrome. Sialidosis is present in an early-onset type between 0 and 10 months and in a late-onset type between 8 and 25 years, both types being due to deficiency of lysosomal sialidase. Myoclonus and seizures are prominent in both types. Galactasialidosis is a combined deficiency of lysosomal sialidase and β-galactosidase due to a deficiency of a protein common to both, which protects these enzymes from intralysosomal breakdown. It presents between birth and 6 years and symptoms largely overlap with pure sialidosis, including cherry-red spots and myoclonus.

Sphingolipidoses that preferentially affect metabolism of myelin (lysosomal leukodystrophies), such as metachromatic leukodystrophy and Krabbe's disease, will eventually cause epilepsy, but epilepsy usually arises some time after the onset of functional regression and treatment is not usually a problem.

SEIZURES IN SOME INHERITED NEURODEGENERATIVE DISORDERS WITHOUT KNOWN BIOCHEMICAL CAUSE

CEROID-LIPOFUSCINOSIS OR BATTEN'S DISEASE

Ceroid-lipofuscinosis or Batten's disease comprises a number of genetically and clinic-

ally different disorders. They are inherited as autosomal recessive disorders. Three childhood types are well defined and some less well known types may represent allelic subtypes or genetically different disorders. The main types are known by their eponymal names as:

Infantile type: Santavuori–Hagberg.
Late-infantile type: Jansky–Bielschowsky.
Juvenile type: Spielmeyer–Vogt.

Other types are:

Late-onset type of Jansky–Bielschowsky, otherwise known as early juvenile type or Lake–Cavanagh.
Late-onset type with granular osmiophilic deposits.

The adult type of ceroid-lipofuscinosis, Kuf's disease, is not included in this review. All infantile and childhood types are associated with neuronal degeneration and storage of a complex protein-lipid-carbohydrate-containing material with autofluorescent properties known as ceroid. Their clinical course is marked by regression, prominence of seizures and myoclonus, especially in the infantile and late-infantile types, and retinal degeneration with extinguished electroretinogram.

Infantile type ceroid-lipofuscinosis (Santavuori–Hagberg type)

The first, almost unnoticed case, was described by Hagberg, Sourander and Svennerholm in 1968. The disorder was later described clinically and pathologically in a large group of patients from Finland, where the disease has the highest incidence in the world (1 : 20 000) (Haltia *et al.*, 1973; Santavuori *et al.*, 1973, 1974), but has been documented in the rest of Europe and the USA. It is characterized by normal early development to 6 months, and decline starting between 8 and 18 months with ataxia, muscle hypotonia followed by spasticity, visual loss, loss of interest, prominent myoclonus, epileptic seizures, and 'knitting' hyperkinesia. Microcephaly is usually present at the onset of the disease, but is progressive. A vegetative state is reached by the age of 3 years. Electroencephalography shows progressive diminution of voltage until the third year, after which the recording becomes isoelectric. Electroretinography is of lowered amplitude, even at an early stage (Santavuori *et al.*, 1973; Pampiglione and Harden, 1974). Optic atrophy with brown discoloration of the macular region is seen later. Death is mostly between 5 and 10 years. Extreme cerebral atrophy lending the macroscopic appearance of a walnut is seen at autopsy, while microscopy will show total disappearance of cortical neurons, storage of autofluorescent material in all remaining neurons, astroglia and large numbers of storage macrophages. The storage material is also seen widely in reticuloendothelial and other cell types outside the CNS. The material is granular and osmiophilic, surrounded by a lysosomal membrane. Diagnosis in biopsies (skin, conjunctiva, skeletal muscle, lymphocytes) should be possible in each case. The disorder is genetically different from the other types. A locus has been found on chromosome 1p by linkage analysis (Järvelä *et al.*, 1992).

Late infantile ceroid-lipofuscinosis (Jansky–Bielschowsky disease)

This disorder has its onset in children between 2 and 4 years of age, with rapidly progressing epilepsy, ataxia, and blindness. Spastic paresis follows. Epilepsy takes the form of generalized tonic-clonic seizures, drop attacks and massive myoclonus. Progression of myoclonus ultimately leads to a permanent myoclonic state which cannot be influenced. Patients usually die before 8 years (Zeman *et al.*, 1970). Optic atrophy and retinopathy develop early in the disease. The electroretinogram is negative at an early age and is a highly suggestive test at the beginning of the disease. Other important neurophysiologic features are a grossly enlarged visual evoked potential and short generalized discharges in the EEG following each flash at low frequency stroboscopy (Harden, Pampiglione and Picton-Robinson, 1973). Storage and atrophy are seen in the brain but are much less severe than in the infantile type. The storage involves so-called curvilinear and other profiles contained within lysosomal membranes. These are widely found in cerebral neurons, but also in various tissues, such as eccrine sweat glands, striated muscle cells, and Schwann cells (Carpenter, Karpati and Andermann, 1972). Lymphocytes also display storage material, but not in all cases (Schuurmans-Stekhoven *et al.*, 1976).

Juvenile ceroid-lipofuscinosis (Spielmeyer–Vogt)

This disorder begins between 4 and 8 years with retinal blindness, later followed by dementia, generalized seizures, regression of motor functions with a Parkinson syndrome and death after 20 years of age. Diagnosis also involves the finding of a negative electroretinogram.

Diagnosis in lymphocytes is usually reliable. Routine bloodsmears stained with Wright–Giemsa will reveal vacuoles in 1–2% of lymphocytes. Electronmicroscopy in peripheral blood cells will show some storage material in the form of fingerprint profiles associated with these vacuoles (Schuurmans-Stekhoven *et al.*, 1977). In contrast to the infantile and late-infantile types, epilepsy is not a major problem in the juvenile type. The juvenile type has been mapped to chromosome 16, and the late-infantile type has been excluded from the same region (Yan *et al.*, 1993). Biochemical analysis has revealed that in the late-infantile and juvenile types but not in the infantile type, a substantial part of the storage product is identical to subunit c of mitochondrial ATP synthase (Palmer *et al.*, 1992).

Other types of ceroid-lipofuscinosis in children

Early juvenile or Lake–Cavanagh type

In this type clinical findings mostly reflect the late-infantile type, but with later onset (Lake and Cavanagh, 1978; Kimura and Goebel, 1987; Santavuori *et al.*, 1993).

Juvenile type with granular osmiophilic material (Carpenter *et al.*, 1973)

This is similar in appearance to the Spielmeyer–Vogt type, but without vacuolated lymphocytes, and inclusion bodies similar to the infantile type.

RETT SYNDROME

The Rett syndrome is a disorder only present in girls. The regression starts after the first birthday, with loss of purposeful hand skills and communicative failure with gait ataxia and apraxia after 2 years, followed by a pseudostationary period, with later wasting and wheelchair dependency after puberty (Hagberg *et al.*, 1983). Epilepsy is usual in this disorder in later stages. Occasionally epilepsy or even status epilepticus is the initial event. This may obscure the otherwise clear symptoms (Hagberg, 1989).

PEHO SYNDROME

PEHO stands for 'progressive encephalopathy with oedema, hypsarrhythmia and optic atrophy'. It represents an early-onset neurodegenerative disorder presenting with therapy-refractory infantile spasms, profound psychomotor retardation, hypotonia and absent visual contact and optic atrophy. The patients develop microcephaly and often show subcutaneous edema of peripheral limbs and face. Neuroradiologic examination shows severe and general cerebellar atrophy and some macroscopic atrophy and myelina-

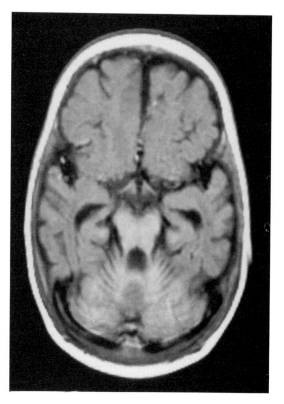

Fig. 4c.7 One-year-old patient with PEHO syndrome. Transverse proton-density magnetic resonance image shows atrophy of temporal lobes and folial atrophy of the cerebellum.

tion delay in the cerebral hemispheres. It was defined as an autosomal recessive disorder in Finland (Salonen *et al.* 1991). Neuropathologic (Haltia and Somer 1993), EEG (Somer and Sainio, 1993), neuroradiologic (Somer *et al.*, 1993a), and ophthalmologic (Somer *et al.*, 1993b) findings give a fairly consistent and recognizable pattern which may be found in some children with severe therapy-refractory epilepsy (Fig. 4c.7). It is not clear whether all patients have the same genetic defect.

REFERENCES

Agamanolis, D.P., Potter, J.L., Herrick, M.K., and Sternberger, N.H. (1982) The neuropathology of glycine encephalopathy: a report of five cases with immunohistochemical and ultrastructural observations. *Neurology*, **32**, 975–85.

Alpers, B.J. (1931) Diffuse cerebral degeneration of the gray matter of the cerebrum. *Archives of Neurology and Psychiatry*, **25**, 469–505.

Arts, W.F.M., Scholte, H.R., Loonen, M.C.B. *et al.* (1987) Cytochrome c oxidase deficiency in subacute necrotizing encephalomyelopathy. *Journal of the Neurological Sciences*, **77**, 103–15.

Aubourg, P., Chaussain, J.L., Dulac, O. and Arthuis, M. (1982) Adrenoleucodystrophie chez l'enfant. A propos de 20 observations. *Archives Francais de Pediatrie (Paris)*, **39**, 663–9.

Aubourg, P., Robain, O., Rocchiccioli, F. *et al.* (1985) The cerebro-hepato-renal (Zellweger) syndrome: lamellar lipid profiles in adrenocortical, hepatic mesenchymal, astrocyte cells and increased levels of very long chain fatty acids and phytanic acid in the plasma. *Journal of the Neurological Sciences*, **69**, 9–25.

Aubourg, P., Scotto, J., Rocchiccioli, F. *et al.* (1986) Neonatal adrenoleukodystrophy. *Journal of Neurology, Neurosurgery and Psychiatry*, **49**, 77–86.

Bankier, A., Turner, M. and Hopkins, I.J. (1983) Pyridoxine-dependent seizures – a wider clinical spectrum. *Archives of Disease in Childhood*, **58**, 415–8.

Barth, P.G., Beemer, F.A., Cats, B.P. *et al.* (1985) Neuropathological findings in a case of combined deficiency of sulphite oxidase and xanthine dehydrogenase. *Virchow's Archiv A, Pathological Anatomy and Histopathology (Berlin)*, **408**, 105–6.

Barth, P.G., Wanders, R.J.A., Schutgens, R.B.H. *et al.* (1990) Peroxisomal β-oxidation defect with detectable peroxisomes. A case with neonatal onset and progressive course in a girl. *European Journal of Pediatrics*, **149**, 722–6.

Bejsovec, M.I.R., Kulenda, Z. and Ponca, E. (1967) Familial intrauterine convulsions in pyridoxine dependency. *Archives of Disease in Childhood*, **42**, 201–7.

Berger, R., Stoker-de Vries, S.A., Wadman, S.K. *et al.* (1984) Dihydropyrimidine dehydrogenase deficiency leading to thymine-uraciluria. An inborn error of pyrimidine metabolism. *Clinica Chimica Acta*, **141**, 227–34.

Bicknese, A.R., May, W., Hickey, W.F. and Dodson, W.E. (1992) Early childhood hepatocerebral degeneration misdiagnosed as valproate hepatotoxicity. *Annals of Neurology*, **32**, 767–75.

Blackwood, W., Buxton, P.H., Cumings, J.N. *et al.* (1963) Diffuse cerebral degeneration in infancy (Alpers' disease). *Archives of Disease in Childhood*, **38**, 193–204.

Bowen, P., Lee, C.S.N., Zellweger, H. and Lindenberg, R. (1964) A familial syndrome of multiple congenital defects. *Bulletin of the Johns Hopkins Hospital*, **114**, 402–14.

Boyd, S.G., Harden, A., Egger, J. and Pampiglione, G. (1986) Progressive neuronal degeneration of childhood with liver disease ('Alpers' disease'): characteristic neurophysiological features. *Neuropediatrics*, **17**, 75–80.

Braakhekke, J.P., Renier, W.O., Gabreëls, F.J.M. *et al.* (1987) Dihydropyrimidine dehydrogenase deficiency. Neurological aspects. *Journal of the Neurological Sciences*, **78**, 71–7.

Brandt, N.J., Gregersen, N., Christensen, E. *et al.* (1979) Treatment of glutaryl-CoA dehydrogenase deficiency (glutaric aciduria). Experience with diet, riboflavin, and GABA analogue. *Journal of Pediatrics*, **94**, 669–73.

Breningstall, G.N. (1986) Neurologic syndromes in hyperammonemic disorders. *Pediatric Neurology*, **2**, 253–62.

Brown, G.K., Scholem, B., Croll, H.B. *et al.* (1989) Sulfite oxidase deficiency: clinical, neuroradiologic, and biochemical features in two new patients. *Neurology*, **39**, 252–7.

Brul, S., Wiemer, E.A.C., Oosthuizen, M. *et al.* (1989) Genetic heterogeneity in inherited disorders with a generalized impairment of peroxisomal functions: visualization by immunofluorescence microscopy of peroxisome assembly after somatic cell fusion of complementary cell lines, in *Molecular Basis of Membrane Associated Disease* (eds N. Azzizi, Z. Drahota and S. Papa), Springer-Verlay, Heidelberg, pp. 420–8.

Cantz, M. and Ulrich-Bott, B. (1990) Disorders of glycoprotein degradation. *Journal of Inherited Metabolic Disease*, **13**, 523–7.

Carpenter, S., Karpati, G. and Andermann, F. (1972) Specific involvement of muscle, nerve, and skin in late infantile and juvenile amaurotic idiocy. *Neurology*, **22**, 170–86.

Carpenter, S., Karpati, G., Wolfe, L.S. and Andermann, F. (1973) A type of juvenile cerebromacular degeneration characterized by granular osmophilic deposits. *Journal of the Neurological Sciences*, **18**, 67–87.

Carson, N.A.J. (1982) Non-ketotic hyperglycinemia – a review of 70 patients. *Journal of Inherited Metabolic Disease*, **5** (suppl 2), 126–8.

Clayton, P.T. (1991) Inborn errors of bile acid metabolism. *Journal of Inherited Metabolic Disease*, **14**, 478–96.

Clayton, P.T., Lake, B.D., Hjelm, M. *et al.* (1988) Bile acid analyses in 'Pseudo-Zellweger' syndrome; clues to the defect in peroxisomal β-oxidation. *Journal of Inherited Metabolic Disease*, **11** (suppl 2), 165–8.

Coker, S.B. (1992) Postneonatal vitamin-B_6-dependent epilepsy. *Pediatrics*, **90**, 221–3.

De Vivo, D.C. (1993) The expanding clinical spectrum of mitochondrial diseases. *Brain and Development*, **15**, 1–22.

De Vivo, D.C., Trifiletti, R.R., Jacobson, R.I. *et al.* (1991) Defective glucose transport across the blood–brain barrier as a cause of persistent hypoglycorrhachia, seizures, and developmental delay. *New England Journal of Medicine*, **325**, 703–9.

Desnick, R.J. and Wang, A.M. (1990) Schindler disease: an inherited neuroaxonal dystrophy due to α-*N*-acetylgalactosaminidase deficiency. *Journal of Inherited Metabolic Disease*, **13**, 549–59.

Dhondt, J-L. (1987) Tetrahydrobiopterin deficiency. Lessons from analysis of 90 patients collected in the international register. *Archives Francaises de Pediatrie*, **44**, 655–9.

Diamantopoulos, N., Painter, M.J., Wolf, B. *et al.* (1986) Biotinidase deficiency: accumulation of lactate in the brain and response to physiologic doses of biotin. *Neurology*, **36**, 1107–9.

DiMauro, S., Servidei, S., Zeviani, M. *et al.* (1987) Cytochrome c oxidase deficiency in Leigh syndrome. *Annals of Neurology*, **22**, 498–506.

Dobyns, W.B. (1989) Agenesis of the corpus callosum and gyral malformations are frequent manifestations of nonketotic hyperglycinemia. *Neurology*, **39**, 817–20.

Duran, M., Beemer, F.A., Van der Heyden, C. *et al.* (1978) Combined deficiency of xanthine oxidase and sulphite oxidase: a defect of molybdenum metabolism or transport? *Journal of Inherited Metabolic Disease*, **1**, 175–8.

Duran, M., Baumgartner, E.R., Suormala, T.M. *et al.* (1993) Cerebrospinal fluid organic acids in biotinidase deficiency. *Journal of Inherited Metabolic Disease*, **16**, 513–6.

Endres, W., Shin, Y.S., Günther, R. *et al.* (1988) Report on a new patient with combined deficiencies of sulphite oxidase and xanthine dehydrogenase due to molybdenum cofactor deficiency. *European Journal of Pediatrics*, **148**, 246–9.

Evrard, P., Caviness, V.S. Jr, Pratts-Vinas, J. and Lyon, G. (1978) The mechanism of arrest of neuronal migration in the Zellweger malformation: an hypothesis based upon cytoarchitectonic analysis. *Acta Neuropathologica (Berlin)*, **41**, 109–17.

Fukuhara, N., Tokiguchi, S., Shirakawa, K. and Tsubaki, T. (1980) Myoclonus epilepsy associated with ragged-red fibres (mitochondrial abnormalities) disease entity or syndrome? Light- and electronmicroscopic studies of two cases and review of the literature. *Journal of the Neurological Sciences*, **47**, 117–33.

Gatfield, P.D., Taller, E., Hinton, G.G. *et al.* (1968) Hyperpipecolatemia: a new metabolic disorder associated with neuropathy and hepatomegaly. *Canadian Medical Association Journal*, **99**, 1215–33.

Gitzelmann, R. and Steinmann, B. (1982) Clinical and therapeutic aspects of non-ketotic hyperglycinemia. *Journal of Inherited Metabolic Disease*, **25**, (suppl 2), 113–6.

Goldfischer, F., Moore, C., Johnson, A. *et al.* (1973) Peroxisomal and mitochondrial defects in the cerebro-hepato-renal syndrome. *Science*, **182**, 62–4.

Goutières, F. and Aicardi, J. (1985) Atypical presentations of pyridoxine dependent seizures: a treatable cause of intractable epilepsy in infants. *Annals of Neurology*, **17**, 117–20.

Govaerts, L., Colon, E., Rotteveel, J. and Monnens, L.A. (1985) Neurophysiological study of children with the cerebro-hepato-renal syndrome of Zellweger. *Neuropediatrics*, **16**, 185–90.

Grove, J., Schechter, P.J., Hanke, N.F. *et al.* (1982) Concentration gradients of free and total γ-aminobutyric acid and homocarnosine in human CSF: comparison of suboccipital and lumbar sampling. *Journal of Neurochemistry*, **39**, 1618–22.

Hagberg, B.A. (1989) Rett syndrome: clinical peculiarities, diagnostic approach, and possible cause. *Pediatric Neurology*, **5**, 75–83.

Hagberg, B., Sourander, P. and Svennerholm, L. (1968) Late infantile progressive encephalopathy with disturbed polyunsaturated fat metabolism. *Acta Paediatrica Scandinavica*, **57**, 495–9.

Hagberg, B.A., Aicardi, J., Dias, K. and Ramos, O. (1983) A progressive syndrome of autism, dementia, ataxia, and loss of purposeful hand use in girls: Rett's syndrome: report of 35 cases. *Annals of Neurology* **14**, 471–9.

Haltia, M., Rapola, J., Santavuori, P. and Keränen, A. (1973) Infantile type of so-called neuronal ceroid-lipofuscinosis. Part 2. Morphological and biochemical studies. *Journal of the Neurological Sciences*, **18**, 269–85.

Haltia, M. and Somer, M. (1993) Infantile cerebello-optic atrophy. Neuropathology of the progressive encephalopathy syndrome with edema, hypsarrhythmia and optic atrophy (the PEHO syndrome). *Acta Neuropathologica (Berlin)*, **85**, 241–7.

Harden, A., Pampiglione, G. and Picton-Robinson, N. (1973) Electroretinogram and visual evoked response in a form of 'neuronal lipidosis' with diagnostic EEG features. *Journal of Neurosurgery and Psychiatry* **36**, 61–7.

Hayasaka, K., Tada, K., Fueki, N. *et al.* (1987) Nonketotic hyperglycinemia: analyses of glycine cleavage system in typical and atypical cases. *Journal of Pediatrics* **110**, 873–7.

Heeley, A., Pugh, R.J.P., Clayton, B.E. *et al.* (1978) Pyridoxol metabolism in vitamin B_6 responsive convulsions of early childhood. *Archives of Disease in Childhood*, **53**, 794–802.

Heymans, H.S.A., v.d. Bosch, H., Schutgens, R.B.H. *et al.* (1984) Deficiency of plasmalogens in the cerebro-hepato-renal (Zellweger) syndrome. *European Journal of Pediatrics*, **142**, 10–5.

Hoffmann, G.F., Trefz, F.K., Barth, P.G. *et al.* (1991) Glutaryl-coenzyme A dehydrogenase deficiency: a distinct encephalopathy. *Pediatrics*, **88**, 1194–203.

Honavar, M., Janota, I., Neville, B.G.R. and Chalmers, R.A. (1992) Neuropathology of biotinidase deficiency. *Acta Neuropathologica (Berlin)*, **84**, 461–4.

Huettner, J.E. (1991) Competitive antagonism of glycine at the *N*-methyl-D-aspartate (NMDA) receptor (Commentary). *Biochemical Pharmacology*, **41**, 9–16.

Hunt, A.D. Jr, Stokes, J., Wallace, W. *et al.* (1954) Pyridoxine dependency: report of a case of intractable convulsions in an infant controlled by pyridoxine. *Pediatrics*, **13**, 140–5.

Huttenlocher, P.R., Solitare, G.B. and Adams, G. (1976) Infantile diffuse cerebral degeneration with hepatic cirrhosis. *Archives of Neurology*, **33**, 186–92.

Hyland, K. (1993) Abnormalities of biogenic amine metabolism. *Journal of Inherited Metabolic Disease*, **16**, 676–90.

Irreverre, F., Mudd, S.H., Heizer, W.D. and Laster, L. (1967) Sulfite oxidase deficiency: studies of a patient with mental retardation, dislocated ocular lenses, and abnormal urinary

excretion of *S*-sulfo-L-cysteine, sulfite and thiosulfate. *Biochemical Medicine*, **1**, 187–217.

Jaeken, J., Corbeel, L., Casaer, P. *et al.* (1977) Dipropylacetate (valproate) and glycine metabolism. *Lancet*, **ii**, 617.

Jaeken, J. Casaer, P., de Cock, P. *et al.* (1984) Gamma-aminobutyric acid-transaminase deficiency: a newly recognized inborn error of neurotransmitter metabolism. *Neuropediatrics*, **15**, 165–9.

Jaeken, J., Casaer, P., Haegele, K.D. and Schechter, P.J. (1990) Review: normal and abnormal central nervous system GABA metabolism in childhood. *Journal of Inherited Metabolic Disease*, **13**, 793–801.

Janota, I. (1974) Spongy degeneration of grey matter in 3 children. *Archives of Disease in Childhood*, **49**, 571–5.

Järvelä, I., Santavuori, P., Puhakka, L. *et al.* (1992) Linkage map of the chromosomal region surrounding the infantile ceroid lipofuscinosis on 1p. *American Journal of Medical Genetics*, **42**, 546–8.

Jellinger, K. and Seitelberger, F. (1979) Spongy glio-neuronal dystrophy in infancy and childhood. *Acta Neuropathologica (Berlin)*, **16**, 125–40.

Kelley, R.I., Datta, N.S., Dobyns, W.B. *et al.* (1986) Neonatal adrenoleukodystrophy: new cases, biochemical studies, and differentiation from Zellweger and related peroxisomal polydystrophy syndromes. *American Journal of Medical Genetics*, **23**, 869–901.

Kimura, S. and Goebel, H.H. (1987) Electron microscopic studies on skin and lymphocytes in early juvenile neuronal ceroid-lipofuscinosis. *Brain and Development*, **9**, 576–80.

Krishnamoorthy, K.S. (1983) Pyridoxine-dependency seizure: report of a rare presentation. *Annals of Neurology*, **13**, 103–4.

Kroll, J.S. (1985) Pyridoxine for neonatal seizures: an unexpected danger. *Developmental Medicine and Child Neurology*, **27**, 377–9.

Kurlemann, G., Löscher, W., Dominick, H.C. and Palm, G.D. (1987) Disappearance of neonatal seizures and low CSF GABA levels after treatment with vitamin B_6. *Epilepsy Research*, **1**, 152–4.

Kyllerman, M. and Steen, G. (1977) Intermittently progressive dyskinetic syndrome in glutaric aciduria. *Neuropädiatrie*, **8**, 397–404.

Kyllerman, M., Blomstrand, S., Månsson, J.E. *et al.* (1990) Central nervous system malformations and white matter changes in pseudo-neonatal adrenoleukodystrophy. *Neuropediatrics*, **21**, 199–201.

Lake, B.D. and Cavanagh, N.P.C. (1978) Early-juvenile Batten's disease – a recognisable subgroup distinct from other forms of Batten's disease. *Journal of Neurological Sciences*, **36**, 265–71.

Lambert, M.A., Marescau, B., Desjardins, M. *et al.* (1991) Hyperargininemia: intellectual and motor improvement related to changes in biochemical data. *Journal of Pediatrics*, **118**, 420–3.

Laurence, K.M. and Cavanagh, J.B. (1968) Progressive degeneration of the cerebral cortex in infancy. *Brain*, **91**, 261–80.

Leibel, R.L., Shih, V.E., Goodman, S.I. *et al.* (1980) Glutaric acidemia: a metabolic disorder causing progressive choreoathetosis. *Neurology*, **30**, 1163–8.

Leigh, D. (1951) Subacute necrotizing encephalomyelopathy. *Journal of Neurology Neurosurgery and Psychiatry*, **14**, 216–21.

Lott, I.T., Coulombe, T., Di Paolo, R.V. *et al.* (1978) Vitamin B_6 dependent seizures: pathology and chemical findings in brain. *Neurology*, **28**, 47–54.

Mandel, H., Berant, M., Aizin, A. *et al.* (1992) Zellweger-like phenotype in two siblings: a defect in peroxisomal β-oxidation with elevated very long-chain fatty acids but normal bile acids. *Journal of Inherited Metabolic Disease*, **15**, 381–4.

Minns, R. (1980) Vitamin B_6 deficiency and dependency. Annotation. *Developmental Medicine and Child Neurology*, **22**, 795–8.

Mises, J., Moussalli-Salefranque, F., Plouin, P. *et al.* (1978) L'E.E.G. dans les hyperglycinémies sans cétose. *Reviews of EEG Neurophysiology*, **8**, 102–6.

Miyabayashi, S., Ito, T., Narisawa, K. *et al.* (1985) Biochemical study in 28 children with lactic acidosis, in relation to Leigh's encephalomyelopathy. *European Journal of Pediatrics*, **143**, 278–83.

Mizutani, N., Maehara, M., Hayakawa, C. *et al.* (1983) Hyperargininemia: clinical course and treatment with sodium benzoate and phenylacetic acid. *Brain and Development*, **5**, 555–63.

Montagna, P., Gallassi, R., Medori, R. *et al.* (1988) MELAS syndrome: characteristic migrainous and epileptic features and maternal transmission. *Neurology*, **38**, 751–4.

Montpetit, V.J.A., Andermann, F., Carpenter, S. *et al.* (1971) Subacute necrotizing encephalomyelopathy. A review and a study of two families. *Brain*, **94**, 1–30.

Morton, D.H., Bennett, M.J., Seargeant, L.E. *et al.* (1991) Glutaric aciduria type I: A common cause of episodic encephalopathy and spastic paralysis in the Amish of Lancaster County, Pennsylvania. *American Journal of Medical Genetics*, **41**, 89–95.

Naidu, S., Hoefler, G., Watkins, P.A. *et al.* (1988) Neonatal seizures and retardation in a girl with biochemical features of X-linked adrenoleukodystrophy: a possible new peroxisomal disease entity. *Neurology*, **38**, 1100–7.

Opitz, J.M., ZuRhein, G.M., Vitale, L. *et al.* (1969) The Zellweger syndrome (cerebro-hepato-renal syndrome). *Birth Defects*, **5**(2), 144–58.

Palmer, D.N., Fearnley, I.M., Walker, J.E. *et al.* (1992) Mitochondrial ATP synthase subunit c storage in the ceroid-lipofuscinoses (Batten disease). *American Journal of Medical Genetics*, **42**, 561–7.

Pampiglione, G. and Harden, A. (1974) An infantile form of neuronal 'storage' disease with characteristic evolution of neurophysiological features. *Brain*, **97**, 355–60.

Pavlakis, S.G., Phillips, P.C., DiMauro, S. *et al.* (1984) Mitochondrial myopathy, encephalopathy, lactic acidosis and strokelike episodes: a distinctive clinical syndrome. *Annals of Neurology*, **16**, 481–8

Pavlakis, S.G., Rowland, L.P., De Vivo, D.C. *et al.* (1988) Mitochondrial myopathies and encephalomyopathies, in *Advances in Contemporary Neurology* (ed. Plum, F.), F.A. Davis, New York, pp. 95–133

Poll-Thé, B.T., Saudubray, J.M., Ogier, H.A.M. *et al.* (1987) Infantile Refsum disease: an inherited peroxisomal disorder. Comparison with Zellweger syndrome and neonatal adrenoleukodystrophy. *European Journal of Pediatrics*, **146**, 477–83.

Poll-Thé, B.T., Roels, F., Ogier, H. *et al.* (1988) A new peroxisomal disorder with enlarged peroxisomes and a specific deficiency of acyl-CoA oxidase (pseudo-neonatal adrenoleukodystrophy). *American Journal of Human Genetics*, **42**, 422–34.

Poulos, A., Sharp, P., Johnson, D.W. and Easton, C. (1988) The occurrence of polyenoic very long chain fatty acids with greater than 32 carbon atoms in molecular species of phophatidylcholine in normal and peroxisome-deficient (Zellweger's syndrome) brain. *Biochemical Journal*, **253**, 645–50.

Powers, J.M., Moser, H.W., Moser, A.B. *et al.*

(1985) Fetal cerebro-hepato-renal (Zellweger) syndrome: dysmorphic, radiologic, biochemical, and pathologic findings in four affected fetuses. *Human Pathology*, **16**, 610–20.

Prick, M.J.J., Gabreëls, F.J.M., Renier, W.O. *et al.* (1981) Progressive infantile poliodystrophy. Association with disturbed pyruvate oxidation in muscle and liver. *Archives of Neurology*, **38**, 767–72.

Prick, M.M.J., Gabreëls, F.J.M., Trijbels, J.M.F. *et al.* (1982) Progressive poliodystrophy (Alpers' disease) with a defect in citric acid cycle activity in liver and fibroblasts. *Neuropediatrics*, **13**, 108–11.

Prick, M.M.J., Gabreëls, F.J.M., Trijbels, J.M.F. *et al.* (1983) Progressive poliodystrophy (Alpers' disease) with a defect in cytochrome aa_3 in muscle: a report of two unrelated patients. *Clinical Neurology and Neurosurgery*, **85**, 57–70.

Rosenblum, W.I. (1968) Neuropathologic changes in a case of sulfite oxidase deficiency. *Neurology*, **18**, 1187–96.

Roth, A., Nogues, C., Monnet, J.P. *et al.* (1985) Anatomopathological findings in a case of combined deficiency of sulphite oxidase and xanthine oxidase with a defect of molybdenum cofactor. *Virchows Archiv A, Pathological Anatomy and Histopathology (Berlin)*, **405**, 379–86.

Sakuta, R., Goto, Y., Horai, S. *et al.* (1992) Mitochondrial DNA mutation and Leigh's syndrome. *Annals of Neurology*, **32**, 597–8.

Salbert, B.A., Pellock, J.M. and Wolf, B. (1993) Characterization of seizures associated with biotinidase deficiency. *Neurology*, **43**, 1351–5.

Salonen, R., Somer, M., Haltia, M. *et al.* (1991) Progressive encephalopathy with edema, hypsarrhythmia, and optic atrophy (PEHO syndrome). *Clinical Genetics*, **39**, 287–93.

Santavuori, P., Haltia, M., Rapola, J. and Raitta, C. (1973) Infantile type of so-called neuronal ceroid-lipofuscinosis. Part 1. A clinical study of 15 patients. *Journal of the Neurological Sciences*, **18**, 257–67.

Santavuori, P., Haltia, M., and Rapola, J. (1974) Infantile type of so-called neuronal ceroid-lipofuscinosis. *Developmental Medicine and Child Neurology*, **16**, 644–53.

Santavuori, P., Rapola, J., Raininko, R. *et al.* (1993) Early juvenile neuronal ceroid-lipofuscinosis or variant Jansky–Bielschowsky disease: Diagnostic criteria and nomenclature. *Journal of Inherited Metabolic Disease*, **16**, 230–2.

Santos, M.J., Imanaka, T., Shio, H. *et al.* (1988) Peroxisomal membrane ghosts in Zellweger syndrome – aberrant organelle assembly. *Science*, **239**, 1536–8.

Santos, M.J., Hoefler, S., Moser, A.B. *et al.* (1992) Peroxisome assembly mutations in humans: structural heterogeneity in Zellweger syndrome. *Journal of Cellular Physiology*, **151**, 103–12.

Sarnat, H.B., Trevenen, C.L. and Darwish, H.Z. (1993) Ependymal abnormalities in cerebro-hepato-renal disease of Zellweger. *Brain and Development* **15**, 270–7.

Scher, M.S., Bergman, I., Ahdab-Barmada, M. and Fria, Th. (1986) Neurophysiological and anatomical correlations in neonatal nonketotic hyperglycinemia. *Neuropediatrics*, **17**, 137–43.

Schmitt, B., Steinmann, B., Gitzelmann, R. *et al.* (1993) Nonketotic hyperglycinemia: clinical and electrophysiologic effects of destromethorphan, an antagonist of the NMDA receptor. *Neurology*, **43**, 421–4.

Schram, A.W., Goldfischer, S., Wanders, R.J.A. *et al.* (1987) A genetic disorder due to the deficiency of the peroxisomal β-oxidation enzyme 3-oxoacyl-CoA thiolase. *Journal of Inherited Metabolic Disease*, **10**(suppl 2), 214–6.

Schulz, H. (1991) Beta oxidation of fatty acids. *Biochimica et Biophysica Acta*, **1081**, 109–20.

Schuurmans-Stekhoven, J.H., van Haelst, U.J.G.M., Joosten, E.M.G. and Gabreëls, F.J.M. (1976) Ultrastructural study of so-called curvilinear bodies and fingerprint structures in lymphocytes in late-infantile amaurotic idiocy. *Acta Neuropathologica (Berlin)*, **35**, 295–306.

Schuurmans-Stekhoven, J.H., van Haelst, U.J.G.M., Joosten, E.M.G. and Loonen, M.C.B. (1977) Ultrastructural study of the vacuoles in the peripheral lymphocytes in juvenile amaurotic idiocy. Juvenile form of generalized ceroid lipofuscinosis. *Acta Neuropathologica (Berlin)*, **38**, 137–42.

Scotto, J.M., Hadchouel, M., Odievre, M. *et al.* (1982) Infantile phytanic acid storage disease, a possible variant of Refsum's disease: three cases, including ultrastructural studies of the liver. *Journal of Inherited Metabolic Disease*, **5**, 83–90.

Seccombe, D.W., James, L. and Booth, F. (1986) L-Carnitine treatment of glutaric aciduria type I. *Neurology*, **36**, 264–7.

Shapira, Y., Cederbaum, S.D., Cancilla, P.A. *et al.* (1975) Familial poliodystrophy, mitochondrial myopathy, and lactate acidemia. *Neurology*, **25**, 614–21.

Shimozawa, N., Suzuki, Y., Orii, T. *et al.* (1993) Standardization of complementation grouping of peroxisome-deficient disorders and the second Zellweger patient with peroxisomal assembly factor-I (PAF-I) defect. *American Journal of Human Genetics*, **52**, 843–84.

Shoffner, J.M., Lott, M.T., Lezza, A.M. *et al.* (1990) Myoclonic epilepsy and ragged-red fiber disease (MERRF) is associated with a mitochondrial DNA tRNA(Lys) mutation. *Cell*, **61**, 931–7.

Shoffner, J.M., Fernhoff, P.M., Krawiecki, N.S. *et al.* (1992) Subacute necrotizing encephalopathy; oxidative phosphorylation defects and ATPase 6 point mutation. *Neurology*, **42**, 2168–74.

Slot, H.M.J., Overweg-Plandsoen, W.C.G., Bakker, H.D. *et al.* (1993) Molybdenum-cofactor deficiency: an easily missed cause of neonatal convulsions. *Neuropediatrics*, **24**, 139–42

Somer, M. and Sainio, K. (1993) Epilepsy and the electroencephalogram in progressive encephalopathy with edema, hypsarrhythmia, and optic atrophy (the PEHO syndrome). *Epilepsia*, **34**, 727–31.

Somer, M., Salonen, O., Pihko, H. and Norio, R. (1993a) PEHO syndrome (Progressive Encephalopathy with Edema, Hypsarrhythmia, and Optic Atrophy) – neuroradiologic findings. *American Journal of Neuroradiology*, **14**, 861-7.

Somer, M., Setala, K., Kivela, T. *et al.* (1993b) The PEHO syndrome (Progressive Encephalopathy with Oedema, Hypsarrhythmia and Optic Atrophy) – ophthalmological findings and differential diagnosis. *Neuro-Ophthalmology*, **13**, 65–74.

Takeda, S., Wakabayashi, K., Ohama, E. and Ikuta, F. (1988) Neuropathology of myoclonus epilepsy associated with ragged-red fibers (Fukuhara's disease). *Acta Neuropathologica (Berlin)*, **75**, 433–40.

Tanaka, R., Okamura, M., Arima, J., Yamakura, S. and Momoi, T. (1992) Pyridoxine dependent seizures: report of a case with atypical clinical features and abnormal MRI scans. *Journal of Child Neurology*, **7**, 24–8.

Terheggen, H.G., Schwenk, A., Lowenthal, A. *et al.* (1969) Argininaemia with arginase deficiency. *Lancet*, **ii**, 748–9.

Thomson, A.M., Walker, V.E. and Flynn, D.M. (1989) Glycine enhances NMDA-receptor mediated synaptic potentials in neocortical slices. *Nature*, **338**, 422–4.

Thurston, J.H. and Hauhart, R.E. (1992) Amelior-

ation of adverse effects of valproic acid on ketogenesis and liver coenzyme A metabolism by cotreatment with pantothenate and carnitine in developing mice: possible clinical significance. *Pediatric Research*, **31**, 419–23.

Tulinius, M.H., Holme, E., Kristiansson, B. *et al.* (1991) Mitochondrial encephalomyopathies in childhood. II. Clinical manifestations and syndromes. *Journal of Pediatrics*, **119**, 251–9.

Ulrich, J., Herschkowitz, N., Heitz, Ph. *et al.* (1978) Adrenoleukodystrophy. Preliminary report of a conatal case. Light- and electron microscopical, immunohistochemical and biochemical findings. *Acta Neuropathologica (Berlin)*, **43**, 77–83.

Van Coster, R., Lombes, A., De Vivo, D.C. *et al.* (1991) Cytochrome *c* oxidase-associated Leigh syndrome: phenotypic features and pathogenetic speculations. *Journal of the Neurological Sciences*, **104**, 97–111.

Van den Bosch, H., Schutgens, R.B.H., Wanders, R.J.A. and Tager, J. (1992) Biochemistry of peroxisomes. *Annual Reviews of Biochemistry*, **61**, 157–97.

Van der Knaap, M.S. and Valk, J. (1991) The MR spectrum of peroxisomal disorders. *Neuroradiology*, **33**, 30–7.

Van Erven, P.M.M., Ruitenbeek, W., Gabreëls, F.J.M. *et al.* (1986) Disturbed oxidative metabolism in subacute necrotizing encephalomyelopathy (Leigh syndrome). *Neuropediatrics*, **17**, 28–32.

Van Erven, P.M.M., Gillessen, J.P.M., Eekhoff, E.M.W. *et al.* (1987) Leigh syndrome. A mitochondrial encephalo(myo)pathy. *Clinical Neurology and Neurosurgery*, **89**, 217–30.

Van Geet, C., Vandenbossche, L., Eggermont, E. *et al.* (1991) Possible platelet contribution to pathogenesis of transient neonatal hyperammonemia syndrome. *Lancet*, **337**, 73–5.

Van Maldergem, L., Espeel, M., Wanders, R.J.A. *et al.* (1992) Neonatal seizures and severe hypotonia in a male infant suffering from a defect in peroxisomal beta-oxidation. *Neuromuscular Disorders*, **2**, 217–24.

Volpe, J.J. and Adams, R.D. (1972) Cerebrohepato-renal syndrome of Zellweger: an inherited disorder of neuronal migration. *Acta Neuropathologica (Berlin)*, **20**, 175–98.

Wadman, S.K., Duran, M., Beemer, F.A. and Cats, B.P. (1983) Absence of hepatic molybdenum cofactor: An inborn error of metabolism leading to a combined deficiency of sulphite oxidase and xanthine dehydrogenase. *Journal of Inherited Metabolic Disease*, **6**, 78–83.

Wallace, D.C. (1992) Diseases of the mitochondrial DNA. *Annual Reviews of Biochemistry*, **61**, 1175–212.

Wanders, R.J.A., van Weringh, G., Schrakamp, J.M. *et al.* (1985) Deficiency of acyl-CoA : dihydroxyacetone phosphate acyltransferase in thrombocytes of Zellweger patients: a simple postnatal test. *Clinica et Chimica Acta*, **151**, 217–21.

Wanders, R.J.A., van Roermund, C.W.T., Schutgens, R.B.H. *et al.* (1990a) The inborn errors of peroxisomal β-oxidation. *Journal of Inherited Metabolic Disease*, **13**, 4–36.

Wanders, R.J.A., van Roermund, C.W.T., Schelen, A. *et al.* (1990b) A bifunctional protein with deficient enzymic activity: identification of a new peroxisomal disorder using novel methods to measure the peroxisomal β-oxidation enzyme activities. *Journal of Inherited Metabolic Disease*, **13**, 375–9.

Wanders, R.J.A., Casteels, M., Mannaerts, G.P. *et al.* (1991) Accumulation and impaired *in vivo* metabolism of di- and trihydroxycholestanoic acid in two patients. *Clinica et Chimica Acta*, **202**, 123–32.

Wanders, R.J.A., van Roermund, C., Brul, S. *et al.* (1992) Bifunctional enzyme deficiency: identification of a new type of peroxisomal disorder in a patient with an impairment in peroxisomal β-oxidation of unknown aetiology by means of complementation analysis. *Journal of Inherited Metabolic Disease*, **15**, 385–8.

Wanders, R.J.A., Schutgens, R.B.H., Barth, P.G.

et al. (1993) Postnatal diagnosis of peroxisomal disorders: a biochemical approach. *Biochimie*, **75**, 269–79.

Watkins, P.A., Chen, W.W., Harris, C.J. *et al.* (1989) Peroxisomal bifunctional enzyme deficiency. *Journal of Clinical Investigation*, **83**, 771–7.

Wijburg, F.A., Wanders, R.J.A., van Lie-Peters, E.M. *et al.* (1991) NADH : Q_1 : oxidoreductase deficiency without lactic acidosis in a patient with Leigh syndrome: implications for the diagnosis of inborn errors of the respiratory chain. *Journal of Inherited Metabolic Disease*, **14**, 297–300.

Willems, P.J., Gatti, R., Darby, J.K. *et al.* (1991) Fucosidosis revisited: a review of 77 patients. *American Journal of Medical Genetics*, **38**, 111–31.

Wolf, B. and Heard, G.S. (1989) Disorders of biotin metabolism, in *The Metabolic Basis of Inherited Disease*, 6th edn (eds C.R. Scriver, A.L. Beaudet, W.S. Sly and D. Valle), McGraw-Hill, New York, pp. 2083–103.

Yan, W., Boustany, R-M.N., Konradi, C. *et al.* (1993) Localization of juvenile, but not late-infantile, neuronal ceroid lipofuscinosis on chromosome 16. *American Journal of Human Genetics*, **52**, 89–95.

Yoshida, T., Tada, K. and Arakawa, T. (1971) Vitamin B6-dependency of glutamic acid decarboxylase in the kidney from a patient with vitamin B6 dependendent convulsions. *Tohuku Journal of Experimental Medicine*, **104**, 195–8.

Zeman, W.S., Donahue, P., Dyken, P. and Green, J. (1970) Neuronal ceroid-lipofuscinosis, in *Leucodystrophies and Poliodystrophies. Handbook of Clinical Neurology*, vol. 10 (eds P.J. Vinken and G.W. Bruyn), North Holland Publ. Cy., Amsterdam, pp. 589–679.

INFECTIONS AND POSTINFECTIVE CAUSES

Mauricio Coelho Neto and Paulo Rogério M. de Bittencourt

INTRODUCTION

Infections, including parasitic diseases, are the commonest associated cause of 'status epilepticus' in children (Aicardi and Chevrie, 1970; Philips and Shanahan, 1989). They constitute possibly the second most common etiology of seizures of recent onset in any age group; but particularly in children, and especially in tropical countries (Axton and Siebert, 1982).

Epidemiologic studies have shown that some 5% of all patients, mostly young children, have epilepsy as a long-term complication of CNS infection (Hauser and Hesdorffer, 1990). In the neonatal period infections account for 12% of seizure disorders (Volpe, 1981), but this percentage may vary significantly with social and environmental factors (Commission on Tropical Diseases, of the International League against Epilepsy, 1994, 1996). In northern Finland, only 3% of 495 cases of brain damage were related to bacterial or viral disease and none were ascribed to parasitic disease (Rantakallio *et al.*, 1986). Conversely in regions where malaria is endemic, it may be the commonest precipitant of febrile seizures (Bittencourt *et al.*, 1988). In other areas acute bacterial meningitis is responsible for 20% of acute seizures in children (Axton and Siebert, 1982).

Infections in the CNS pose special diagnostic and management problems related to the blood–brain and other physical barriers between the site of disease and the therapeutic agents. Knowledge of the distribution of the most probable etiologies responsible for specific clinical pictures is relevant at the bedside, so that early therapy and planning of prophylaxis can be instituted and CNS sequelae avoided. In the neonate and infant infections frequently lead to later morbidity characterized by mental and motor disability, with or without concomitant seizure disorders. Early effective etiologic therapy may make the difference between total health and chronic neurologic disability. A summary of useful investigations is given in Chapter 21.

RELATIONSHIP BETWEEN ACTIVITY OF THE INFECTION AND THE SEIZURE DISORDER

The Commission on Epidemiology and Prognosis of the International League Against Epilepsy (1993) has defined seizure disorders as acute symptomatic and remote symptomatic. The former indicates seizures taking place during active disease, and the latter those occurring as sequelae. In infections such as acute bacterial meningitis this distinction is clear, whereas in, for example, neurocysticercosis and HIV encephalopathy the terms may overlap (Commission on Tropical Diseases of the International League against Epilepsy, 1994, 1996). In neurocysticercosis seizures tend to be more severe during the

Epilepsy in Children. Edited by Sheila Wallace. Published in 1996 by Chapman & Hall, London. ISBN 0 412 56860 8

Table 4d.1 List of CNS infections that may lead to acute symptomatic seizure disorders (acute phase) and particularly to remote symptomatic epilepsy (chronic phase)

Acute phase
  Schistosomiasis
  Hydatidosis
  Cysticercosis
  Malaria
  Cerebral malaria
  Toxoplasmosis (HIV)
  Acute meningitis
  Acute encephalitis

Chronic phase
  Cysticercosis
  Toxoplasmosis (HIV)
  Hydatidosis
  HIV

active disease but nonetheless occur during the inactive lifelong period of calcification (Bittencourt *et al.*, 1988). Table 4d.1 shows diseases that will manifest prominent seizure disorders during their acute or chronic phases.

The risk for the development of spontaneous seizures is related to the bacterial or viral etiology and to the extent of cerebral involvement; it is also related to the occurrence of acute symptomatic seizures, as shown in the epidemiologic study of Annegers *et al.* (1988). These authors demonstrated that the 20-year risk for remote symptomatic epilepsy was 22% in viral encephalitis with and 10% without acute seizures. Similarly, the risk was 13% in patients with bacterial meningitis with and 2.4% in those without acute seizures.

PATHOPHYSIOLOGY

Most acute infective causes will lead to epilepsies with localization, i.e. with partial or secondary generalized seizures (Bittencourt *et al.*, 1988; Pomeroy *et al.*, 1990). In many cases there will be a flurry of seizures and sometimes partial or generalized status epilepticus (Bittencourt *et al.*, 1988). The main exceptions are cerebral malaria and AIDS encephalopathy. In the former, seizures are tonic-clonic, and in the latter they tend to be myoclonic or absences. In AIDS, when seizures are partial in their origin, a secondary infection is more likely (Commission on Tropical Diseases of the International League against Epilepsy, 1994, 1996).

In African trypanosomiasis, because of the typical basal meningitic process with relatively little involvement of epileptogenic areas in the cerebral hemispheres, seizures are rare until the final stages of the disease (Commission on Tropical Diseases of the International League against Epilepsy, 1996). In cerebral malaria the encephalopathy is acute and typically hemispherical: 28% have generalized tonic-clonic sezures (Bittencourt *et al.*, 1988). Remote symptomatic epilepsy is less frequent, occurring in some 10% (Brewster *et al.*, 1990). A severe acute symptomatic seizure disorder during cerebral malaria is a risk factor for chronic neurologic sequelae, the commonest of which are hemiplegia, cortical blindness, aphasia, and ataxia (Brewster *et al.*, 1990).

The mechanisms of epileptogenesis in CNS infections are multiple (Table 4d.2). The seizures of subacute sclerosing panencephalitis (Dixit *et al.*, 1981) and of HIV, typically

Table 4d.2 Mechanisms of epileptogenesis in infections of the CNS

Mechanism	Seizure type	Disease
Fever	Febrile	Malaria
Multifactorial	Generalized	Cerebral malaria
Vasculitis	Localized	Cysticercosis
Inflammation		Tuberculosis
Mass effect		Cryptococcus
		Toxoplasmosis
		Bacterial meningitis
Cortical damage	Myoclonus	HIV, other viruses
	Absence (?)	
	Tonic-clonic	
Systemic toxemia	Tonic-clonic	Shigellosis

generalized and myoclonic, appear to be due to direct neuronal damage in diffuse areas of the cortex (Commission on Tropical Diseases of the International League against Epilepsy, 1996). The mechanisms in herpes simplex and other more focal encephalitides, characterized by localized seizure disorders, may be similar, as the pathologic process is much the same (Menkes, 1977).

In a highly selected population of candidates for epilepsy surgery, Marks *et al.* (1992) found that encephalitis usually led to neocortical epileptogenic foci, while meningitis tended to be associated with mesial temporal lobe damage. The age of onset of encephalitis was predicitive of the type of epileptogenic lesion: only disease before 4 years of age was strongly associated with mesial temporal sclerosis.

DIAGNOSIS

Systemic symptoms may be confined to fever and malaise in acute viral or bacterial diseases. In subacute or chronic infections, e.g. tuberculosis and cryptococcal meningitis, neurologic signs may be prominent, including intracranial hypertension, meningeal involvement, disturbances of behavior and conciousness, with or without focal signs. In infants, acute bacterial and viral infections may present only with malaise and seizures (Bell *et al.*, 1982).

The first investigation in these young patients should be a full blood count and an erythrocyte sedimentation rate (ESR). As a rule the ESR is high in bacterial and a few viral diseases, and normal in parasitic and most viral infections (Bittencourt *et al.*, 1985).

The role of CT has become more important with increasing availability and rapid examination times, allowing early examination of all but the most agitated children. In general hospitals this will be the first investigation, a practice which avoids the rare instances of complications of lumbar puncture (Fishman, 1980; Lee *et al.*, 1987). CT will show focal

areas of low attenuation, with peripheral enhancement, in a variety of granulomatous disorders, including toxoplasmosis, neurocysticercosis, and tuberculosis (Lee *et al.*, 1987; Bittencourt *et al.*, 1988). Signs compatible with vasculitis, from irregular 'fluffy' enhancement to frank infarction, may take place in bacterial, viral, and parasitic diseases. Finally, many infections present with hydrocephalus, frequently obstructive (Lee *et al.*, 1987). In later stages of the disease, magnetic resonance imaging (MRI) may give more detailed information (Lee *et al.*, 1987). Arteriography is confined to specific cases when a diagnosis such as sinus thrombosis needs to be established, although this may be possible with CT or MRI.

The critical decision is when to perform a lumbar puncture. There is little doubt that one should wait for the CT when there is intracranial hypertension and signs of a focal lesion. In order for the lumbar puncture to be risk-free, CT should show lack of blockage of flow through the ventricular system (Fishman, 1980). Highly specialized advice may be required, even for a suboccipital tap, in cases where CT shows obstruction of CSF flow.

CSF should be obtained in children presenting with seizures and fever below 18, or at most 24 months (Ouelette, 1974; Illingworth, 1980; Wallace, 1985), when meningeal signs and fever may take longer to appear. Jaffe *et al.* (1981) suggested in addition that CSF should be obtained in children with seizures lasting more than 15 minutes, with a focal nature, occurring more than 12 hours after the onset of fever, and when the temperature is less than 38.5 °C. Rossi *et al.* (1986) were more conservative and concluded that all children younger than 6 months presenting with fever and a seizure should have their CSF examined. Some of these concepts may need to be changed in view of the yield of CT and MRI, but a definitive study of the role of neuroimaging in decision-making is not yet available.

Electroencephalography can be useful in

Table 4d.3 Main etiologic agents of acute bacterial meningitis according to Centers of Disease Control, and ages and conditions of peak incidence of each etiology (Benson *et al.*, 1988, modified)

Etiologic agent	Percentage of all cases	Most frequent ages or associated features
Hemophilus influenzae b	48	6 months–6 years
Neisseria meningitidis	20	5–20 years
Streptococcus pneumoniae	13	1st year, 30+ years
Gram-negative		Systemic infection, alcohol, trauma, immune
Listeria monocytogenes	13	depression, surgery, neonates, elderly
Streptococcus B		
Staphylococcus		
Other bacteria	6	–

the definition of seizure type, diagnosis of encephalitis, and in the follow-up of severe encephalopathies (Vas and Cracco, 1990). In patients with acute bacterial meningitis there is a correlation between the late development of epilepsy and the acute finding of focal slowing and sharp waves during the infection (Pomeroy *et al.*, 1990).

BACTERIAL DISEASE OF THE CNS

The etiologies of acute bacterial meningitis in children are well established (Benson *et al.*, 1988), but they may vary with environmental factors. Table 4d.3 lists the frequencies of the various etiologies in the general population and the ages of peak frequency of each etiology.

There are few published reports of the characteristics of seizures and epilepsy in the context of acute bacterial meningitis. Pomeroy and colleagues (1990), in a prospective study of 185 children followed up for up to 9 years after the acute infection, found *Hemophilus influenzae* in 64%, *Streptococcus pneumoniae* in 16%, *Neisseria meningitidis* in 11%, and other organisms in 4%. Thirty-one per cent of the children developed seizures during the infection, and in 67% there was a partial onset. Seven per cent of the 185 children developed seizures between 0.1 and 96 months after the initial disease; of these 13 cases, 12 had partial-onset seizures; 10 had had meningitis due to *H. influenzae* and three

secondary to *S. pneumoniae*. Ten of the 13 patients, that is some 5.4% of the whole population, developed remote symptomatic epilepsy: six were refractory to pharmacologic therapy, and seven had an accompanying motor or mental deficit. It is concluded that acute bacterial meningitis will lead to chronic epilepsy in some 5% of cases that survive, and these will usually be patients with additional mental or motor deficits.

In a placebo-controlled, double-blind comparison of two groups of children, 75% of whom had *H. influenzae* meningitis, Odio *et al.* (1991) found that those who received 0.6 mg/kg dexamethasone had significantly less cerebral damage on CT scan. Only two of 51 children on dexamethasone had seizures, compared to seven of 48 who received antimicrobial therapy only.

Cerebral abscess is an important cause of chronic epilepsy (Nielsen *et al.*, 1983). Some 28% of 200 adults and children presented with seizures as an acute symptom. Of 67 patients who participated in a study between 3 and 40 years after surgery, 21 were below 15 years of age at the time of operation. Eleven of these children developed epilepsy after surgery; some three-quarters in the first two years. Seizures were generalized tonic-clonic in 60%, simple partial in 14%, and complex partial with or without secondary generalization in 21%. Epilepsy and mental deficiency were commoner sequelae in children than in adults suffering from cerebral abcesses; epilepsy occurred in 20 and 9%, and mental deficits in 33 and 13% respectively.

Subdural empyemas, a complication of sinusitis, meningitis, or neurosurgical procedures, are a rarer cause of seizures acutely, and perhaps of chronic epilepsy (Kaufman *et al.*, 1975).

The organisms found in 39 cases of cerebral abcesses and subdural empyema in a recent study (Brook, 1992) were anerobic in 56%, aerobic in 18%, and mixed anaerobic and aerobic in 26%. The predominant anaerobes were gram-positive *Bacteroides* species and *Fusobacterium* species. Although the predominant aerobes were gram-positive, a significant number were *Hemophilus* species.

Tuberculosis of the CNS is possibly an important cause of acute symptomatic seizures, but its specific role is not clear, much less as a cause of remote symptomatic epilepsy. As a general rule, seizures will arise when there are tuberculomata, or arteritis in the cerebral hemispheres; seizures will be more frequent acutely than after successful therapy (Commission on Tropical Diseases of the International League against Epilepsy, 1994).

Epidemiologic studies (Miller *et al.*, 1981; Bellman *et al.*, 1983; Stetler *et al.*, 1985) have demonstrated that pertussis immunization can be associated with neurologic complications, including seizures and West's syndrome, but is unlikely to be causative. Immunization should be deferred until infants have been shown not to have an evolving neurologic disease (Stetler *et al.*, 1985).

PARASITIC DISEASES

Malaria may lead to seizures by two distinct mechanisms: malaria, caused by *Plasmodium vivax*, is possibly the commonest cause in the world of fever precipitating febrile seizures (Commission on Tropical Diseases of the International League against Epilepsy, 1994). Cerebral malaria, caused by *P. falciparum*,

leads to acute symptomatic seizures during the severe encephalopathy, and to remote symptomatic epilepsy, more rarely (Bittencourt *et al.*, 1988; Brewster *et al.*, 1990).

Toxoplasmosis leads to remote symptomatic epilepsy in the congenital form (Bittencourt *et al.*, 1988). Special attention should be given to reports that congenital infection may be subclinical and treatment may be delayed if this diagnosis is not considered (Wilson *et al.*, 1980). In adults toxoplasmosis is a frequent cause of localized symptomatic seizures during HIV infection (Bittencourt *et al.*, 1988).

Neurocysticercosis may occur in children, and frequently leads to seizure disorders (Bittencourt *et al.*, 1988; Commission on Tropical Diseases of the International League against Epilepsy, 1994). Seizures are of partial onset, and simple partial status is common. Acute symptomatic seizures are as common as remote symptomatic epilepsy, but there is much easier control of seizures after the active phase of the disease has passed (Commission on Tropical Diseases of the International League against Epilepsy, 1996).

VIRAL DISEASES

The most severe viral encephalitis leading to acute symptomatic seizures and to remote symptomatic epilepsy is herpes simplex encephalitis. Seizures are usually partial and very frequent in the acute phase, and there may be remote symptomatic refractory simple or complex partial seizures. In neonates partial motor seizures start, on average, 5.4 days after the initial lethargy and low grade fever (Arvin *et al.*, 1982).

Seizures have been observed in 10–20% of children with HIV encephalopathy. They tend to be generalized and associated with spike-waves on the EEG, sometimes with a cortical myoclonic component. When there is secondary infection, seizures may be focal (Labar, 1992; Commission on Tropical Diseases of the International League against

Epilepsy, 1996). The more advanced the encephalopathy, the more severe and frequent the seizures.

Cytomegalovirus (CMV) is a cause of epilepsy in congenital infection, as part of a severe encephalopathy with mental retardation, microcephaly and deafness (Bale, 1984). Patients with clinical encephalopathy at birth have a significant risk of developing West's syndrome, and, conversely, some 5% of patients with West's syndrome have congenital or immediate postnatal CMV encephalopathy (Riikonen, 1978) (see Chapter 11b).

The encephalitis of measles leads to acute symptomatic seizures in some 50% of cases, but only one in 10 continue to have remote symptomatic seizures (Aarli, 1974). Seizures with a localized onset are of poor prognostic significance for the development of subsequent epilepsy.

Exanthema subitum due to human herpes 6 may lead to encephalitis with abnormalities in the EEG and CT scan (Suga *et al.*, 1993). All 21 cases studied had seizures in the febrile pre-eruptive phase of the disease. Acute symptomatic generalized tonic or tonic-clonic seizures were observed in 15 and lateralized seizures in six. Of four patients who developed clear encephalopathy or encephalitis defined by CT and EEG, one developed remote symptomatic epilepsy and one died. The role of viral infection in the precipitation of febrile seizures is considered in Chapter 10.

SYSTEMIC DISEASES

Seizures may be the result of multifactorial involvement of the CNS without actual direct damage. As a general rule, tonic-clonic seizures are a symptom of toxic-metabolic insults common in severe systemic infections, as in septicemia, hepatic or renal failure. When seizures are focal, as determined clinically or by EEG, imaging studies are likely to show direct cerebral involvement.

The reports of seizures associated with childhood shigellosis are probably all of febrile convulsions and unrelated epilepsy. Of 153 cases studied by Ashkenazi *et al.* (1987), all had seizures with fever, 75% with temperatures above 39°C, 20% had a positive family history, 23% had a previous history of seizures, and 87% were younger than 5 years. Furthermore, 80% were brief tonic-clonic seizures. All 34 patients who had lumbar punctures had normal CSF.

ACKNOWLEDGMENTS

The authors are grateful for the use of the computerized literature searches provided by the National Epilepsy Library (Epilepsy Foundation of America, Maryland), Biogalênica Quimica e Farmacêutica Ltda (Ciba of Brazil, São Paulo), and the Library of the Sector of Health Sciences of the Federal University of Parana (Curitiba). Dr Sérgio Mazer (Computed Tomography Unit, Hospital Nossa Senhora das Graças, Curitiba) helped with his expertise in the area of neuroimaging. Ms Ieda Carlins helped in printing the manuscript.

REFERENCES

Aarli, J.A. (1974) Nervous system complications of measles: clinical manifestations and prognosis. *European Neurology*, **12**, 79–93.

Aicardi, J. and Chevrie, J.J. (1970) Convulsive status epilepticus in infants and children. *Epilepsia*, **11**, 187–97.

Annegers, J.F., Hauser, W.A., Beghi, E. *et al.* (1988) The risk of unprovoked seizures after encephalitis and meningitis. *Neurology*, **38**, 1407–10.

Arvin, A.M., Yeager, A.S., Bruhn, F.W. *et al.* (1982) Neonatal herpes simplex infection in the absence of mucocutaneous lesions. *Journal of Pediatrics*, **100**, 715–21.

Ashkenazi, S., Dinari, G., Zevulunov, A. *et al.* (1987) Convulsions in childhood shigellosis: clinical and laboratory features in 153 children. *American Journal of Diseases of Children*, **141**, 208–10.

Axton, J.H.M. and Siebert, S.L. (1982) Aetiology

of convulsions in Zimbabwe children three months to eight years old. *Central African Journal of Medicine*, **28**(10), 246–9.

Bale Jr, J.F. (1984) Human cytomegalovirus infection and disorders of the nervous system. *Archives of Neurology*, **41**, 310–20.

Bell, W.E., Chun, R.W.M., Jabbour J.T. *et al.* (1982) Infections of the brain and spinal cord, in *The Practice of Pediatric Neurology*, 2nd edn (eds K.F. Swaiman and F.S. Wright), C.V. Mosby, St Louis, pp. 659–764.

Bellman, M.H., Ross, E.M. and Miller, D.L. (1983) Infantile spasms and pertussis immunisation. *Lancet*, **i**, 1031–3.

Benson, C.A., Harris, A.A., and Levin, S. (1988) Acute bacterial meningitis: general aspects, in *Handbook of Clinical Neurology*, vol 52 (8) (eds P.J. Vinken, G.W. Bruyn and A.A. Harris), Elsevier Science, Amsterdam, pp. 1–19.

Bittencourt, P.R.M., Moraes, L.M., Bernardes, A.B.S. *et al.* (1985) Meningite viral benigna: criterios para diagnostico. *Revista Medica do Parana*, **51**, 70–3.

Bittencourt, P.R.M., Gracia, M.C. and Lorenzana, P. (1988) Epilepsy and parasitosis of the central nervous system, in *Recent Advances in Epilepsy – No. 4*, 1st edn (eds T.A. Pedley and B.S. Meldrum), Churchill Livingstone, London, pp. 123–159.

Brewster, R.D., Kwiatrowski, D., White, N.J. *et al.* (1990) Neurological sequelae of cerebral malaria in children. *Lancet*, **336**, 1039–43.

Brook, I. (1992) Aerobic and anaerobic bacteriology of intracranial abscesses. *Pediatric Neurology*, **81**, 210–14.

Commission on Epidemiology and Prognosis of the International League Against Epilepsy (1993) Guidlines for epidemiology studies on epilepsy. *Epilepsia*, **34**, 592–6.

Commission on Tropical Diseases of the International League Against Epilepsy (1994) The relationship of epilepsy and tropical disease. *Epilepsia*, **35**, 89–93.

Commission on Tropical Diseases of the International League Against Epilepsy (1996) Epilepsy in the tropics. (in press).

Dixit, V.M., Hettiaratchi, E.S.G., Muoka, T. *et al.* (1981) A study of subacute sclerosing panencephalitis in Kenya. *Developmental Medicine and Child Neurology*, **23**, 208–16.

Fishman, R.A. (1980) Clinical examination of cerebrospinal fluid, in *Cerebrospinal Fluid in Diseases of the Nervous System*, 1st edn (ed. R.A. Fishman), W.B. Saunders Company, Philadelphia, pp. 141–67.

Hauser, W.A. and Hesdorffer, D.C. (1990). Risk factors, in *Epilepsy: Frequency, Causes and Consequences* (eds W.A. Hauser and D.C. Hesdorffer), Demos, New York, pp. 53–91.

Illingworth, R. (1980) Lumbar puncture in children who have had fever and a convulsion. *Lancet*, **ii**, 208.

Jaffe, M., Bar-Joseph, G., Tirosh, E. *et al.* (1981) Fever and convulsion – indications for laboratory investigation. *Pediatrics*, **67**, 729–31.

Kaufman, D.M., Miller, M.H. and Steigbigel, N.H. (1975) Subdural empyema: analysis of 17 recent cases and review of the literature. *Medicine*, **54**, 485–98.

Labar, D.R. (1992) Seizures and HIV infection, in *Recent Advances in Epilepsy*, 1st edn (eds T.A. Pedley and B.S. Meldrum), Churchill Livingstone, New York, pp. 119–26.

Lee, S.H. and Rao, K.C.G. (1987) Infectious diseases, in *Cranial Computed Tomography and MRI*, 2nd ed (eds S.H. Lee *et al.*), MacGraw-Hill Book Company, New York, pp. 557–68.

Marks, D.A., Kim, J., Spencer, D.D. *et al.* (1992) Characteristics of intractable seizures following meningitis and encephalitis. *Neurology*, **42**, 1513–8.

Menkes, J.H. (1977) Viral neurologic infection in children. *Hospital Practice*, **12**, 100–9.

Miller, D.L., Ross, E.M., Alderslade, R. *et al.* (1981) Pertussis immunisation and serious acute neurological illness in children. *British Medical Journal*, **282**, 1595–9.

Nielsen, H., Harmsen, A. and Gyldensted, C. (1983) Cerebral abscess: a long-term follow-up. *Acta Neurologica Scandinavica*, **67**, 330–7.

Odio, C.M., Faingezicht, I., Paris, M. *et al.* (1991) The benefical effects of early dexamethasone administration in infants and children with bacterial meningitis. *New England Journal of Medicine*, **324**, 1525–31.

Ouelette, E.M. (1974) The child who convulses with fever. *Pediatric Clinics of North America*, **21**, 467–81.

Phillips, A.S. and Shanahan, J.R. (1989) Etiology and mortality of status epilepticus in children – a recent update. *Archives of Neurology*, **46**, 74–6.

Pomeroy, L.S., Homes, J.S., Dodge, P.R. *et al.* (1990) Seizures and other neurologic sequelae of bacterial meningitis in children. *New England Journal of Medicine*, **323**, 1651–7.

Rantakallio, P., Leskinen, M. and Von Wendt, L.

(1986) Incidence and prognosis of central nervous system infections in a birth cohort of 12 000 children. *Scandinavian Journal of Infectious Diseases*, **18**, 287–94.

Riikonen, R. (1978) Cytomegalovirus infection and infantile spasms. *Developmental Medicine and Child Neurology*, **20**, 570–9.

Rossi, L.N., Brunelli, G., Duzioni, N. *et al.* (1986) Lumbar punture and febrile convulsions. *Helvetica Paediatrica Acta*, **41**, 19–24.

Stetler, H.C., Orenstein, W.A., Bart, K.J. *et al.* (1985) History of convulsions and use of pertussis vaccine. *Journal of Pediatrics*, **107**, 175–9.

Suga, S., Yoshikawa, T., Asano, Y. *et al.* (1993) Clinical and virological analyses of 21 infants with exanthem subitum (roseola infantum) and

central nervous system complications. *Neurology*, **33**, 597–603.

Vas, G.A. and Cracco, J.B. (1990) Diffuse encephalopathies, in *Current Practice of Clinical Electroencephalography*, 2nd edn, Raven Press, New York, pp. 371–99.

Volpe, J.J. (1981) in *Epilepsy in Children*, 1st edn (ed. J. Aicardi), Raven Press, New York, p. 193.

Wallace, S.J. (1985) Convulsions and lumbar puncture. *Developmental Medicine and Child Neurology*, **27**, 69–71.

Wilson, C.B., Remington, J.S., Stagno, S.C. and Reynolds, D.W. (1980) Development of adverse sequelae in children born with subclinical congenital toxoplasmosis infection. *Pediatrics*, **66**, 767–74.

5

PATHOLOGY OF CHILDHOOD EPILEPSY

Harry V. Vinters and Claude G. Wasterlain

There have been few studies of the neuropathology associated with epilepsy in childhood. In the first report associating brain damage with epileptic seizures, Bouchet and Cazauvielh (1825) noted acute hippocampal softening in two of their 18 autopsied patients. Norman (1964) studied 11 children after status epilepticus. All of them showed the classic 'ischemic nerve cell change' of Spielmeyer (1927) with narrow, triangular neurons with pyknotic nuclei and eosinophilic cytoplasm, establishing that these changes were the result of status epilepticus or of associated events. Such changes were found in the CA_1 (Sommer) sector in all patients, in the end-folium (CA_3 and dentate hilus) in most, in the thalamus in nine of 11, in the amygdala in six, and in the striatum and cerebellum in five.

Margerison and Corsellis (1966) found Ammon's horn sclerosis in 65–75% of patients with temporal lobe epilepsy, many of whom were below the age of 20 years. Corsellis and Bruton (1983) studied the brains of 20 patients who died during or shortly after status epilepticus. Some children showed the presence of acute neuronal necrosis, which was more severe in CA_1, but was also seen in other hippocampal regions, in the middle layers of cerebral cortex, the thalamus, striatum, and cerebellum. All six patients who died in infancy showed acute changes which must have resulted from the seizures themselves or from associated pathology.

Sagar and Oxbury (1987) found reduced neuronal counts in CA_1, end-folium, and dentate gyrus of the resected temporal lobes of patients who had their first convulsion before the age of 3 years and were operated upon for intractable epilepsy.

Represa et al., (1989) studied high-affinity binding sites for kainate autoradiographically. Increased binding was seen in the hippocampi of epileptic children, especially in CA_3. Other studies on the resected hippocampi of children with intractable seizures showed evidence of cell loss in the dentate gyrus and of aberrant mossy fiber sprouting in the inner molecular layer of the fascia dentata (Mathern et al., 1993, 1994).

This chapter will briefly review some of the experimental evidence relating brain damage to epilepsy in the immature brain, and will provide a description of the range and type of neuropathology observed in a surgical program for intractable childhood epilepsy (see also Chapter 23d).

EXPERIMENTAL EVIDENCE

There are unfortunately no animal models of the 'catastrophic epilepsies of childhood' which make up a high proportion of patients operated on in childhood for intractable epilepsy. Many cases of childhood epilepsy

Epilepsy in Children. Edited by Sheila Wallace. Published in 1996 by Chapman & Hall, London. ISBN 0 412 56860 8

leading to corticectomy or hemispherectomy are associated with extrahippocampal lesions, and the effects of these lesions on the immature brain have received little attention. Therefore this discussion of the experimental literature is limited to three topics:

1. The relationship between hippocampal sclerosis and epilepsy.
2. The relative vulnerability of the immature brain to seizure-induced damage (or lack thereof).
3. The effect of seizures occurring in the immature brain on brain growth and the establishment of neuronal connections.

The mechanism of disorders of neuronal migration (see Chapter 4a), which are associated with a large number of intractable childhood epilepsies, will not be covered, though relevant neuropathologic findings are described below.

IS HIPPOCAMPAL SCLEROSIS THE CAUSE OR THE CONSEQUENCE OF EPILEPSY?

Experimental seizures-induced hippocampal sclerosis

In 1880, Sommer described the loss of CA_1 hippocampal pyramidal cells which has become associated with his name. This pattern has been found in the brains of many patients with chronic epilepsy or with a history of status epilepticus, with minor modifications such as a more widespread distribution of damage affecting most hippocampal sectors, and more extensive lesions in CA_3. Sommer was convinced that this lesion was the cause of his patients' epilepsy. In the same year, Pfleger (1880) described hemorrhagic lesions in the temporal lobes of patient dying shortly after status epilepticus, and concluded that hippocampal lesions were the result of metabolic or local circulatory disturbances caused by the seizures. The controversy has persisted to the present, but it is now clear that both Sommer and Pfleger were

correct. Human material has continued to provide evidence of a strong association between status epilepticus and hippocampal lesions. Norman (1964) described acute hippocampal lesions in every one of 11 children (age 1–6 years) after status epilepticus, Margerison and Corsellis (1966) found hippocampal lesions in nearly three-quarters of patients with temporal lobe epilepsy, and Falconer, Serafetindes and Corsellis (1964) reported an association between those lesions and a history of febrile seizures (Chapter 10). However, clinical data cannot provide final proof of causality in complex clinical situations such as status epilepticus. The occurrence of associated events such as hypoxia or hypotension could confuse the picture. Only experimental data can provide definitive answers.

The classic studies of Meldrum and associates in pubescent baboons proved that electrographic seizures can damage the brain in the absence of behavioral convulsions or of systemic complications (Meldrum and Brierley, 1973). Flurothyl-induced seizures in paralyzed oxygen-ventilated rats in good metabolic balance produce neuronal necrosis and 'hypermetabolic' infarction of the substantia nigra (Nevander *et al.*, 1985). Focal penicillin seizures in rat neocortex induce thalamic lesions in synaptically connected sites (Collins and Olney, 1982). Limbic status epilepticus induced by kainic acid (Olney, Rhee and Ho, 1974), by muscarinic cholinergic agents (Honchar, Olney and Sherman, 1983; Olney, de Gubarett and Labruyere, 1983) and by electrical stimulation (McIntyre, Nathason and Edson, 1982; Buterbaugh, Michelson and Keyser, 1986; Strain and Tasker, 1991; Lothman and Bertram, 1993) causes both hippocampal lesions and widespread extrahippocampal damage. This neuronal damage depends on synaptic activation (Ben-Ari, 1985) and the hippocampal lesions closely resemble hippocampal sclerosis in human epileptic brain.

Electrical stimulation of the perforant path

for 2–24 hours leads to ipsilateral neuronal necrosis of hilar interneurons (end-folium sclerosis) and of CA_3 pyramidal cells (Sloviter, 1983). This necrosis closely resembles that caused by intraventricular injection of glutamate or aspartate (Sloviter and Dempster, 1985), suggesting an excitotoxic mechanism. A subpopulation of hilar interneurons containing neuropeptide Y is selectively preserved by the non-NMDA blocker NBQX (Penix, Thompson and Wasterlain 1994), while a separate population of hilar interneurons including some of the somatostatin-immunopositive cells are protected by the NMDA blocker MK-801 (Penix, Thompson and Wasterlain, 1994). These data establish that even focal status epilepticus in the absence of any systemic changes produces a pattern of hippocampal damage resembling hippocampal sclerosis through glutamatergic excitotoxic mechanisms.

Experimental hippocampal lesions leading to chronic epilepsy

Clinically, there is a strong association between status epilepticus and later development of chronic epilepsy, but clinical material is too varied and complex to provide definitive evidence of a cause and effect relationship. To take just a few examples, Aicardi and Chevrie (1983) reported that when status epilepticus develops in children without a prior history of seizures, it is followed by chronic epilepsy in 21% of cases. In the prospective study of Maytal *et al.*, (1989) this percentage was 25%, and Annegers *et al.*, (1987) found that in children without a previous history of epilepsy, severe febrile convulsions with complex seizures carried a risk of subsequent chronic epilepsy three time higher than that of simple febrile convulsions. Of course this association does not establish causality, and Maytal *et al.* (1989) have actually argued that in their cases status epilepticus is simply the first manifestation of a developing chronic epilepsy.

In animals which have developed hippocampal sclerosis-like changes as a result of status epilepticus induced by kainic acid (Lothman and Collins, 1981; Nadler, Perry and Cotman, 1978; Ben-Ari, 1985) or pilocarpine (Cavalheiro, Riche and La Gal la Salle, 1982), spontaneous limbic-like seizures develop after a period of 3–4 weeks (Cavalheiro, Riche and Le Gal la Salle, 1982; Cepeda *et al.* 1982; Pisa *et al.* 1982; Tanaka *et al.*, 1985). This delay has given rise to several hypotheses, including the possibility that it might reflect the time needed for sprouting to establish a recurrent excitatory pathway from granule cell to granule cell (Tauck and Nadler, 1985; Cronin and Dudek, 1988; Sutula *et al.*, 1988; Babb *et al.* 1991) and the 'filter hypothesis', which postulates the loss of an inhibitory filter that prevents kindling in response to physiologic events (Wasterlain, Farber and Fairchild, 1986). Loss of that filter would lead to spontaneous kindling over the next few weeks.

Following electrically induced self-sustaining limbic status epilepticus, Lothman *et al.* (1990) and Lothman and Bertram (1993) showed chronic interictal spikes and electrographic seizures. Over 75% of the animals displayed spontaneous recurring seizures as sequelae of self-sustaining limbic status epilepticus. In all of these models, the association between spontaneous seizures and hippocampal damage is very tentative, because they all produce widespread neuronal loss at many extrahippocampal sites in addition to hippocampal sclerosis, and the precise origin of spontaneous seizures is impossible to determine.

Using the Sloviter (1983) model of perforant path stimulation, we have recently demonstrated that in many rats the damage induced by this type of focal status epilepticus is restricted to the hilus of the hippocampus ipsilateral to the stimulation. Most of those animals display spontaneous seizures and all of them have vastly accelerated kindling rates (Shirasaka and Wasterlain, 1994). While we cannot completely rule out the possibility that the seizures actually originated from a part of the brain which shows no histologic lesions, these data establish a proven link between the sequelae of status epilepticus and the later development of spontaneous seizures, and a probable link between end-folium sclerosis and lesions of interneurons in the hilus of the dentate gyrus, and epileptogenicity. Gowers' statement (1881) that 'seizures beget seizures' has finally received experimental proof.

IS THE IMMATURE BRAIN VULNERABLE TO SEIZURE-INDUCED DAMAGE?

Studies in humans show a strong association between severe seizures in infancy or childhood and brain damage, but the significance of that association is highly controversial. Studies suggesting that the mildest seizures can have serious consequences (Schiottz–Christensen and Bruhn, 1973) coexist with other studies which emphasize the benign nature of status epilepticus (Maytal *et al.*, 1989). Recent studies of neonatal seizures using strict EEG criteria show a normal outcome in only a third of patients and development of chronic epilepsy in 56% (Scher *et al.*, 1989; Clancy and Legido, 1991; Legido, Clancy and Berman, 1991). However, studies done outside the neonatal intensive care unit show a much better prognosis, related mostly to etiology (Andre, Matisse and Vert, 1990). Aicardi and Chevrie (1970, 1983) and Chevrie and Aicardi (1978) found a high incidence of serious sequelae after status epilepticus in children, and these tended to be more severe in younger patients. Mental retardation followed status epilepticus in 48% and other neurologic deficits were found in 37%. They documented the development of hemiatrophy following unilateral status epilepticus. Maytal *et al.* (1989) found 9% of neurologic deficits after status epilepticus, and sequelae were more common at younger ages. Yager, Cheang and Seshia (1988) found

developmental deficits in 30% of children after status epilepticus. Holmes *et al.* (1988) found deficits on tests of memory, learning, and behavior after status epilepticus. Fujiwara *et al.* (1979) and Dodrill and Wilenski (1990) also found a strong association between poor outcome and status epilepticus in early life. However, the latter authors pointed out that prospective studies did not find as many sequelae as the older, retrospective studies.

In contrast to these clinical results, many animal studies emphasize the lack of brain damage following status epilepticus in the immature brain. Albala, Moshé and Okada (1984) emphasize the benign outcome of status epilepticus induced by kainic acid in 15–16-day-old rats. Mortality was 90%, but survivors showed no brain damage. Several investigators have confirmed these results (Nitecka *et al.*, 1984; Holmes and Thompson, 1988; Sperber *et al.*, 1991). Following pilocarpine status epilepticus, Cavalheiro *et al.*, (1987) found hippocampal lesions in only five of 14 rats between the ages of 10 and 21 days, and in their recent reviews have emphasized the lack of lesions in the majority of subjects, although the presence of extrahippocampal lesions and that of hippocampal pathology in a third of the animals might point in the opposite direction. Franck and Schwartzkroin (1984) found extensive hippocampal damage, most severe in CA_1, in newborn rabbits after kainic acid status epilepticus, raising the possibility that the resistance of the immature rat to kainic acid status epilepticus might be seizure or species specific.

Our recent studies used the Sloviter method of perforant path stimulation in 14–16-day-old rats (Sloviter, 1987, 1991; Penix, Thompson and Wasterlain, 1994). We found loss of frequency-dependent and short interstimulus interval-dependent paired pulse inhibition in the hippocampi of stimulated animals, and a pattern of neuronal cell loss characterized by unilateral damage to hilar interneurons in all animals, with the majority of rats also showing bilateral lesions in CA_3, mild damage in CA$_1$ and subiculum, and bilateral neuronal necrosis in pyriform cortex. These results show that the resistance of the immature rat brain to seizure-like activity is not absolute, but do not resolve the problem of its clinical relevance or of its incidence in milder forms of seizures or status epilepticus.

DO SEIZURES OCCURRING AT CRITICAL STAGES OF DEVELOPMENT ALTER BRAIN GROWTH AND THE ESTABLISHMENT OF SYNAPTIC CONNECTIONS?

The immature brain has unique metabolic adaptations to seizures: its slower metabolic rate (Vannucci and Duffy, 1975) delays the occurrence of energy failure in spite of a relative increase in metabolic rate as impressive as that of the adult (Fujikawa *et al.*, 1989), but the difficulty in transporting glucose across the immature blood–brain barrier (Morin *et al.*, 1988) accelerates energy failure (Dwyer and Wasterlain, 1985). Inhibition of protein synthesis (Dwyer and Wasterlain, 1984; Fujikawa *et al.*, 1988), DNA synthesis (Wasterlain, 1976), and mitotic rates (Suga and Wasterlain, 1980) by seizure activity have adverse effects on brain growth at critical stages of development if seizures are sufficiently severe (Wasterlain, 1976). In the immature rat, neonatal seizures reduce cell numbers, whereas later seizures reduce cell size, myelin markers, and synaptic markers, suggesting a curtailment of synaptic connections (Wasterlain and Sankar, 1993). However, the relevance of these experimental data in rodents to human epilepsy or even to brain development in nonhuman primates is unexplored.

ROLE OF THE NEUROPATHOLOGIST IN ASSESSING 'EPILEPTOGENIC' TISSUE

This section will deal with clinicopathologic issues relevant to 'pediatric epilepsy', accepting the heterogeneity and lack of precision of this term. It will describe neuropathologic findings in the brains of infants and children who have intractable seizure disorders. Until recently, these abnormalities (including malformative and inflammatory lesions) were usually assessed at necropsy (Friede, 1989), by which time 'secondary' changes (brain structural abnormalities *resulting from* a protracted seizure disorder rather than contributing to its cause) were likely to have complicated the neuropathologic findings. In recent years, however, the surgical treatment of pediatric epilepsy has evolved into an acceptable alternative to the medical management of intractable seizures in children (Chugani *et al.*, 1993; Shields, Duchowny and Holmes, 1993). The result has been that neuropathologists have had the opportunity to assess brain lesions (associated with seizures in infants and children) in a relatively pristine state, allowing for more reasonable clinicopathologic correlations than were possible in the past using only autopsy tissues.

Modern histochemical, ultrastructural and immunoultrastructural, biochemical, molecular, and pharmacologic techniques can also be applied more accurately and reproducibly to surgical specimens than to autopsy materials, allowing for analyses of human (in this case pediatric) brain tissues comparable in sophistication to those previously possible only in experimental animal studies. This frequently allows for rapid extrapolation of novel findings in experimental paradigms to the comparable human situation, and in general more meaningful communication between basic scientists interested in pediatric epilepsy and neurologists, neurosurgeons, and neuropathologists involved in the treatment of seizure disorders in infants and children. Many examples will be provided below of how this interaction has shed light on basic mechanisms and the pathophysiology of pediatric epilepsy.

As long as care is taken to standardize tissue-processing parameters, surgically resected 'epileptic' brain can provide a wealth of neurobiologic information that may not be available in necropsy material. Immunostaining of tissues can be carried out to search for novel antigens, e.g. structural (cytoskeletal) proteins or those associated with cell proliferation (De Rosa *et al.*, 1992a; Duong *et al.*, 1994). In situ hybridization may be used to detect unique gene sequences or mRNA transcripts within the tissue (Valentino *et al.*, 1987). Using the polymerase chain reaction (PCR), unique genes can be isolated, amplified, and further studied, sometimes even using paraffin-embedded tissue blocks as a starting material (Vinters, Wang and Wiley, 1993). In situ hybridization and PCR methodology have been combined to allow for gene and mRNA amplification and visualization in tissue sections (Nuovo *et al.*, 1993). Messenger RNA isolated from freshly resected brain tissue can be used to construct cDNA libraries that may then be used to look for new genes (including epilepsy-associated genes) in the CNS. Epileptic brain tissue can be used for electrophysiologic measurements and subsequently studied morphologically (Wuarin *et al.*, 1990) by injecting tracer dyes into the cell bodies of neurons from which recordings have been made.

Whilst morphologic studies of brain tissue from epileptic patients (examined either at the time of surgery or at autopsy) are recognized as being inherently valuable in helping to understand the pathogenesis of human seizures, care must be taken not to overinterpret brain lesions as being causal, rather than simply associated with, a given epileptic disorder (Vinters *et al.*, 1993). For example, in brain tissue from patients with cortical dysplasia/neuronal migration disorders (see below), the finding of severely disorganized cortex, though it suggests deranged movement of neurons from the germinal matrix to their normal location in the neocortex during intrauterine life and thus extremely abnormal cortical 'wiring', does not necessarily explain the genesis of the abnormal electrical activity within the brain that presumably underlies the generation of the seizures themselves.

UNIQUE FEATURES OF NEUROPATHOLOGIC FINDINGS IN INFANTS/CHILDREN WITH EPILEPSY

Pediatric epilepsy, particularly in its most severe manifestations in infants and children with intractable and catastrophic forms of seizure disorder such as infantile spasms, is associated with unique types of neuropathologic abnormality (Vinters, Mah and Shields, 1990; Farrell *et al.*, 1992; Vinters *et al.*, 1992; Robain and Vinters, 1994) that in general are hypothesized to reflect either

1. Abnormal migration of neurons to their 'usual' location in the neocortex (i.e. neuron migration disorders, NMD), or
2. Sequelae of destructive brain lesions that occur *in utero* or in the perinatal period.

The patterns of neuropathologic change identified are different than those seen in the brains of patients with primary generalized seizures (PGS) or temporal lobe epilepsy (TLE).

There is debate about the significance of subtle cortical cytoarchitectural abnormalities ('microdysgenesis') identified in the CNS of patients with PGS, i.e. seizures *not* associated with a structural lesion such as a neoplasm or encephalitis. Whereas some authors believe that regional microdysgenesis is a lesion of possible etiologic importance for the genesis of seizures (Meencke and Janz, 1984), others contend that such abnormalities are so commonly identified in neurologically normal controls that they do not have a causal role in producing PGS disorders (Lyon and Gastaut, 1985). Nevertheless, extratemporal corticectomies, lobectomies, and functional hemispherectomies performed for the treatment of chronic drug-resistant epilepsy in the second and third decades of life show a variety of less subtle structural abnormalities, including glioneuronal and vascular malformations (with or without hamartomas), lesions suggestive of pre- or perinatal brain necrosis (e.g. ulegyria, porencephaly), low-grade glial neoplasms or infectious/inflammatory disorders (Robitaille *et al.*, 1992; Wolf *et al.*, 1993b). Though these abnormalities occur or become symptomatic somewhat later in life than those associated with catastrophic infantile or pediatric seizure disorders, they clearly overlap with morphologic alterations noted in resected brain tissues from infants and younger children with intractable epilepsy, and highlight the importance of common pathophysiologic mechanisms.

TLE is commonly associated with hippocampal or Ammon's horn sclerosis (HS, see above) or neoplasms, including gangliogliomas and dysembryoplastic neuroepithelial tumors (DNET), though other types of neuropathologic change observed include metabolic diseases and phakomatoses, cortical dysplasias or NMDs, vascular malformations, and sequelae of cerebrovascular disease, trauma, or infectious/inflammatory disorders (Armstrong, 1993; Plate *et al.*, 1993; Wolf *et al.*, 1993a). Even in patients whose resected temporal lobe shows the expected lesion of HS, extrahippocampal lesions may often be present (Levesque *et al.*, 1991), emphasizing the need to precisely define the 'true epileptogenic area' before surgical treatment of TLE is undertaken. Low-grade tumors are commonly encountered in temporal lobectomy specimens from children with TLE (Adelson *et al.*, 1992).

CEREBRAL LESIONS ASSOCIATED WITH INFANTILE/PEDIATRIC EPILEPSY

Imaging and EEG diagnostic techniques have reached such a level of sophistication that the location and gross anatomy of many of the structural abnormalities to be described can be predicted prior to surgical resection (Adams *et al.*, 1992; Chapter 20). In young patients studied as part of the UCLA Pediatric Epilepsy Surgery Program the 'zone of cortical abnormality' (ZCA) putatively linked to a given seizure disorder is defined by a combination of methodologies, including MRI, EEG, and positron emission tomography (PET). Following tissue resection, it becomes the task of the neuropathologist to further define the cellular and (when possible) molecular substrates of the lesion(s). In the discussion that follows, we will describe only non-neoplastic lesions associated with infantile/pediatric epilepsy.

DESTRUCTIVE LESIONS

The developing CNS is at risk of structural damage caused by inadequate oxygenation of the fetus *in utero*, in the intrapartum, and early perinatal periods, the latter particularly if a baby is born prematurely (for reviews see Norman, 1978; Fenichel, 1983; Rorke, 1989; Guzzetta, 1991; Rorke 1992; Younkin, 1992). The lesions that result can be envisioned simplistically as infantile 'strokes', though the range of resultant infarcts and hemorrhages seen by the neuropathologist is even greater than the spectrum of 'stroke' in the adult or aging brain, possibly because the 'insult' producing a structural anomaly will produce different results depending on the developmental stage of the affected CNS. The descriptive terms applied to the involved brain reflect the heterogeneity of the lesions encountered. The best characterized (though still poorly understood) of these include germinal matrix hemorrhages, multicystic encephalopathy, periventricular leukomalacia and hydranencephaly (Rorke, 1992).

That these lesions, variable though they are, can produce epilepsy in infants and children is suggested by the experience of encountering them in cerebral cortical resection specimens from infants and children with a history of infantile spasms or West's syndrome (IS) (Vinters *et al.*, 1992; Robain and Vinters, 1994). In our initial experience with specimens from 13 such patients, destructive brain lesions were encountered in four. We have used the generic term 'cystic encephalomalacia' to describe these, though the spectrum of neuropathologic change has been broad, ranging from cortical and white matter infarcts identical in appearance to those seen in adults with large vessel occlusions, to large cysts lined by astrocytes that are confined to the white matter (Vinters, 1994). Hemosiderin at the edges of some foci of encephalomalacia reflects a hemorrhagic component. In some instances, only intense cortical astrogliosis of apparent anoxic–ischemic origin is identified (Farrell *et al.*, 1992).

Figure 5.1A illustrates an example of one of the more severely affected cases from this category, with glial cysts in the white matter and 'mushroom-like' gyri best described by the term ulegyria. Figure 5.1B, on the other hand, illustrates a destructive lesion essentially confined to the subcortical white matter; a lesion that conceivably arose by mechanisms akin to those that produce periventricular infarcts/leukomalacia in infants (Vinters, 1994). Many of the encephalomalacic lesions have been extensively calcified, reflecting the propensity of infant brain to show dystrophic calcification in areas of injury, often regardless of the inciting event. In one case, the regions of punctate calcification showed a strong resemblance to bradyzoites of *Toxoplasma gondii*, though immunohistochemical studies demonstrated an absence of toxoplasmosis in the affected tissue.

MALFORMATIVE–HAMARTOMATOUS LESIONS

These are among the more biologically intriguing anomalies observed in a surgical neuropathologic practice (Cochrane, Poskitt and Norman, 1991; Hirabayashi *et al.*, 1993). The variability of the precise nature and severity of the morphologic alterations in the CNS fails to obscure the fact that certain neuropathologic 'themes' pointing to deranged histogenesis of the neocortex recur upon review of the clinicopathologic material.

Furthermore, the cellular and molecular pathologic changes seen in some forms of neocortical malformation, best characterized by the terms cortical dysplasia (CD) or neuron(al) migration disorders (NMD), and initially described by Taylor *et al.* (1971), often bear a striking resemblance to brain lesions seen in patients with tuberous sclerosis (TS). Among cortical resections (including hemispherectomies) performed as part of the therapy of intractable childhood epilepsy at the UCLA Medical Center, malformations (with or without associated hamartomas) have been encountered as frequently as encephalomalacic lesions (Farrell *et al.*, 1992), and are especially common in infants and very young children who present with the clinical and electroencephalographic features of West's syndrome (Vinters, DeRosa and Farrell, 1993; Robain and Vinters, 1994).

Here, somewhat arbitrarily, cortical/white matter malformations have been subclassified into three main types, while accepting the fact that in a given cortical resection specimen there may be a mix of the specific neuropathologic features. These are best characterized as:

1. Polymicrogyria (Friede, 1989).
2. Heterotopic collections of neurons and individual ectopic neurons in the subcortical white matter.
3. Cortical dysplasia (with severe disorganization of the normal laminar pattern), often with associated neuronal cytomegaly and cytoskeletal disorganization and the presence of collections of 'balloon cells' resembling gemistocytic astrocytes. The latter are commonly situated in the deep cortex or the superficial subcortical white matter, though they may be present throughout the involved cerebral hemisphere.

The lesions in subcategory 3 most closely resemble those of TS. Children with hemimegalencephaly (HME) often show within the malformed cerebral hemisphere two or

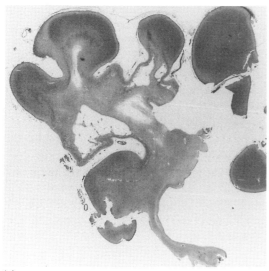

Fig. 5.1 Cystic-gliotic encephalopathy. (a) A resection specimen from a child with severe epilepsy shows multiple cysts within the subcortical white matter. Tissue destruction has resulted in some of the gyri taking on a 'mushroom-like' appearance. (Hematoxylin & eosin, × 5.) (b) Another specimen (from a different patient) shows cribriform area of cystic encephalomalacia confined to the subcortical white matter. (Stained with Kluver–Barrera. × 4.5.) ((b) Reproduced with permission fron Vinters (1994).)

(a)

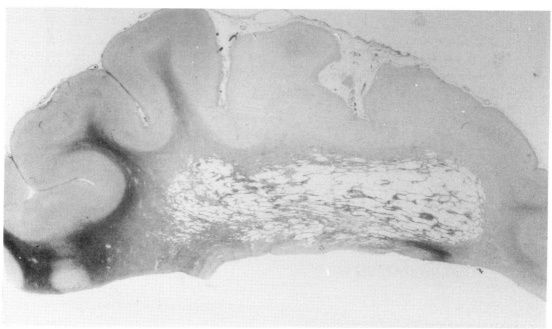

(b)

three of the different types of abnormality in various regions, as discussed in greater detail below.

Cortical malformations can often be seen on cut sections of the fixed brain, where they may be quite focal and thus most easily appreciated in contrast to the adjacent un-

involved neocortical ribbon and underlying homogeneous white matter (Farrell *et al.*, 1992). Even in a grossly normal cortical resection specimen, the presence of different patterns of CD will become readily apparent on superficial inspection of whole mount sections, especially those stained with a technique (e.g. Kluver-Barrera) that highlights differences between cortical gray matter and underlying myelinated fibers, as illustrated in Fig. 5.2.

The cellular pathology of CD can further be stratified depending on whether or not certain specific microscopic abnormalities are noted in a given specimen. In a review of over 70 examples of CD (Mischel, Nguyen and Vinters, 1995) from patients who underwent hemispherectomy or partial lobectomy, eight major histopathologic features were scored as being present or absent in each specimen. The specific light microscopic changes sought (and the relative percentage of cases in which they were found) were:

1. Cortical laminar disorganization (a defining feature of CD and hence present in all specimens).
2. Single ectopic neurons within the deep white matter or molecular layer (layer I) of cortex (94.4%).
3. Neuronal cytomegaly (63.9%).
4. Neuronal cytoskeletal abnormalities, often resembling neurofibrillary tangles found in Alzheimer's disease brain (Duong *et al.*, 1994) (55.6%).
5. Macroscopically visible neuronal heterotopias, usually in the subcortical white matter (40.3%).
6. Foci of polymicrogyria (PMG) (13.9%).
7. Neuroglial excrescences in the subarachnoid space (13.9%).
8. Balloon cell change, consisting of gemistocytic astrocyte-like cells with variable glial fibrillary acidic protein (GFAP) cytoplasmic immunoreactivity (18.1%).

Based on the presence or absence of various combinations of these histologic features, individual cases could be subclassified as being mild, moderate, or severe (Mischel, Nguyen and Vinters, 1995). Preliminary correlation of the severity of CD with clinical severity of the seizure disorder has shown that mean preoperative seizure frequency correlated well with the histologic grade, and children with moderate or severe degrees of CD were more likely to have shown a preoperative neurologic deficit. Obviously, the predictive value of this primarily morphologic grading system will need to be validated by careful prospective and quantitative analyses of the patients' clinical course in relation to neuropathologic abnormalities in the resected brain tissue.

A large and rapidly growing body of literature deals with the spectrum of CD/NMD and its role in pediatric and adult epilepsy, including the methods by which it can be visualized (e.g. using magnetic resonance imaging or CT scan techniques) (Moreland *et al.*, 1988; Marchal *et al.*, 1989; Kuzniecky *et al.*, 1991; Palmini *et al.*, 1991a,b). An understanding of the basic neurobiology that underlies the pathogenesis of CD/NMD will emerge as the mysteries of normal human brain development are unravelled using modern immunohistochemical and molecular techniques (McConnell, 1988; Rakic, 1988; Sarnat, 1991) that illuminate key events in neuronal migration from the germinal matrix to the neocortex and synaptogenesis (Becker, 1991). Even with our present level of knowledge about human brain embryogenesis and maturation, hypotheses can be formulated about when 'insults' must impact the developing brain to produce specific types of CD/NMD (Barth, 1987; Kazee *et al.*, 1991; Palmini *et al.*, 1993). In our experience, one of the key questions that will require a coherent answer is: why are manifestations of CD/NMD so often strikingly unilateral?

An example of the latter phenomenon is encountered in a subset of CD/NMD, best described as 'hemimegalencephaly' (HME). In this rare malformation (Fig. 5.3), which may be amenable to surgical treatment by hemispherectomy (King *et al.*, 1985), a malformed cerebral hemisphere shows various combinations of neuropathologic change that range from hemilissencephaly to polymicrogyria to hamartomatous malformation (Manz *et al.*, 1979; DeRosa *et al.*, 1992b; Robain

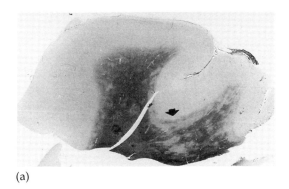

(a)

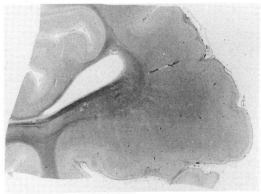

(b)

Fig. 5.2 Patterns of CD/NMD (for details, see text) from pediatric cortical resection specimens. All sections have been stained with the Kluver–Barrera technique, which highlights the cortex–white matter junction and stains deep white matter more darkly than cortex, and have been photographed at low magnification to highlight neuropathologic abnormalities. (a) Poorly demarcated cortex–white matter junction, with obvious collections of 'gray matter' within the deep white matter (e.g. indicated by arrow). (b) A more diffuse pattern of CD, with virtual absence of well-defined cortex–white matter distinction in much of the region of cortex illustrated. Note also that the gyri show an unusually thick and broad appearance. (c) Relatively well-defined cortex–white matter junction, but hyperconvoluted cortex (arrow) in one region indicative of focal polymicrogyria. ((a) × 6; (b), (c) × 5.)

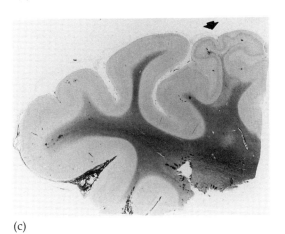

(c)

et al., 1988; Robain, Chiron and Dulac, 1989; Barkovich and Chuang, 1990). Most of the eight cellular features of CD described above are seen in variable numbers and various combinations. Morphometric data (DeRosa *et al.*, 1992b) have shown significant increases (above autopsy controls) in neuronal profile area and (sometimes) increase in neuronal cell density in HME brain.

TUBEROUS SCLEROSIS

Tuberous sclerosis (TS) is a syndrome, components of which include regions of malformed/dysplastic cerebral neocortex (tubers) with hamartomatous proliferation of neuroectodermal (undifferentiated/dedifferentiated) cells, subependymal giant cell astrocytomas, cutaneous and visceral manifestations, the latter usually hamartomas or neoplasms of the heart (rhabdomyomas) and kidneys (angiomyolipomas), though other organ systems are frequently involved (Critchley and Earl, 1932). CD/NMD often shows the cellular features of cerebral TS, i.e. disorganized cortex with enlarged neuronal cell bodies sometimes showing marked cytoskeletal and cytoplasmic abnormalities (Hirano, Tuazan and Zimmerman, 1968). The balloon cells often seen with severe CD are identical to their variably GFAP-immunoreactive counterparts in neocortical tubers of TS (Bender and Yunis, 1980). Ultrastructural and immunocytochemical features of the cells seen in

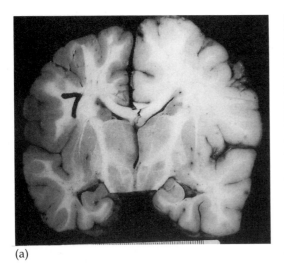
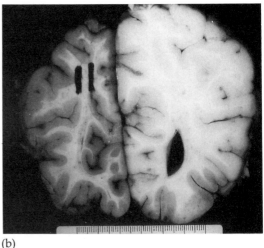

(a)   (b)

Fig. 5.3 (a), (b) Hemimegalencephaly. Autopsy specimen from a 7-month-old child with severe seizures. Note diffuse enlargement of the right cerebral hemisphere, widening of the gyri and blurring of the cortex–white matter junction throughout the affected hemisphere. Deep central gray structures are relatively well preserved.

tubers support the view that they are 'uncommitted' cells that have features of both neurons and astrocytes (Ribadeau Dumas, Poirier and Escourolle, 1973; Bender and Yunis, 1980). In this regard, they are similar to some of the cell types seen in CD cortex (from patients *without* visceral manifestations of TS) (Vinters *et al.*, 1992). Studies using markers of cellular proliferation (DeRosa *et al.*, 1992a) show that balloon cells in CD constitute a largely nonproliferating cell population.

TS may be seen in very young children and even premature infants (Thibault and Manuelidis, 1970; Probst and Ohnacker, 1977). It is inherited as an autosomal dominant condition with variable expression (Northrup *et al.*, 1993). Genetic linkage studies of the disorder suggest that more than one gene may be associated with it. Most recently, TS loci have been identified on chromosomes 9 (9q34) and 16 (16p13.3); the latter may function as a tumor suppressor gene (Harris *et al.*, 1993; Nellist *et al.*, 1993; Green, Smith and Yates, 1994). Tubers appar-

ently causing epilepsy may be removed neurosurgically, though they constitute a relatively rare type of specimen in comparison to destructive lesions and CD/NMD.

CHRONIC (RASMUSSEN TYPE) ENCEPHALITIS (Chapter 15b)

Though the clinicopathologic features of this syndrome, first recognized by Theodore Rasmussen in the late 1950s, are remarkably stereotyped, its etiology is unknown (Rasmussen, Olszewski and Lloyd-Smith, 1958; Aguilar and Rasmussen, 1960; Rasmussen, 1978). It produces seizures in young children who have, until the time of onset of the epileptic disorder, usually developed normally. The seizures may present as epilepsia partialis continua (Zupanc *et al.*, 1990), and are associated with a progressive hemiparesis reflecting neuropathologic abnormalities in one cerebral hemisphere. The pathologic change encountered when the 'epileptogenic' hemisphere is resected shows the features of a chronic, patchy and severe encephalitis,

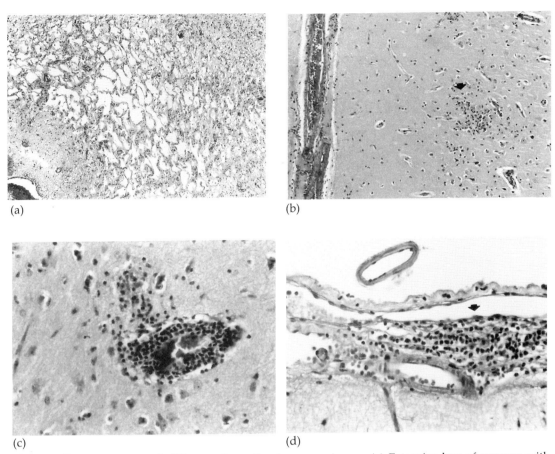

Fig. 5.4 Rasmussen encephalitis seen in corticectomy specimens. (a) Extensive loss of neurons with microcystic change but relatively minimal inflammation. (b) In contrast to (a), this shows a relatively intact cortex with a single inflammatory (microglial) nodule in mid-cortex, indicated by arrow. (c) Mononuclear inflammatory cells infiltrating the wall of a cortical microvessel, and extending into surrounding brain parenchyma. (d) A leptomeningeal venule with focal infiltration of its wall (arrow) by mononuclear inflammatory cells. (All sections, hematoxylin & eosin. (a) × 85; (b), × 225; (c), × 590; (d), × 600.)

with evidence of chronic inflammation, astrocytic gliosis, microcystic change, and a prominent microvascularity (Gray *et al.*, 1987; Piatt *et al.*, 1988; Robitaille, 1991; Gordon, 1992) (Fig. 5.4). The value of hemispherectomy (as opposed to less radical neurosurgical intervention) in the treatment of these patients has been discussed by Honavar, Janota and Polkey (1992).

Despite the neuropathologic features of RE, which strongly suggest that the causal agent is viral, no consistent data implicating a single pathogen or group of pathogens had, until recently, emerged. For instance, no viral inclusions could consistently be identified in RE brain. However, several reports over the past 5 years have implicated herpesviruses, especially cytomegalovirus (CMV) and Epstein–Barr virus (EBV), in the pathogenesis of RE (Walter *et al.*, 1989; Power *et al.*, 1990), though molecular probe studies attempting to localize these viral genes in chronic encephalitis (RE) brain tissue were not consistently positive (Farrell *et al.*, 1991). Recently, PCR methodology has been utilized to examine DNA extracted from RE tissues for genes specific to human herpesviruses (Vinters, Wang and Wiley, 1993). Low levels of CMV and EBV were detected in some RE brain tissue, but were also found less frequently in non-RE brain, e.g. from patients with CD/NMD. Evidence for (low level) infection of the brain by human herpesvirus 6 (HHV-6) was found in a single specimen. The results of the study suggest that herpesvirus infection of the CNS does not *directly* result in RE, though the possibility that it triggers an autoimmune response that is of pathogenetic importance cannot be ruled out.

STURGE–WEBER–DIMITRI SYNDROME (ENCEPHALOTRIGEMINAL ANGIOMATOSIS) (Chapter 16)

This is encountered in surgical specimens from infants/children with intractable epilepsy much less commonly than destructive and malformative/hamartomatous lesions already described at length. Clinicopathologic reports describe the association of the cerebral lesion, usually localized to the occipital cortex, with facial nevus flammeus, and provide excellent accounts of the natural history of the disorder (Venes and Linder, 1989; Oakes, 1992; Wohlwill and Yakovlev, 1957). Visceral angiomas may be encountered in some patients (Bentz *et al.*, 1982).

Neuropathologic abnormalities in cortical resection specimens are easily appreciated at low magnification (Fig. 5.5), and soft tissue radiographs of the sliced specimen may show the characteristic 'tram-track' pattern of neocortical calcification. The leptomeninges show a dense angiomatosis, characterized by some authors as a venous angioma (Wohlwill and Yakovlev, 1957). The cortex itself shows calcifications centred on microvessels (Fig. 5.5), with associated neuronal loss and astrocytic gliosis that is assumed to result from ischemic phenomena secondary (at least in part) to the meningeal angiomatosis. Ultrastructural studies of the parenchymal calcifications in Sturge–Weber brain have suggested that the earliest calcium deposits occur within perithelial cells of small blood vessels, and

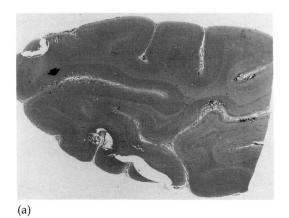

(a)

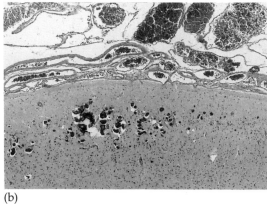

(b)

Fig. 5.5 Sturge–Weber–Dimitri syndrome. (a) Whole mount of occipital cortex from cortical resection specimen shows variable but focally prominent linear calcifications (e.g. arrow) in superficial cortical laminae. (Hematoxylin & eosin.) (b) Histologic section from the specimen shows leptomeningeal angiomatosis and concretions of calcium in the superficial cortex. (× 80.) (Reproduced with permission from Vinters (1994).)

that the underlying cause of the calcification may be anoxic injury to endothelial, perithelial, and glial mitochondria due to stasis and abnormally increased vascular permeability of vessels in the hemangioma (Guseo, 1975; Norman and Schoene, 1977).

FUTURE DIRECTIONS

The neuropathologist, especially in collaboration with his/her clinical and basic research colleagues, is in a unique position to contribute to an understanding of the morphologic substrates of basic cellular mechanisms of epilepsy (Dichter and Ayala, 1987; Dichter, 1989). While investigations into the etiology/pathogenesis of each of the subtypes of neuropathologic change encountered will require distinctive neurobiologic approaches, the tools of immunocytochemistry, pharmacology, and molecular biology can be brought to bear on a more complete understanding of how and why the structurally abnormal brain generates seizures. An even more pertinent question might be: why do seizures occur in one individual with a given type of brain lesion, but *not* in another patient with the otherwise identical abnormality? A neuropathologist who deals with lesions discovered in the course of hemispherectomy or unihemispheral cortical resections cannot help but be struck by another peculiarity of these lesions – their occurrence predominantly/exclusively on one side of the brain. The latter observation suggests a very specific insult that 'scars' one cerebral hemisphere *in utero* (in the case of CD/NMD and encephalomalacic lesions) or during development (in RE). Attempting to understand these peculiarities of 'epileptogenic' brain will be certain to yield insights into the most basic questions of human neurobiology.

ACKNOWLEDGMENTS

Work in H.V.V.'s laboratory was supported in part by US Public Health Service Grant NS 28383. Long-term collaborators in this work include Dr Michael Farrell (Dublin, Ireland), Dr Michael DeRosa (UCLA), and Dr Robin Fisher (UCLA). Outstanding technical assistance was provided by Diana Lenard Secor, Laurel Reed, Alex Brooks, and Yan Cheng. We are indebted to the clinicians involved with the UCLA Pediatric Epilepsy Surgery Program.

REFERENCES

Adams, C., Hwang, P.A., Gilday, D.L. *et al.* (1992) Comparison of SPECT, EEG, CT, MRI, and pathology in partial epilepsy. *Pediatric Neurology,* **8,** 97–103.

Adelson, P.D., Peacock, W.J., Chugani, H.T. *et al.* (1992) Temporal and extended temporal resections for the treatment of intractable seizures in early childhood. *Pediatric Neurosurgery,* **18,** 169–78.

Aguilar, M.J. and Rasmussen, T. (1960) Role of encephalitis in pathogenesis of epilepsy. *Archives of Neurology,* **2,** 663–76.

Aicardi, J. and Chevrie, J.J. (1970) Convulsive status epilepticus in infants and children: a study of 239 cases. *Epilepsia,* **11,** 187–97.

Aicardi, J. and Chevrie, J.J. (1983) Consequences of status epilepticus in infants and children. *Advances in Neurology,* **34,** 115–25.

Albala, B.J., Moshé, S.L. and Okada R. (1984) Kainic acid-induced seizures: a developmental study. *Developmental Brain Research,* **13,** 139–48.

André, M., Matisse, N. and Vert, P. (1990) Prognosis of neonatal seizures, in *Neonatal Seizures,* (eds C.G. Wasterlain and P. Vert), Raven Press, New York, pp. 61–7.

Annegers, J.F., Hauser, W.A., Shirts, S.B. and Kurland, L.T. (1987) Factors prognostic of unprovoked seizures after febrile convulsions. *New England Journal of Medicine,* **316,** 493–8.

Armstrong, D.D. (1993) The neuropathology of temporal lobe epilepsy. *Journal of Neuropathology and Experimental Neurology,* **52,** 433–43.

Babb, T.L., Kupfer, W.R., Pretorius, J.K. *et al.* (1991) Synaptic reorganization by mossy fibers in human fascia dentata. *Neuroscience,* **42,** 351–62.

Barkovich, A.J. and Chuang, S.H. (1990) Unilateral megalencephaly: correlation of MR imaging and pathologic characteristics. *American Journal of Neuroradiology,* **11,** 523–31.

Barth, P.G. (1987) Disorders of neuronal migration. *Canadian Journal of Neurological Sciences*, **14**, 1–16.

Becker, L.E. (1991) Synaptic dysgenesis. *Canadian Journal of Neurological Sciences*, **18**, 170–80.

Ben-Ari, Y. (1985) Limbic seizures and brain damage produced by kainic acid: mechanisms and relevance to human temporal lobe epilepsy. *Neuroscience*, **14**, 375–403.

Bender, B.L. and Yunis, E.J. (1980) Central nervous system pathology of tuberous sclerosis in children. *Ultrastructural Pathology*, **1**, 287–99.

Bentz, M.S., Towfighi, J., Greenwood, S. and Zaino, R. (1982) Sturge–Weber syndrome. A case with thyroid and choroid plexus hemangiomas and leptomeningeal melanosis. *Archives of Pathology and Laboratory Medicine*, **106**, 75–8.

Bouchet, C. and Cazauvielh, J.B. (1825) De l'epilepsie considerée dans ses rapports avec l'alienation mentale. *Archives of General Medicine*, **9**, 510–42.

Buterbaugh, G.G., Michelson, H.B. and Keyser, D.O. (1986) Status epilepticus facilitated by pilocarpine in amygdala-kindled rats. *Experimental Neurology*, **94**, 91–102.

Cavalheiro, E.A., Riche, D.A. and Le Gal la Salle, G. (1982) Long-term effects of intrahippocampal kainic acid injection in rats; a method for inducing spontaneous recurrent seizures. *Electroencephalography and Clinical Neurophysiology*, **53**, 581–9.

Cavalheiro, E.A., Silva, D.F., Turski, W.A. *et al.* (1987) The susceptibility of rats to pilocarpine-induced seizures is age-dependent. *Developments in Brain Research*, **37**, 43–58.

Cepeda, C., Tanaka, T., Riche, D. and Naquet, R. (1982) Limbic status epilepticus behavior and sleep alterations after intra-amygdaloid kainic acid microinjections in Papio baboons. *Electroencephalography and Clinical Neurophysiology*, **54**, 603–13.

Chevrie, J.J. and Aicardi, J. (1978) Convulsive disorder in the first year of life: neurological and mental outcome and mortality. *Epilepsia*, **19**, 67–74.

Chugani, H.T., Shewmon, D.A., Shields, W.D. *et al.* (1993) Surgery for intractable infantile spasms: neuroimaging perspectives. *Epilepsia*, **34**, 764–71.

Clancy, R.R. and Legido, A. (1991) Postnatal epilepsy after EEG-confirmed neonatal seizures. *Epilepsia*, **32**, 69–76.

Cochrane, D.D., Poskitt, K.J. and Norman, M.G. (1991) Surgical implications of cerebral dysgenesis. *Canadian Journal of Neurological Sciences*, **18**, 181–95.

Collins, R. C. and Olney, J. W. (1982) Focal cortical seizures cause distant thalamic lesions. *Science*, **218**, 177–9.

Corsellis, J.A.N. and Bruton, C.J. (1983) Neuropathology of status epilepticus in humans. *Advances in Neurology*, **34**, 129–39.

Critchley, M. and Earl, C.J.C. (1932) Tuberose sclerosis and allied conditions. *Brain*, **55**, 311–46.

Cronin, J. and Dudek, F.E. (1988) Chronic seizures and collateral sprouting of dentate mossy fibers after kainic acid treatment in rats. *Brain Research*, **474**, 181–4.

DeRosa, M.J., Farrell, M.A., Burke, M.M. *et al.* (1992a) An assessment of the proliferative potential of 'balloon cells' in focal cortical resections performed for childhood epilepsy. *Neuropathology and Applied Neurobiology*, **18**, 566–74.

DeRosa, M.J., Secor, D.L., Barsom, M. *et al.* (1992b) Neuropathologic findings in surgically treated hemimegalencephaly: immunohistochemical, morphometric, and ultrastructural study. *Acta Neuropathologica*, **84**, 250–60.

Dichter, M.A. (1989) Cellular mechanisms of epilepsy and potential new treatment strategies. *Epilepsia*, **30** (suppl. 1), S3–S12.

Dichter, M.A. and Ayala, G.F. (1987) Cellular mechanisms of epilepsy: a status report. *Science*, **237**, 157–64.

Dodrill, C.B. and Wilenski, A.J. (1990) Intellectual impairment as an outcome of status epilepticus. *Neurology*, **40** (suppl. 2), 23–7.

Duong, T., DeRosa, M.J., Poukens, V., Vinters, H.V. and Fisher, R.S. (1994) Neuronal cytoskeletal abnormalities in human cerebral cortical dysplasia. *Acta Neuropathologica*, **87**, 493–503.

Dwyer, B.E. and Wasterlain, C.G. (1984) Selective focal inhibition of brain protein synthesis during generalized bicuculline seizures in newborn marmoset monkeys. *Brain Research*, **308**, 109–21.

Dwyer, B.E. and Wasterlain, C.G. (1985) Neonatal seizures in monkeys and rabbits: brain glucose depletion in the face of normoglycemia, prevention by glucose loads. *Pediatric Research*, **19**, 992–5.

Falconer, M.A., Serafetindes, E.A. and Corsellis, J.A.N. (1964) Etiology and pathogenesis of temporal lobe epilepsy. *Archives of Neurology*, **10**, 233–48.

Farrell, M.A., Cheng, L., Cornford, M.E. *et al.*

(1991) Cytomegalovirus and Rasmussen's encephalitis. *Lancet*, **337**, 1551–2.

Farrell, M.A., DeRosa, M.J., Curran, J.G. *et al.* (1992) Neuropathologic findings in cortical resections (including hemispherectomies) performed for the treatment of intractable childhood epilepsy. *Acta Neuropathologica*, **83**, 246–59.

Fenichel, G.M. (1983) Hypoxic-ischemic encephalopathy in the newborn. *Archives of Neurology*, **40**, 261–6.

Franck, J.E. and Schwartzkroin, P.A. (1984) Immature rabbit hippocampus is damaged by systemic but not intraventricular kainic acid. *Developments in Brain Research*, **13**, 219–27.

Friede, R.L. (1989) *Developmental Neuropathology*, 2nd revised and expanded edition, Springer-Verlag, Berlin.

Fujikawa, D.G., Vannucci, R.C., Dwyer, B.E. and Wasterlain, C.G. (1988) Generalized seizures deplete brain energy reserves in normoxemic newborn monkeys. *Brain Research*, **454**, 51–9.

Fujikawa, D.G., Dwyer, B.E., Lake, R.R. and Wasterlain, C.G. (1989) Local cerebral glucose utilization during status epilepticus in newborn primates. *American Journal of Physiology*, **256** (Cell. Physiol. 25), C1160–7.

Fujiwara, T., Ishida, S., Miyakoshi, M. *et al.* (1979) Status epilepticus in childhood: a retrospective study of initial convulsive status and subsequent epilepsies. *Folia Psychiatrica Neurologica Japonica*, **33**, 337–44.

Gordon, N. (1992) Chronic progressive epilepsia partialis continua of childhood: Rasmussen syndrome. *Developmental Medicine and Child Neurology*, **34**, 182–5.

Gowers, W.R. (1881) *Epilepsy and Other Chronic Convulsive Diseases*, J.A. Churchill, London.

Gray, F., Serdaru, M., Baron, H. *et al.* (1987) Chronic localised encephalitis (Rasmussen's) in an adult with epilepsia partialis continua. *Journal of Neurology, Neurosurgery and Psychiatry*, **50**, 747–51.

Green, A.J., Smith, M. and Yates, J.R.W. (1994) Loss of heterozygosity on chromosome 16p13.3 in hamartomas from tuberous sclerosis patients. *Nature Genetics*, **6**, 193–6.

Guseo, A. (1975) Ultrastructure of calcification in Sturge–Weber disease. *Virchows Archiv. A. Pathological Anatomy and Histopathology*, **366**, 353–6.

Guzzetta, F. (1991) Ischemic and hemorrhagic cerebral lesions of the new-born. Current concepts. *Child's Nervous System*, **7**, 417–24.

Harris, R.M., Carter, N.P., Griffiths, B. *et al.* (1993) Physical mapping within the tuberous sclerosis linkage group in region 9q32–q34. *Genomics*, **15**, 265–74.

Hirabayashi, S., Binnie, C.D., Janota, I. and Polkey, C.E. (1993) Surgical treatment of epilepsy due to cortical dysplasia: clinical and EEG findings. *Journal of Neurology, Neurosurgery and Psychiatry*, **56**, 765–70.

Hirano, A., Tuazon, R. and Zimmerman, H.M. (1968) Neurofibrillary changes, granulovacuolar bodies and argentophilic globules observed in tuberous sclerosis. *Acta Neuropathologica*, **11**, 257–61.

Holmes, G.L. and Thomson, J.L. (1988) Effects of kainic acid on seizure susceptibility in the developing brain. *Developments in Brain Research*, **39**, 51–9.

Holmes, G.L., Thompson, J.L., Marchi, T. and Feldman, D.S. (1988) Behavioral effects of kainic acid administration on the immature brain. *Epilepsia*, **29**, 721–30.

Honavar, M., Janota, I. and Polkey, C.E. (1992) Rasmussen's encephalitis in surgery for epilepsy. *Developmental Medicine and Child Neurology*, **34**, 3–14.

Honchar, M.P., Olney, J.W. and Sherman, W.R. (1983) Systemic cholinergic agents induce seizures and brain damage in lithium-treated rats. *Science*, **20**, 323–5.

Kazee, A.M., Lapham, L.W., Torres, C.F. and Wang, D.D. (1991) Generalized cortical dysplasia. Clinical and pathologic aspects. *Archives of Neurology*, **48**, 850–3.

King, M., Stephenson, J.B.P., Ziervogel, M. *et al.* (1985) Hemimegalencephaly – a case for hemispherectomy? *Neuropediatrics*, **16**, 46–55.

Kuzniecky, R., Garcia, J.H., Faught, E. and Morawetz, R.B. (1991) Cortical dysplasia in temporal lobe epilepsy: magnetic resonance imaging correlations. *Annals of Neurology*, **29**, 293–8.

Legido, A., Clancy, R.R. and Berman, P.H. (1991) Neurologic outcome after electroencephalographically proven neonatal seizures. *Pediatrics*, **88**, 583–96.

Levesque, M.F., Nakasato, N., Vinters, H.V. and Babb, T.L. (1991) Surgical treatment of limbic epilepsy associated with extrahippocampal lesions: the problem of dual pathology. *Journal of Neurosurgery*, **75**, 364–70.

Lothman, E.W. and Bertram, E.H. (1993) Epileptogenic effects of status epilepticus. *Epilepsia*, **34**, S59–S70.

Lothman, E.W. and Collins, R.C. (1981) Kainic acid induced limbic seizures: metabolic, behavioral, electroencephalographic and neuropathological correlates. *Brain Research*, **218**, 299–318.

Lothman, E.W., Bertram, E.H., Kapur, J. and Stringer, J.L. (1990) Recurrent spontaneous hippocampal seizures in the rat as a chronic sequela to limbic status epilepticus. *Epilepsy Research.*, **6**, 110–8.

Lyon, G. and Gastaut, H. (1985) Considerations on the significance attributed to unusual cerebral histological findings recently described in eight patients with primary generalized epilepsy. *Epilepsia*, **26**, 365–7.

Manz, H.J., Phillips, T.M., Rowden, G. and McCullough, D.C. (1979) Unilateral megalencephaly, cerebral cortical dysplasia, neuronal hypertrophy, and heterotopia: cytomorphometric, fluorometric cytochemical, and biochemical analyses. *Acta Neuropathologica*, **45**, 97–103.

Marchal, G., Andermann, F., Tampieri, D. *et al.* (1989) Generalized cortical dysplasia manifested by diffusely thick cerebral cortex. *Archives of Neurology*, **46**, 430–4.

Margerison, J.H. and Corsellis, J.A.N. (1966) Epilepsy and the temporal lobes. *Brain*, **84**, 499–530.

Mathern, G.W., Leite, J.P., Pretorius, J.K. *et al.* (1993) Evidence for progressive hippocampal neuron loss and mossy fiber sprouting from children under 2 years of age with seizures since birth. *Epilepsia*, **34** (suppl. 6), 53 (abstr).

Mathern, G.W., Leite, J.P., Pretorius, J.K. *et al.* (1994) Severe seizures in young children are associated with hippocampal neuron losses and aberrant mossy fiber sprouting during fascia dentata postnatal development. *Epilepsy Research*, (suppl.), (in press).

Maytal, J., Shinnar, S., Moshé, S.L. and Alvarez, L.A. (1989) Low morbidity and mortality of status epilepticus in children. *Pediatrics*, **83**, 323–31.

McConnell, S.K. (1988) Development and decision-making in the mammalian cerebral cortex. *Brain Research Reviews*, **13**, 1–23.

McIntyre, D.C., Nathanson, D. and Edson, N. (1982) A new model of partial status epilepticus based on kindling. *Brain Research*, **250**, 53–63.

Meencke, H.-J. and Janz, D. (1984) Neuropathological findings in primary generalized epilepsy: a study of eight cases. *Epilepsia*, **25**, 8–21.

Meldrum, B.S. and Brierley, J.B. (1973) Prolonged epileptic seizures in primates: ischemic cell change and its relation to ictal physiological events. *Archives of Neurology*, **28**, 10–17.

Mischel, P.S., Nguyen, L.P. and Vinters, H.V. (1995) Cerebral cortical dysplasia associated with pediatric epilepsy. Review of neuropathologic features and proposal for a grading system. *Journal of Neuropathology and Experimental Neurology*, **54**, 137–53.

Moreland, D.B., Glasauer, F.E., Egnatchik, J.G. *et al.* (1988) Focal cortical dysplasia. Case report. *Journal of Neurosurgery*, **68**, 487–90.

Morin, A.M., Dwyer, B.E., Fujikawa, D.G. and Wasterlain, C.G. (1988) Low [^{3}H]-cytochalasin B binding in the cerebral cortex of newborn rat. *Journal of Neurochemistry*, **51**, 206–11.

Nadler, J.V., Perry, B.W. and Cotman, C.W. (1978) Intraventricular kainic acid preferentially destroys hippocampal pyramidal cells. *Nature*, **271**, 676–7.

Nellist, M., Brook-Carter, P.T., Connor, J.M. *et al.* (1993) Identification of markers flanking the tuberous sclerosis locus on chromosome 9 (TSC 1). *Journal of Medical Genetics*, **30**, 224–7.

Nevander, G., Ingvar, M., Auer, R. and Siesjø, B.K. (1985) Status epilepticus in well-oxygenated rats causes neuronal necrosis. *Annals of Neurology*, **19**, 281–90.

Nitecka, L., Tremblay, E., Charton, G. *et al.* (1984) Maturation of kainic acid seizure-brain damage syndrome in the rat. II. Histopathological sequelae. *Neuroscience*, **13**, 1073–94.

Norman, M.G. (1978) Perinatal brain damage. *Perspectives in Pediatric Pathology*, **4**, 41–92.

Norman, M.G. and Schoene, W.C. (1977) The ultrastructure of Sturge–Weber disease. *Acta Neuropathologica*, **37**, 199–205.

Norman, R.M. (1964) The neuropathology of status epilepticus. *Medicine, Science and the Law*, **4**, 46–51.

Northrup, H., Wheless, J.W., Bertin, T.K. and Lewis, R.A. (1993) Variability of expression in tuberous sclerosis. *Journal of Medical Genetics*, **30**, 41–3.

Nuovo, G.J., Forde, A., MacConnell, P. and Fahrenwald, R. (1993) *In situ* detection of PCR-amplified HIV-1 nucleic acids and tumor necrosis factor cDNA in cervical tissues. *American Journal of Pathology*, **143**, 40–8.

Oakes, W.J. (1992) The natural history of patients with the Sturge–Weber syndrome. *Pediatric Neurosurgery*, **18**, 287–90.

Olney, J.W., de Gubareff, T. and Labruyere, J. (1983) Seizure-related brain damage induced by cholinergic agents. *Nature (London)*, **301**, 520–2.

Olney, J.W., Rhee, V. and Ho, O.L. (1974) Kainic acid: a powerful neurotoxic analogue of glutamate. *Brain Research*, **77**, 507–12.

Palmini, A., Andermann, F., de Grissac, H. *et al.* (1993) Stages and patterns of centrifugal arrest of diffuse neuronal migration disorders. *Developmental Medicine and Child Neurology*, **35**, 331–9.

Palmini, A., Andermann, F., Olivier, A. *et al.* (1991a) Focal neuronal migration disorders and intractable partial epilepsy: results of surgical treatment. *Annals of Neurology*, **30**, 750–7.

Palmini, A., Andermann, F., Olivier, A. *et al.* (1991b) Focal neuronal migration disorders and intractable partial epilepsy: a study of 30 patients. *Annals of Neurology*, **30**, 741–9.

Penix, L.P., Thompson, K. and Wasterlain, C.G. (1994) Selective vulnerability to perforant path stimulation: role of NMDA and non-NMDA receptors. *Epilepsy Research*, (in press).

Pfleger, L. (1880) Beobachtunge uber Schrumpfung and Sklerose des Ammons–Horns bei Epilepsie. *Allg. Z. Psychiatric.*, **35**, 359–65.

Piatt, J.H. Jr, Hwang, P.A., Armstrong, D.C. *et al.* (1988) Chronic focal encephalitis (Rasmussen syndrome): six cases. *Epilepsia*, **29**, 268–79.

Pisa, M., Sanberg, P.R., Corcoran, M.E. and Fibiger, H.C. (1982) Spontaneously recurrent seizures after intracerebral injections of kainic acid in rat: a possible model of human temporal lobe epilepsy. *Brain Research*, **200**, 481–7.

Plate, K.H., Wieser, H-G., Yasargil, M.G. and Wiestler, O.D. (1993) Neuropathological findings in 224 patients with temporal lobe epilepsy. *Acta Neuropathologica*, **86**, 433–8.

Power, C., Poland, S.D., Blume, W.T. *et al.* (1990) Cytomegalovirus and Rasmussen's encephalitis. *Lancet*, **336**, 1282–4.

Probst, A. and Ohnacker, H. (1977) Sclérose tubereuse de Bourneville chez un prématuré. Ultrastructure des cellules atypiques: présence de microvillosités. *Acta Neuropathologica*, **40**, 157–61.

Rakic, P. (1988) Defects of neuronal migration and the pathogenesis of cortical malformations. *Progress in Brain Research*, **73**, 15–37.

Rasmussen, T. (1978) Further observations on the syndrome of chronic encephalitis and epilepsy. *Applied Neurophysiology*, **41**, 1–12.

Rasmussen, T., Olszewski, J. and Lloyd-Smith, D. (1958) Focal seizures due to chronic localized encephalitis. *Neurology*, **8**, 435–45.

Represa, A., Robain, O., Tremblay, E. and Ben-Ari, Y. (1989) Hippocampal plasticity in childhood epilepsy. *Neuroscience Letters*, **99**, 351–5.

Ribadeau Dumas, J.L., Poirier, J. and Escourolle, R. (1973) Ultrastructural study of cerebral lesions in tuberous sclerosis. *Acta Neuropathologica*, **25**, 259–70.

Robain, O. and Vinters, H.V. (1994) Neuropathologic studies in West syndrome, in *Infantile Spasms and West Syndrome*, (eds O. Dulac, H.T. Chugani and B. Dalla Bernardina), W.B. Saunders, London, pp. 99–117.

Robain, O., Chiron, C. and Dulac, O. (1989) Electron microscopic and Golgi study in a case of hemimegalencephaly. *Acta Neuropathologica*, **77**, 664–6.

Robain, O., Floquet, Ch., Heldt, N. and Rozenberg, F. (1988) Hemimegalencephaly: a clinicopathological study of four cases. *Neuropathology and Applied Neurobiology*, **14**, 125–35.

Robitaille, Y. (1991) Neuropathologic aspects of chronic encephalitis, in *Chronic Encephalitis and Epilepsy, Rasmussen's Syndrome*, (ed. F. Andermann), Butterworth-Heinemann, Oxford, pp. 79–110.

Robitaille, Y., Rasmussen, T., Dubeau, F. *et al.* (1992) Histopathology of nonneoplastic lesions in frontal lobe epilepsy. Review of 180 cases with recent MRI and PET correlations. *Advances in Neurology*, **57**, 499–513.

Rorke, L.B. (1989) Pathology of cerebral vascular disease in children and adolescents, in *Cerebral Vascular Disease in Children and Adolescents*, (eds M.S.B. Edwards and H. J. Hoffman), Williams & Wilkins, Baltimore, pp. 95–138.

Rorke, L.B. (1992) Anatomical features of the developing brain implicated in pathogenesis of hypoxic-ischemic injury. *Brain Pathology*, **2**, 211–21.

Sagar, H.J. and Oxbury, J.M. (1987) Hippocampal neuron loss in temporal lobe epilepsy: correlation with early childhood convulsions. *Annals of Neurology*, **22**, 334–40.

Sarnat, H.B. (1991) Cerebral dysplasias as expressions of altered maturational processes. *Canadian Journal of Neurological Sciences*, **18**, 196–204.

Scher, M.S., Painter, M.J., Bergman, I. *et al.* (1989) EEG diagnoses on neonatal seizures: clinical correlations and outcome. *Pediatric Neurology*, **5**, 17–24.

Schiottz-Christensen, E. and Bruhn, P. (1973) Intelligence, behaviour and scholastic achievement subsequent to febrile convulsions: an analysis of discordant twin-pairs. *Developmental Medicine and Child Neurology*, **15**, 565–75.

Shields, W.D., Duchowny, M.S. and Holmes, G.L. (1993) Surgically remediable syndromes of infancy and early childhood, in *Surgical Treatment of the Epilepsies*, 2nd edn, (ed. J. Engel Jr), Raven Press, New York, pp. 35–48.

Shirasaka, Y. and Wasterlain, C.G. (1994) Chronic epileptogenicity following focal status epilepticus. *Brain Research*, (in press).

Sloviter, R. S. (1983) 'Epileptic' brain damage in rats induced by sustained electrical stimulation of the perforant path. I. Acute electrophysiological light microscopic studies. *Brain Research Bulletin*, **10**, 675–97.

Sloviter, R.S. (1987) Decreased hippocampal inhibition and a selective loss of interneurons in experimental epilepsy. *Science*, **235**, 73–6.

Sloviter, R.S. (1991) Permanently altered hippocampal structure, excitability and inhibition after experimental status epilepticus in the rat: the 'dormant basket cell' hypothesis and its possible relevance to temporal lobe epilepsy. *Hippocampus*, **1**, 41–66.

Sloviter, R.S. and Dempster, D.W. (1985) 'Epileptic' brain damage is replicated qualitatively in the rat hippocampus by central injection of glutamate or aspartate but not by GABA or acetylcholine. *Brain Research Bulletin*, **15**, 39–60.

Sommer, W. (1880) Erkrankung des Ammonshornes als aetiologisches Monment der Epilepsie. *Arch. Psychiatr. Nervenkr.*, **10**, 631–75.

Sperber, E.F., Stanton, P.K., Haas, K.Z. *et al.* (1991) Resistance of the immature brain to hippocampal damage following flurothyl-induced status epilepticus. *Annals of Neurology*, **30**, 495.

Spielmeyer, W. (1927) Die Pathogenese des epileptischen Krämpfes. *Z. Ges. Neurol. Psychiatric.*, **109**, 501–20.

Strain, F.M. and Tasker, R.A.R. (1991) Hippocampal damage produced by domoic acid in mice. *Neuroscience*, **44**, 343–52.

Suga, S. and Wasterlain, C.G. (1980) Effects of neonatal seizures or anoxia on cerebellar mitotic activity in the rat. *Experimental Neurology*, **67**, 573–80.

Sutula, T., Xiao-Xian, H., Cavazos, J. and Scott, G. (1988) Synaptic reorganization in the hippocampus induced by abnormal functional activity. *Science*, **239**, 1147–50.

Tanaka, T., Kaijima, M., Yonemasa, Y. and Cepeda, C. (1985) Spontaneous secondarily generalized seizures induced by a single microinjection of kainic acid into unilateral amygdala in cats. *Electroencephalography and Clinical Neurophysiology*, **61**, 422–9.

Tauck, D.L. and Nadler, J.V. (1985) Evidence of functional mossy fiber sprouting in hippocampal formation of kainic acid-treated rats. *Journal of Neuroscience*, **5**, 1016–22.

Taylor, D.C., Falconer, M.A., Bruton, C.J. and Corsellis, J.A.N. (1971) Focal dysplasia of the cerebral cortex in epilepsy. *Journal of Neurology, Neurosurgery and Psychiatry*, **34**, 369–87.

Thibault, J.H. and Manuelidis, E.E. (1970) Tuberous sclerosis in a premature infant. Report of a case and review of the literature. *Neurology*, **20**, 139–46.

Valentino, K.L., Eberwine, J.H. and Barchas, J.D. (eds) (1987) *In situ Hybridization. Applications to Neurobiology*, Oxford University Press, Oxford.

Vannucci, R.C. and Duffy, T.E. (1975) Oxidative and energy metabolism of fetal and neonatal rats during anoxia and during recovery. *American Journal of Physiology*, **230**, 1269–75.

Venes, J.L. and Linder, S. (1989) Sturge–Weber–Dimitri syndrome. Encephalotrigeminal angiomatosis, in *Cerebral Vascular Disease in Children and Adolescents*, (eds M.S.B. Edwards and H.J. Hoffman), Williams & Wilkins, Baltimore, pp. 337–341.

Vinters, H.V. (1994) Vascular diseases, in *Pediatric Neuropathology*, (ed. S. Duckett), Williams & Wilkins, Baltimore, pp. 302–33.

Vinters, H.V., DeRosa, M.J. and Farrell, M.A. (1993) Neuropathologic study of resected cerebral tissue from patients with infantile spasms. *Epilepsia*, **34**, 772–9.

Vinters, H.V., Mah, V. and Shields, W.D. (1990) Neuropathologic correlates of pediatric epilepsy. *Journal of Epilepsy*, **3** (suppl.), 227–35.

Vinters, H.V., Wang, R. and Wiley, C.A. (1993) Herpesviruses in chronic encephalitis associated with intractable childhood epilepsy. *Human Pathology*, **24**, 871–9.

Vinters, H.V., Armstrong, D.L., Babb, T.L. *et al.* (1993) The neuropathology of human symptomatic epilepsy, in *Surgical Treatment of the Epilepsies*, 2nd edn, (ed. J. Engel Jr), Raven Press, New York, pp. 593–608.

Vinters, H.V., Fisher, R.S., Cornford, M.E. *et al.* (1992) Morphological substrates of infantile spasms: studies based on surgically resected cerebral tissue. *Child's Nervous System*, **8**, 8–17.

Walter, G.F., Renella, R.R., Hori, A. and Wirnsberger, G. (1989) Nachweis von Epstein–Barr–Viren bei Rasmussen's Enzephalitis. *Nervenarzt*, **60**, 168–70.

Wasterlain, C.G. (1976) Effects of neonatal status epilepticus on rat brain development. *Neurology*, **26**, 975–86.

Wasterlain, C.G. and Sankar, R. (1993) Excitotoxicity and the developing brain, in *Epileptogenic and Excitotoxic Mechanisms*, (eds G. Avanzini, R. Fariello, U. Heinemann and R. Mutani), John Libbey, London, pp. 131–151.

Wasterlain, C.G., Farber, D.B. and Fairchild, M.D. (1986) Synaptic mechanisms in the kindled epileptic focus: a speculative synthesis, in *Basic Mechanisms of the Epilepsies*, (eds A. V. Delgado-Escueta, A.A. Ward, D.M. Woodbury *et al.*), Raven Press, New York, pp. 411–33.

Wohlwill, F.J. and Yakovlev, P.I. (1957) Histopathology of meningo-facial angiomatosis (Sturge–Weber's disease). *Journal of Neuropathology and Experimental Neurology*, **16**, 341–64.

Wolf, H.K., Campos, M. G., Zentner, J. *et al.* (1993a) Surgical pathology of temporal lobe epilepsy: experience with 216 cases. *Journal of Neuropathology and Experimental Neurology*, **52**, 499–506.

Wolf, H.K., Zentner, J., Hufnagel, A. *et al.* (1993b) Surgical pathology of chronic epileptic seizure disorders: experience with 63 specimens from extratemporal corticectomies, lobectomies and functional hemispherectomies. *Acta Neuropathologica*, **86**, 466–72.

Wuarin, J.-P., Kim, Y.I., Cepeda, C. *et al.* (1990) Synaptic transmission in human neocortex removed for treatment of intractable epilepsy in children. *Annals of Neurology*, **28**, 503–11.

Yager, J.Y., Cheang, M. and Seshia, S.S. (1988) Status epilepticus in children. *Canadian Journal of Neurological Sciences*, **15**, 402–5.

Younkin, D.P. (1992) Hypoxic-ischemic brain injury of the newborn – statement of the problem and overview. *Brain Pathology*, **2**, 209–10.

Zupanc, M.L., Handler, E.G., Levine, R.S. *et al.* (1990) Rasmussen encephalitis: epilepsia partialis continua secondary to chronic encephalitis. *Pediatric Neurology*, **6**, 397–401.

CELLULAR MECHANISMS OF EPILEPSY PATHOGENESIS

6

John G.R. Jefferys and Roger D. Traub

DEFINITION OF EPILEPSY IN CELLULAR TERMS

What defines epileptic activity? It is not simple to provide an adequate definition, in cellular terms, that both encompasses the clearly abnormal and also excludes the normal. The reason is that synchronous firing of populations of neurons – a standard basis for defining the epileptic – is a *sine qua non* of normal brain function, from high-frequency rhythms during visual attention (Gray and Singer, 1989) to physiologic sharp waves recorded in the hippocampus of immobile rats (Buzsáki, 1986). The most extreme example of apparently normal synchronized bursting (and in some neurons even afterdischarge-like potentials) occurs in the neocortex during slow-wave sleep in the cat, where as many as 85% of neurons participate in slow waves at frequencies of 0.3 Hz and less (Steriade, Nuñez and Amzica, 1993). We propose, then, the following tentative criteria as defining an epileptic event:

1. Paroxysmal – emerging quickly out of, and returning quickly toward, relatively normal brain activity.
2. Disruptive of normal brain function.
3. Involving all or most of the neurons in a defined brain region.
4. Associated with increased firing rate in many of the neurons in the involved region.

These criteria are difficult to apply simultaneously. For example, in an *in vitro* preparation, one can determine if activity is paroxysmal, how many neurons are involved and what the firing patterns are, but it is impossible to define normal brain function. On the other hand, in an awake animal, or in a patient, disruption of brain function may be recognized, but criteria (3) and (4) are indeterminate. Furthermore, it is hard to know when normal brain function is being disrupted during sleep. Nevertheless, the criteria serve to define a class of neuronal events that can occur in the brains of human patients or of animals, events that often can be imitated, with greater or lesser faithfulness, in ***in vitro* systems**. In the *in vitro* system, experiments can be performed that define conditions under which epileptic events happen, and that clarify exactly what the cells are doing during the event itself.

We shall analyze some of the experimental epilepsies and relate their cellular mechanisms to the developing brain wherever possible. These are complex issues and will occupy the bulk of the chapter. Their application to clinical issues is starting to become apparent, and we will discuss some of these in the final sections. We shall concentrate on *in vitro* models, with the dual aims of elucidating pathophysiology and of illustrating aspects of neuroscience where basic research can contribute to solving clinical

Epilepsy in Children. Edited by Sheila Wallace. Published in 1996 by Chapman & Hall, London. ISBN 0 412 56860 8

problems. As Osler once asserted that to understand syphilis was to understand medicine, so we would claim that to understand epilepsy is to understand the brain. More anatomical aspects of pathology are found in Chapter 5, an overview of brain development is given in Chapter 4a, and aspects of pathology of epilepsy of particular relevance to surgery are reviewed in Chapter 23d. Cellular mechanisms are particularly important with reference to status epilepticus (Chapter 18) and febrile seizures (Chapter 10); and, to the development and efficacy of drugs for epilepsy (Chapters 22 and 23a).

REVIEW OF ELECTROPHYSIOLOGY PERTINENT TO EPILEPTOGENESIS

No understanding of epilepsy is possible without consideration of the respective roles of intrinsic cell properties and of synaptic circuitry. We shall review some of these matters for two brain regions, the hippocampal CA3 region (Fig. 6.1) and the complex of intrinsic thalamic nuclei and nucleus reticularis thalami (NRT). Of all cortical regions, the organization of connections between pyramidal neurons is best understood in CA3; at the same time, the principles that apply in CA3 appear to apply, at least in a general way, to other cortical regions. Hippocampal and other cortical regions together, of course, are involved in the majority of seizures, so that the properties of their principle neurons are of special relevance. The thalamic/NRT complex is likely to be critical in the generation of the so-called corticoreticular epilepsies, including absence seizures.

SINGLE NEURON PHYSIOLOGY

Pyramidal cells

What does it mean to understand (better yet, to have a quantitative model of) a neuron? One must at least know the time course of

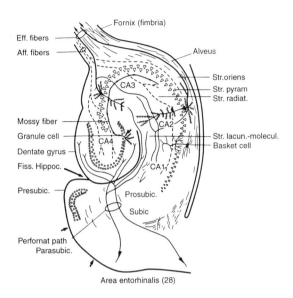

Fig. 6.1 Schematic illustration of some of the synaptic interconnections within the hippocampus, along with some of the afferent and efferent pathways. Recurrent excitatory connections between CA3 pyramidal neurons are not shown. (Reproduced with permission of Oxford University Press from Brodal (1981).)

synaptic inputs to which a neuron is exposed and how it transposes those inputs into axonal output – this at the minimum. In addition (but of uncertain significance for epilepsy), cells may produce 'outputs' not necessarily reflected in axonal output; examples include dendritic transmitter release, and transient intradendritic accumulations of Ca^{2+} ions (Callaway, Ross and Lasser-Ross, 1992). One usually begins with a phenomenologic description of the neuron obtained from its response to current injections into the soma and, if possible, the dendrites. In the case of CA3 hippocampal pyramidal neurons, the cell responds to injection of small depolarizing currents into the soma with **intrinsic bursts**, repeated rhythmically at higher frequency the stronger the current, a pattern that occurs at frequencies up to about 3 Hz *in vitro*. The intrinsic burst (so called

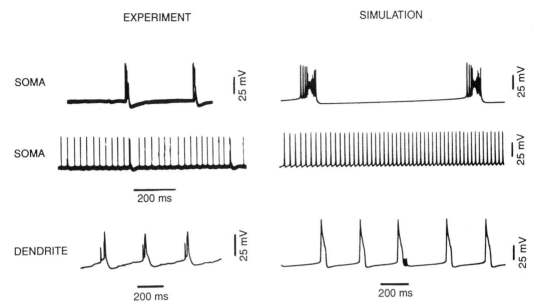

EXPERIMENT   SIMULATION

SOMA

SOMA

200 ms

DENDRITE

200 ms   200 ms

Fig. 6.2 Firing patterns in CA3 pyramidal neurons depend on the site, as well as the strength, of the stimulation. Somatic stimulation with steady depolarizing currents produces first rhythmic intrinsic bursts (top traces), then (as the soma become more depolarized) rhythmic single-action potentials. Currents passed into the apical dendrites can evoke fast and slow action potentials, the latter presumably Ca-mediated (bottom traces). Experiments are from guinea-pig neurons *in vitro* (Wong and Prince (1981) for somatic stimuli, R. Miles (unpublished data) for dendritic stimulation – see also Traub, Miles and Jefferys, 1993). Simulations use a cell model described in Traub *et al.* 1991. (Reproduced with permission of IOP Publishing from Traub *et al.*, 1992.)

because it can be generated by the cell without synaptic inputs) consists of a series of three or more action potentials riding on a depolarizing envelope, often succeeded by one or more broadened action potentials (Fig. 6.2). The intrinsic burst is followed by a long (hundreds of milliseconds to seconds) after-hyperpolarization (AHP). Intrinsic bursts have been recorded intracellularly *in vivo* (Kandel, Spencer and Brinley, 1961) in anesthetized animals, and their extracellular correlates are regularly detectable with wire electrodes in unanesthetized animals, particularly during immobility (Ranck, 1973). As CA3 pyramidal cells are depolarized further, at the cell body, their firing behavior evolves, first to spike doublets and brief bursts, then to rhythmic single action potentials (Wong and Prince, 1981) (Fig. 6.2). The transition from slower

bursting to faster single action potentials is also observed at some sites in apical dendrites (R. Miles, R.D. Traub and J.G.R. Jefferys, unpublished data), but other sites in the apical dendrites produce a quite different behavior in response to rather large injected currents (over 1 nA) – broad, presumably Ca-mediated action potentials, at frequencies of 5 to about 8 Hz, a type of electrogenesis thought to be critical in the shaping of epileptic afterdischarges (Traub, Miles and Jefferys, 1993) (Fig. 6.2).

Intrinsic bursts in other cell types

CA1 pyramidal cells rarely respond to somatic stimulation with a burst, but dendritic stimulation, by injected current, often evokes a localized burst (Wong, Prince and Basbaum, 1979; Masukawa and Prince, 1984; Wong and

Stewart, 1992). The differentiation of cell response in CA1 neurons, by stimulus localization, may possibly be explained in part by the narrower apical dendritic shaft of these cells compared with CA3 cells (Lorente de Nó, 1934; R.D. Traub, J.G.R, Jefferys and R. Miles, unpublished data). A significant minority of neocortical pyramidal cells, particularly in the deeper cortical layers, generate intrinisic bursts in response to somatic current injections (Agmon and Connors, 1989). Data are beginning to accumulate on the dendritic responses of neocortical cells (Amitai *et al.*, 1993). In many of these cases, the classification of cells as 'intrinsic bursting' or 'repetitively firing' may not be absolute; for example, the tendency of a cell to burst can be modified by extracellular K concentration (M.A. Whittington and J.G.R. Jefferys, unpublished data). Likewise, dendritic inhibition can, if properly timed, prevent a burst or alter its form (R. Miles, R.D. Traub and J.G.R. Jefferys, unpublished data; Wong, Prince and Basbaum, 1979).

In order to make sense of the cellular response to current injection (and to be able to predict the responses to synaptic inputs), one must consider the properties of the intrinsic membrane conductances, and the way the conductances are distributed over different portions of the cell membrane (soma, proximal dendrites, distal dendrites, etc.). As some of the currents are gated by internal Ca ions, as well as transmembrane potential, the factors regulating the control of intracellular Ca, on a millisecond time scale, are also critical (Miyakawa *et al.*, 1992). (Intracellular Ca concentrations are altered in interrelated ways by transmembrane flux and release of intracellular stores under the control of both $[Ca^{2+}]_i$ itself and second messengers gated by metabotropic glutamate receptors, a complex subject not reviewed here (MacDermott and Miles, 1991).) We may conveniently divide the intrinsic conductances in pyramidal neurons (and probably most neurons) into four groups. Conduct-ances are conventionally denoted by 'g', a measure of the ease of ion flux through specific channels in the neuronal membrane. Thus, we have:

1. Action potential-generating, g_{Na} and $g_{K(DR)}$ (DR stands for delayed rectifier). It is likely (but not proven) that these conductances are co-localized in the membrane.

2. Calcium spike-generating, g_{Ca} (in mature pyramidal cells, predominantly high-voltage-activated, of several different subtypes; in thalamocortical relay neurons and some other cell types, low-threshold 'T' channels), and Ca-gated K currents, $g_{K(C)}$ and $g_{K(AHP)}$, where the relatively fast C-conductance is both voltage- and Ca-gated. Again, it would seem likely that Ca and Ca-gated conductances should co-localize.

3. Other K conductances, including the rapid transient A-conductance, (Numann, Wadman and Wong, 1987), the muscarinically regulated M-conductance (Halliwell and Adams, 1982), and the slow transient D-conductance (Storm, 1988).

4. Other inward conductances, including the hyperpolarization-activated H-conductance (Maccaferri *et al.*, 1993), the Ca-activated cation conductance (Caeser *et al.*, 1993), and, at least in some neurons, a persistent Na conductance.

Conductances in **axons** differ from the soma-dendritic membrane in certain ways. First, the fast action-potential-generating g_{Na} in axons probably is a different channel type than on the soma (Westenbroek, Merrick and Catterall, 1989), with density also thought to be higher than on the soma. Second, unmyelinated axons are believed to possess significant g_K that repolarizes the action potential, whereas the node of Ranvier in myelinated axons appears to lack g_K, with action potential repolarization taking place by Na inactivation and a large leak conductance (Kocsis, Malenka and Waxman, 1980; Kocsis and Waxman, 1980). Immature peripheral axons generate bursts in the presence of 4-aminopyridine (4AP) (Kocsis, Ruiz and Waxman, 1983), suggesting the localization there of still other conductances. The electrical properties of axons are not idle curiosities but have specific relevance to epilepsy: the way in which neurons communicate with each other determines in part what sort of population activities can be supported. For example, $[K^+]_o$ increases during seizures, and this can either enhance axonal conduction or block it, depending on concentration and axonal properties. In addition, the anticonvulsants phenytoin and carbamazepine appear to work via an action on Na channels (Willow, Gonoi and Catterall, 1985). As these experiments are typically done on somatic Na channels, it is of interest to know if the drugs exert similar effects on central axonal Na channels. Finally, cortical epileptogenic foci are associated with 'back-firing' of axons, the spontaneous generation of ectopic action potentials in the axon or presynaptic terminals (Gutnick and Prince, 1972; Stasheff, Mott and Wilson, 1993). Ectopic axonal action potentials also occur in the presence of the K-channel blocker 4AP (Flores-Hernández *et al.*, 1993). In both of these cases, axons contribute to the spread of excitability.

The **dendrites** of pyramidal neurons (also Purkinje neurons and perhaps all central neurons) likewise have distinctive properties *vis-à-vis* the soma. Here the difference is not, so far as is known, in channel properties so much as in channel densities. Specifically, Ca-mediated action potentials tend to be larger in the dendrites than at the soma, while the reverse is true for Na-mediated action potentials (Wong, Prince and Basbaum, 1979; Llinás and Sugimori, 1980a, 1980b; Masukawa and Prince, 1984; Amitai *et al.*, 1993). The distribution of membrane conductances has two profound consequences:

1. The very large active dendritic conductances influence synaptic integration and provide interesting and novel ways for dendritic inhibition to combine with excitation (Midtgaard, 1992; Callaway, Ross and Lasser-Ross, 1992; Traub *et al.*, 1994).

2. The interactions between dendritic and somatic conductances shape the patterns of cellular response to excitatory inputs, from single intrinsic bursts to the trains of bursts seen during epileptic afterdischarges. In particular, the spatial distribution of the conductances, along with knowledge of channel kinetic properties, allows one to explain the differential responses of the cell to current injections at different sites (Wong and Prince, 1981; Traub *et al.*, 1991; Traub, Miles and Jefferys, 1993) (see also below).

Developmental aspects

Immature and dedifferentiated pyramidal cells appear to have somewhat different membrane properties from those in mature cells, differences that may be of significance for epileptogenesis. We give three examples. First, very immature cells do not generate full action potentials (Johansson, Friedman and Århem, 1992). Second, individual neurons in microcultures can develop large and prolonged depolarizations independent of synaptic input and of Ca conductances, and so presumably possess a large noninactivating Na conductance (Segal, 1993). Finally, immature CA3 pyramidal cells exhibit a much larger current through low-threshold 'T' Ca channels than do mature cells (Thompson and Wong, 1991). It is possible, therefore, but not proven, that many of the details of epileptic afterdischarge generation in the immature brain are different from those in the adult.

Inhibitory interneurons (i.e. GABAergic cells)

These are vital to any understanding of epileptogenesis or of normal brain function: selective loss of interneuron subpopulations or of their innervation (Sloviter, 1987, 1991), and time-dependent (Wong and Watkins, 1982) or neuromodulator-induced (Madison and Nicoll, 1988) decreases in inhibition are likely to be critical to the generation of certain seizure types. In addition, GABA may serve (paradoxically) as an excitatory neurotransmitter and possibly as a growth factor in the developing brain (Cherubini, Gaiarsa and Ben-Ari, 1991). The classification of interneurons is an active research area, and no straightforward 'taxonomy' is yet available. The reason is that the correlations between various observed properties of interneurons (e.g. are all parvalbumin-containing cells excited by recurrent axons?) are not always known. The classification is, however, important not only for understanding function but because selective subpopulations of interneurons (somatostatin-containing) appear to be lost after experimental electrically induced seizures (Sloviter, 1987); the circuitry patterns both of the disappearing and of the remaining interneurons might help to explain this pattern. In the hippocampus, some of the properties relevant to a classification of interneurons are these:

1. Location of the cell body (stratum oriens, pyramidale, etc.) (Knowles and Schwartz-kroin, 1981; Lacaille *et al.*, 1987)
2. Major postsynaptic sites on pyramidal cells: basilar and/or proximal or distal apical dendrites, somata, axon initial segment (Gulyás *et al.*, 1993).
3. Postsynaptic actions: $GABA_A$ or $GABA_B$ receptors (Segal, 1990) or, possibly, both (M. M. Segal, personal communication).
4. Peptide staining, possibly representing co-released substances (e.g. somatostatin, cholecystokinin (CCK), neuropeptide Y, etc.) (Sloviter and Nilaver, 1987).
5. Presynaptic cells whose axons impinge on the interneuron (local or distant principal neurons, septal neurons, other interneurons, etc.) and synaptic receptors used

(AMPA, NMDA, ACh, serotonin, GABA, etc.) (e.g. Freund and Antal, 1988).
6. Ca-binding proteins, including parvalbumin and calbindin (Katsumaru *et al.*, 1988; Sloviter *et al.*, 1991).
7. Dendritic branching pattern (Schlander and Frotscher, 1986).
8. Dendritic gap junctions (Kosaka, 1983).
9. Intrinsic membrane properties, with many interneurons exhibiting nonadapting trains of narrow action potentials, but some showing adaptation, intrinsic bursts, or subthreshold oscillations (Schwartzkroin and Mathers, 1978; Kawaguchi and Hama, 1987; Miles, 1990a; Fraser and MacVicar, 1991).

Thalamus

We now consider some of the principle neurons of the **diencephalon**, the excitatory thalamocortical relay cells (TCR cells) of the intrinsic thalamic nuclei, and the GABAergic neurons of the nucleus reticularis thalami (NRT) and homologous ventral lateral geniculate nucleus. These neurons are not only fascinating in their own right, but their properties are clearly relevant to EEG patterns (such as sleep spindles) and probably to the generation of absence seizures (Steriade and Deschênes, 1984; Steriade and Llinás, 1988). As is the case for CA3 pyramidal cells, the firing properties of the individual diencephalic cells are strongly dependent on the membrane potential, although the ionic mechanisms underlying this dependence are not the same as in CA3. Again, TCR and NRT cells fire repetitive single spikes when relatively depolarized (Deschênes *et al.*, 1984; Jahnsen and Llinás 1984a, 1984b; Avanzini *et al.*, 1989), a firing mode relevant to information transfer through the thalamus in the waking state. A variety of oscillatory patterns occur at more hyperpolarized potentials, including slow rhythmic bursts and spindles (up to about 10 Hz) that may be interspersed with silent intervals. Spindles and delta frequency oscillations are related to collective oscillations in these structures (and in the cortex) during sleep when diencephalic neurons are relatively hyperpolarized, probably because of modulatory inputs from brainstem and/or basal forebrain (Steriade and Llinás, 1988; McCormick, 1992). The critical ionic mechanism in both sets of neurons is the low threshold 'T' channel that inactivates when the membrane is relatively depolarized (hence the tonic firing only in this potential range), but whose inactivation can be removed when the cell is held hyperpolarized long enough (hence the ability of properly timed inhibitory inputs to allow the cells to oscillate). TCR cells possess another interesting conductance, called the H (for hyperpolarization) conductance, that is activated by hyperpolarization and that helps to drive T channels toward threshold (Huguenard and McCormick, 1992; McCormick and Huguenard, 1992). Oscillations in NRT cells depend in large part on the interaction between T channels and a Ca-gated K current (Avanzini *et al.*, 1989; Bal and McCormick, 1993). The ability of diencephalic cells to oscillate collectively and **synchronously** (a requirement for their ability to drive spindles and probably also absence seizures) depends on the synaptic interactions between these neurons: excitatory from TCR to NRT, and inhibitory between NRT cells and from NRT to TCR. NRT-to-TCR connections probably involve both $GABA_A$ and $GABA_B$ receptors (Thomson, 1988). There are, of course, also connections to and from the cortex, but these latter may not be critical to the oscillations, as the oscillations can – in certain preparations – occur in slices lacking cortex (von Krosigk, Bal and McCormick, 1993). Collective oscillations probably arise from the interaction between:

1. Synchronized inhibitory postsynaptic potentials (IPSPs) that are relatively long-lasting (80 ms to several hundred ms), and
2. The T-channel-induced rebound bursting

properties of TCR and NRT neurons (Jahnsen and Llinás, 1984b; von Krosigk, Bal and McCormick, 1993; Destexhe, McCormick and Sejnowski, 1993; Wang, 1993).

SYNAPTIC INTERACTIONS IN THE HIPPOCAMPUS

Synapses allow groups of connected neurons to perform useful computational work. Under special conditions – epilepsy – they also allow groups of neurons to express abnormal synchronized oscillations or other collective phenomena that we call seizures. Synaptic receptors are targets for certain convulsant drugs (e.g. picrotoxin), as well as anticonvulsant drugs, both used (barbiturates) and contemplated (NMDA blockers).

Synaptic transmission

Receptors for bioactive transmitters and modulators (small amino acids, amines, purines, peptides) are found on diverse parts of neuronal membranes: presynaptic terminals, axon initial segments, cell bodies and dendrites. A given molecule (such as glutamate) may interact with different receptor types having significantly different actions. Receptors for the same molecule may be co-localized (Bekkers and Stevens, 1989) or not. In some cases ('ionotropic' receptors), the receptor and a selective membrane channel form a single large molecular complex, so that receptor binding causes a rapid-onset, rapidly declining specific ionic current (e.g. $GABA_A$). In other cases, receptor binding is coupled to membrane ionic fluxes through biochemical steps inside the membrane of the postsynaptic cell, so-called second messengers (e.g. $GABA_B$ receptors are coupled to a particular K conductance). An alternative action is for the second messenger to be coupled not to (or not **just** to) a special channel but rather to a membrane channel that is also gated by membrane potential and/or intracellular Ca concentration (e.g. acetylcholine and norepinephrine both reduce the conductance of Ca-gated AHP channels). Finally, ligand binding may be coupled, through second messengers, to Ca release from intracellular stores (e.g. the metabotropic glutamate receptor). As a result of ligand-gated ionic currents and channel conductance alterations, electric properties of the cell are temporarily modified: cells may then fire more or fewer action potentials, dendrites may or may not generate Ca spikes, presynaptic terminals release more or less transmitter. (Cholinergic, opiate, muscarinic, $GABA_B$, and adenosine receptors all, among others, regulate transmitter release in the brain – Pitler and Alger, 1992b; Scanziani *et al.*, 1992, 1993.) Because the behaviour of neuronal membranes is so highly nonlinear, the effect of one packet of transmitter generally cannot be predicted without knowing the state of the membrane, i.e. how activated or inactivated the voltage-gated conductances are, as well as the actions of other simultaneously present transmitters.

Why are there so many different transmitters and transmitter actions (any and all of which are of possible significance for epileptogenesis)? The transmitter diversity allows neurons to influence each other in a variety of ways (turning on or off this or that conductance), on a wide spectrum of time scales (milliseconds to minutes). (Interestingly, action-potential Na conductances seem not to be so regulated.) It is likely that single neurons can affect different postsynaptic target cells in different ways (Traub and Miles, 1991; Thomson, Deuchars and West, 1993; Thomson and West, 1993). Transmitter release properties themselves can be regulated, and postsynaptic receptor properties are time dependent (by virtue of desensitization, modification by phosphorylation and intracellular Ca, etc. (Numann and Wong, 1984; Chen *et al.*, 1990)). Thus, there exists an interlocking knot of nonlinear controls that it seems hopeless to disentangle quantitatively. Nevertheless, by concentrating on seizure phenomena *in vitro*, that occur on time scales of only a few hundred milliseconds and seem to involve only four transmitter

actions in a critical way, we can present an intelligible (if still incomplete) story. For *in vitro* epileptogenesis, the most critical receptor types are, for glutamate, the AMPA/kainate and NMDA receptors (named for experimentally used agonist compounds – AMPA is α-amino-3-hydroxy-5-methyl-4-isoxazole propionic acid, NMDA is *N*-methyl-D-aspartic acid). For GABA, they are the so-called A and B receptors. Each receptor 'type' is itself diverse, a result of the fact that ligand receptors, like many macromolecules, are constructed by assembling together pieces, and each piece can exist in different molecular forms, providing Nature the opportunity to express various 'flavors' of receptor at different stages of development, or in response to yet undefined biological needs. (Analogies with hemoglobin spring to mind.) We summarize a few of the relevant details:

1. AMPA/kainate glutamate receptors provide for EPSCs (excitatory postsynaptic currents) of rapid onset and decay (both within a few milliseconds). The conductance is independent of membrane potential over most of the physiologic range. Various subtypes of these receptors are rectifying (i.e. pass current solely in one direction) or not, at depolarized potentials. The rectifying channels are more likely to be Ca-permeable and to be found on interneurons (Audinat *et al.*, 1993). The AMPA receptors desensitize quickly (Trussel and Fischbach, 1989) while kainate receptors do not; unfortunately, there are no specific blockers to distinguish the subtypes, although blockers of the general AMPA/kainate class exist. The EPSPs on interneurons are larger and faster than on pyramidal cells (Miles, 1990a), but it is not known if this reflects receptor pharmacology or other postsynaptic membrane properties. The AMPA/kainate receptors are probably the main means by which principal neurons in the cortex communicate with one another (Collingridge Herron

and Lester, 1988) and with interneurons (Miles, 1990a).

2. NMDA glutamate receptors have many interesting properties. The underlying conductance is of slower onset than for the AMPA receptor (perhaps 5–8 ms compared with 1 or 2 ms (Hestrin *et al.*, 1990)), and the conductance decays much more slowly, with a time constant of about 100 ms. NMDA receptors possess unique forms of regulation that occur on rapid time scales and are of immediate physiologic relevance: the channel conductance is regulated by transmembrane potential (being greater at depolarized potentials), and this regulation is itself modified by Mg ions (the higher the external Mg concentration, the lower the conductance at any membrane potential); this is the basis of one epilepsy model, to be discussed. The channel is also regulated at distinct sites by drugs (e.g. ketamine), polyamines, and protein kinase C. A site on the NMDA receptor called the glycine-binding site, that is strychnine-insensitive, actually binds to a number of small amino acids (including serine and alanine) in a way that appears to control receptor desensitization, a process that is typically incomplete and that proceeds over several hundreds of milliseconds (Clark, Clifford and Zorumski, 1990; Vyklicky, Benveniste and Mayer, 1990). NMDA receptors also exist in different molecular subtypes. NMDA-mediated currents have a faster decay on interneurons than on pyramidal cells (Perouansky and Yaari, 1993). NMDA receptors are involved in long-term potentiation, in development of the brain, and in several, but not all, experimental epilepsies. Some fraction of the ionic flux through these channels is carried by Ca, and it is thought that this Ca acts as a second messenger in the mediation of the long-term effects of receptor activation. As synaptic NMDA receptors (at least in pyramidal neurons) are generally on dendritic spines, and as Ca in spines can be sequestrated (Guthrie, Segal and Kater, 1991; Müller and Connor, 1991), it is possible that NMDA conductances and voltage-gated Ca conductances (on dendritic shafts) could have distinct second-messenger actions. There are some data to suggest that NMDA regulation by divalent cations, including Ca and Mg, is different in earlier stages of development than later, with relative Mg insensitivity in the immature brain (Brady, Smith and Swann, 1991; Kleckner and Dingledine, 1991), but some of this has been called into question (Bregestovski *et al.*, 1993). NMDA receptors are also believed to contribute to normal information processing.

3. $GABA_A$ receptors exert at least two ionotropic actions: a Cl^- flux of rapid onset and decay that shunts the membrane and is therefore inhibitory – whether this flux is hyperpolarizing, depolarizing, or nonpolarizing depends on the cell type and experimental conditions (i.e. the cell's resting potential compared with the Cl reversal potential); and a depolarizing action that is dendritic and shunting/inhibitory in pyramidal cells but which may be (at least under special circumstances) **excitatory** in interneurons (Michelson and Wong, 1991). The depolarizing action of GABA is most significant in the apical dendrites and is especially prominent in the presence of 4AP, a drug believed to enhance transmitter release; thus, it is possible that these receptors are extrasynaptic. Hyperpolarizing $GABA_A$ responses also occur in the dendrites, where their kinetics have a slower time course than on the cell body (Pearce, 1993), a fact that may be relevant to the proposed role of this dendritic inhibition in suppressing Ca spikes (Traub *et al.*, 1994). $GABA_A$ conductances are regulated – generally **decreased** – by a bewildering variety of physiologic factors (reviewed in Thompson, 1994), including extracellular

$[K^+]_o$ increases (Thompson and Gähwiler, 1989), receptor desensitization (Numann and Wong, 1984), decreased transmitter release (due to presynaptic $GABA_B$ receptors (Thompson and Gähwiler, 1992), as well as **post**synaptic Ca increases (Pitler and Alger, 1992a), and postsynaptic receptor modifications (Chen *et al.*, 1990). These properties are almost certainly relevant to the ability of strong repetitive stimulation to induce seizures. $GABA_A$-mediated IPSPs are the fundamental means by which extreme synchronization of firing is prevented (see below), and presumably are used by the brain for computational purposes. These receptors (both hyperpolarizing and depolarizing) can be blocked with drugs (penicillin, picrotoxin, bicuculline), with the depolarizing response being more sensitive (Wong and Watkins, 1982). The net conductance is enhanced and/or prolonged by various benzodiazepines and barbiturates, presumably the basis of their anticonvulsant action. Interestingly, early in development, $GABA_A$-mediated responses are generally depolarizing, even to the point of allowing synchronous bursting of neurons (Ben-Ari *et al.*, 1989), an effect that may be relevant to brain development.

4. $GABA_B$ receptors produce IPSPs that are of slower onset and decay than $GABA_A$ receptors (Otis, De Koninck and Mody, 1993; Thalmann, 1984). The conductance is mediated by K channels rather than Cl channels, the K channels being activated via a second messenger (a so-called G protein). Because of the channel type, these IPSPs are more hyperpolarizing than $GABA_A$ IPSPs, as a rule; they are also predominantly dendritic (Newberry and Nicoll, 1984). The threshold for activating these IPSPs by orthodromic stimuli tends to be higher than for $GABA_A$ IPSPs; the reason for this is not known – it may reflect distinctive properties of the respective presynaptic neurons, or a requirement for prolonged GABA release before $GABA_B$ IPSPs can develop. $GABA_B$ IPSPs have a clear 'braking' role in limiting the duration of afterdischarges, at least in low Mg epileptogenesis (J.G.R. Jefferys and M.A. Whittington, unpublished data). The role of this form of inhibition in normal physiologic states is less clear.

Synaptic connectivity

Receptor pharmacology is necessary but not sufficient for the complete analysis of seizures. Another important domain is connectivity (Traub and Miles, 1991). Connectivity has several aspects:

1. For each neuron, **how many** cells does it contact, and of what types (pyramidal, interneuron etc.).
2. How are the postsynaptic cells distributed in space, i.e. what is the **axonal branching pattern**.
3. **Where** on the postsynaptic cells are contacts made, and, for each pair of connected cells, how many synaptic transmitter release sites are there?

These parameters determine, in part, what influence one cell has on others, as they affect which intrinsic conductances will be engaged, along with the probability of transmitter release failures. In order to make these considerations more concrete, we shall review data from the hippocampal CA3 region of the guinea-pig and rat, a brain area both intensively studied and readily expressing epileptic afterdischarges.

1. **CA3 pyramidal cell → CA3 pyramidal cell**. The axonal length from a single neuron along the long axis of the hippocampus is at least 4 mm (Tamamaki, Watanabe and Nojyo, 1984); consistent with this, compound excitatory postsynaptic potentials (EPSPs) can be recorded *in vitro* in longitudinal slices up to 5 mm away from a stimulus (Miles, Traub and Wong, 1988). It is estimated that a single

CA3 pyramidal cell axon has up to 1785 release sites in a 400 μm thick slice (Ishizuka, Weber and Amaral, 1990) and 60,000 sites *in vivo* (Li *et al.*, 1993). While most of these release sites are in CA1, it is likely that hundreds of release sites are in the CA3 region of a slice and many thousands in the CA3 region in the whole animal. Unfortunately, the number of release sites per connected pair of cells is not yet known, but quantal analysis (Traub and Miles, 1991) and anatomical data on CA3 $\rightarrow$ CA1 connections (Sorra and Harris, 1993) suggest that this number may be small, perhaps less than five. Physiologic evidence using dual intra-cellular recordings indicates a connection probability of a few percent (Miles and Wong, 1986, 1987a; Traub and Miles, 1991), which would be a lower bound on the true connectivity. Interestingly, in the CA3 region of immature animals, the connectivity is significantly higher than for mature animals (Swann, Smith and Brady, 1991). Such high connectivity could explain both the ease of initiation of seizures in slices from immature animals and their long duration. Collaterals of CA3 axons appear to contact both basilar and apical dendrites, in patterns that depend on the subregion of the presynaptic cell (Ishizuka, Weber and Amaral, 1990; Li *et al.*, 1993). In longitudinal slices, the connectivity declines with distance from the presynaptic neuron (Miles, Traub and Wong, 1988), but it is not known if this is true *in vivo*. Based on indirect evidence, both AMPA and NMDA receptors exist at recurrent CA3 synapses (Traub, Jefferys and Whittington, 1994). Both in the CA3 region, and indeed in all cortical regions, the recurrent excitatory connections are probably **the most critical element** for epileptogenesis.

2. **CA3 pyramidal cell $\rightarrow$ CA3 interneuron (stratum pyramidale)**. This connection is remarkable both for its physiologic properties and for the fact that it involves only one release site, 80–250 μm from the soma (Gulyás *et al.*, 1993). The variation of connection probability with distance is not known. Pharmacologic data indicate that AMPA/kainate receptors are used at this synapse (Miles, 1990a), and indirect evidence also suggests the presence of NMDA receptors (Traub, Jefferys and Whittington, 1994).

3. **CA3 interneuron (stratum pyramidale) $\rightarrow$ CA3 pyramidal cell**. The axon of inter-neurons is more restricted (500–1700 μm in slices) than for pyramidal cells, but within the arborization of a single inter-neuron contacts appear to be made with a large fraction of the pyramidal cells there residing (Gulyás *et al.*, 1993); the number of release sites per connection is estimated to be five to nine. Depending on the interneuron, contacts might be made selectively onto initial segment, soma and proximal dendrites, or more distal dend-rites (Gulyás *et al.*, 1993). Apparently, the lability of synaptic inhibition in the brain does not result from a small number of release sites, but rather from other factors. The relative spreads of excitatory and inhibitory axons determine, in part, the pattern of the 'inhibitory surround' about a focal interictal spike (Traub, Jefferys and Miles, 1993).

Synaptic function in the hippocampus

Now that we have considered briefly the chemistry of synapses (receptors, transmit-ters) and the 'wiring diagram', it is necessary to examine functional aspects. What effect does a single action potential (or a burst) in one neuron have on the electrical behavior of connected neurons? Such **unitary synaptic** effects will be critical in understanding the initiation of epileptic discharges from the firing of small numbers of neurons under special circumstances. In contrast, during an epileptic discharge, many cells are firing at high rates; one must therefore consider the synaptic effects of the simultaneous firing of many presynaptic neurons. These effects may introduce new properties not apparent from unitary synaptic interactions, effects including receptor saturation and desensitization. Extrapolation from unitary interactions to the population are further complicated by the following:

1. As the dendritic membranes of pyramidal neurons contain active conductances, and many possible sites of action potential initiation, there is no simple relation between unitary EPSP size and the number of EPSPs necessary to induce firing.

2. Repetitive presynaptic firing, especially of many neurons simultaneously, increases the probability of transmitter release failures and probably of conduction failures in axons. The simultaneous firing of many neurons is also expected to lead to receptor saturation (because of the finite number of postsynaptic receptors) and receptor desensitization, although these effects are hard to demonstrate by direct experiment.

In spite of these complexities, the data on unitary synaptic interactions in CA3 have led to some important insights. Some pertinent facts are these:

1. **Pyramidal cell → pyramidal cell** (Miles and Wong, 1986, 1987a; Traub and Miles, 1991). The unitary EPSP is about 1 mV at the soma. Release failures occur, suggesting a relatively small number of release sites. The EPSP peak is slow, at 5–12 ms after the presynaptic action potential, probably a result of the passive dendritic membrane properties. It is rare for a single presynaptic action potential to induce a postsynaptic action potential (except in slices from immature animals (Swann, Smith and Brady, 1991)).

2. **Pyramidal cell → interneuron** (Miles, 1990a; Traub and Miles, 1991). The unitary EPSP is larger (2 mV not being unusual) and of faster rise time than for pyramidal neurons. Transmission failures occur, consistent with the small number of release sites (only one in examples so far studied (Gulyás *et al.*, 1993)). The peak of the EPSP is within 3 or 4 ms and an action potential often occurs after a single presynaptic action potential. Given that the synapse is in the dendrites, this rapid signal transduction suggests that interneuron dendrites might also be electrically excitable.

3. **Interneuron (stratum pyramidale, GABA$_A$) → pyramidal cell.** Typical IPSP amplitudes are 1 or 2 mV, but there is an approximately eight-fold range in amplitudes, depending on the interneuron (Miles, 1990b). The latency is only a few milliseconds (Miles and Wong, 1984). Transmission failures are rare.

4. **Disynaptic inhibition (pyramidal cell → interneuron → pyramidal cell)** (Miles and Wong, 1984, 1987a). The latencies are such, and the pyramidal cell → interneuron synapse powerful enough, that disynaptic inhibition develops **faster** than the unitary EPSP peaks. Multiple disynaptic inhibitory paths also exist between pyramidal cells (Miles and Wong, 1987a), a consequence in part of the rich density of the interneuron axonal arborization. For this reason, recurrent inhibition is well designed to limit the development of synchronized firing. Feed-forward inhibition in the hippocampus also develops **faster** than does excitation from afferents, at least for the dentate → CA3 pathway (Miles and Wong, 1987a), a fact that likely helps to limit the spread of synchronized firing from one region to another (Mesher and Schwartzkroin, 1980).

5. **Pyramidal cell → pyramidal cell when the presynaptic cell bursts** (Miles and Wong, 1986, 1987a; Traub and Miles, 1991). In this case, there is some probability (about 0.3) that the postsynaptic cell also bursts, with a latency in the tens of milliseconds.

Several mechanisms contribute to this burst-propagation property that is most important for the initiation of synchrony. First, the first few EPSPs potentiate, before synaptic depression sets in (Miles and Wong, 1987a). Dendritic Ca conductances may provide further amplification, but this is uncertain. Modeling studies suggest that the CA3 pyramidal burst is initiated when the dendritic depolarization induces a somatic/initial segment action potential that then propagates in a retrograde manner into the dendrites leading to a depolarizing afterpotential (from g_{Ca}), and a second or third action potential. Eventually, a full dendritic Ca spike occurs in the dendrites, if the latter are not inhibited (Wong and Prince, 1981; Traub *et al.*, 1991, 1994). In summary, early amplification of synaptic excitation is provided by presynaptic factors (facilitation) and postsynaptic membrane properties (depolarizing afterpotentials, dendritic Ca spikes). Later **attenuation** is also provided presynaptically (synaptic depression – see also Thomson and West, 1993) and postsynaptically (the AHP). There are few data on the effects of pyramidal cell bursts on interneurons, but based on data from the neocortex, synaptic facilitation seems possible (Thomson, Deuchars and West, 1993).

Generality of ideas of synaptic interrelationships in other cortical regions

There is a rich network of excitatory local axon collateralization throughout the cortex, with most synaptic excitation on pyramidal cells coming from other pyramidal cells. The quantitative details of synaptic transmission seem different than in CA3 (Mason, Nicoll and Stratford, 1991; Thomson and West, 1993), and we are not aware of the demonstration of spread of repetitive firing from single neuron to single neuron. Our hypothesis, based on the similarity of afterdischarge patterns in different cortical regions, is that

synaptic inputs to pyramidal neurons are quite similar, throughout the cortex, when a large enough number of nearby neurons are firing; but that the detailed neuronal computations may be very different in normal states when far fewer cells are simultaneously firing. Further experiments will prove or disprove this idea.

Some developmental aspects of synaptic transmission

Unitary CA3 EPSPs are significantly larger in immature animals, with 3 mV EPSPs possible (Smith, Turner and Swann, 1988), an effect likely to be synergistic with the high connectivity in increasing seizure susceptibility. As mentioned above, GABA$_A$ potentials are depolarizing in sufficiently young animals (e.g. the 6-day-old rabbit – Mueller, Taube and Schwartzkroin, 1984); there are also differences with respect to this property in CA3 vs. CA1, so that in the 6-day-old rat CA3 GABA-mediated potentials are hyperpolarizing, but CA1 GABA-mediated potentials are depolarizing (Swann, Brady and Martin, 1989).

EXPERIMENTAL EPILEPSIES

EXPERIMENTAL EPILEPSIES IN THE HIPPOCAMPUS *IN VITRO*

We shall discuss several different experimental epilepsies that can be induced (most readily, at least) in the CA3 region *in vitro*. As these different experimental models involve distinctive underlying synaptic mechanisms (Table 6.1), it is possible that their similarity in electrical pattern implies a common underlying mechanism for *in vivo* (including human) limbic seizures. We shall consider **initiation** (how does the synchronized discharge grow out of the background activity) and **shaping** (why does a sustained discharge take the form of a synchronized population oscillation, typically at about 5–15 Hz). In addition, we must analyze temporal aspects

Table 6.1 Summary of some epilepsy mechanisms in cortical local circuits

	Epilepsy paradigm		
	GABA$_A$ blockade	**Low Mg**	**4AP**
GABA$_A$ (synaptic inhibition)	Blocked	Reduced	Probably increased
AMPA/kainate (fast synaptic excitation)	Required for synchrony	Not essential	Required for synchrony and later bursts
NMDA (slow synaptic excitation)	Required for later bursts	Required for any synchrony	Not required
Intrinsic properties	—	↑ Excitability	↑ Excitability
	High K	**Tetanic stimulation**	**Low Ca**
GABA$_A$ (synaptic inhibition)	Reduced	Reduced	Reduced or blocked
AMPA/kainate (fast synaptic excitation)	Required	Not tested	Reduced or blocked
NMDA (slow synaptic excitation)	Not required for synchrony (later bursts may be similar to 0 Ca)	Not required	Reduced or blocked
Intrinsic	↑ Excitability	↑ Excitability	↑ Excitability

References: Haas and Jefferys, 1984; Taylor and Dudek, 1984; Miles and Wong, 1987a; Chamberlin, Traub and Dingledine, 1990; Roper, Obenaus and Dudek, 1993; Stasheff, Mott and Wilson, 1993; Traub, Miles and Jefferys, 1993; Traub and Jefferys, 1994; Traub, Jefferys and Whittington, 1994; Whittington, Traub and Jefferys, 1995.

(how the form of the discharge is shaped in a local neuronal population) and spatial aspects (how the discharge propagates). The data do not allow a complete analysis of all these aspects for all the experimental epilepsies; the data are most complete for the case of GABA$_A$ blockade.

In all of the experimental epilepsies to be considered in this section, two basic types of event are seen:

1. In the first type of event, most or all of the neurons fire a single **synchronized burst** (Fig. 6.3), followed by a long AHP. By an abuse of terminology we sometimes refer to such events as **interictal spikes**, considering them to be analogous to the *in vivo* naturally occurring epileptiform events. Single synchronized bursts *in vitro* often occur spontaneously and repeatedly, with interburst intervals depending on the experimental model: sometimes hundreds of ms in 4AP, typically a few seconds in GABA$_A$ blockade, possibly minutes in low Mg.

2. The second type of event is a so-called **afterdischarge** (Fig. 6.4), actually a series of synchronized population bursts, the initial burst typically longer than the succeeding bursts, with interburst intervals from about 50 ms to hundreds of milliseconds (depending on the experimental model), and the whole event lasting from a few hundred milliseconds to over a minute. Afterdischarges may themselves repeat spontaneously, again with intervals depending on the model, shorter in 4AP, longer in low Mg, with the interval for GABA$_A$ blockade in between.

Table 6.1 lists some means by which the underlying synaptic mechanisms of the different experimental epilepsies can be distinguished. Note in particular, that GABA$_A$ inhibition is only slightly decreased (by 5–30 %) in low Mg (Whittington, Traub and

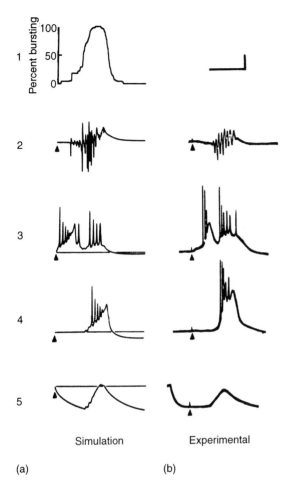

Fig. 6.3 (a), (b) Synchronization of pyramidal cell firing by recurrent excitatory synapses. The simulation was of a 100-cell network, randomly interconnected, with connections powerful enough that a burst in one cell would evoke bursts in postsynaptic cells. The experimental records are from the CA2 region of a guinea-pig hippocampal slice bathed in penicillin to block GABA$_A$ receptors. (a) Rapid build up of firing in the model after stimulating four cells. Row 2: field potentials. Note the long latency after the shock (triangle) to peak of the response. Row 3 (intracellular): initially firing cells may be re-excited to a second burst. Row 4: typical cells are silent and then exhibit a long-latency burst. Row 5: hyperpolarization of the cells reveals a large underlying EPSP. Calibrations: 50 ms (simulation), 60 ms (experiment), 4 mV (A2, B2), 25 mV (A3, A4, A5), 20 mV (B3, B4, B5). (Reproduced with permission of AAAS from Traub and Wong (1982).)

Jefferys, 1995) and is thought to be **increased** in 4AP. Hence, disinhibition is not the *sine qua non* in these experimental models. Nor is the NMDA receptor: during GABA$_A$ blockade, single synchronized bursts occur during NMDA blockade, but not the complete afterdischarge; in low Mg, no synchronized activity occurs in NMDA blockade; but in 4AP, NMDA blockade has little effect, and afterdischarges can still be recorded (Traub, Jefferys and Whittington, 1994; Traub, Colling and Jefferys, 1995).

Initiation

In all of the experimental models in Table 6.1 (except low Ca), we believe that events are initiated by spread of firing along local excitatory collaterals, as simultaneous blockade of both AMPA/kainate receptors and NMDA receptors uniformly prevents synchronous firing (Lee and Hablitz, 1989; Traub, Miles and Jefferys, 1993; Traub, Jefferys and Whittington, 1994; B. Strowbridge, personal communication). Experimentally, events can be triggered during disinhibition (Miles and Wong, 1983) or in low Mg (Neuman, Cherubini and Ben-Ari, 1989) by stimulating a single neuron. Such a phenomenon can be viewed as a chain reaction. A chain reaction is able to occur when an event (burst) in one cell can induce a corresponding event in more than one other cell, with the next generation proceeding likewise. Certainly, the synaptic divergence is high enough (each CA3 neuron contacting at least 20 others within 200 μm *in vitro*) for this to happen, and bursting can then propagate from neuron to neuron. Even if burst propagation occurs with probability only 0.3, the **expected** number of bursting followers per neuron is at least 6. Normally, inhibition would quickly shut this process off, but not in the presence of GABA$_A$ blockers. The spread of bursting from neuron to neuron takes tens of milliseconds; let us say that 20 ms is typical. The number of generations of

EXPERIMENT   SIMULATION

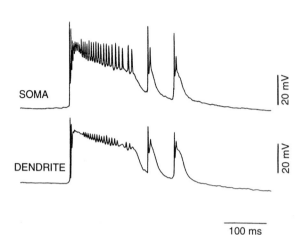
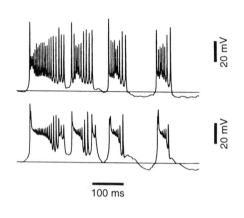

Fig. 6.4 Synchronized after-discharges during blockade of GABA$_A$ inhibitory synapses. The experimental recordings are from presumed pyramidal cells in the CA3 region of a transverse guinea-pig hippocampal slice, bathed in 50 μM picrotoxin. The somatic and dendritic recordings were from different cells. The simulation was performed in a model of 100 19-compartment neurons, each receiving excitatory synaptic input from 20 other randomly chosen neurons. At each excitatory synapse, both AMPA and NMDA types of glutamate receptors were simulated. (Reproduced with permission of the Physiological Society from Traub, Miles and Jefferys (1993).)

spread from 1 neuron to 1000 neurons is at most n, where $6^n = 1000$, so that n = $3/\log_{10}(6) = 3.86$, corresponding to about 80 ms. This is a very reasonable figure experimentally. A model based on the chain reaction concept (Fig. 6.3) (Traub and Wong, 1982) could account for the time lag from small stimulus to the epileptiform field potential, the occasional finding of cells that burst early, and the large EPSP coincident with the epileptiform event (Johnston and Brown, 1981). Note that GABA$_B$ IPSPs peak slowly and probably have onset still further delayed by the relatively high threshold for their activation (Thalmann, 1984). Hence, during disinhibition the synchronization process can 'outrun' the slow inhibition (Traub and Miles, 1991).

When GABA$_A$ inhibition is present, synchrony could, in principle, nevertheless proceed provided recurrent excitation were sufficiently enhanced. We believe that this is

the way initiation proceeds in others of this class of experimental epilepsies (low Mg, 4AP, high K, etc.) In low Mg, the enhancement of recurrent excitation occurs via the increased conductance of NMDA receptors believed to be present at recurrent excitatory synapses (Ascher, Bregestovski and Nowak, 1988; Jahr and Stevens, 1990; Traub, Jefferys and Whittington, 1994). Based on analogy with the electroplax organ and the squid giant synapse (Llinás, Walton and Bohr, 1976; Muller, 1986), as well as data from mammalian axons (Kocsis, Ruiz and Waxman, 1983), there are at least two (not mutually exclusive) mechanisms by which 4AP could increase the gain of recurrent excitation:

1. Prolongation of transmitter release from the presynaptic terminal, thereby increasing the peak conductance and the duration of postsynaptic events.

2. Ectopic action potentials (Traub, Colling and Jefferys, 1995; see also Gutnick and Prince, 1972), either as spontaneous events, or converting single orthodromic action potentials into axonal bursts.

The proposed mechanism of synchronization – enhanced recurrent excitation when inhibition remains present – involves certain complexities that only experiments can resolve: conditions that increase synaptic 'gain' between pyramidal cells are expected to recruit more powerfully inhibitory neurons. Inhibitory neurons appear to possess glutamate receptors (AMPA/kainate, NMDA, and metabotropic) (Miles, 1990a; Sah, Hestrin and Nicoll, 1990; Miles and Poncer, 1993; Traub, Jefferys and Whittington, 1994), as do pyramidal cells, although certain differences do exist:

1. Repetitive stimulation has different effects on interneurons than on pyramidal cells (Thomson, Deuchars and West, 1993; Thomson and West, 1993).
2. The mean open time of interneuron NMDA receptors is shorter than for pyramidal cells (Perouansky and Yaari, 1993).

Net population effects will then depend on how many parameters in the system are tuned, something that cannot be predicted *a priori* (Traub, Jefferys and Whittington, 1994). Interneurons also do not behave uniformly: in the $GABA_A$ blocker penicillin, some interneurons fire in prolonged bursts far outlasting pyramidal cell firing, while others fire in a brief burst succeeded by a deep AHP (Domann, Dorn and Witte, 1991).

Shaping of the afterdischarge

This issue is easiest to understand in the case of afterdischarges induced by $GABA_A$ blockade (Fig. 6.4). There are, we believe, two critically relevant experiments. First, passage of a large depolarizing current via an electrode into the apical dendrites of CA3

pyramidal cells can evoke rhythmic bursts, with underlying events that appear to be Ca spikes. Second, NMDA blockers abolish the later bursts in the afterdischarge but not the initial burst. A detailed simulation model of CA3 circuitry is able to account for the available experiments (Traub, Miles and Jefferys, 1993). It predicts that once synchronized firing is underway, NMDA receptors on the pyramidal cells are powerfully excited, driving the intrinsic dendritic oscillators. This produces the afterdischarge in the separate neurons; synchrony is maintained because the neurons remain coupled together by short-acting AMPA receptors (a detail which is, however, hard to confirm by direct experiment).

The data on low Mg epilepsy are consistent with a similar model, provided recurrent inhibition is not too powerful (Traub, Jefferys and Whittington, 1994). Here, NMDA blockade is not available as an experimental test (as NMDA blockade abolishes all synchronized firing in low Mg), but other manipulations are consistent, including the prolongation of the afterdischarge by L-alanine, a compound believed to reduce desensitization of the NMDA receptor (Benveniste *et al.*, 1990). One hypothesis, consistent with known 4AP actions, that would explain the 4AP-induced afterdischarge, is this: sufficiently prolonged glutamate release could cause the non-desensitizing kainate receptors to behave functionally like NMDA receptors, i.e. to stay open for tens or hundreds of milliseconds; of course, such kainate receptors would lack the voltage dependence of the NMDA receptor, but that may not be critical. This idea would explain why NMDA blockade has so little effect on 4AP epileptogenesis (Avoli *et al.*, 1993; H. Michelson and R.K.S. Wong, personal communication; B. Strowbridge, personal communication). Thus, NMDA receptors may not be essential in all cortical epilepsies. This issue has potential clinical consequence as NMDA blockers have been considered as anticonvulsant drugs. NMDA receptors are also not required during electrically induced seizures in the isolated guinea-pig brain (Federico and MacVicar, 1993).

In summary, the basic mechanisms in experimental afterdischarges are

1. Recurrent excitatory synaptic connections, a feature of the entire cortex.
2. The ability of pyramidal neuron dendrites to generate, by intrinsic mechanisms, repetitive bursts, something demonstrated directly for CA3 pyramidal neurons (Traub, Miles and Jefferys, 1993) and some cortical pyramidal cells (Amitai *et al.*, 1993), and plausible for pyramidal cells in general.
3. Prolonged activation of the recurrent synapses so as to recruit the intrinsic oscillation, either through NMDA receptors, sustained glutamate release, or perhaps via some other means.

Spatial aspects of epileptic events *in vitro*

The spread of epileptic activity (Table 6.2) is obviously of great clinical relevance, and some of the underlying physiologic mechanisms are amenable to analysis *in vitro*. The details of spatial aspects can be rather complicated even in slices, at least for certain parts of the brain, including the pyriform cortex and underlying endopyriform nucleus (Hoffman and Haberly, 1991), or the neocortex, in which jumps in propagation followed by retrograde movement occur (Chervin, Pierce

and Connors, 1988). We shall confine our discussion, therefore, to the longitudinal CA3 slice, which contains a uniform population of neurons, at least approximately.

The simplest epileptic phenomenon with spatial aspects is the so-called inhibitory surround, originally described in the penicillin focus *in vivo* (Prince, 1968; Dichter and Spencer, 1969). In this case, inhibition (GABA$_A$) is blocked locally, allowing synchronous bursting or afterdischarges to occur in the region of blockade. Cells immediately adjacent to the focus exhibit sequences of IPSPs followed by firing, then followed by hyperpolarization; while cells several millimetres away exhibit large IPSPs with admixed EPSPs, but generally no action potentials. We have been able to account for this behavior with the known axonal anatomy and synaptic properties in the CA3 region: the long-ranging pyramidal axons excite not only other pyramidal cells outside the focus, but also interneurons. As the pyramidal → interneuron synapses are so powerful, the interneurons are recruited and generate IPSPs in nearby cells before the pyramidal cells can be excited to burst (Traub, Jefferys and Miles, 1993).

We have discussed above a hypothesis for the generation of the temporal pattern of an afterdischarge in a local population of neurons. A stringent test of this hypothesis is to account for some of the observed properties of afterdischarge propagation in the longit-

Table 6.2 How might seizure activity spread?

Mechanism	Expected velocity	Comments
Along local axon collaterals with synaptic integration	0.1–0.3 m/s *in vitro*, faster *in vivo*	Tissue invaded at or near epileptogenic threshold
Wave of $\uparrow [K^+]_0$	0.001–0.01 m/s	?Jacksonian march (at 0.005 m/s: 10 s to spread 5 cm)
Repetitive activity causing disinhibition and other effects in normal tissue	Perhaps several s per synaptic relay (but repetitive activity also elevates $[K^+]_0$)	? 2^0 generalization of focal seizure

References: Haas and Jefferys, 1984; Konnerth, Heinemann and Yaari, 1984; Knowles, Traub and Strowbridge, 1987; Jensen and Yaari, 1988; Miles and Wong, 1987a; Traynelis and Dingledine, 1988; Traub, Jefferys and Miles, 1993.

udinal slice, a preparation about 1 cm long and containing an estimated 10 000–20 000 pyramidal neurons. In this preparation, both the initial burst and the later bursts propagate (usually about 0.1–0.2 m/s) from a stimulus along the slice, at a velocity significantly slower than the axon conduction velocity, about 0.5 m/s (Miles, Traub and Wong, 1988). The propagation velocity can be explained by the fact that *in vitro* axonal connections are relatively localized, so that continuous synaptic integration must take place. Of great interest is the observation that both in transverse slices (Knowles, Traub and Strowbridge, 1987) and in longitudinal slices, there can be a **preferred direction** for the secondary bursts: the initial burst always propagates away from a shock, but the secondary bursts propagate in a certain fixed direction independent of the site of the shock. We have found that this behavior is replicated when there is an inhomogeneity in some synaptic property (e.g. NMDA conductance, AMPA conductance, connection density) (Traub, Jefferys and Miles, 1993); we suspect that connection density gradients are the true explanation (Li *et al.*, 1993), but this remains an open question. The model also predicted correctly that NMDA blockade would slow afterdischarge propagation in the slice. The clinical relevance of these facts are not clear, depending as they do on the *in vitro* nature of the preparation, but the facts remain important as they increase confidence in the model of afterdischarge generation, and the model is important for suggesting new experiments and perhaps therapeutic approaches.

Another experimental system with important spatial aspects is the electrically evoked limbic seizure, either *in vivo* (Stringer and Lothman, 1992), in the isolated guinea-pig brain (Pare, de Curtis and Llinás, 1992), or in entorhinal/hippocampal combined slices (Rafiq, DeLorenzo and Coulter, 1993); intracellular recording is possible in the latter two cases. Repetitive stimulation in, say, the entorhinal cortex evokes population spikes, with appropriate phase lags, in the dentate gyrus, CA3, CA1, and subiculum. Eventually, sustained afterdischarges occur, at frequencies of 4–10 Hz in the isolated brain, corresponding, it is believed, to failure of inhibition in the dentate/hilar region. This gives the appearance of re-entrant cyclic activity, but it is not yet proven experimentally that cyclic activation around the limbic loop is indeed crucial for the afterdischarge to occur in the whole brain (M. de Curtis, personal communication); it is conceivable that local increases in $[K^+]_o$, loss of $GABA_A$-mediated inhibition, etc. lead to afterdischarges locally, with propagation around the loop taking place simply because the synaptic connections are there. Such a notion would be consistent with the known ability of repetitive electrical stimulation to induce afterdischarges in the CA3 region *in vitro* in the absence of a limbic loop (Stasheff, Bragdon and Wilson, 1985; Miles and Wong, 1987b). On the other hand, Rafiq, DeLorenzo and Coulter (1993), working *in vitro*, showed that cutting mossy fibers prevented their delayed afterdischarges; this observation indicates that re-entrant activity could indeed be critical. These are extremely pertinent questions with respect to epilepsy surgery, specifically temporal lobectomy for intractable partial complex seizures of medial temporal origin: if 're-entrant' seizures actually can occur in humans, then the notion of a 'seizure focus' becomes ill defined, just as an ectopic focus is not defined in certain cardiac tachyarrhythmias (e.g. Wolff–Parkinson–White syndrome). The conventional idea of seizure focus (that is, first produce temporally sustained afterdischarges in a local region, then allow the afterdischarge to propagate in space) would be more analogous to an ectopic ventricular focus in the heart. Further experiments in the isolated brain preparation may shed light on these issues.

EXPERIMENTAL EPILEPSIES ASSOCIATED WITH SPIKE-WAVE OR 2–4 HZ OSCILLATIONS

Data on experimental preparations that may be relevant to certain human epileptic syndromes, including typical and atypical absence, are considered briefly. Some of the data come from *in vivo* experimental models; there are also exciting *in vitro* data that build on earlier studies of the electrophysiology of TCR and NRT cells. Two types of *in vivo* model can be discussed: generalized penicillin epilepsy (Fisher and Prince, 1977a, 1977b; reviewed in Gloor and Fariello, 1988) in which penicillin is administered parenterally or diffusely over the cortex at low concentrations, in normal cats (i.e. cats without known genetic epileptic tendencies), and inherited absence-like syndromes in rodents, including GAERS (Genetic Absence Epilepsy Rats from Strasbourg, Vergnes *et al.*, 1982) and the stargazer mouse (Qiao and Noebels, 1993). In both model types, a diffuse cortical spike-wave-like EEG occurs, generally at frequencies higher than in human absence, along with behavioral arrest, staring, and possible facial myoclonus. In generalized penicillin epilepsy, Gloor and colleagues (Pellegrini and Gloor, 1979; Gloor, Quesney and Zumstein, 1977; Gloor, Pellegrini and Kostopoulos, 1979; Musgrave and Gloor, 1980; Avoli and Gloor, 1981, 1982) found that:

1. An intact thalamus is necessary to initiate a run of spike-wave.
2. Injection of penicillin into the thalamus is not sufficient.
3. Diffuse application of penicillin to the cortex, along with physiologic synaptic inputs from the thalamus, is sufficient for spike-wave to occur. Penicillin application to isolated cortex produces a different type of epileptiform activity that does not resemble spike-wave (Prince and Tseng, 1993).

In the GAERS model, the nucleus reticularis thalami is required for expression of the spike-wave (Avanzini *et al.*, 1993). While we are not aware of data on a specific cortical abnormality in GAERS, it has been shown that the low-threshold Ca conductance of NRT neurons is increased in these animals (H.-C. Pape and M. de Curtis, personal communication).

In *in vitro* studies, a slice preparation has been developed that expresses spindle-like oscillations: the ferret dorsal and ventral lateral geniculate slice (ventral lateral geniculate is homologous to NRT) (von Krosigk, Bal and McCormick, 1993). Both dorsal and ventral lateral geniculate components are required. Interestingly, $GABA_A$ blockade in this preparation transforms the higher frequency spindle population oscillation to a lower frequency 2–4 Hz oscillation, in which more spikes per population burst occur than in the spindle. Further addition of a $GABA_B$ blocker suppresses all oscillatory activity, presumably because now the ventral lateral geniculate cells are uncoupled both from each other and from dorsal lateral geniculate cells (von Krosigk, Bal and McCormick, 1993). It is known furthermore that in hippocampal slices, partial blockade of $GABA_A$-mediated inhibition causes population oscillations at about 2 Hz (Schneiderman, 1987).

Taken together, these data suggest that some degree of $GABA_A$ blockade can allow both diencephalic and cortical structures to oscillate at 2–4 Hz *in vitro*, perhaps faster *in vivo* (Table 6.3). When interconnected, these structures perhaps can resonate diffusely. In contrast, *in vitro* afterdischarges, at least under conditions of normal NMDA efficacy, normal $[K^+]_o$, and so on, require rather complete blockade of $GABA_A$ inhibition for their expression.

FIELD BURSTS

Hippocampal structures, including CA1, CA3, and the dentate, are able to express a remarkable type of epileptic activity *in vitro*

Table 6.3 Comparison of *in vitro* hippocampal afterdischarges and diencephalic 3 Hz oscillations

	Hippocampal AD	*Diencephalic 3 Hz*
Cellular oscillator	High-threshold g_{Ca}, $I_{K(C)}$	Low-threshold g_{Ca}, H-current, $I_{K(AHP)}$ (NRT)
Membrane potential in which cellular oscillations occur	Depolarized (dendrites)	Hyperpolarized
GABA$_A$ block	Enhances	Enhances
GABA$_B$ block	Further enhances	Appears to block
Critical synaptic interactions	Excitatory between pyramidal cells	Excitatory TCR→NRT Inhibitory NRT→NRT, NRT→TCR

H-current = hyperpolarization-activated cation current; TCR = thalamocortical relay; NRT = nucleus reticularis thalami
References: Traub, Miles and Jefferys, 1993; van Krosigk, Bal and McCormick, 1993.

under conditions where synaptic transmission appears to be completely blocked, as in media lacking Ca ions (Haas and Jefferys, 1984; Taylor and Dudek, 1984). These events, called field bursts, can also occur, with similar morphology, in certain conditions, such as elevated $[K^+]_o$, in which some degree of synaptic transmission may be preserved (Traynelis and Dingledine, 1988; Jensen and Yaari, 1988). A field burst may last several seconds or longer. It is associated with a DC field shift, negative in stratum pyramidale, with high-frequency firing of action potentials. In most cases, the firing is tightly time-locked between different cells, so that trains of large (several mV) population spikes occur; the population spikes need not always occur, however (Konnerth, Heinemann and Yaari, 1984). The occurrence of field bursts is favored by ionic changes that increase cellular excitability (high extracellular K concentration, low extracellular Ca concentration), as well as by hypo-osmolarity of the medium, with cell swelling and increased extracellular resistivity (Traynelis and Dingledine, 1989; Dudek, Obenaus and Tasker, 1990). The field burst is a true collective phenomenon that paroxysmally involves thousands of neurons and that itself can propagate through the tissue at rather low velocity (0.001–0.01 m/ms Haas and Jefferys, 1984) (see also Table 6.2). When large population spikes are seen, the synchronization mechanism is believed to involve current flow through the extracellular medium, so-called 'field effects' (Haas and Jefferys, 1984; Taylor and Dudek, 1984; Traub *et al.*, 1985).

The clinical correlates of field bursts are unclear, but they could underlie:

1. Seizures induced by hypo-osmolar states or hypocalcemia.
2. The tonic phase of generalized tonic-clonic convulsions.
3. The electrodecremental response sometimes recorded during infantile spasms (see below).

Significant changes in extracellular ion concentrations occur in the course of seizures in the photosensitive baboon *Papio papio*, and it has been argued that field bursts might occur in those animals (Pumain *et al.*, 1985).

IMPLICATIONS OF CELLULAR WORK FOR HUMAN EPILEPSY

The interictal spike

The synchronized burst *in vitro* is almost certainly an analog of isolated EEG spikes. Intracellular potentials during *in vivo* interictal spikes are quite similar to those *in vitro*, with the difference that in epilepsy models other than disinhibition, some neurons can be found in the 'spike focus' that hyperpolarize during the EEG paroxysmal wave (Goldensohn and Purpura, 1963). Unit recordings in humans also indicate a high probability of increased firing rate in temporal correlation with the EEG wave (Wyler, Ojemann and Ward, 1982). The cellular mechanisms for generating synchronized bursts in neocortical, entorhinal and olfactory cortical slices appear to be quite similar to the hippocampal slice, even though only a minority of neocortical pyramidal cells have intrinsic burst-generating properties (at least upon somatic stimulation) (Connors, Gutnick and Prince, 1982; Jones and Lambert, 1990; Hoffman and Haberly, 1991).

Correlates of *in vitro* afterdischarges

EEG polyspike-and-wave is a possible human correlate of a brief *in vitro* afterdischarge, but we are not aware of intracellular recordings that would confirm this directly. Rats with encephalopathy consequent to intrahippocampal tetanus toxin injection exhibit limbic seizures with EEG spikes and sharp waves at 2 Hz and above (Hawkins and Mellanby, 1987); hippocampal slices from these animals exhibit spontaneous afterdischarges quite similar in form to picrotoxin-induced afterdischarges, although the frequency of secondary bursts is lower in the tetanus toxin-injected animals (5–10 Hz vs. 10–15 Hz) (Jefferys, 1989). There are several examples of experimental seizure types in animals in which EEG waves occur at frequencies of 5–20 Hz, wherein action potentials or bursts in presumed pyramidal neurons are time-locked to the local EEG waves. Examples include locally applied penicillin to neocortex (Matsumoto and Ajmone Marsan, 1964a, 1964b) and electrically induced seizures in neocortex (Sawa, Nakamura and Naito, 1968) or limbic system (Kandel and Spencer, 1961; Paré, de Curtis and Llinás, 1992). It is reasonable to guess (but needs to be checked) that any seizure whose EEG correlate is rhythmic waves at, say, 4–20 Hz is associated with rhythmic bursting of pyramidal neurons and has underlying cellular mechanisms similar to *in vitro* afterdischarges. An example would

be certain tonic seizures correlated with fast EEG rhythms (Brenner and Atkinson, 1982).

Electrodecremental response

One of the puzzling aspects of infantile spasms (Chapter 11b) is that behavioral paroxysms may associated with paroxysmal 'flattening' of the EEG (e.g. see figure 24 of Saunders and Westmoreland, 1979). Field bursts (see above) are an example of *in vitro* epileptic activity whose field potentials have only high frequencies (caused by action potential firing that may be at hundreds of Hz) and very low frequencies associated with ionic concentration changes, particularly $[K^+]$. Of course, for technical reasons, both of these field potential changes would be undetectable in scalp EEG recordings. If the mechanism of the electrodecremental response really is a widespread field burst, one should seek to determine whether the brains of affected children are predisposed to large changes in $[Ca^{2+}]_o$ and/or $[K^+]_o$, factors known to predispose to field bursts.

Absence (Chapter 13a)

Extrapolations from experimental studies to the human disorder are complicated by the fact that both diencephalic and cortical structures participate in this seizure type, and one or the other is manipulated (probably disinhibited) in various experimental models: predominantly cortex in generalized penicillin epilepsy *in vivo* and diencephalic neurons *in vitro* (von Krosigk, Bal and McCormick, 1993). In slice studies, it appears to be easier to induce spontaneous 3-Hz oscillations in diencephalic slices than in neocortical slices, nor are we aware of 3-Hz oscillations in undercut cortex. Perhaps this oscillation requires that the neocortex be in a particular 'state' (partially disinhibited?) and that it be rhythmically driven. One type of antiepileptic drug effective in absence, ethosuximide, has been shown to diminish, in voltage-

Table 6.4 Some developmental aspects of brain relevant to epileptogenesis

Mechanism	Possible consequences
Peak in recurrent excitatory connectivity	Favors rapid development of synchrony, and large total excitatory conductance/neuron (which should sustain afterdischarges)
Predominance of depolarizing action of $GABA_A$ receptors on pyramidal cells	Favors GABA-dependent synchronized firing
Possible altered regulation of NMDA receptors by voltage or divalent cations	Favors ↑ NMDA currents (could prolong afterdischarges)

Other developmental features of the immature brain that might be important include generation of an initial excess of neurons, disruptions of neuronal migration, temperature sensitivity of neuronal membrane kinetics, K homeostasis, and osmotic sensitivity of immature brain.

dependent fashion, the low-threshold Ca conductance g_T in thalamic neurons (Coulter, Huguenard and Prince, 1989a, 1989b). This observation is now especially interesting, given the apparent increase in g_T in the GAERS model (H-C. Pape and M. de Curtis, personal communication).

Regulation of NMDA receptor conductance

In the rare inherited disorder nonketotic hyperglycinemia, CSF glycine concentrations are greatly increased (Gerritsen, Kavoggia and Waisman, 1965; Chapter 4c). NMDA receptors possess a strychnine-insensitve glycine-binding site that appears to regulate desensitization. An increase in local glycine concentrations could, possibly, cause prolongation and enhancement of NMDA-induced currents and contribute to the myoclonus and seizures occurring in this illness (McDonald and Johnson, 1990). Changes in NMDA receptors during postnatal development may alter the expression of epilepsies (Table 6.4).

Implications for the development of antiepileptic drugs

It is essential to determine what cellular activities occur only during seizures and never during normal brain states, so that one may focus attention on particular cellular or synaptic 'targets'. The goal would be finding

antiepileptic drugs without cerebral side effects (drowsiness, ataxia, hyperactivity, disrupted learning and so on). To the extent that epileptic activities (such as afterdischarges) appear to overlap or blend into normal cerebral electrophysiology (as appears to be the case for slow wave sleep (Steriade, Nuñez and Amzica, 1993)) this task becomes more difficult. Another example of such overlap concerns the accepted anticonvulsant action of phenytoin, increasing accommodation of high-frequency trains of Na spikes (Macdonald and McLean, 1982). Such an action is expected to interfere with cells firing high-frequency trains of action potentials under normal conditions, such as the neurons that generate saccadic eye movements, or cerebellar Purkinje cells, an effect of likely relevance to the nystagmus and ataxia associated with phenytoin. We have proposed (Traub, Miles and Jefferys, 1993) an attempt to prevent the trains of high-threshold Ca spikes that appear to underlie afterdischarges *in vitro*. If, as now seems likely, such trains occur in pyramidal neurons (at least some of them) during slow wave sleep (Steriade, Nuñez and Amzica, 1993), or Purkinje cells during tracking movements (K. Hepp, personal communication), this hypothetical drug might have side effects as well. Another complication is the development of Ca-blocking that affects postsynaptic Ca channels but not presynaptic ones (or vice

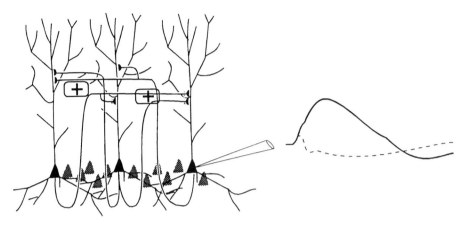

Fig. 6.5   The connectivity of CA3 and other cortical regions holds the key to epileptic synchronization. The connectivity may change in chronic epileptic foci (+) sufficiently to recruit neurons into synchronous epileptic discharges (shown as the solid trace, from which action potentials have been omitted). At normal connectivity, inhibition prevents this recruitment (broken trace). Anatomic evidence exists for sprouting of mossy fibers, but not (yet) for pyramidal cells.

versa), something that may be impossible in principle – both presynaptic and postsynaptic sites appear to use combinations of the same sorts of Ca channels (Takahashi and Momiyama, 1993; Markram, Sakmann and Helm, 1994).

Abnormalities of excitatory connectivity

One of the interesting suggestions of the network simulations is that increased excitatory connectivity (Fig. 6.5), if of sufficient degree, may by itself lead to afterdischarges (R.D. Traub, J.G.R. Jefferys, R. Miles, unpublished data). There are two general clinical settings in which this observation might apply. First are the many disorders of cortical neuron migration, including heterotopias, often associated with seizures and likely (but not proven) to involve abnormal synaptic connectivity (Engel *et al.*, 1992, Chapter 4a). Second are post-traumatic lesions that have been shown to involve axonal sprouting (Sutula *et al.*, 1988; Cronin et al., 1992; Nadler, Perry and Cotman, 1980). In this context, it would be useful to have a rapid method for assessing connectivity in brain tissue. Dual intracellular recording, probably

the definitive technique, is difficult and time consuming, and likely to yield at most a few neuronal pairs in any one tissue sample. The glutamate microdrop technique is an alternative, but still requires intracellular recording in living tissue (Christian and Dudek, 1988). As always in electrophysiologic studies of human tissue, normal controls are a difficulty.

Epileptic brain damage and possible consequent spontaneous seizures

Limbic seizures, as well as sustained electrical stimulation of the perforant path, have been shown to cause loss of hilar neurons, including selected subtypes of GABAergic interneurons (Sloviter, 1987). There is not, in general, a total loss of interneurons. It has been proposed that the remaining inhibitory cells, while viable, are not activated in normal fashion by excitatory pathways, the 'dormant interneuron hypothesis', for which there is some electrophysiologic evidence (Sloviter, 1991; Bekenstein and Lothman, 1993; see also Empson and Jefferys, 1993; Whittington and Jefferys, 1994) (Fig. 6.6). The dentate/hilar region is the last part of the 'limbic loop' to

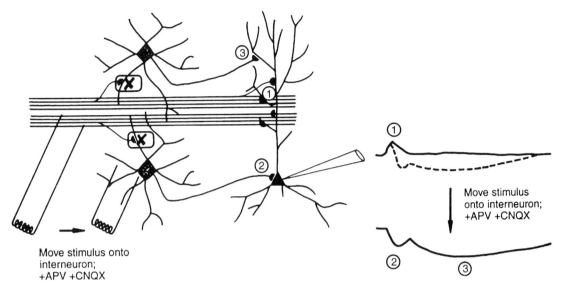

Fig. 6.6 A cartoon of hippocampal circuitry showing the response to stimulation of the afferent input. Normally (broken trace to the right) this evokes an EPSP followed by fast and slow IPSPs. In certain experimental epilepsies, the inhibitory interneurons fail to respond (crosses near synapses in cartoon), so that the response from pyramidal cells is a simple EPSP ①. Fast ② and slow ③ IPSPs can then be revealed when the experimenter adjusts the stimulus site (arrow) and strength to stimulate interneurons directly, and also uses drugs such as APV and CNQX to block epileptic discharge that would otherwise mask the IPSP.

participate in electrically evoked afterdischarges (Paré, de Curtis and Llinás, 1992; Stringer and Lothman, 1992) and has been suggested to act as a gate or brake. Functionally abnormal inhibition in this region might therefore predispose to seizures. These ideas have been proposed to account both for part of the mesial temporal sclerosis lesion and for the delayed development of complex partial seizures following complicated febrile seizures (among other insults) (Sloviter, 1991). In principle, this idea is testable in human dentate/hilar tissue.

ACKNOWLEDGMENTS

We thank Drs Robert K.S. Wong, Richard Miles, Frances Jensen, Marco de Curtis, Michael M. Segal, and Miles A. Whittington for helpful discussions. This work was supported by the IBM Corporation and the Wellcome Trust. J.G.R.J. is a Wellcome Trust Senior Lecturer.

REFERENCES

Agmon, A. and Connors, B.W. (1989) Repetitive burst-firing neurons in the deep layers of mouse somatosensory cortex. *Neuroscience Letters*, **99**, 137–41.

Amitai, Y., Friedman, A., Connors, B.W. and Gutnick, M.J. (1993) Regenerative activity in apical dendrites of pyramidal cells in neocortex. *Cerebral Cortex*, **3**, 26–38.

Ascher, P., Bregestovski, P. and Nowak, L. (1988) N-methyl-D-aspartate-activated channels of mouse central neurones in magnesium-free solutions. *Journal of Physiology*, **399**, 207–26.

Audinat, E., Bochet, P., Lambolez, B. *et al.* (1993) Subunit composition of calcium permeable AMPA receptor-channels at the single cell level. *Society for Neuroscience Abstracts*, **19**, 625.

Avanzini, G., de Curtis, M., Panzica, F. and Spreafico, R. (1989) Intrinsic properties of the nucleus reticularis thalami neurones of the rat studied *in vitro. Journal of Physiology*, **416**, 111–22.

Avanzini, G., Vergnes, M., Spreafico, R. and Marescaux, C. (1993) Calcium-dependent regulation of genetically determined spike and waves by the reticular thalamic nucleus of rats. *Epilepsia*, **34**, 1–7.

Avoli, M. and Gloor, P. (1981) The effects of transient functional depression of the thalamus on spindles and on bilateral synchronous epileptic discharges of feline generalized penicillin epilepsy. *Epilepsia*, **22**, 443–52.

Avoli, M. and Gloor, P. (1982) Interaction of cortex and thalamus in spike and wave discharges of feline generalized penicillin epilepsy. *Experimental Neurology*, **76**, 196–217.

Avoli, M., Psarropoulou, C., Tancredi, V. and Fueta, Y. (1993) On the synchronous activity induced by 4-aminopyridine in the CA3 subfield of juvenile rat hippocampus. *Journal of Neurophysiology*, **70**, 1018–29.

Bal, T. and McCormick, D.A. (1993) Mechanisms of oscillatory activity in guinea-pig nucleus reticularis thalami *in vitro*: a mammalian pacemaker. *Journal of Physiology*, **468**, 669–91.

Bekenstein, J.W. and Lothman, E.W. (1993) Dormancy of inhibitory interneurons in a model of temporal lobe epilepsy. *Science*, **259**, 97–100.

Bekkers, J.M. and Stevens, C.F. (1989) NMDA and non-NMDA receptors are co-localized at individual excitatory synapses in cultured rat hippocampus. *Nature*, **341**, 230–3.

Ben-Ari, Y., Cherubini, E., Corradetti, R. and Gaiarsa, J.-L. (1989) Giant synaptic potentials in immature rat CA3 hippocampal neurones. *Journal of Physiology*, **416**, 303–25.

Benveniste, M., Clements, J., Vyklicky, L., Jr and Mayer, M.L. (1990) A kinetic analysis of the modulation of N-methyl-D-aspartic acid receptors by glycine in mouse cultured hippocampal neurones. *Journal of Physiology*, **428**, 333–57.

Brady, R.J., Smith, K.L. and Swann, J.W. (1991) Calcium modulation of the N-methyl-D-aspartate (NMDA) response and electrographic seizures in immature hippocampus. *Neuroscience Letters*, **124**, 92–6.

Bregestovski, P., Khazipov, R., Ragozzino, D. *et al.* (1993) Magnesium block of NMDA channels in hippocampal slices does not change during development. *Society for Neuroscience Abstracts*, **19**, 625.

Brenner, R.P. and Atkinson, R. (1982) Generalized paroxysmal fast activity: electroencephalographic and clinical features. *Annals of Neurology*, **11**, 386–90.

Brodal, A. (1981) *Neurological Anatomy in Relation to Clinical Medicine*, Oxford University Press, Oxford

Buzsáki, G. (1986) Hippocampal sharp waves: their origin and significance. *Brain Research*, **398**, 242–52.

Caeser, M., Brown, D.A., Gähwiler, B.H. and Knöpfel, T. (1993) Characterization of a calcium-dependent current generating a slow afterdepolarization of CA3 pyramidal cells in rat hippocampal slice cultures. *European Journal of Neuroscience*, **5**, 560–9.

Callaway, J.C., Ross, W.N. and Lasser-Ross, N. (1992) IPSPs strongly inhibit climbing fiber activated $[Ca^{2+}]_i$ increases in the dendrites of cerebellar Purkinje neurons. *Society for Neuroscience Abstracts*, **18**, 1343.

Chamberlin, N.L., Traub, R.D. and Dingledine, R. (1990) Role of EPSPs in initiation of spontaneous synchronized burst firing in rat hippocampal neurons bathed in high potassium. *Journal of Neurophysiology*, **64**, 1000–8.

Chen, Q.X., Kay, A.R., Stelzer, A. *et al.* (1990) $GABA_A$-receptor function is regulated by phosphorylation in acutely dissociated guinea-pig hippocampal neurones. *Journal of Physiology*, **420**, 207–21.

Cherubini, E., Gaiarsa, J.L. and Ben-Ari, Y. (1991) GABA: an excitatory transmitter in early postnatal life. *Trends in Neurosciences*, **14**, 515–19.

Chervin, R.D., Pierce, P.A. and Connors, B.W. (1988) Periodicity and directionality in the propagation of epileptiform discharges across neocortex. *Journal of Neurophysiology*, **60**, 1695–713.

Christian, E.P. and Dudek, F.E. (1988) Characteristics of local excitatory circuits studied with glutamate microapplication in the CA3 area of rat hippocampal slices. *Journal of Neurophysiology*, **59**, 90–109.

Clark, G.D., Clifford, D.B. and Zorumski, C.F. (1990) The effect of agonist concentration, membrane voltage and calcium on N-methyl-D-aspartate receptor desensitization. *Neuroscience*, **39**, 787–97.

Collingridge, G.L., Herron, C.E. and Lester, R.A.J. (1988) Synaptic activation of N-methyl-D-aspartate receptors in the Schaffer collateral-commissural pathway of rat hippocampus. *Journal of Physiology*, **399**, 283–300.

Connors, B.W., Gutnick, M.J. and Prince, D.A. (1982) Electrophysiological properties of neocortical neurons *in vitro*. *Journal of Neurophysiology*, **48**, 1302–20.

Coulter, D.A., Huguenard, J.R. and Prince, D.A. (1989a) Specific petit mal anticonvulsants reduce calcium currents in thalamic neurons. *Neuroscience Letters*, **98**, 74–8.

Coulter, D.A., Huguenard, J.R. and Prince, D.A. (1989b) Characterization of ethosuximide reduction of low-threshold calcium current in thalamic neurons. *Annals of Neurology*, **25**, 582–93.

Cronin, J., Obenaus, A., Houser, C.R. and Dudek, F.E. (1992) Electrophysiology of dentate granule cells after kainate-induced synaptic reorganization of the mossy fibers. *Brain Research*, **573**, 305–10.

Deschênes, M., Paradis, M., Roy, J.P. and Steriade, M. (1984) Electrophysiology of neurons of lateral thalamic nuclei in cat: resting properties and burst discharges. *Journal of Neurophysiology*, **51**, 1196–219.

Destexhe, A., McCormick, D.A. and Sejnowski, T.J. (1993) A model for 8–10 Hz spindling in interconnected thalamic relay and reticularis neurons. *Biophysical Journal*, **65**, 2473–7.

Dichter, M. and Spencer, W.A. (1969) Penicillin-induced interictal discharges from the cat hippocampus. I. Characteristics and topographical features. *Journal of Neurophysiology*, **32**, 649–62.

Domann, R., Dorn, T. and Witte, O.W. (1991) Afterpotentials following penicillin-induced paroxysmal depolarizations in rat hippocampal CA1 pyramidal cells *in vitro*. *Pflügers Archiv*, **417**, 469–78.

Dudek, F.E., Obenaus, A. and Tasker, J.G. (1990) Osmolality-induced changes in extracellular volume alter epileptiform bursts independent of chemical synapses in the rat: importance of non-synaptic mechanisms in hippocampal epileptogenesis. *Neuroscience Letters*, **120**, 267–70.

Empson, R.M. and Jefferys, J.G.R. (1993) Synaptic inhibition in primary and secondary chronic epileptic foci induced by intrahippocampal tetanus toxin in the rat. *Journal of Physiology*, **465**, 595–614.

Engel, J., Jr, Wasterlain, C., Cavalheiro, E.A. *et al.* (1992) *Molecular Neurobiology of Epilepsy*, Elsevier, Amsterdam.

Federico, P. and MacVicar, B.A. (1993) The role of glutamate receptor subtypes in the induction and propagation of seizure activity in the hippocampus and olfactory cortex of the guinea-pig isolated whole brain. *Society for Neuroscience Abstracts*, **19**, 1032.

Fisher, R.S. and Prince, D.A. (1977a) Spike-wave rhythms in cat cortex induced by parenteral penicillin. I. Electroencephalographic features. *Electroencephalography and Clinical Neurophysiology*, **42**, 608–24.

Fisher, R.S. and Prince, D.A. (1977b) Spike-wave rhythms in cat cortex induced by parenteral penicillin. II. Cellular features. *Electroencephalography and Clinical Neurophysiology*, **42**, 625–39.

Flores-Hernández, J., Galarraga, E., Pineda, J.C. and Bargas, J. (1993) Spontaneous synaptic potentials induced by 4-aminopyridine in neostriatal neurons. *Society for Neuroscience Abstracts*, **19**, 977.

Fraser, D.D. and MacVicar, B.A. (1991) Low-threshold transient calcium current in rat hippocampal lacunosum-moleculare interneurons: kinetics and modulation by neurotransmitters. *Journal of Neuroscience*, **11**, 2812–20.

Freund, T.F. and Antal, M. (1988) GABA-containing neurons in the septum control inhibitory interneurons in the hippocampus. *Nature*, **336**, 170–3.

Gerritsen, T., Kaveggia, E. and Waisman, H.A. (1965) A new type of hyperglycinemia with hypooxaluria. *Pediatrics*, **36**, 882–91.

Gloor, P. and Fariello, R.G. (1988) Generalized epilepsy: some of its cellular mechanisms differ from those of focal epilepsy. *Trends in Neurosciences*, **11**, 63–8.

Gloor, P., Pellegrini, A. and Kostopoulos, G.K. (1979) Effects of changes in cortical excitability upon the epileptic bursts in generalized penicillin epilepsy of the cat. *Electroencephalography and Clinical Neurophysiology*, **46**, 274–89.

Gloor, P., Quesney, L.F. and Zumstein, H. (1977) Pathophysiology of generalized penicillin epilepsy in the cat: the role of cortical and subcortical structures. II. Topical application of penicillin to the cerebral cortex and to subcortical structures. *Electroencephalography and Clinical Neurophysiology*, **43**, 79–94.

Goldensohn, E.S. and Purpura, D.P. (1963) Intracellular potentials of cortical neurons during focal epileptogenic discharges. *Science*, **139**, 840–2.

Gray, C.M. and Singer, W. (1989) Stimulus-specific neuronal oscillations in orientation columns of cat visual cortex. *Proceedings of the National Academy of Sciences, USA*, **86**, 1698–702.

Gulyás, A.I., Miles, R., Hajos, N. and Freund, T.F. (1993) Precision and variability in postsynaptic target selection of inhibitory cells in the hippocampal CA3 region. *European Journal of Neuroscience*, **5**, 1729–51.

Gulyás, A.I., Miles, R., Sik, A. *et al.* (1993) Hippocampal pyramidal cells excite inhibitory neurons through a single release site. *Nature*, **366**, 683–7.

Guthrie, P.B., Segal, M. and Kater, S.B. (1991) Independent regulation of calcium revealed by imaging dendritic spines. *Nature*, **3**, 76–80.

Gutnick, M.J. and Prince, D.A. (1972) Thalamo-cortical relay neurons: antidromic invasion of spikes from a cortical epileptogenic focus. *Science*, **176**, 424–6.

Haas, H.L. and Jefferys, J.G.R. (1984) Low-calcium field burst discharges of CA1 pyramidal neurones in rat hippocampal slices. *Journal of Physiology*, **354**, 185–201.

Halliwell, J.V. and Adams, P.R. (1982) Voltage-clamp analysis of muscarinic excitation in hippocampal neurons. *Brain Research*, **250**, 71–92.

Hawkins, C.A. and Mellanby, J.H. (1987) Limbic epilepsy induced by tetanus toxin: a longitudinal electroencephalographic study. *Epilepsia*, **28**, 431–44.

Hestrin, S., Nicoll, R.A., Perkel, D.J. and Sah, P. (1990) Analysis of excitatory synaptic action in pyramidal cells using whole-cell recording from rat hippocampal slices. *Journal of Physiology*, **422**, 230–25.

Hoffman, W.H. and Haberly, L.B. (1991) Bursting-induced epileptiform EPSPs in slices of piriform cortex are generated by deep cells. *Journal of Neuroscience*, **11**, 2021–31.

Huguenard, J.R., and McCormick, D.A. (1992) Simulation of the currents involved in rhythmic oscillations in thalamic relay neurons. *Journal of Neurophysiology*, **68**, 1373–83.

Ishizuka, N., Weber, J. and Amaral, D.G. (1990) Organization of intrahippocampal projections originating from CA3 pyramidal cells in the rat. *Journal of Comparative Neurology*, **295**, 580–623.

Jahnsen, H. and Llinás, R. (1984a) Electrophysiological properties of guinea-pig thalamic neurones: an *in vitro* study. *Journal of Physiology*, **349**, 205–26.

Jahnsen, H. and Llinás, R. (1984b) Ionic basis for the electroresponsiveness and oscillatory properties of guinea-pig thalamic neurones *in vitro*. *Journal of Physiology*, **349**, 227–47.

Jahr, C.E. and Stevens, C.F. (1990) Voltage dependence of NMDA-activated macroscopic conductances predicted by single-channel kinetics. *Journal of Neuroscience*, **10**, 3178–82.

Jefferys, J.G.R. (1989) Chronic epileptic foci *in vitro* in hippocampal slices from rats with the tetanus toxin epileptic syndrome. *Journal of Neurophysiology*, **62**, 458–68.

Jensen, M.S. and Yaari, Y. (1988) The relationship between interictal and ictal paroxysms in an *in vitro* model of focal hippocampal epilepsy. *Annals of Neurology*, **24**, 591–8.

Johansson, S., Friedman, W. and Arhem, P. (1992) Impulses and resting membrane properties of small cultured rat hippocampal neurons. *Journal of Physiology*, **445**, 129–40.

Johnston, D. and Brown, T.H. (1981) Giant synaptic potential hypothesis for epileptiform activity. *Science*, **211**, 294–97.

Jones, R.S. and Lambert, J.D. (1990) Synchronous discharges in the rat entorhinal cortex *in vitro*: site of initiation and the role of excitatory amino acid receptors. *Neuroscience*, **34**, 657–70.

Kandel, E.R. and Spencer, W.A. (1961) Excitation and inhibition of single pyramidal cells during hippocampal seizure. *Experimental Neurology*, **4**, 162–179.

Kandel, E.R., Spencer, W.A. and Brinley, F.J., Jr. (1961) Electrophysiology of hippocampal neurons. I. Sequential invasion and synaptic organization. *Journal of Neurophysiology*, **24**, 225–42.

Katsumaru, H., Kosaka, T., Heizmann, C.W. and Hama, K. (1988) Immunocytochemical study of GABAergic neurons containing the calcium-binding protein parvalbumin in the rat hippocampus. *Experimental Brain Research*, **72**, 347–62.

Kawaguchi, Y. and Hama, K. (1987) Two subtypes of non-pyramidal cells in rat hippocampal formation identified by intracellular recording and HRP injection. *Brain Research*, **411**, 190–5.

Kleckner, N.W. and Dingledine, R. (1991) Regulation of hippocampal NMDA receptors by magnesium and glycine during development. *Molecular Brain Research*, **11**, 151–9.

Knowles, W.D. and Schwartzkroin, P.A. (1981) Local circuit synaptic interactions in hippocampal brain slices. *Journal of Neuroscience*, **1**, 318–22.

Knowles, W.D., Traub, R.D. and Strowbridge, B.W. (1987) The initiation and spread of epileptiform bursts in the *in vitro* hippocampal slice. *Neuroscience*, **218**, 441–445.

Kocsis, J.D. and Waxman, S.G. (1980) Absence of potassium conductance in central myelinated axons. *Nature*, **287**, 348–9.

Kocsis, J.D., Malenka, R.C. and Waxman, S.G. (1980) Effects of 4-aminopyridine on the frequency following properties of the parallel fibers of the cerebellar cortex. *Brain Research*, **195**, 511–6.

Kocsis, J.D., Ruiz, J.A. and Waxman, S.G. (1983) Maturation of mammalian myelinated fibers: changes in action-potential characteristics following 4-aminopyridine application. *Journal of Neurophysiology*, **50**, 449–63.

Konnerth, A., Heinemann, U. and Yaari, Y. (1984) Slow transmission of neural activity in hippocampal area CA1 in absence of active chemical synapses. *Nature*, **307**, 69–71.

Kosaka, T. (1983) Gap junctions between non-pyramidal cell dendrites in the rat hippocampus (CA1 and CA3 regions). *Brain Research*, **271**, 157–61.

Lacaille, J.-C., Mueller, A.L., Kunkel, D.D. and Schwartzkroin, P.A. (1987) Local circuit interactions between oriens/alveus interneurons and CA1 pyramidal cells in hippocampal slices: electrophysiology and morphology. *Journal of Neuroscience*, **7**, 1979–93.

Lee, W.-L. and Hablitz, J.J. (1989) Involvement of non-NMDA receptors in picrotoxin-induced epileptiform activity in the hippocampus. *Neuroscience Letters*, **107**, 129–34.

Li, X.-G., Somogyi, P., Ylinen, A. and Buzsáki, G. (1993) The hippocampal CA3 network: an *in vivo* intracellular labeling study. *Journal of Comparative Neurology*, **33**, 1–29.

Llinás, R. and Sugimori, M. (1980a) Electrophysiological properties of *in vitro* Purkinje cell somata in mammalian cerebellar slices. *Journal of Physiology*, **305**, 171–95.

Llinás, R. and Sugimori, M. (1980b) Electrophysiological properties of *in vitro* Purkinje cell dendrites in mammalian cerebellar slices. *Journal of Physiology*, **305**, 197–213.

Llinás, R., Walton, K. and Bohr, V. (1976) Synaptic transmission in squid giant synapse after potassium conductance blockage with external 3-, and 4-aminopyridine. *Biophysical Journal*, **16**, 83–6.

Lorente de Nó, R. (1934) Studies on the structure of the cerebral cortex II. Continuation of the study of the Ammonic system. *Journal of Psychology and Neurology*, **46**, 113–77.

Maccaferri, G., Mangoni, M., Lazzari, A. and DiFrancesco, D. (1993) Properties of the hyperpolarization-activated current in rat hippocampal CA1 pyramidal cells. *Journal of Neurophysiology*, **69**, 2129–36.

McCormick, D.A. (1992) Neurotransmitter action in the thalamus and cerebral cortex and their role in neuromodulation of thalamocortical activity. *Progress in Neurobiology*, **39**, 337–88.

McCormick, D.A. and Huguenard, J.R. (1992) A model of the electrophysiological properties of thalamocortical relay neurons. *Journal of Neurophysiology*, **68**, 1384–400.

MacDermott, A.M. and Miles, R. (1991) Calcium currents in the regulation of patterns of cellular activity, in *The Calcium Channel: Biophysics, Physiology, Pharmacology and Clinical Implications*, (eds L. Hurwitz, L.D. Partridge and J.K. Leach), Telford Press, NJ.

McDonald, J.W. and Johnson, M.V. (1990) Nonketotic hyperglycinemia: pathophysiological role of NMDA-type excitatory amino acid receptors. *Annals of Neurology*, **27**, 449–50.

Macdonald, R.L. and McLean, M.J. (1982) Cellular bases of barbiturate and phenytoin anticonvulsant drug action. *Epilepsia*, **23**, (Suppl.), S7–18.

Madison, D.V. and Nicoll, R.A. (1988) Enkephalin hyperpolarizes interneurones in the rat hippocampus. *Journal of Physiology*, **398**, 123–30.

Markram, H., Sakmann, B. and Helm, P.J. (1994) Dendritic action potentials trigger discrete calcium transients through multiple calcium channel-types in rat layer V neocortical cells, *Journal of Physiology*, **475**, 146P.

Mason, A., Nicoll, A. and Stratford, K. (1991) Synaptic transmission between individual pyramidal neurons of the rat visual cortex *in vitro Journal of Neuroscience*, **11**, 72–84.

Masukawa, L.M. and Prince, D.A. (1984) Synaptic control of excitability in isolated dendrites of hippocampal neurons. *Journal of Neuroscience*, **4**, 217–27.

Matsumoto, H. and Ajmone Marsan, C. (1964a) Cortical cellular phenomena in experimental epilepsy: interictal manifestations. *Experimental Neurology*, **9**, 286–304.

Matsumoto, H. and Ajmone Marsan, C. (1964b) Cortical cellular phenomena in experimental epilepsy: ictal manifestations. *Experimental Neurology*, **9**, 305–26.

Mesher, R.A. and Schwartzkroin, P.A. (1980) Can CA3 epileptiform burst discharge induce bursting in normal CA1 hippocampal neurons? *Brain Research*, **183**, 472–6.

Michelson, H.B. and Wong, R.K.S. (1991) Excitatory synaptic responses mediated by GABA$_A$ receptors in the hippocampus. *Science*, **253**, 1420–3.

Midtgaard, J. (1992) Stellate cell inhibition of

Purkinje cells in the turtle cerebellum *in vitro.* *Journal of Physiology,* **457,** 355–67.

Miles, R. (1990a) Synaptic excitation of inhibitory cells by single CA3 hippocampal pyramidal cells of the guinea-pig *in vitro. Journal of Physiology,* **428,** 61–77.

Miles, R. (1990b) Variation in strength of inhibitory synapses in the CA3 region of guinea-pig hippocampus *in vitro. Journal of Physiology,* **431,** 659–76.

Miles, R. and Poncer, J.-C. (1993) Metabotropic glutamate receptors mediate a post-tetanic excitation of guinea-pig hippocampal inhibitory neurones. *Journal of Physiology,* **463,** 461–73.

Miles, R. and Wong, R.K.S. (1983) Single neurones can initiate synchronized population discharge in the hippocampus. *Nature,* **306,** 371–3.

Miles, R. and Wong, R.K.S. (1984) Unitary inhibitory synaptic potentials in the guinea-pig hippocampus *in vitro. Journal of Physiology,* **356,** 97–113.

Miles, R. and Wong, R.K.S. (1986) Excitatory synaptic interactions between CA3 neurones in the guinea-pig hippocampus. *Journal of Physiology,* **373,** 397–418.

Miles, R. and Wong, R.K.S. (1987a) Inhibitory control of local excitatory circuits in the guinea-pig hippocampus. *Journal of Physiology,* **388,** 611–29.

Miles, R. and Wong, R.K.S. (1987b) Latent synaptic pathways revealed after tetanic stimulation in the hippocampus. *Nature,* **329,** 724–6.

Miles, R., Traub, R.D. and Wong, R.K.S. (1988) Spread of synchronous firing in longitudinal slices from the CA3 region of the hippocampus. *Journal of Neurophysiology,* **60,** 1481–96.

Miyakawa, H., Ross, W.N., Jaffe, D. *et al.* (1992) Synaptically activated increases in Ca^{2+} concentration in hippocampal CA1 pyramidal cells are primarily due to voltage-gated Ca^{2+} channels. *Neuron,* **9,** 1163–73.

Mueller, A.L., Taube, J.S. and Schwartzkroin, P.A. (1984) Development of hyperpolarizing inhibitory postsynaptic potentials and hyperpolarizing response to γ-aminobutyric acid in rabbit hippocampus studied *in vitro. Journal of Neuroscience,* **4,** 860–7.

Müller, D. (1986) Potentiation by 4-aminopyridine of quantal acetylcholine release at the *Torpedo* nerve–electroplaque junction. *Journal of Physiology,* **379,** 479–93.

Müller, W. and Connor, J.A. (1991) Dendritic spines as individual neuronal compartments for synaptic Ca^{2+} responses. *Nature,* **354,** 73–6.

Musgrave, J. and Gloor, P. (1980) The role of the corpus callosum in bilateral interhemispheric synchrony of spike and wave discharge in feline generalized penicillin epilepsy. *Epilepsia,* **21,** 369–78.

Nadler, J.V., Perry, B.W. and Cotman, C.W. (1980) Selective reinnervation of hippocampal area CA1 and the fascia dentata after destruction of CA3–CA4 afferents with kainic acid. *Brain Research,* **182,** 1–9.

Neuman, R.S., Cherubini, E. and Ben-Ari, Y. (1989) Endogenous and network bursts induced by N-methyl-D-aspartate and magnesium free medium in the CA3 region of the hippocampal slice. *Neuroscience,* **28,** 393–9.

Newberry, N.R. and Nicoll, R.A. (1984) A bicuculline-resistant inhibitory post-synaptic potential in rat hippocampal pyramidal cells *in vitro. Journal of Physiology,* **348,** 239–54.

Numann, R. and Wong, R.K.S. (1984) Voltage-clamp study on GABA response desensitization in single pyramidal cells dissociated from the hippocampus of adult guinea pigs. *Neuroscience Letters,* **47,** 289–94.

Numann, R.E., Wadman, W.J. and Wong, R.K.S. (1987) Outward currents of single hippocampal cells obtained from the adult guinea-pig. *Journal of Physiology,* **393,** 331–53.

Otis, T.S., De Koninck, Y. and Mody, I. (1993) Characterization of synaptically elicited GABA$_B$ responses using patch-clamp recordings in rat hippocampal slices. *Journal of Physiology,* **463,** 391–407.

Paré, D., de Curtis, M. and Llinás, R. (1992) Role of the hippocampal-entorhinal loop in temporal lobe epilepsy: extra- and intracellular study in the isolated guinea pig brain *in vitro. Journal of Neuroscience,* **12,** 1867–81.

Pearce, R.A. (1993) Physiological evidence for two distinct GABA$_A$ responses in rat hippocampus. *Neuron,* **10,** 189–200.

Pellegrini, A. and Gloor, P. (1979) Effects of bilateral partial diencephalic lesions on cortical epileptic activity in generalized penicillin epilepsy in the cat. *Experimental Neurology,* **66,** 285–308.

Perouansky, M. and Yaari, Y. (1993) Kinetic properties of NMDA receptor-mediated synaptic currents in rat hippocampal pyramidal cells *versus* interneurones. *Journal of Physiology,* **465,** 223–44.

Pitler, T.A. and Alger, B.E. (1992a) Postsynaptic spike firing reduces synaptic GABA$_A$ responses in hippocampal pyramidal cells. *Journal of Neuroscience*, **12**, 4122–32.

Pitler, T.A. and Alger, B.E. (1992b) Cholinergic excitation of GABAergic interneurons in the rat hippocampal slice. *Journal of Physiology*, **450**, 127–42.

Prince, D.A. (1968) Inhibition in 'epileptic' neurons. *Experimental Neurology*, **21**, 307–21.

Prince, D.A. and Tseng, G.-F. (1993) Epileptogenesis in chronically injured cortex: *in vitro* studies. *Journal of Neurophysiology*, **69**, 1276–91.

Pumain, R., Menini, C., Heniemann, U. *et al.* (1985) Chemical synaptic transmission is not necessary for epileptic seizures to persist in the baboon *Papio papio. Experimental Neurology*, **89**, 250–8.

Qiao, X. and Noebels, J.L. (1993) Developmental analysis of hippocampal mossy fiber outgrowth in a mutant mouse with inherited spike-wave seizures. *Journal of Neuroscience*, **13**, 4622–35.

Rafiq, A., DeLorenzo, R.J. and Coulter, D.A. (1993) Generation and propagation of epileptiform discharges in a combined entorhinal cortex/hippocampal slice. *Journal of Neurophysiology*, **70**, 1962–74.

Ranck, J.B., Jr (1973) Studies on single neurons in dorsal hippocampal formation and septum in unrestrained rats. Part I. Behavioral correlates and firing repertoire. *Experimental Neurology*, **40**, 461–555.

Roper, S.N., Obenaus, A. and Dudek, F.E. (1993) Increased propensity for nonsynaptic epileptiform activity in immature rat hippocampus and dentate gyrus. *Journal of Neurophysiology*, **70**, 857–62.

Sah, P., Hestrin, S. and Nicoll, R.A. (1990) Properties of excitatory postsynaptic currents recorded *in vitro* from rat hippocampal interneurones. *Journal of Physiology*, **430**, 605–16.

Saunders, M.G. and Westmoreland, B.F. (1979) The EEG in evaluation of disorders affecting the brain diffusely, in *Current Practice of Clinical Electroencephalography*, (eds D.W. Klass and D.D. Daly), Raven, New York, pp. 343–79.

Sawa, M., Nakamura, K. and Naito, H. (1968) Intracellular phenomena and spread of epileptic seizure discharges. *Electroencephalography and Clinical Neurophysiology*, **24**, 146–54.

Scanziani, M., Gähwiler, B.H. and Thompson, S.M. (1993) Presynaptic inhibition of excitatory synaptic transmission mediated by α adrenergic receptors in area CA3 of the rat hippocampus *in vitro. Journal of Neuroscience*, **13**, 5393–401.

Scanziani, M., Capogna, M., Gähwiler, B.H. and Thompson, S.M. (1992) Presynaptic inhibition of miniature excitatory synaptic currents by baclofen and adenosine in the hippocampus. *Neuron*, **9**, 919–27.

Schlander, M. and Frotscher, M. (1986) Nonpyramidal neurons in the guinea pig hippocampus. A combined Golgi–electron microscope study. *Anatomy and Embryology*, **174**, 35–47.

Schneiderman, J.H. (1987) 'Slow' field potentials in penicillin-perfused hippocampal slices. *Brain Research*, **403**, 162–6.

Schwartzkroin, P.A. and Mathers, L.H. (1978) Physiological and morphological identification of a nonpyramidal hippocampal cell type. *Brain Research*, **157**, 1–10.

Segal, M. (1990) A subset of local interneurons generate slow inhibitory postsynaptic potentials in hippocampal neurons. *Brain Research*, **511**, 163–4.

Segal, M.M. (1993) Phenytoin attenuates seizure-associated plateau bursts in solitary hippocampal neurons. *Society for Neuroscience Abstracts*, **19**, 20.

Sloviter, R.S. (1987) Decreased hippocampal inhibition and a selective loss of interneurons in experimental epilepsy. *Science*, **235**, 73–6.

Sloviter, R.S. (1991) Permanently altered hippocampal structure, excitability, and inhibition after experimental status epilepticus in the rat: the 'dormant basket cell' hypothesis and its possible relevance to temporal lobe epilepsy. *Hippocampus*, **1**, 41–66.

Sloviter, R.S. and Nilaver, G. (1987) Immunocytochemical localization of GABA-cholecystokinin-, vasoactive intestinal polypeptide-, and somatostatin-like immunoreactivity in the area dentata and hippocampus of the rat. *Journal of Comparative Neurology*, **256**, 42–60.

Sloviter, R.S., Sollas, A.L., Barbaro, N.M. and Laxer, K.D. (1991) Calcium-binding protein (calbindin-D28K) and parvalbumin immunocytochemistry in the normal and epileptic human hippocampus. *Journal of Comparative Neurology*, **308**, 381–96.

Smith, K.L., Turner, J. and Swann, J.W. (1988) Paired intracellular recordings reveal mono- and polysynaptic excitatory interactions in immature hippocampus. *Society of Neuroscience Abstracts*, **14**, 883.

Sorra, K.E. and Harris, K.M. (1993) Occurrence

and three-dimensional structure of multiple synapses between individual radiatum axons and their target pyramidal cells in hippocampal area CA1. *Journal of Neuroscience*, **13**, 3736–48.

Stasheff, S.F., Bragdon, A.C. and Wilson, W.A. (1985) Induction of epileptiform activity in hippocampal slices by trains of electrical stimuli. *Brain Research*, **344**, 296–302.

Stasheff, S.F., Mott, D.D. and Wilson, W.A. (1993) Axon terminal hyperexcitability associated with epileptogenesis *in vitro*. II. Pharmacological regulation by NMDA and GABA$_A$ receptors. *Journal of Neurophysiology*, **70**, 976–84.

Steriade, M. and Deschênes, M. (1984) The thalamus as a neuronal oscillator. *Brain Research Reviews*, **8**, 1–63.

Steriade, M. and Llinás, R.R. (1988) The functional states of the thalamus and the associated neuronal interplay. *Physiological Reviews*, **68**, 649–739.

Steriade, M., Nuñez., A. and Amzica, F. (1993) Intracellular analysis of relations between the slow (<1 Hz) neocortical oscillation and other sleep rhythms of the electroencephalogram. *Journal of Neuroscience*, **13**, 3266–83.

Storm, J.F. (1988) Temporal integration by a slowly inactivating K$^+$ current in hippocampal neurons. *Nature*, **336**, 379–81.

Stringer, J.L. and Lothman, E.W. (1992) Reverberatory seizure discharges in hippocampal–parahippocampal circuits *Experimental Neurology*, **116**, 198–203.

Sutula, T., Xiao-Xian, H., Cavazos, J. and Scott, G. (1988) Synaptic reorganization in the hippocampus induced by abnormal functional activity. *Science*, **239**, 1147–50.

Swann, J.W., Brady, R.J. and Martin, D.L. (1989) Postnatal development of GABA-mediated synaptic inhibition in rat hippocampus. *Neuroscience*, **28**, 551–61.

Swann, J.W., Smith, K.L. and Brady, R.J. (1991) Age-dependent alterations in the operations of hippocampal neural networks. *Annals of the New York Academy of Sciences*, **627**, 264–76.

Takahashi, T. and Momiyama, A. (1993) Different types of calcium channels mediate central synaptic transmission. *Nature*, **366**, 156–8.

Tamamaki, N., Watanabe, K. and Nojyo, Y. (1984) A whole image of the hippocampal pyramidal neuron revealed by intracellular pressure-injection of horseradish peroxidase. *Brain Research*, **307**, 336–40.

Taylor, C.P. and Dudek, F.E. (1984) Synchronization without active chemical synapses during hippocampal afterdischarges. *Journal of Neurophysiology*, **52**, 143–55.

Thalmann, R.H. (1984) Reversal properties of an EGTA-resistant late hyperpolarization that follows synaptic stimulation of hippocampal neurons. *Neuroscience Letters*, **46**, 103–8.

Thompson, S.M. (1994) Modulation of inhibitory synaptic transmission in the hippocampus. *Progress in Neurobiology*, **42**, 576–609.

Thompson, S.M. and Gähwiler, B.H. (1989) Activity-dependent disinhibition. I. Repetitive stimulation reduces both IPSP driving force and conductance in the hippocampus *in vitro*. *Journal of Neurophysiology*, **61**, 501–11.

Thompson, S.M. and Gähwiler, B.H. (1992) Comparison of the actions of baclofen at pre- and postsynaptic receptors in the rat hippocampus *in vitro*. *Journal of Physiology*, **451**, 329–45.

Thompson S.M. and Wong R.K.S. (1991) Development of calcium current subtypes in isolated rat hippocampal pyramidal cells. *Journal of Physiology*, **439**, 671–89.

Thomson, A.M. (1988) Biphasic responses of thalamic neurons to GABA in isolated brain slices – II. *Neuroscience*, **25**, 503–12.

Thomson, A.M. and West, D.C. (1993) Fluctuation in pyramid-pyramid excitatory postsynaptic potentials modified by presynaptic firing pattern and postsynaptic membrane potential using paired intracellular recordings in rat neocortex. *Neuroscience*, **54**, 329–346.

Thomson, A.M., Deuchars, J. and West, D.C. (1993) Single axon excitatory postsynaptic potentials in neocortical interneurons exhibit pronounced paired pulse facilitation. *Neuroscience*, **54**, 347–60.

Traub, R.D. and Jefferys, J.G.R. (1994) Are there unifying principles underlying the generation of epileptic afterdischarges *in vitro*? *Progress in Brain Research*, **102**, 371–82.

Traub, R.D. and Miles, R. (1991) *Neuronal Networks of the Hippocampus*, Cambridge University Press, New York.

Traub, R.D. and Miles, R. (1992) Modeling hippocampal circuitry using data from whole cell patch clamp and dual intracellular recordings *in vitro*. *Seminars in the Neurosciences*, **4**, 27–36.

Traub, R.D. and Wong, R.K.S. (1982) Cellular mechanism of neuronal synchronization in epilepsy. *Science*, **216**, 745–7.

Traub, R.D., Colling, S.B. and Jefferys, J.G.R. (1995) Cellular mechanisms of 4-aminopyridine-induced synchronized afterdischarges in the rat hippocampal slice. *Journal of Physiology* (in press).

Traub, R.D., Jefferys, J.G.R. and Miles, R. (1993) Analysis of the propagation of disinhibition-induced after-discharges in the guinea-pig hippocampal slice *in vitro*. *Journal of Physiology*, **472**, 267–87.

Traub, R.D., Jefferys, J.G.R. and Whittington, M.A. (1994) Enhanced NMDA conductance can account for epileptiform activity induced by low magnesium in the rat hippocampal slice. *Journal of Physiology*, **478**, 379–93.

Traub, R.D., Miles, R. and Jefferys, J.G.R. (1993) Synaptic and intrinsic conductances shape picrotoxin-induced synchronized afterdischarges in the guinea-pig hippocampal slice. *Journal of Physiology*, **461**, 525–47.

Traub, R.D., Dudek, F.E., Taylor, C.P. and Knowles, W.D. (1985) Simulation of hippocampal afterdischarges synchronized by electrical interactions. *Neuroscience*, **14**, 1033–8.

Traub, R.D., Wong, R.K.S., Miles, R. and Michelson, H. (1991) A model of a CA3 hippocampal pyramidal neuron incorporating voltage-clamp data on intrinsic conductances. *Journal of Neurophysiology*, **66**, 635–50.

Traub, R.D., Miles, R., Muller, R.V. and Gulyás, A.I. (1992) Functional organization of the hippocampal CA3 region: implications for epilepsy, brain waves and spatial behavior. *Network*, **3**, 1–24.

Traub, R.D., Jefferys, J.G.R., Miles, R. *et al.* (1994) A branching dendritic model of a guinea-pig CA3 pyramidal neurone. *Journal of Physiology*, **481**, 79–95.

Traynelis, S.F. and Dingledine, R. (1988) Potassium-induced spontaneous electrographic seizures in the rat hippocampal slice. *Journal of Neurophysiology*, **59**, 259–76.

Traynelis, S.F. and Dingledine, R. (1989) Role of extracellular space in hyperosmotic suppression of potassium-induced electrographic seizures. *Journal of Neurophysiology*, **61**, 927–38.

Trussel, L.O. and Fischbach, G.D. (1989) Glutamate receptor desensitization and its role in synaptic transmission. *Neuron*, **3**, 209–18.

Vergnes, M., Marescaux, C., Micheletti, G. *et al.* (1982) Spontaneous paroxysmal electroclinical patterns in rat: a model of generalized non-convulsive epilepsy. *Neuroscience Letters*, **33**, 97–101.

von Krosigk, M., Bal, T. and McCormick, D.A. (1993) Cellular mechanisms of a synchronized oscillation in the thalamus. *Science*, **261**, 361–4.

Vyklicky, L., Jr, Benveniste, M. and Mayer, M.L. (1990) Modulation of *N*-methyl-D-aspartic acid receptor desensitization by glycine in mouse cultured hippocampal neurones. *Journal of Physiology*, **428**, 313–31.

Wang, X.-J. (1993) Ionic basis for intrinsic 40 Hz neuronal oscillations. *Neuroreport*, **5**, 221–40.

Westenbroek, R.E., Merrick, D.K. and Catterall, W.A. (1989) Differential subcellular localization of the R_I and R_{II} Na^+ channel subtypes in central neurons. *Neuron*, **3**, 695–704.

Whittington, M.A. and Jefferys, J.G.R. (1994) Epileptic activity outlasts disinhibition after intrahippocampal tetanus toxin in the rat. *Journal of Physiology*, **481**, 593–604.

Whittington, M.A., Traub, R.D. and Jefferys, J.G.R. (1995) Erosion of inhibition contributes to the progression of low magnesium bursts in rat hippocampal slices. *Journal of Physiology*, **486**, 723–34.

Willow, M., Gonoi, T. and Catterall, W.A. (1985) Voltage clamp analysis of the inhibitory actions of diphenylhydantoin and carbamazepine on voltage-sensitive sodium channels in neuroblastoma cells. *Molecular Pharmacology*, **27**, 549–58.

Wong, R.K.S. and Prince, D.A. (1981) Afterpotential generation in hippocampal pyramidal cells. *Journal of Neurophysiology*, **45**, 86–97.

Wong, R.K.S. and Stewart, M. (1992) Different firing patterns generated in dendrites and somata of CA1 pyramidal neurones in guinea-pig hippocampus. *Journal of Physiology*, **457**, 675–87.

Wong, R.K.S. and Watkins, D.J. (1982) Cellular factors influencing GABA response in hippocampal pyramidal cells. *Journal of Neurophysiology*, **48**, 938–51.

Wong, R.K.S., Prince, D.A. and Basbaum, A.I. (1979) Intradendritic recordings from hippocampal neurons. *Proceedings of the National Academy of Science, USA*, **76**, 986–90.

Wyler, A.R., Ojemann, G.A. and Ward, A.A. Jr (1982) Neurons in human epileptic cortex: correlation between unit and EEG activity. *Annals of Neurology*, **11**, 301–8.

7

CLASSIFICATION OF SEIZURES AND EPILEPSIES

Olaf Henriksen

In a textbook on epilepsy, special attention must be given to the classification of seizures as well as to the classification of epileptic syndromes. Several other chapters will deal with specific syndromes, while this chapter will present a 'skeleton' facilitating the classification of each case. In doing so, however, it is important to recognize that some syndromes are well defined and very useful, while others are more vaguely defined; and, for many patients, the seizures and accompanying symptomatology will be accorded to categories which can hardly be called syndromes.

During the past 100 years there have been several attempts to classify epileptic seizures and epilepsy syndromes; thus, several terms have evolved, which, with our present knowledge, have become misleading. Labels such as grand mal and petit mal were used to describe seizures as well as syndromes. Whereas petit mal originally denoted the absence seizure, it was later defined as the epileptic syndrome consisting of absences with generalized bilaterally synchronous 3 Hz spike and wave complexes in the EEG. Despite decades with this definition, petit mal continues frequently to be used to describe any kind of 'small' seizure. A minor seizure with loss of consciousness with or without automatisms resembling an absence would thus be called a petit mal seizure. Specialists dealing with epilepsy have learned that an EEG is necessary to differentiate between an absence (a generalized seizure) and a focal (partial) seizure. People who treat epilepsy infrequently still sometimes use the term petit mal for every seizure which they find unworthy of calling a grand mal seizure. While Lennox (1945) defined the petit mal triad, Janz (1969) used the term petit mal for various age-related syndromes with 'minor seizures', adding to confusion in the use of this label.

Another example of a term, initially a description of a seizure, but ending up as a syndrome, is the psychomotor seizure, which was thought to originate in the temporal lobe, and therefore became synonymous with a temporal lobe seizure, and thus a seizure typical of 'temporal lobe epilepsy'. Recent neurophysiologic studies and experience from epilepsy surgery have demonstrated that such seizures may originate in areas of the brain outside the temporal lobe, especially the frontal lobes. Evidently a need for a new and better classification has been demonstrated.

Classification is necessary for communication and for pooling of data, both for clinicians and researchers. It is of practical importance, since medication is chosen according to seizure type. In addition, for further development and research, a uniform terminology is necessary. This terminology must be based on simple, well-defined facts

Epilepsy in Children. Edited by Sheila Wallace. Published in 1996 by Chapman & Hall, London. ISBN 0 412 56860 8

which are retrievable, understandable, and acceptable to everyone. The epilepsies may be classified according to seizure type and EEG findings – partial or generalized, or according to etiology – idiopathic or primary and symptomatic or secondary epilepsy; or they may be classified according to the anatomic origin of the seizure; for example temporal lobe, frontal lobe, rolandic region or occipital lobe. Precipitating factors, as well as age, may also be of importance.

CLASSIFICATION OF SEIZURES

Increased knowledge and improved diagnostic tools have led to much effort being put into the development of an international classification. Although it would be preferable to categorize all patients according to a syndrome classification, our knowledge is too limited and the diversity and complexity of the epilepsies so large that it has proved necessary to start with a classification of the epileptic seizures. As a result of several workshops organized by the International League Against Epilepsy, the present seizure classification was accepted at the World Congress in Kyoto in 1981 (Commission on Classification and Terminology of the International League Against Epilepsy, 1981). This classification is based on the clinical seizure type and ictal and interictal EEG data. In the previous classification (Gastaut, 1970), the anatomic substrate, as well as etiology and age, were also included. Since both anatomic substrate and etiology may frequently be uncertain, it was decided to omit these criteria and to rely on the clinical picture of the seizure and the EEG data. The development of video-telemetry made it possible to study the various seizures thoroughly, paving the way for a seizure classification which is well defined and universally acceptable.

The classification separates seizures into two main categories: partial and generalized. Partial seizures are divided into simple and complex, depending upon whether con-

sciousness is preserved or not. This has caused debate, partly because complex previously meant that the symptomatology of the seizure was complex, i.e. consisted of several consecutive symptoms often including automatisms. Another major objection has been the problem of evaluating the state of consciousness in each particular seizure. If a patient can respond during a seizure, the consciousness is said to be undisturbed. However, to assess this, an interaction with the patient during a seizure by a specially trained person is required.

Partial seizures are further subdivided according to various symptoms, both subjective and objective. The subjective symptoms will be related by the patient, usually after a seizure, but sometimes also during a seizure, and consist of somatosensory or special sensory symptoms or psychic symptoms. When followed by a complex partial seizure, such an event, which represents a simple partial seizure, is called an aura.

The objective signs may consist of motor symptoms or just impairment of consciousness or a combination of these. Other objective signs may be autonomic symptoms or automatisms. A seizure is often characterized by an evolution of symptoms correlated not only to its origin, but also the route of spread. Guided by the clinical symptoms and the EEG findings precise localization of the epileptogenic source is desirable. As a result of many observations, particularly those obtained in relation to epilepsy surgery (Penfield and Jasper, 1954), and intracranial recordings including stereotactically placed depth electrodes (Munari and Bancaud, 1985), detailed knowledge of cortical representation of various modalities has been obtained. While some seizures may be typical for a certain localization, other seizures, although they may arise from various parts of the frontal lobes or even the temporal lobes, may be clinically indistinguishable. More knowledge about the various 'frontal lobe seizures' has emerged during recent years (Chauvel *et al.*,

1992). When detailed studies of clinical seizures, including video-telemetry, are compared with results of epilepsy surgery and all data are gathered and pooled in a uniform manner, it may some day, be possible to include the anatomic substrate in the seizure classification. With the development of new diagnostic methods, for instance magneto-encephalography (MEG) and magnetic resonance spectroscopy (MRS), improvement of position emission tomography (PET) and single photon emission computed tomography (SPECT), this goal may be reached earlier than anticipated, but for the time being the present classification of epileptic seizures (Commission on Classification and Terminology of the International League Against Epilepsy, 1981) based on the clinical seizure and ictal as well as interictal EEG findings, will have to suffice.

INTERNATIONAL CLASSIFICATION OF EPILEPTIC SEIZURES

Partial (focal, local) seizures

A. *Simple partial seizures*
   (Consciousness not impaired)
   1. With motor signs
      a. Focal motor without march
      b. Focal motor with march (Jacksonian)
      c. Versive
      d. Postural
      e. Phonatory (vocalization or arrest of speech)
   2. With somatosensory or special-sensory symptoms (simple hallucinations, e.g., tingling, light flashes, buzzing)
      a. Somatosensory
      b. Visual
      c. Auditory
      d. Olfactory
      e. Gustatory
      f. Vertiginous
   3. With autonomic symptoms or signs (including epigastric sensation, pallor, sweating, flushing, piloerection and pupillary dilatation)
   4. With psychic symptoms (disturbance of higher cerebral function). These symptoms rarely occur without impairment of consciousness and are much more commonly experienced as complex partial seizures
      a. Dysphasic
      b. Dysmnesic (e.g. déjà-vu)
      c. Cognitive (e.g. dreamy states, distortions of time sense)
      d. Affective (fear, anger, etc.)
      e. Illusions (e.g. macropsia)
      f. Structured hallucinations (e.g. music, scenes)

B. *Complex partial seizures*
   (With impairment of consciousness; may sometimes begin with simple symptomatology)
   1. Simple partial onset followed by impairment of consciousness
      a. With simple partial features (A.1–A.4) followed by impaired consciousness
      b. With automatisms
   2. With impairment of consciousness at onset
      a. With impairment of consciousness only
      b. With features as in A.1–4.
      c. With automatisms

C. *Partial seizures evolving to secondarily generalized seizures*
   (This may be generalized tonic-clonic, tonic, or clonic)
   1. Simple partial seizures (A) evolving to generalized seizures
   2. Complex partial seizures (B) evolving to generalized seizures
   3. Simple partial seizures evolving to complex partial seizures evolving to generalized seizures

II. Generalized seizures (convulsive or non-convulsive)

Clinical seizure type

A. 1. *Absence seizures*
   a. Impairment of consciousness only
   b. With mild clonic components
   c. With atonic components
   d. With tonic components
   e. With automatisms
   f. With autonomic components
   (b through f may be used alone or in combination)
2. *Atypical absence.*
   May have:
   a. Changes in tone that are more pronounced than in A.1
   b. Onset and/or cessation that is not abrupt

B. *Myoclonic seizures*
   Myoclonic jerks (single or multiple)
C. *Clonic seizures*
D. *Tonic seizures*
E. *Tonic-clonic seizures*
F. *Atonic seizures* (Astatic)
   (Combinations of the above may occur, e.g. B and F, C and D)

III. Unclassified epileptic seizures

This category includes all seizures that cannot be classified because of inadequate or incomplete data and some that defy classification in hitherto described categories. This includes some neonatal seizures, e.g. rhythmic eye movements, chewing, and swimming movements. The classification of neonatal seizures is addressed in detail in Chapter 9.

Not all seizures are satisfactorily described by the current classification. Everyone knows what is meant by salaam seizures or infantile spasms, yet these terms do not exist in the classification. This is just one example of many seizures in children and infants, particularly those occurring in the neonatal period, which are difficult to describe using the current classification. A classification of neonatal seizures based on studies with video-EEG recordings has been suggested by Mizrahi and Kellaway (1987) and Volpe (1989). The International League Against Epilepsy (ILAE) Commission on classification is concerning itself with the development of a proposal for a classification of seizures in infants and neonates.

In spite of its limitations, various authors report on the usefulness of the classification in children (Viani *et al.*, 1988; Eslava-Cobos and Nariño, 1989; Ohtsuka *et al.*, 1993). Most seizures can be classified easily; some categories are sometimes so large and heterogeneous, that the classification hardly serves much more than to separate a partial seizure from a generalized seizure. The vast category of complex partial seizures must be subdivided as much as possible according to the initial symptoms and the anatomic substrate. To keep the old misleading term psychomotor seizure, as suggested by some authors (Wyllie and Lüders, 1993), is not recommended.

Several generalized seizures are actually secondarily generalized, and it could be debatable whether they should be classified as generalized seizures or as partial seizures with secondary generalization.

CLASSIFICATION OF SYNDROMES

It is quite clear that with present knowledge and needs, a precise classification, which could not only act as a guide in the choice of medical and surgical treatment, but also include etiology and prognostic factors, is desirable. Such a classification of the epilepsies and epileptic syndromes was proposed by the ILAE in Hamburg in 1985. Since then the Commission on Classification and Terminology of the ILAE has revised the proposal in the light of findings and suggestions emanating from experience with the 1985 scheme (Commission on Classification and Terminology of the International League Against Epilepsy, 1989).

An epileptic syndrome is an epileptic disorder characterized by a cluster of signs and symptoms customarily occurring together. Some syndromes are specific, while other syndromes are rather poorly defined and composed of a heterogeneous group of patients. In the proposed classification of the epilepsies from 1989 (Commission on Classification and Terminology of the International League Against Epilepsy, 1989), some syndromes are categorized according to the anatomic substrate with limited specificity while other syndromes are more clearly defined, with age-related seizures combined with other symptoms. Such syndromes are especially well documented among the epilepsies in childhood. A workshop in Marseilles in 1983 resulted in a book on epileptic syndromes in infancy, childhood, and adolescence in 1985; a second edition was published in 1992 (Roger *et al.*, 1985, 1992). These are considered in detail in Chapters 11–15.

The International Classification of Epilepsies and Epileptic Syndromes is presented below (see also Dreifuss and Henriksen, 1992; Dreifuss, 1993).

Two divisions are used in the classification of the epilepsies. The first separates epilepsies with generalized seizures (generalized epilepsy) from epilepsies with partial or focal seizures (localization-related, partial or focal epilepsies). The other separates epilepsies of known etiology (symptomatic or 'secondary' epilepsies) from those with unknown etiology, presumably genetic epilepsy (idiopathic or primary epilepsy). Cryptogenic epilepsy suggests a secondary epilepsy, but the causation remains hidden.

INTERNATIONAL CLASSIFICATION OF EPILEPSIES AND EPILEPTIC SYNDROMES

1.0 Localization-related (focal, local, partial) epilepsies and syndromes
  1.1 *Idiopathic.* (with age-related onset)
    a. Benign childhood epilepsy with centrotemporal spikes
    b. Childhood epilepsy with occipital paroxysms
  1.2 *Symptomatic.* This category comprises syndromes of individual variability, and is mainly based on anatomic localization, clinical features, seizure types, and etiologic factors (if known).
    1.2.1 Epilepsy characterized by simple partial seizures with the characteristics of seizures:
      a. Arising from frontal lobes
      b. Arising from parietal lobes
      c. Arising from temporal lobes
      d. Arising from occipital lobes
      e. Arising from multiple lobes
      f. Locus of onset unknown
    1.2.2 Characterized by complex partial seizures, that is, attacks with alteration of consciousness often with automatisms
      a. Arising from frontal lobes
      b. Arising from parietal lobes
      c. Arising from temporal lobes
      d. Arising from occipital lobes
      e. Arising from multiple lobes
      f. Locus of onset unknown
    1.2.3 Characterized by secondarily generalized seizures with seizures:
      a. Arising from frontal lobes
      b. Arising from parietal lobes
      c. Arising from temporal lobes
      d. Arising from occipital lobes
      e. Arising from multiple lobes
      f. Locus of onset unknown
  1.3 *Cryptogenic.* Unknown as to whether the syndrome is idiopathic or symptomatic

2.0 Generalized epilepsies and syndromes
  2.1 *Idiopathic* (with age-related onset – listed in order of age)
    a. Benign familial neonatal convulsions (Chapter 9)
    b. Benign neonatal convulsions (Chapter 9)

c. Benign myoclonic epilepsy in infancy (Chapter 11d)
d. Childhood absence epilepsy (pyknolepsy) (Chapter 13a)
e. Juvenile absence epilepsy (Chapter 14a)
f. Juvenile myoclonic epilepsy (impulsive petit mal) (Chapter 14b)
g. Epilepsy with grand mal (GTCS) seizures on awakening (Chapter 14c)

Other generalized idiopathic epilepsies, if they do not belong to one of the above syndromes, can still be classified as generalized idiopathic epilepsies.

2.2 *Cryptogenic or symptomatic* (in order of age)
  a. West syndrome (infantile spasms, Blitz–Nick–Salaam Krampfe) (Chapter 11b)
  b. Lennox–Gastaut syndrome (Chapter 12a)
  c. Epilepsy with myoclonic-astatic seizures (Chapter 12b)
  d. Epilepsy with myoclonic absences (Chapter 13b)

2.3 *Symptomatic*
  2.3.1 Nonspecific etiology
    a. Early myoclonic encephalopathy (Chapter 11a)
  2.3.2 Specific syndromes
    Epileptic seizures may complicate many disease states. Under this heading are included those diseases in which seizures are a presenting or predominant feature (see Chapter 4c, especially)

3.0 Epilepsies and syndromes undetermined whether focal or generalized
  3.1 With both generalized and focal seizures
    a. Neonatal seizures (Chapter 9)
    b. Severe myoclonic epilepsy in infancy (Chapter 11e)
    c. Epilepsy with continuous spike-waves during slow wave sleep (Chapter 13d)
    d. Acquired epileptic aphasia (Landau–Kleffner syndrome) (Chapter 13d)
    e. Other undetermined epilepsies not defined above
  3.2 Without unequivocal generalized or focal features.
    All cases with generalized tonic-clonic seizures in which clinical and EEG findings do not permit classification as clearly generalized or localization-related such as in many cases of generalized seizures occurring during sleep.

4.0 Special syndromes
  4.1 Situation-related seizures (Gelegenheitsanfälle)
    a. Febrile convulsions (Chapter 10)
    b. Isolated seizures or isolated status epilepticus
    c. Seizures occurring only when there is an acute metabolic or toxic event due to factors such as alcohol, drugs, eclampsia, nonketotic hyperglycinemia, uremia, etc. (see especially Chapters 4c and 21).

SYMPTOMATIC EPILEPSIES WITH LOCALIZATION-RELATED SEIZURES

The etiology is very variable. The common feature is the presence of a focal epileptogenic abnormality.

Seizures arising from the temporal lobe

General characteristics (features strongly suggestive of the diagnosis):

1. Simple partial seizures typically characterized by autonomic and/or psychic symptoms and certain sensory phenomena, such as olfactory, gustatory, auditory (including illusions), and vertiginous

seizures. Most common is an epigastric, often rising, sensation.

2. Complex partial seizures often but not always beginning with motor arrest, typically followed by oroalimentary automatism. Reactive automatisms frequently follow. Postictal confusion usually occurs. The duration is typically more than 1 minute followed by amnesia. There is frequently a history of febrile seizures and a family history of seizures is common. Memory deficits may occur. Hypometabolism is frequently seen in temporal lobe lesions. Unilateral or bilateral temporal spikes are common on EEG. Onset is usually in childhood or young adulthood. Seizures may progress to become generalized tonic-clonic.

Hippocampal (mesiobasal limbic or primary rhinencephalic psychomotor) epilepsy

This is the most common form of epilepsy arising in the temporal lobe, and the symptoms are those described in the previous paragraphs except that auditory and vertiginous symptoms may not occur. Seizures are characterized by rising epigastric discomfort, nausea, marked autonomic signs and other symptoms, including borborygmia, belching, pallor, fullness of the face, flushing of the face, arrest of respiration, pupillary dilatation, fear, panic, and olfactory–gustatory hallucinations. Seizures occur in clusters at intervals or randomly, and are of about 2 minutes duration. Generalized tonic-clonic seizures may follow progressive propagation of discharges. The interictal EEG typically shows medial or mesial anterior temporal sharp waves.

Lateral temporal epilepsy

Seizures are characterized by auras of auditory hallucinations or illusions or dreamy states; visual perceptual hallucinations or language disorder, in the case of a language-dominant hemisphere focus. The symptoms may progress to complex partial seizures if propagation to mesial temporal structures occurs. The surface EEG shows unilateral or bilateral mid-temporal or posterior-temporal spikes which are most prominent in the lateral derivations.

Seizures arising from the frontal lobe

General characteristic (features that are strongly suggestive of the diagnosis): frequent short attacks with impairment of consciousness; complex partial seizures with minimal or no postictal confusion; presentations similar to nonepileptic attack disorder; rapid secondary generalization; frequent status epilepticus; prominent motor manifestations; automatisms which are complex, stereotyped and gestural at onset; urinary incontinence; and drop attacks.

Supplementary motor seizures

Here the seizure patterns are postural, simple focal tonic, with localization, speech arrest, fencing postures, and complex focal features.

Cingulate

Seizure patterns are complex partial with complex motor gestural automatisms at the onset. Vegetative signs are common, as are changes in mood and affect.

Anterior frontopolar region

Seizure patterns include initial loss of contact, versive movements of head and eyes, axial clonic jerks and falls and autonomic signs. Secondary generalization is especially common.

Orbitofrontal

Seizure patterns are complex partial with initial motor and gestural automatisms, olfactory hallucinations, and illusions and autonomic signs.

Dorsolateral

The seizure patterns may be tonic or less commonly clonic with versive eye and head movements and speech arrest.

Opercular (perisylvian, insular)

Characteristics include mastication, salivation, swallowing, laryngeal symptoms, epigastric aura with fear, and vegetative phenomenon. Simple partial seizures, particularly partial clonic facial seizures, are common. If secondary sensory change occurs, numbness may be a symptom, particularly in the hands. Bilateral movement of the upper extremities may be seen.

Epilepsies of the motor cortex (perirolandic)

These are mainly characterized by simple partial seizures, and their localization depends on the side and topography of the area involved. In cases of the lower prerolandic area, there may be speech arrest, vocalization or dysphasia, tonic-clonic movements of the face on the contralateral side, or swallowing. Generalization of the seizure frequently occurs. In the rolandic area, partial motor seizures without march or jacksonian seizures, particularly beginning in the contralateral upper extremities, occur. The nature of the attack is determined by the direction of the seizure propagation. In the case of seizures involving the paracentral lobule, tonic movements of the ipsilateral foot may occur, in addition to the expected contralateral leg movements. Postictal or Todd's paralysis is frequent. It should be noted that some epilepsies are difficult to assign to specific lobes. Such epilepsies include central epilepsy, which includes pre- and postcentral symptomatology, as in perirolandic seizures. Such overlap to adjacent anatomic regions is also seen in opercular epilepsy.

Parietal lobe epilepsies

Seizures are predominantly sensory attacks with many characteristics. Positive phenomena consist of tingling and a feeling of electricity, which may be localized or may spread in a jacksonian manner. There may be a desire to move a body part, or a sensation as if a part were being moved. Muscle tone may be lost. The parts most frequently involved are those with the largest cortical representation, for example, the hand, arm, and face. There may be tongue sensations of crawling, stiffness, or coldness, and facial sensory phenomena may occur bilaterally. Occasionally, an intraabdominal sensation of sinking, choking or nausea may occur, particularly in cases of inferior and lateral parietal lobe involvement. Rarely, there may be pain, and this may take the form of a superficial burning dysesthesia or a vague, very severe, episodic painful sensation. Parietal lobe visual phenomena may occur as photopsias or as hallucinations of a formed variety. Metamorphopsia with distortions, foreshortenings, and elongations may occur; and are more frequently seen with non-dominant hemisphere discharges. Negative phenomena include numbness, feeling as if a body part were absent, and a loss of awareness of a part or a half of the body, known as asomatognosia. This is particularly the case in right-sided attacks. Severe vertigo or disorientation in space may be indicative of inferior parietal lobe seizures. Dominant parietal seizures result in a variety of receptive or conductive speech disturbances. Well-lateralized genital sensations suggest paracentral involvement. Rotatory or postural motor phenomena may occur. Seizures of the paracentral lobule have a tendency to become secondarily generalized.

Occipital lobe epilepsy

The clinical seizure manifestations usually, but not exclusively, include visual manifestations. Elementary visual seizures are characterized by fleeting visual manifestations that may be either negative (scotoma, hemianopsia, amaurosis) or, more commonly, positive (sparks or flashes, phosphenes). Such sensations appear in the visual field contralateral to the discharge in the specific visual cortex, but spread to the whole visual field. Perceptive illusions, in which the objects appear to be distorted, may occur. The following varieties can be distinguished: a change in size – macropsia or micropsia; a change in distance; an inclination of objects in a given plane of space; and, distortion of objects or a sudden change of shape (metamorphopsia). Visual hallucinatory seizures are occasionally characterized by complex visual perceptions, e.g., colourful scenes of varying complexity. In some cases, the scene is distorted or made smaller and, in rare instances, the subject sees his own image (autoscopy). Such illusional and hallucinatory visual seizures involve epileptic discharge in the temporo-parieto-occipital junction. The initial signs may also include clonic and/or tonic contraversion of the eyes and head or the eyes only (oculoclonic or oculogyric deviation), palpebral jerks, and forced closure of the eyelids. A sensation of ocular oscillation or of the whole body may occur, as may headache or migraine. The discharge may spread to the temporal lobe, producing seizure manifestations of either lateral posterior temporal or hippocampo-amygdala epilepsies. When the primary focus is located in the supracalcarine area, the discharge can spread forward on the suprasylvian convexity or the mesial surface, leading to seizures mimicking those of parietal lobe or frontal motor seizures. Occasional secondary generalization occurs.

Based on the workshop in Marseille in 1985, several epileptic syndromes in children have been defined. The definitions do not imply a complete and unanimous agreement, but only a general consensus based on a compromise (Roger *et al.*, 1985, 1992). These syndromes are included under 2, 3 and 4 above. In addition, benign partial epilepsies

(Chapters 13c, and 14e) have been delineated.

Epilepsia partialis continua is examined in more detail in Chapter 15. Briefly, in type I (Kojewnikow), partial motor seizures are well localized. The EEG shows a normal background and focal paroxysmal disturbances. The onset is at any age. An etiology is frequently demonstrable – tumour, vascular. No progressive evolution occurs except that of the causal lesion.

In type II (Rasmussen) onset is at 2–10 years (peak at 6). Partial motor seizures predominate, often associated with others, e.g. myoclonus. There is a progressive motor deficit. Mental retardation is usual. The EEG shows an abnormal background which is asymmetric and slow and there are ictal discharges. Any anatomic lesion, when present, is diffuse and progressive. Viral etiology is strongly suspected. Treatment may be by hemispherectomy.

These attempts at a classification of epileptic syndromes in childhood will be elaborated as increasing knowledge of the etiology of these syndromes is attained. Hopefully this will be derived from a better recognition of the syndromes, coupled with modern research in molecular biology and genetics. The specificity of the various syndromes will increase, with resultant impacts on future antiepileptic therapy. While an optimal classification of the epilepsies is the ultimate goal, it is important currently to rely on a uniform utilization of the International Classification of Seizures, as one of the cornerstones in the diagnosis and treatment of the epilepsies, as well as a basis for the future development of epileptology.

REFERENCES

Chauvel, P., Delgado-Escueta, A.V., Hallgren, E. and Bancaud, J. (eds) (1992) Frontal lobe seizures and epilepsies, in *Advances in Neurology*, Vol. 57, Raven, New York, pp. 59–88.

Commission on Classification and Terminology of the International League Against Epilepsy

(1981) Proposal for revised clinical and electroencephalographic classification of epileptic seizures. *Epilepsia*, **22**, 489–501.

Commission on Classification and Terminology of the International League Against Epilepsy (1989) Proposal for revised classification of epilepsies and epileptic syndromes. *Epilepsia*, **30**, 389–99.

Dreifuss, F.E. (1993) Classification of epilepsies in childhood, in *Paediatric Epilepsy, Diagnosis and Therapy*, (eds E. Dodson and J.M. Pellock), Demos, New York, pp. 45–56.

Dreifuss, F.E. and Henriksen, O. (1992) Classification of epileptic seizures and the epilepsies. *Acta Neurologica Scandinavica* **86** (Suppl. 140), 8–17.

Eslava-Cobos, J. and Nariño, D. (1989) Experience with the International League Against Epilepsy proposals for classification of epileptic seizures and the epilepsies and epileptic syndromes in a pediatric outpatient clinic. *Epilepsia*, **30**, 112–5.

Gastaut, H. (1970) Clinical and electroencephalographic classification of epileptic seizures. *Epilepsia*, **11**, 102–13.

Janz, D. (1969) *Die Epilepsien*, Thieme, Stuttgart.

Lennox, W.G. (1945) The petit mal syndrome. *Journal of the American Medical Association*, **129**, 1069–73.

Mizrahi, E.M. and Kellaway, P. (1987) Characterization and classification of neonatal seizures. *Neurology*, **37**, 1837–44.

Munari, C. and Bancaud, J. (1985). The role of stereoelectroencephalography (SEEG) in the evaluation of partial epileptic seizures, in *The Epilepsies*, (eds R.J. Porter and P.L. Morselli), Butterworths, London, pp. 267–306.

Ohtsuka, Y., Ohno, S., Oka, E. and Ohtahara, S. (1993) Classification of epilepsies and epileptic syndromes of childhood according to the 1989 ILAE Classification. *Journal of Epilepsy*, **6**, 272–6.

Penfield, W. and Jasper, H. (1954) *Epilepsy and the Functional Anatomy of the Human Brain*, Little, Brown, Boston.

Roger, J., Dravet, C., Bureau, M. *et al.* (eds) (1985) *Epileptic Syndromes in Infancy, Childhood and Adolescence*, John Libbey Eurotext, Paris.

Roger, J., Bureau, M., Dravet, Ch. *et al.* (1992) *Epileptic Syndromes in Infancy, Childhood and Adolescence*, 2nd edn, John Libbey, Paris.

Viani, F., Beghi, E., Atza, G. and Gulotta, M.P. (1988) Classification of epileptic syndromes: advantages and limitations for evaluation of childhood epileptic syndromes in clinical practice. *Epilepsia*, **29**, 440–5.

Volpe, J.J. (1989) Neonatal seizures: current concepts and revised classification. *Pediatrics*, **84**, 422–8.

Wyllie, E. and Lüders, H., (1993) Classification of seizures, in *The Treatment of Epilepsy, Principles and Practice*, (ed. E. Wyllie), Lea & Febiger, Philadelphia, pp. 359–68.

Genetics

8

R. Mark Gardiner

INTRODUCTION

Unequivocal evidence exists for a genetic contribution to the etiology of certain human and animal epilepsies. Inherited human epilepsies probably account for about 20% of all patients with epilepsy: the proportion is even higher in children. The familial clustering of human epilepsy has long been recognized, and numerous investigations in the last 50 years, including twin and family studies, have clarified the varieties of epilepsy in which inheritance is a factor.

The human genetic epilepsies can be most conveniently categorized into those displaying a mendelian pattern of inheritance and therefore determined by mutations in a single gene, and those in which the pattern is non-mendelian or 'complex' and which can therefore be assumed to arise from the interaction of several genes together with environmental factors. In the former, epilepsy is usually one component of a complex neurologic phenotype, whereas in the latter recurrent seizures often occur in individuals who have no other apparent neurologic abnormality. Over 150 mendelian disorders are associated with epilepsy, but they are individually rare and collectively account for no more than 1% of patients with epilepsy. The familial, non-mendelian epilepsies are in contrast quite common and often show age-dependent penetrance with peak onset in childhood. Epilepsy as part of a phenotype arising from mutations in the mitochondrial genome displays, of course, a maternal pattern of inheritance; affected males never pass the disease to their offspring.

The molecular genetic basis of the inherited epilepsies is almost entirely unknown. It is true that the molecular basis of many of the mendelian disorders complicated by epilepsy is understood, but in these the mechanism of seizure generation, for example an alteration in the circulating levels of metabolites such as ammonia or an amino acid or gross structural abnormality of the brain as occurs in tuberous sclerosis, is often indirect. Although it is reasonable to assume that the genes involved play some direct role in the control of neuronal excitability, the fundamental molecular basis of the more common familial epilepsies remains obscure. The prospect that the revolution in molecular genetic techniques will allow these epilepsies to be understood at a molecular level is responsible for the current revival of interest in the genetics of the epilepsies.

The genetic aspects of the epilepsies have been the subject of several recent reviews (Bird, 1992; Dichter and Buchhalter, 1993). In this chapter the strategies now available for investigation of the molecular genetic basis of the epilepsies will be reviewed. The genetics of childhood epilepsies will then be considered, with particular emphasis on the evidence for a genetic contribution to etiology; and, on those epilepsies for which progress has been made towards identification of their genetic bases. Finally, aspects of

Epilepsy in Children. Edited by Sheila Wallace. Published in 1996 by Chapman & Hall, London. ISBN 0 412 56860 8

genetic counselling for the familial epilepsies of childhood are briefly enumerated.

STRATEGIES FOR MOLECULAR GENETIC ANALYSIS OF CHILDHOOD EPILEPSY

Recent advances have allowed the fusion of classic genetic methodology and molecular biological techniques, providing new approaches to the investigation of the molecular basis of human inherited diseases. These have been applied with most spectacular success to mendelian disorders, but recent advances encourage the hope and expectation that it will also be possible to dissect those disorders displaying a complex, nonmendelian pattern of inheritance.

The strategies available can be broadly divided into positional cloning and candidate gene analysis, although there is considerable overlap between the two. In the former, the map localization of the locus responsible for a disease trait is first established by linkage analysis. The interval containing the disease gene is subsequently refined to an interval – usually about 1cM or one million base pairs – which is amenable to molecular cloning techniques. In the latter, a candidate gene is selected on the basis of knowledge of the pathophysiology of the disease and directly analysed for sequence variation. There is considerable overlap between the two approaches. As the transcriptional map of the human genome becomes more complete, an obvious 'candidate' gene may already be known to be located within the genetic interval to which a disease locus is mapped by linkage.

Moreover, linkage analysis represents one method by which the role of a particular candidate gene in a disease can be investigated.

POSITIONAL CLONING

In the last decade, the development of methods for detecting polymorphism at the DNA level has revolutionized linkage analysis as a method for mapping disease genes in man. The genetic marker map of the human genome has been transformed from a handful of protein polymorphisms to almost complete coverage with several thousand highly polymorphic DNA-based polymorphic loci (NIH/CEPH collaborative mapping group 1992; Weissenbach *et al*, 1992).

This strategy has been applied with great success to mendelian disorders, and carried to a successful conclusion – isolation of the disease gene – especially in those disorders, such as neurofibromatosis type 1, in which gross chromosomal rearrangements have provided a 'short-cut' to the gene (Collins, 1992). Successful mapping of two mendelian epilepsies, benign familial neonatal convulsions (Chapter 9) and progressive myoclonic epilepsy of Unverricht and Lundborg (Chapter 15a), (see below) has been achieved, but the genes have yet to be isolated.

Linkage analysis is of course much more difficult to apply to diseases which do not display mendelian segregation. These include all the more common human diseases with a genetic component in their etiology: asthma, diabetes mellitus, cardiovascular disease, major psychoses, and the epilepsies. The problems involved may conspire to generate both false-positive and false-negative results and in general reduce the statistical power provided by a given family resource (Lander, 1989; Ott, 1990; Risch, 1990). The increased resolution and informativeness of the current genetic maps allow hope that dissection of the genetic basis of these nonmendelian disorders will prove feasible.

CANDIDATE GENE ANALYSIS

The role of a candidate gene in the etiology of a genetic disease can be directly examined either by linkage analysis or by direct mutational analysis of the gene in affected individuals.

Linkage analysis is carried out in appropriate families using an intragenic or close polymorphism. In nonmendelian disorders uncertainty concerning the mode of inheritance and penetrance of disease alleles reduces the power of this approach. Such polymorphism can also be used in association studies, comparing the frequency of particular alleles in affected individuals with that in members of a control population.

The polymerase chain reaction has rendered direct analysis of a gene a more feasible approach, and the statistical basis of such analysis has recently been considered (Sobell, Heston and Sommer, 1992). Functionally important regions of the gene are examined in order to detect a Variation Affecting Protein Structure or Expression (VAPSE analysis). Various methodologies are available to achieve this, including single-strand conformation polymorphism (SSCP), heteroduplex analysis or direct di-deoxy sequencing. If a sequence variation is identified its significance can be evaluated by considering its functional consequences (such as alteration of a highly conserved amino acid) and determining whether it is significantly associated with the disease trait both in family-based linkage studies and population-based association studies.

The recent explosion of work in molecular neurobiology has led to cloning of a host of candidate epilepsy genes. Although the molecular and cellular basis of the common genetic epilepsies is entirely unknown, it is reasonable to propose that a disturbance of neuronal excitability must occupy a central role in seizure generation.

Of the 30 000 or so genes expressed in neurones, those encoding membrane proteins directly mediating neuronal excitability can therefore be regarded as candidates for the site of mutations which could be expected to result in an epilepsy phenotype. Ion channel proteins are a prominent class of such genes. These can be conveniently divided into the ligand-gated and voltage-gated ion channels. Amongst the former,

genes encoding subunits of excitatory amino acid receptors (McNamara, 1992) and the principal inhibitory receptor, the $GABA_A$ receptor (Cutting *et al.*, 1992), have been isolated and mapped. Of the latter, at least one human brain-specific voltage-gated K^+ channel has been cloned (Grupe *et al.*, 1990).

Mutations in skeletal muscle sodium and chloride ion channels have recently been shown to cause the human diseases hyperkalemic periodic paralysis and paramyotonia congenita (Rojas *et al.*, 1991; McClatchey *et al.*, 1992), and Thomsen's disease (Koch *et al.*, 1992). Most recently, mutations in the $\alpha 1$ subunit of the glycine receptor have been described in familial hyperekplexia (Shiang *et al.*, 1993). The reasonable proposition that ion channel mutations may at least account for some of the genetic epilepsies is now, at last, amenable to testing.

GENETICS OF CHILDHOOD EPILEPSIES

The major epilepsies of childhood with a genetic basis are described in this section. Their clinical features are considered elsewhere, and the focus in this section is on studies of their inheritance.

MENDELIAN GENETIC EPILEPSIES

There are 163 mendelian disorders listed in McKusick (1990), which include epilepsy as a component of the phenotype. A significant proportion of these may present with recurrent seizures during childhood. The diagnosis is usually revealed by associated features or on imaging or biochemical investigations. There may of course be no affected relatives. A selection of these conditions is considered, including in particular those in which recent advances have occurred in our understanding of their genetic basis.

Benign familial neonatal convulsions (BFNC) (Chapter 9)

This rare autosomal dominant idiopathic epilepsy was first described by Rett and

Teubel (1964). Since that time at least 20 pedigrees have been reported (Plouin, 1992). In most cases seizures start during the first week. The seizures may be generalized tonic-clonic or focal. The newborn infants are otherwise healthy – the perinatal history is unremarkable and investigations including neuroimaging are unremarkable. Although seizures usually remit within a few months, afebrile seizures recur in infancy or childhood in about 10%.

Segregation in well-documented families (Zonana, Silvey and Strimling, 1984) revealed a 41% incidence in at-risk individuals and no male-to-male transmission, suggesting autosomal dominant inheritance with high but not complete penetrance.

BFNC was the first epileptic syndrome to be localized by linkage analysis. A large, four generation family with 19 affected individuals was studied by Leppert *et al.* (1989). A random genome search was undertaken. Two marker loci on the long arm of chromosome 20 were found to be linked: D20S20 and D20S19. The maximum lod score with the two loci combined was 5.64, unequivocal evidence that the disease locus was in that region.

This localization has subsequently been replicated in additional pedigrees, but evidence for genetic (locus) heterogeneity in this condition has also emerged. Ryan and colleagues (1991) studied two further families segregating for BFNC. The individual pedigrees were too small to give independent statistically significant results, but a positive lod score was only obtained in one family, in which recurrent seizures had persisted to age 1 year in several affected individuals. Most recently, linkage has been identified to a marker on chromosome 8q, D8S88, in a BFNC family unlinked to the markers on 20q (Lewis *et al.*, 1993).

Work now in progress is aimed at positional cloning of the disease gene. This task is rendered difficult by the rarity of the disease,

incomplete penetrance, and locus heterogeneity.

Huntington's disease

This is an autosomal dominant disorder characterized by degeneration of neurons most prominently in the caudate nucleus and putamen. The characteristic involuntary movements are accompanied by psychiatric symptoms and progressive dementia. Although seizures occur in only a minority (approx 10%) of male adult-onset patients, they are more frequent in those few subjects with onset of symptoms before age 10 years.

Huntington's disease (HD) was the first genetic disorder to be mapped by linkage analysis using a restriction fragment length polymorphism (Gusella *et al.*, 1983). HD was mapped to chromosome 4 by linkage to the marker D4S10 – one of the first 13 DNA markers tested. No crossovers were detected between HD and this marker in a large section of a very extensive Venezuelan pedigree or in an independent American HD family with 14 affected members.

After a further decade of effort, the HD gene was identified in 1993 (Huntington's Disease Collaborative Research Group, 1993). Analysis of patients with Wolf–Hirschorn syndrome, caused by heterozygous deletion on 4p, localized D4S10 to the terminal 4p16 band. Progress was hindered by the absence of chromosomal deletions or translocations, which can serve to position precisely the disease gene. Saturation mapping and haplotype analysis indicated the existence of multiple independent HD mutations and a most likely location between D4S180 and D4S182 (Gusella and MacDonald, 1993).

Transcripts within this region were identified using exon trapping, and one of these, ITI5, contained an expanded (CAG)n trinucleotide repeat which was present in all 150 HD families tested. The ITI5 mRNA encodes a protein, called Huntingtin, of

>3130 amino acids with no clear resemblance to any known protein. The length of the trinucleotide repeat on HD chromosomes shows an inverse correlation with the age of onset.

Tuberous sclerosis

About 90% of patients with tuberous sclerosis complex (TSC) have epilepsy which may be manifest by generalized or partial seizures. Infantile spasms occur in 30% of those with seizures (Gomez, 1988). Typical clinical findings include mental retardation, facial angiofibromata, depigmented skin patches and hamartomatous tumours in organs including the brain, retina, kidney and heart (Chapter 16).

Inheritance is autosomal dominant with reduced penetrance and a probable high new mutation rate. Linkage studies have identified genetic (locus) heterogeneity with loci for tuberous sclerosis complex (TSC) on human chromosomes 9q and 16p.

Linkage between TSC and the ABO blood group locus on distal 9q was first reported in a study of 19 UK families, with a lod score of 3.85 at $\theta = 0$ (Fryer *et al.*, 1987). Subsequently, families unlinked to this 9q region were identified, and evidence was obtained for additional TSC loci on chromosomes 11q and 12q (Smith *et al.*, 1990; Fahsold, Rott and Lorenz, 1991).

The situation was clarified by a study collating phenotypic and genotypic information on 1622 members of 128 families, following reassessment of affection status using uniform diagnostic criteria. One locus (TSC1), accounting for approximately half of the families, was found to map in the region of D9S10 on 9q34, but no evidence in support of major loci on 11q or 12q was found (Sampson *et al.*, 1992). Soon afterwards a TSC locus was identified near the region of PKD 1 on chromosome 16p13 (Kandt *et al.*, 1992). Work is in progress to clone these two genes which cause TSC.

Neurofibromatosis type 1 (NF1)

NF-1 (von Recklinghausen's disease) is characterized by *cafe-au-lait* spots, cutaneous neurofibromata, axillary freckling, mental retardation, skeletal defects, and several types of intracranial tumours including neurofibromata, neuromata, gliomata, and meningiomata (Chapter 16).

Epilepsy is documented in around 30% of children with NF-1. Recurrent seizures are presumably related to the intracranial hamartomata and heterotopias of neurons and glial cells.

The NF1 gene was localized to chromosome 17 by linkage analysis in 1987 (Barker *et al.*, 1987) and the disease gene region subsequently narrowed to about 3 cM of 17q11.2. Data from two NF1 patients with balanced translocations in this region further narrowed the candidate interval, and the NF1 gene was cloned simultaneously by two groups in 1990 (Cawthon *et al.*, 1990; Wallace *et al.*, 1990). NF1 is a tumour-suppressor gene, the product of which acts upstream of *ras*. The NF1 gene encodes a ubiquitous protein homologous to p120^{GAP}, the GTPase activating protein (GAP), for the products of the *ras* protooncogenes. There is a high mutation rate and most NF1 patients have unique mutations, restricting opportunities for DNA diagnostics.

The neuronal ceroid lipofuscinoses

The neuronal ceroid lipofuscinoses (NCL) are a group of inherited neurodegenerative disorders, several types of which have their onset in childhood. Inheritance of these childhood forms is autosomal recessive. They are characterized by the accumulation of autofluorescent lipopigment (with features of both ceroid and lipofuscin – hence the name) in neurons and other cell types. Three main subtypes are recognized on the basis of age of onset and ultrastructural features: infantile (Haltia–Santuavori disease, CLN1), late-infantile (Jansky–Bielschowsky disease, locus CLN2), and juvenile (Spielmeyer–Sjögren–

Vogt, Batten's disease, locus CLN3). More details are given in Chapters 4c and 15a.

A positional cloning strategy was initiated for these diseases several years ago and the chromosomal location of CLN1 and CLN3 has been determined.

Infantile NCL is enriched in the Finnish population with an incidence of 1 in 20 000. Onset is age 8–20 months with seizures, visual failure, ataxia, and choreoathetosis. Granular osmiophilic deposits are seen on electronmicroscopy. Linkage to a marker on chromosome 1p, D1S57, was established (Jarvela *et al.*, 1991) using 26 Finnish families.

The map localization has subsequently been refined by the identification of allelic association with haplotypes formed by alleles at the loci D16S62 and L-MYC (Hellsten *et al.*, 1993). Prenatal diagnosis has been carried out using linked DNA markers and work is in progress to clone the disease gene.

Juvenile-onset NCL (Batten's disease) presents in the latter half of the first decade with visual failure followed by seizures and dementia. Lymphocytes are vacuolated on light microscopy and so-called 'finger-print' profiles are the characteristic ultrastructural feature.

Linkage to the haptoglobin locus using 26 families allowed assignment of CLN3 to chromosome 16 (Eiberg, Gardiner and Moberg, 1989). Localization was subsequently refined to the region 16p12 by a combination of linkage analysis using additional families and markers combined with physical mapping using somatic cell hybrid analysis and in situ hybridization (Callen *et al.*, 1991). Subsequent studies using 15 highly informative microsatellite loci in a total of 70 families has identified three loci (D16S288, D16S298 and D16S299) in strong allelic association with CLN3, suggesting that CLN3 lies within 1 cM of this group of loci. Haplotype analysis indicates a strong founder effect, with the majority of CLN3 chromosomes having a common origin (Mitchison *et al.*, 1993).

Classic late-infantile NCL is characterized by the onset of seizures and progressive dementia at the age of 2–4 years. The typical ultrastructural appearance is that of 'curvilinear profiles'. This variety has been shown not to be an allelic variant of either the juvenile or infantile subtypes (Williams *et al.*, 1993). A genome search is underway and to date approximately 40% of the genome has been excluded as the site of the CLN2 locus.

Progressive myoclonic epilepsy – Unverricht–Lundborg type

Several varieties of so-called progressive myoclonic epilepsy (PME) have been recognized in which neurologic deterioration is associated with both sporadic nonepileptic myoclonus and epileptic seizures. These are reviewed in Chapter 15a and include Lafora body disease, Unverricht–Lundborg disease (ULD), Baltic myoclonus epilepsy (Koskiniemi, 1986), and Mediterranean myoclonus (Genton *et al.*, 1990). Current evidence suggests that the latter three types are genetically homogeneous.

PME Unverricht–Lundborg type is one of the diseases enriched in the Finnish population, with a prevalence of 1 in 20 000 births. Onset is usually between 6 and 15 years with severe incapacitating stimulus-sensitive myoclonus. Mild mental deterioration, ataxia and dysarthia evolve associated with nonspecific histologic changes. Lafora bodies are not found. In so-called Baltic myoclonus the seizures are more varied and phenytoin produces an acceleration of neurologic deterioration.

In a group of 107 Finnish patients with ULD the proportion of affected siblings was 26% (Norio and Koskiniemi, 1979) and a high degree of consanguinity was noted. Inheritance is autosomal recessive.

This disease locus has been mapped to chromosome 21 (Lehesjoki *et al.*, 1991). After testing 64 DNA markers in a group of 11 families including 26 affected individuals, linkage was identified with multipoint analysis giving a maximal lod score of 10.08 with three markers in 21q22.3. Refined mapping of this locus, designated EPM1, allowed its assignment to a region of 20 cM with a maximum multipoint lod score of 11.04 at loci PFKL-D21S154 (Lehesjoki *et al.*, 1992). The localization has been further refined by conventional recombinational mapping using microsatellite loci to a region of 7 cM and by so-called linkage disequilibrium mapping to a region of 0.3 cM. This represents a physical distance of approximately 300 Kb, and work is in progress to clone this gene.

Myoclonic epilepsy-ragged red fibers (MERRF)

It is now well recognized that mutations in the mitochondrial genome (mt DNA) cause human disease. The mitochondrial genome is a circular DNA molecule, 16 569 bp long, present in up to 10 copies per mitochondrion. It encodes just 13 mRNAs specifying components of the inner mitochondrial membrane respiratory chain, two ribosomal RNAs, and 22 transfer RNAs. mtDNA is maternally inherited.

Point mutations and major structural alterations (deletions and duplications) in mtDNA have been documented in association with human disease. Two mitochondrial disorders with CNS involvement manifested in part as epilepsy have been described, which appear to be caused by point mutations in mitochondrial tRNA genes. These are myoclonic epilepsy with ragged red fibers (MERRF) and mitochondrial encephalomyopathy, lactic acidosis and stroke-like episodes (MELAS). The characteristics of the epileptic manifestations are reviewed in Chapter 15a.

The classic features of MERRF include epilepsy, intention myoclonus, muscle weakness, progressive ataxia, and deafness. Shofner *et al.* (1990) described an A to G transition mutation at nucleotide pair 8344 in the pseudouridyl loop of the tRNA^{lys} gene in three unrelated MERRF families. The patients were heteroplasmic, that is to say both normal and mutated mtDNA populations were present. The altered nucleotide is highly conserved, the base change was not observed in 75 controls, and this mutation has now been demonstrated in most MERRF families. These observations have provided the first confirmation that epilepsy can be caused by deficiencies in mitochondrial energy production, and raise the question of whether mutations in mtDNA could explain, at least in part, the well-recognized but unexplained maternal influence on seizure susceptibility.

NONMENDELIAN GENETIC EPILEPSIES

Most common familial epilepsies do not display a pattern of inheritance of a mendelian nature. The incidence of epilepsy in relatives of probands is generally much lower than occurs in mendelian disorders, and segregation analysis does not allow the phenotype to be attributed to the action of mutant alleles, either recessive or dominant, at a single locus. This pattern of inheritance is usually described as 'complex', and the assumption is made that the trait arises from the interaction of alleles at several loci (oligogenic or polygenic inheritance depending on the number). If environmental factors are also invoked, the inheritance pattern is described as 'multifactorial'. In several epileptic syndromes segregation studies have provided conflicting results, or at least results consistent with several different interpretations. Once a mendelian pattern is lost, formal segregation analysis may lack the power to distinguish between several possible underlying mechanisms of inheritance. The difficulties are compounded in the genetic analysis of the epilepsies by uncertainties concerning phenotype definition and age-dependent penetrance. Such uncertainties are hardly surprising in a trait or phenotype which involves transitory disturbances in an organ as complex as the mammalian brain.

Common familial epileptic syndromes of childhood which have been extensively studied and for which there is good evidence for a genetic contribution to etiology include juvenile myoclonic epilepsy (JME), childhood absence epilepsy (CAE), and benign childhood epilepsy with centrotemporal spikes (BCECTS). These are considered here.

Juvenile myoclonic epilepsy

This is a common idiopathic generalized epilepsy (IGE) with a significant genetic component in its etiology (see Chapter 14b). It was first delineated as a distinct clinical and electrophysiologic syndrome by Janz and Christian (1957). The age of onset is between 8 and 26 years. The characteristic clinical feature is myoclonic seizures which are brief muscle contractions usually involving the upper limbs symmetrically. They commonly occur on awakening and consciousness is retained. Generalized tonic-clonic seizures also occur in the majority, and absence seizures in a minority.

The characteristic, but not pathognomonic, EEG abnormality is bilateral and symmetric polyspike and wave complexes. The disorder is nonprogressive and usually responds to continued therapy with antiepilepsy drugs.

The mode of inheritance of JME is uncertain, although several studies have demonstrated an increased incidence of JME and other idiopathic generalized epilepsies in relatives of probands with JME. In the studies by Janz (1969), Tsuboi and Christian (1973), and Sundqvist (1990) a family history of epilepsy was present in up to 25% of patients. Evidence has been obtained for autosomal dominant (Delgado-Escueta *et al.*, 1990), autosomal recessive (Panayiotopolous and Obeid, 1989), two-locus (Greenberg *et al.*, 1989), and multifactorial (Andermann, 1982) models of inheritance. These observations may reflect genuine variation in the mode of inheritance in different kindreds or merely differences in criteria for phenotype definition. EEG abnormalities, for example, may be observed in asymptomatic relatives and it is, of course, unknown whether these are a subclinical expression of the JME trait.

Evidence for linkage of a locus predisposing to JME (designated EJM1) to the HLA region of chromosome 6p was first reported by Greenberg and his colleages (1988). Classical markers, properdin factor B, and HLA typing were informative in 18 of 33 families studied. Linkage analysis was carried out using various models of inheritance, penetrance and phenotype definition. A maximum lod score was obtained of 3.78 (θm + f, 0.01) assuming autosomal dominant inheritance, 90% penetrance and a definition of affectedness which included relatives who were asymptomatic individuals. Analysis of a subset of these families using HLA-DQ restriction fragment length polymorphisms gave similar results (Durner *et al.*, 1991).

More recently, a maximum lod score of 5.5 for HLA-Bf in 24 informative families assuming AD inheritance and 90% penetrance has been reported (Liu *et al.*, 1992). Taken together these studies provide evidence to support the existence of a locus (EJM1), located on 6p in the HLA region, which predisposes to JME and other IGEs. However, some doubt exists concerning the exact statistical significance of lod scores which have been 'maximized' over several different parameters for mode of inheritance and penetrance.

Linkage analysis has been carried out in a third distinct set of families including a patient with JME and at least one first-degree relative with IGE. Pairwise and multipoint linkage analysis was undertaken in these 25 kindreds using eight loci on chromosome 6p and assuming either AD or AR inheritance and age-dependent high or low penetrance (Whitehouse *et al.*, 1993b). No significant evidence in favour of linkage was obtained.

These conflicting results raise the possibility of genetic (locus) heterogeneity within this phenotype. The small size of the kindreds ascertained renders this a difficult question to resolve, but work is in progress to assemble the necessary extensive family resource.

Childhood absence epilepsy (Chapter 13a)

This is a relatively uncommon form of idiopathic generalized epilepsy with an incidence of between 6.0 and 8.0 per 100 000 children in the age range 0–15 years. Peak age of onset is at 6–7 years and girls are more frequently affected than boys. The typical absence seizures are of abrupt onset, short duration and involve a temporary cessation of awareness. Generalized tonic-clonic seizures develop in about 40% of patients, but most patients are cognitively and neurologically intact. The characteristic EEG pattern is a bilateral, symmetrical and synchronous discharge of regular 3 Hz spike and wave complexes on a normal background activity.

There is good evidence for a genetic predisposition to CAE. The concordance rate for monozygotic twins with absence epilepsy is 75% (Lennox, 1951; Gedda and Tatarelli, 1971) and is 84% if 3 Hz spike-wave EEG is included as evidence of affectedness (Lennox, 1951). The mode of inheritance is uncertain. Interpretation of results is complicated by variations in phenotype definition and uncertainty as to whether EEG changes are a reliable subclinical marker for the trait. Evidence for autosomal dominant (Metrakos and Metrakos, 1972) and autosomal recessive (Serratosa, Weissbecker and Delgado-Escueta, 1990) modes of inheritance has been obtained. Preliminary linkage studies with marker loci on human chromosome 6p have given negative results, suggesting that there is no locus in this region predisposing to absence epilepsy.

Benign childhood epilepsy with centrotemporal spikes (Chapter 13c)

The first description of this condition was by Nayrac and Beaussart (1957). Synonyms include benign focal epilepsy of childhood and benign rolandic epilepsy (BRE). Onset is usually between 5 and 10 years of age. The seizures occur during awakening or very soon thereafter, and consist of speech arrest, focal facial twitching and salivation, but consciousness is retained. Characteristic EEG changes form part of the phenotype. Interictally, monomorphic spike discharges maximal in, or often confined to, the centrotemporal region are recorded.

Patients with this syndrome have a family history of seizures in up to 68% of cases, and one or more asymptomatic relatives with sharp waves in the EEG in 30%. However, the spectrum of seizures and EEG changes found in relatives creates uncertainty as to how the trait should be defined for the purposes of genetic analysis. Two studies (Bray and Wiser, 1965; Heijbel *et al.*, 1975) suggested that centrotemporal foci were inherited as an autosomal dominant trait with age-dependent penetrance. More recently, a positive family history of epilepsy – including individuals with generalized seizures and febrile convulsions – was found in 40% of 43 probands (Degen and Degen, 1990).

Linkage analysis has been carried out in families of probands with benign rolandic epilepsy and marker loci from the HLA region on 6p and the FRAX region. Genetic linkage analysis was undertaken in 11 families with probands with benign rolandic epilepsy and one or more first degree relatives with focal sharp waves on EEG with or without BRE, using a polymorphic marker within the HLA region. Negative lod scores were obtained excluding the putative EJM1 gene as a locus contributing to this disorder. (Whitehouse *et al.*, 1993a).

As seizures occur in a significant proportion of individuals with the fragile X syndrome, in association with EEG abnormalities comparable to those found in BRE (Musumecci *et al.*, 1991), the (remote) possibility of a common genetic basis for these disorders was investigated by linkage analysis. Six pedigrees with probands with benign childhood epilepsy with centrotemporal spikes were analysed using a marker locus DXS548 close to fra (X). The results excluded FMR-1 and genes in the region of FMR-1 as the locus responsible for benign childhood epilepsy with centrotemporal spikes and the associated focal sharp wave trait segregating in these families (Rees *et al.*, 1993).

GENETIC COUNSELING

Specific and detailed advice concerning genetic counseling appropriate for all circumstances is beyond the scope of this chapter. Readers are referred to reviews in Bundey (1992) and Blandfort, Tsuboi and Vogel (1987). Rapid advances in molecular genetics are occurring, and where relevant the availability of DNA-based information must be determined at the time of counseling.

It is clear that the epilepsies from a heterogeneous group of disorders, and the first imperative is to make a specific diagnosis in affected individuals and to construct a pedigree. Physical examination should include a search for signs which might allow a specific diagnosis of, for example, one of the neurocutaneous syndromes. Investigations required may include intracranial imaging, EEG, ophthalmologic examination, and a host of biochemical investigations depending on the exact clinical context. It may be necessary and appropriate to examine other family members who may be asymptomatic carriers of, for example, the TSC gene. Genetic counseling is particularly difficult in a family with just one child affected with TSC. Although it is not possible to absolutely exclude TSC however many additional studies are done, the parents should be examined under UV light, undergo retinal examination with an indirect ophthalmoscope and consideration should be given to renal ultrasound and cranial CT or MRI examination. If neither parent has evidence of TSC, a 2–3% recurrence risk remains, allowing for gonadal mosaicism or reduced penetrance. Antenatal presumptive diagnosis may be made by ultrasound visualization of cardial rhabdomyomas, and of course linkage analysis is possible in any well-studied family known to harbor TSC at a specific locus.

Diagnosis of an epilepsy or epileptic syndrome displaying mendelian inheritance allows fairly precise prediction of recurrence risks, but variable penetrance introduces an element of uncertainty. The availability of a closely linked marker or cloned gene may of course allow presymptomatic diagnosis of individuals at risk. In the more common familial epilepsy recurrence risks are empirical, based on the literature and should be modified for families in which there are many affected members.

The approximate risks for the common familial epileptic syndromes discussed above are as follows. Siblings and children of an individual with childhood absence epilepsy have a risk of developing this syndrome of about 10% (Beck-Mannagetta *et al.*, 1989; Doose and Baier, 1989). Siblings and children of an individual with other idiopathic generalized epilepsies, including juvenile myoclonic epilepsy, have a recurrence risk of between 3 and 7% (Janz *et al.*, 1989); this should be manipulated to 10% or higher in families with several affected members. The sibling of a child with benign childhood epilepsy with centrotemporal spikes has a risk of about 15% (Heijbel *et al.*, 1975). It should be remembered that each individual in the general population has a 1–2% risk of developing a non-febrile seizure by the age of 40 years.

REFERENCES

Andermann, E. (1982) Multifactorial inheritance of generalised and focal epilepsy, in *Genetic Basis of the Epilepsies*, (eds V.E. Anderson, W.A. Hauser, J.K. Penry *et al.*), Raven Press, New York, pp. 355–74.

Barker, D., Wright, E., Nguyen, K. *et al.*, (1987) Gene for von Recklinghausen neurofibromatosis is in the pericentromeric region of chromosome 17. *Science*, **236**, 1100–2.

Beck-Mannagetta, G., Janz, D., Hoffmeister, U. *et al.*, (1989) Morbidity risk for seizures and epilepsy in offspring of patients with epilepsy, in *Genetics of the epilepsies*, (eds G. Beck-Mannagetta, V.E. Anderson, H. Doose and D. Janz), Springer-Verlag, Berlin, pp. 119–26.

Bird, T.D. (1992) Epilepsy, in *The Genetic Basis of Common Diseases*, (eds R.A. King, J.I. Rotter and A.G. Motulsky), Oxford University Press, Oxford, pp. 732–52.

Blandfort, M., Tsuboi, T. and Vogel, F. (1987) Genetic counseling in the epilepsies. *Human Genetics*, **76**, 303–31.

Bray, P. and Wiser, W.C. (1965) Hereditary characteristics of familial temporal-central focal epilepsy. *Paediatrics*, **36**, 207–11.

Bundey, S. (1992) *Genetics and Neurology*, 2nd edn, Churchill Livingstone, Edinburgh

Callen, D.F., Baker, E., Lane, S. *et al.*, (1991) Regional mapping of the Batten disease locus (CLN3) to human chromosome 16p12. *American Journal of Human Genetics*, **49**, 1372–7.

Cawthon, R.M., Weiss, R., Xu, G. *et al.*, (1990) A major segment of the neurofibromatosis type 1 gene: cDNA sequence, genomic structure, and point mutations. *Cell*, **62**, 193–201.

Collins, F.S. (1992) Positional cloning: let's not call it reverse anymore. *Nature Genetics*, **1**, 3–6.

Cutting, G.R., Curristin, S., Zoghbi, H. *et al.*, (1992) Identification of a putative GABA receptor subunit rho_2 cDNA and colocalisation of the genes encoding rho_2 and rho_1 to human chromosome 6q 14–q21 and mouse chromosome 4. *Genomics*, **12**, 801–6.

Degen, R. and Degen, H.E. (1990) Some genetic aspects of rolandic epilepsy: waking and sleeping EEGs in siblings. *Epilepsia*, **31**, 795–801.

Delgado-Escueta, A.V., Greenberg, D., Weissbecker, K. *et al.*, (1990) Gene mapping in the idiopathic generalised epilepsies. *Epilepsia*, **31**, (suppl. 3), 519–29.

Dichter, M.A. and Buchhalter, J.R. (1993) The genetic epilepsies, in *The Molecular and Genetic Basis of Neurological Disease*, (eds R.N. Rosenberg, S.B. Prusiner, S. DiMauro *et al.*), Butterworth, Boston, pp. 925–48.

Doose, H. and Baier, W.K. (1989) Absences, in *Genetics of the Epilepsies*, (ed. G.B. Managetta, V.E. Anderson, H. Doose, D. Janz *et al.*), Springer-Verlag, Berlin, pp. 34–42.

Durner, M., Sander, T., Greenberg, D.A. *et al.*, (1991) Localisation of idiopathic generalised epilepsy on chromosome 6p in families of juvenile myoclonic epilepsy patients. *Neurology*, **41**, 1651–5.

Eiberg, H., Gardiner, R.M. and Mohr, J. (1989) Batten disease (Spielmeyer–Sjögren disease) and haptoglobins (HP): indication of linkage and assignment to chromosome 16. *Clinical Genetics*, **36**, 217–8.

Fahsold, R., Rott, H.D. and Lorenz, P. (1991) A third gene locus for tuberous sclerosis is closely linked to the phenylalanine hydroxylase locus. *Human Genetics*, **88**, 85–90.

Fryer, A.E., Chalmers, A., Connor, J.M. *et al.*, (1987) Evidence that the gene for tuberous sclerosis is on chromosome 9. *Lancet*, **i**, 659–61.

Gedda, L. and Tatarelli, R. (1977) Essential isochronic epilepsy in MZ twin pairs. *Acta Genetica Medica*, **20**, 380–3.

Genton, P., Michelucci, R., Tassinari, C.A. *et al.*, (1990) The Ramsay–Hunt syndrome revisited: Mediterranean myoclonus versus MERRF and Baltic myoclonus. *Acta Neurologica Scandinavia*, **81**, 8–15.

Gomez, M.R. (1988) *Tuberous Sclerosis*, 2nd edn, Raven Press, New York.

Greenberg, D.A., Delgado-Escueta, A.V., Widelitz, H. *et al.*, (1988) Juvenile myoclonic epilepsy may be linked to the BF and HLA loci on human chromosome 6. *American Journal of Medical Genetics*, **31**, 185–92.

Greenberg, D.A., Delgado-Escueta, A.V., Maldonado, H.M. *et al.*, (1989) Segregation analysis of juvenile myoclonic epilepsy, in *Genetics of the Epilepsies*, (eds G. Beck-Mannagetta, V.E. Anderson, H. Doose *et al.*), Springer-Verlag, Berlin, pp. 53–61.

Grupe, A., Schroter, K.H., Ruppersberg, J.P. *et al.* (1990) Cloning and expression of a human voltage-gated potassium channel. A novel member of the RCK potassium channel family. *EMBO Journal*, **9**, 1749–56.

Gusella, J.F. and MacDonald, M.E. (1993) Hunting for Huntington's disease, in *Molecular Genetic Medicine*, Vol 3, (ed. T. Friedmann), Academic Press, London, pp. 139–58.

Gusella, J.F., Wexler, N.S., Conneally, P.M. *et al.*, (1983) A polymorphic DNA marker genetically linked to Huntington's disease. *Nature*, **306**, 234–8.

Heijbel, J., Blom, S., Rasmuson, M. *et al.*, (1975) Benign epilepsy of childhood with centro-temporal EEG foci: a genetic study. *Epilepsia*, **16**, 285–93.

Hellsten, E., Vesa, J., Speer, M.C. *et al.* (1993) Refined assignment of the infantile neuronal ceroid lipofuscinosis (INCL, CLN1) locus at 1p32: incorporation of linkage disequilibrium in multipoint analysis. *Genomics*, **16**, 720–5.

Huntington's Disease Collaborative Research Group (1993) A novel gene containing a tri-nucleotide repeat that is expanded and unstable on Huntington's disease chromosomes. *Cell*, **72**, 971–83.

Janz, D. (1969) *Die Epilepsien*, Stuttgart, Thieme.

Janz, D. and Christian, W. (1957) Impulsiv-petit mal. *Journal of Neurology*, **176**, 346–86.

Janz, D., Durner, M., Mannagetta, G.B. *et al.* (1989) Family studies on the genetics of juvenile myoclonic epilepsy (epilepsy with impulsive petit mal), in *Genetics of the Epilepsies*, (eds B.G. Mannagetta, V.E. Anderson, H. Doose and D. Janz), Springer-Verlag, Berlin, pp. 43–52.

Jarvela, I., Schleutker, J., Haataja, L. *et al.* (1991) Infantile form of neuronal ceroid-lipofuscinosis (CLN1) maps to the short arm of chromosome 1. *Genomics*, **9**, 170–3.

Kandt, R.S., Haines, J.L., Smith, M. *et al.* (1992) Linkage of an important gene locus for tuberous sclerosis to a chromosome 16 marker for poly-cystic kidney disease. *Nature Genetics*, **2**, 37–40.

Koch, M.C., Steinmeyer, K., Lorenz, C. *et al.* (1992) The skeletal muscle chloride channel in dominant and recessive human myotonia. *Science*, **257**, 797–800.

Koskiniemi, M.L. (1986) Baltic myoclonus, in *Myoclonus*, Raven Press, New York, pp. 57–64.

Lander, E.S. (1989) Mapping complex genetic traits in humans, in *Genome Analysis – A Practical Approach*, (ed. K.E. Davies), Oxford University Press, Oxford, pp. 171–91.

Lehesjoki, A.E., Koskiniemi, M., Sistonen, P. *et al.* (1991) Localisation of a gene for progressive myoclonus epilepsy to chromosome 21q22. *Proceedings of the National Academy of Sciences USA*, **88**, 3696–9.

Lehesjoki, A.E., Koskiniemi, M., Sistonen, P. *et al.* (1992) Linkage studies in progressive myoclonic epilepsy: Unverricht–Lundborg and Lafora disease. *Neurology*, **42**, 1545–50.

Lennox, W.G. (1951) Heredity of epilepsy as told by relatives and twins. *Journal of the American Medical Association*, **146**, 529–36.

Leppert, M., Anderson, V.E., Quattlebaum, T. *et al.* (1989) Benign familial neonatal convulsions linked to genetic markers on chromosome 20. *Nature*, **337**, 647–8.

Lewis, T.B., Leach, R.J., Ward, K. *et al.* (1993) Genetic heterogeneity in benign familial neo-natal convulsions: identification of a new locus on chromosome 8q. *American Journal of Human Genetics*, **53**, 670–5.

Liu, A.W.H., Delgado-Escueta, A.V., Weiss-becker, K. *et al.* (1992) Chromosome 6p Markers and Juvenile Myoclonic Epilepsy, Abstract presented at 1st International Workshop on chromosome 6.

McClatchey, A.I., McKenna-Yasek, D., Cros, D. *et al* (1992) Novel mutations in families with unusual and variable disorders of the skeletal muscle sodium channel. *Nature Genetics*, **2**, 148–52.

McKusick, V.A. (1990) *Mendelian Inheritance in Man*, 9th edn, The John Hopkins University Press, Baltimore.

McNamara, J.O. (1992) The neurobiological basis of epilepsy. *Trends in Neurosciences*, **2**, 148–52.

Metrakos, J.D. and Metrakos, K. (1972) Genetic factors in the epilepsies, in *The Epidemiology of Epilepsy: A Workshop*, US Government Printing Office, Washington DC, pp. 97–102.

Musumeci, S.A., Ferri, R., Elia, M. *et al.* (1991) Epilepsy and fragile X syndrome: a follow up study. *American Journal of Medical Genetics*, **38**, 511–13.

Mitchison, H.M., Thompson, A.D., Mulley, J.C. *et al.* (1993) Fine genetic mapping of the Batten disease locus (CLN3) by haplotype analysis and demonstration of allelic association with chromosome 16p microsatellite loci. *Genomics*, **16**, 455–60.

Nayrac, P. and Beaussart, M. (1957) Les pointes-ondes prerolandique: expression EEG très particulière. Etude electroclinique de 21 cas. *Reviews of Neurology*, **99**, 201–6.

NIH/CEPH collaborative mapping group (1992) A comprehensive genetic linkage map of the human genome. *Science*, **258**, 67–86.

Norio, R. and Koskiniemi, M. (1979) Progressive myoclonic epilepsy: genetic and nosological aspects with special reference to 107 Finnish patients. *Clinical Genetics*, **15**, 382–98.

Ott, J. (1990) Cutting a Gordian Knot in the linkage

analysis of complex human traits. *American Journal of Medical Genetics*, **46**, 219–21.

Panayiotopoulos, C.P. and Obeid, T. (1989) Juvenile myoclonic epilepsy: an autosomal recessive disease. *Annals of Neurology*, **25**, 440–3.

Plouin, P. (1992) Benign idiopathic neonatal convulsions, in *Epileptic Syndromes in Infancy, Childhood and Adolescence*, 2nd edn, (eds J. Roger, M. Bureau, C. Dravet *et al.*), Libby, London, pp. 3–11.

Rees, M., Diebold, U., Parker, K. *et al.* (1993) Benign childhood epilepsy with centrotemporal spikes and the focal sharp wave trait is not linked to the fragile X region. *Neuropediatrics*, **24**, 211–3.

Rett, A and Teubel, R. (1964) Neugeborenenkrämpfe im rahmen einer epileptisch belasteten Familie. *Wiener Klinische Wochenschrift*, **76**, 609–13.

Risch, N. (1990) Genetic linkage and complex diseases with special reference to psychiatric disorders. *Genetic Epidemiology*, **7**, 3–16.

Rojas, C.V., Wang, J.Z., Schwartz, L.S. *et al.* (1991) A met-to-val mutation in a skeletal muscle Na channel alpha subunit in hyperkalaemic periodic paralysis. *Nature*, **354**, 387–89.

Ryan, S.G., Wiznitzer, M., Hollman, C. *et al.* (1991) Benign familial neonatal convulsions: evidence for clinical and genetic heterogeneity. *Annals of Neurology*, **29**, 469–73.

Sampson, J.R., Jannssen, L.A.J., Sandkuijl, L.A. *et al.* (1992) Linkage investigation of three putative tuberous sclerosis determinant loci on chromosomes 9q, 11q and 12q. *Journal of Medical Genetics*, **29**, 861–6.

Serratossa, J., Weissbecker, K. and Delgado-Escueta, A. (1990) Childhood absence epilepsy: an autosomal recessive disorder? *Epilepsia*, **31**, 651.

Shiang, R., Ryan, S.G., Zhu, Y. *et al.* (1993) Mutations in the α_1 subunit of the inhibitory glycine receptor cause the dominant neurologic disorder, hyperekplexia. *Nature Genetics*, **5**, 351–7.

Shofner, J.M., Lott, M.T., Lezza, A.M.S. *et al* (1990) Myoclonic epilepsy and ragged red fibre disease (MERRF) is associated with a mitochondrial DNA tRNA lysine mutation. *Cell*, **61**, 931–7.

Smith, M., Smalley, S., Cantor, R. *et al.* (1990) Mapping of a gene determining tuberous sclerosis to human chromosome 11q14–q23. *Genomics*, **6**, 105–14.

Sobell, J.L., Heston, L.L. and Sommer, S.S. (1992) Delineation of genetic predisposition to multifactoral disease: a general approach on the threshold of feasibility. *Genomics*, **12**, 1–6.

Sundqvist, A. (1990) Juvenile myoclonic epilepsy: events before diagnosis. *Journal of Epilepsy*, **3**, 189–92.

Tsuboi, T. and Christian, W. (1973) On the genetics of primary generalised epilepsy with sporadic myoclonus of impulsive petit-mal type. *Humangenetik*, **19**, 155–82.

Wallace, M.R., Marchuk, D.A., Andersen, L.B. *et al.* (1990) Type 1 neurofibromatosis gene: identification of a large transcript disrupted in three NF1 patients. *Science*, **249**, 181–6.

Weissenbach, J., Gyapay, G., Dib, C. *et al.* (1992) A second-generation linkage map of the human genome. *Nature*, **359**, 794–801.

Whitehouse, W., Diebold, U., Rees, M. *et al.* (1993a) Exclusion of linkage of genetic focal sharp waves to the HLA region on chromosome 6p in families with benign partial epilepsy with centrotemporal sharp waves. *Neuropediatrics*, **24**, 208–10.

Whitehouse, W.P., Rees, M., Curtis, D. *et al.* (1993b) Linkage analysis of idiopathic generalised epilepsy and marker loci on chromosome 6p in families of patients with juvenile myoclonic epilepsy: no evidence for an epilepsy locus in the HLA region. *American Journal of Human Genetics*, **53**, 652–62.

Williams, R., Vesa, J., Jarvela, I. *et al.* (1993) Genetic heterogeneity in neuronal ceroid lipofuscinosis (NCL): evidence that the late-infantile subtype (Jansky–Bielschowsky disease; CLN2) is not an allelic form of the juvenile or infantile subtypes. *American Journal of Human Genetics*, **53**, 93–5.

Zonana, J., Silvey, K. and Strimling, B. (1984) Familial neonatal and infantile seizures: an autosomal-dominant disorder. *America Journal Medical Genetics*, **18**, 455–9.

SEIZURES IN THE NEONATE

9

Eli M. Mizrahi

INTRODUCTION

CLINICAL SIGNIFICANCE

The occurrence of seizures in a newborn infant is a significant clinical event with specific diagnostic, therapeutic, and prognostic implications. Seizures may be the most frequent clinical signs of CNS dysfunction in the neonate, and their presence requires a thorough investigation for potentially treatable causes of the underlying disorder. Depending upon type, duration, recurrence, and severity, the seizures themselves may require treatment with antiepileptic drugs (AED).

PROBLEMS OF DIAGNOSIS AND MANAGEMENT

Despite the clinical significance and almost universal acknowledgement of their importance, there are a number of problems in the diagnosis and management of neonatal seizures (Mizrahi, 1987). It may often be difficult to accurately identify clinical seizures. Recent studies indicate that clinical events historically thought to be neonatal seizures may be generated by different pathophysiologic mechanisms – either epileptic or nonepileptic (Mizrahi and Kellaway, 1987; Kellaway and Mizrahi, 1990). The natural history of acute seizures is not well known. Traditional diagnostic criteria of some major etiologic factors (such as hypoxic-ischemic encephalo-

pathy) associated with neonatal seizures are currently being reexamined (Nelson and Leviton, 1991), and the role of diagnostic studies such as EEG and EEG/video monitoring have been reevaluated (Hrachovy, Mizrahi and Kellaway, 1990). The requirements of AED therapy have been reconsidered (Moshé, 1987; Mizrahi, 1989) and the clinical efficacy of standard AED in controlling neonatal seizures has been called into question (Painter *et al.*, 1994). New therapies devised to protect the brain from further injury, rather than to arrest seizures, are being tested. In addition, the prognostic significance of neonatal seizures has been linked more closely to the underlying etiologic factors, rather than to the occurrence of the seizures themselves (Kellaway and Mizrahi, 1987).

The once relatively static field of the study of neonatal seizures is now more dynamic, as fundamental clinical questions are reexamined. What are neonatal seizures? What are their characteristic features? How can they best be diagnosed? What are the diagnostic criteria of important etiologic factors? What is the best therapeutic strategy? What determines prognosis of newborns with seizures? What is the role of EEG and EEG/video monitoring in diagnosis and management? These questions will be considered here in relation to current clinical practice and to the findings of recent clinical and basic research.

Epilepsy in Children. Edited by Sheila Wallace. Published in 1996 by Chapman & Hall, London. ISBN 0 412 56860 8

INCIDENCE

METHODOLOGICAL CONSIDERATIONS

The methods of determining incidence of neonatal seizures differ considerably among studies. There may be variability in the definitions and in the methods of seizure identification: clinical observation only, clinical observation correlated with interictal EEG, or clinical observation correlated with bedside EEG. In addition, the level and quality of care of newborns has dramatically improved since early epidemiologic studies. As a result, some associated risk factors or etiologies have become less important and may have altered the incidence of seizures. Some studies consider all neonates as a single population, without consideration of conceptional age – although the incidence of seizures may vary if premature newborns are compared to term infants. Some studies are prospective while others are retrospective – based upon chart reviews and notations of observers with varying levels of diagnostic skill and training. In addition, most studies report the incidence of seizures which occur during the newborn's initial hospitalization, but may not include infants who have seizures following discharge, or who are readmitted to the hospital but are still within the neonatal age period.

REPORTS OF INCIDENCE

It has been reported that seizures occur in between 0.15% and 0.5% of all live births (Eriksson and Zetterström, 1979; Holden, Mellits and Freeman, 1982; Spellacy *et al.*, 1987). Scher and colleagues (1993) have reported the incidence to be 2.3% in all infants cared for in an intensive care setting, 1.5% in premature neonates older than 30 weeks conceptional age (CA), and 3.9% in those less than 30 weeks CA. The relationship between CA and incidence of seizures requires further study, since some investigators question whether the brain of a very premature infant can initiate and propagate epileptogenic activity which can be clinically manifested as seizures (Hrachovy, Mizrahi and Kellaway, 1990).

CHARACTERIZATION

CLINICAL INVESTIGATIONS OF SEIZURE CHARACTERIZATION

The main consideration in the characterization of clinical seizures in neonates, has been the recognition that seizures of the immature brain may be significantly different from those of older children or adults. This is thought to be due to the rapid rate of brain development near term, and to the types and the number of etiologic factors that may be responsible for brain injury during the neonatal period.

Neonatal seizures have been traditionally characterized as either: stereotypic motor activity; anarchic or atypical behaviours, or phenomena thought secondary to activation of the autonomic nervous system. Early investigators recognized both clonic and tonic, but not generalized tonic-clonic seizures (Minkowski *et al.*, 1955; Dreyfus-Brisac and Monod, 1964). In addition, ocular movements, oral-buccal-lingual movements, and limb and body movements of progression were characterized as neonatal seizures (Minkowski and Sainte-Anne-Dargassies, 1956; Dreyfus-Brisac and Monod, 1964). Eventually, myoclonic movements of limb and trunk were identified as seizures (Lombroso, 1974). Sudden changes in clinical signs mediated by the autonomic nervous system (ANS) have also been considered to be manifestations of neonatal seizures. These signs include: changes in heart rate, respiration and systemic blood pressure; vasomotor changes such as flushing, and pupillary dilatation and excessive salivation (Cadilhac, Passouant and Ribstein 1959; Schulte, 1966; Lou and Friis-Hansen, 1979; Fenichel, Olson and Fitzpatrick, 1980; Goldberg *et al.*, 1982).

Later, Volpe designated a group of behaviours and clinical signs as 'subtle' seizures (Volpe, 1973). This group included ocular signs, oral-buccal-lingual movements, progression movements (rowing, stepping, and pedalling limb movements), and some signs referable to autonomic nervous system (ANS) function activation. The application of the term 'subtle seizures' to these events helped to further advance the concept that neonatal seizures had unique features which warranted distinct diagnostic criteria.

RECENT INVESTIGATIONS OF SEIZURE
CHARACTERIZATION

Unlike previous clinical investigations, recent studies of the characterization of neonatal seizures have been based upon time-synchronized, EEG/polygraphic/video monitoring of newborns experiencing clinical seizures (Mizrahi and Kellaway, 1987; Kellaway and Mizrahi, 1990). All of the clinical types of motor and behavioral seizures previously described by others were recorded. Each type was further characterized. The clonic seizures were noted to be unifocal, multifocal, alternating, migratory, or hemiconvulsive. Tonic seizures were observed to be either generalized or focal. The generalized seizures were observed to be either symmetric or asymmetric. Ocular signs were characterized as either random movements or sustained tonic deviation. Movements of progression included stepping or pedalling of the legs and swimming or rowing movements of the arms. Myoclonic seizures were described as generalized, focal, or fragmentary (multifocal).

The findings of these EEG/video monitoring clinical investigations suggested that not all of these clinical events were of epileptic origin. Some types of spontaneous clinical events could be provoked by stimulation of the infant, could be suppressed by light restraint of the infant and did not consistently occur with simultaneously recorded EEG seizure activity. This led to the consideration that clinical seizures would eventually be characterized and classified as either seizures of epileptic or nonepileptic origin.

CLASSIFICATION

CLASSIFICATION SYSTEMS

The most widely utilized classification system is one initially proposed and updated by Volpe (1973, 1989). The last revision takes into account the possibility that some seizure types may occur in the absence of simultaneous EEG seizure activity and expands the categories of clinical seizures.

Another classification system has been proposed by Mizrahi and Kellaway (first in 1984 and later revised), which has been developed from findings of their EEG/video monitoring studies (Table 9.1) (Mizrahi and Kellaway, 1984, 1987; Kellaway and Mizrahi, 1990; Mizrahi, 1994). This system recognizes the possibility that not all neonatal seizures may be initiated or generated by an epileptic process – it is a classification system based upon the presumed pathophysiology of the clinical events. Because of the pathophysiology-based scheme, the term 'motor automatisms' has been proposed to designate some of the events currently classified as 'subtle seizures'.

ANALYSIS OF THE SYSTEMS

Regardless of the system utilized, the clinician will easily conclude that each classification scheme has limitations. For example, there is a lack of specific data concerning paroxysmal changes in heart rate, respirations and systemic blood pressure. Early investigations suggested these changes could be clinical seizure activity. However, the precise relationship between these clinical signs, other motor seizure phenomena which may occur simultaneously, and electric seizure activity has not been specifically determined. While early studies suggested

Table 9.1 Classification of neonatal seizures based upon electroclinical findings and presumed pathophysiology

A. Clinical seizures with a consistent
   electrocortical signature
   Pathophysiology – epileptic
   Focal clonic
     Unifocal
     Multifocal
     Hemiconvulsive
     Axial
   Focal tonic
     Asymmetric truncal posturing
     Limb posturing
     Sustained eye deviation
   Myoclonic
     Generalized
     Focal

B. Clinical seizures without a consistent
   electrocortical signature
   Pathophysiology – presumed nonepileptic
   Myoclonic
     Generalized
     Focal
     Fragmentary
   Generalized tonic
   Motor automatisms
     Oral-buccal-lingual movements
     Ocular signs
     Progression movements

C. Electric seizures without clinical seizure
   activity
   Pathophysiology – epileptic

that apnea may be a seizure manifestation, others have not found apnea as a seizure phenomena unless accompanied by other signs such as clonic or tonic seizures (Mizrahi and Kellaway, 1987). Further investigations are required to more completely understand paroxysmal tachycardia, hypertension or tachypnea as features of clinical seizures.

Another limitation of the classification systems is their emphasis upon a single seizure type, since many infants will experience several seizure types. In one study, 22% of neonates with seizures experienced more than one type of seizure (Mizrahi and Kellaway, 1987). Therefore, classification schemes

for neonatal seizures are best utilized in the same manner as classification schemes for older children and adults – as a basis for designation of individual seizure types.

Another feature not specifically addressed in the classification of clinical seizures, is the occurrence of electric seizure activity in the absence of any clinical signs. This may represent an important clinical problem and will be discussed more fully below.

Overall, the most accurate application of seizure classification is a three-staged process. First, the clinical events should be precisely described as observed. Based upon this characterization, the clinical events can be classified. The seizures can be further classified according to pathophysiology responsible for their initiation, and this will be discussed more completely below.

CONSIDERATIONS OF NEONATAL SEIZURE NOSOLOGY

The most controversial aspect of nosology of neonatal seizures concerns the application of the terms 'epileptic' and 'nonepileptic'. It has been proposed that the term 'seizure' be utilized for all abnormal paroxysmal clinical events currently considered to be seizures in the newborn. Some types of clinical events may be generated by paroxysmal, hypersynchronous neuronal discharges characteristic of epileptogenesis. These seizures are referred to as epileptic seizures, and include: focal and multifocal clonic, focal and asymmetrical tonic, and some myoclonic seizures. Other clinical seizures may be generated and propagated by nonepileptic mechanisms and can be referred to as nonepileptic seizures. These include generalized symmetrical tonic posturing, some myoclonic events and the motor automatisms of progression movements, ocular signs and oral-buccal-lingual movements. Undoubtedly, nosology will continue to evolve and will soon be studied in detail by the International League Against Epilepsy Commission on Terminology.

PATHOPHYSIOLOGY

PATHOPHYSIOLOGIC MECHANISMS

As noted above, studies of neonatal seizures utilizing EEG/video monitoring suggest that seizures may be generated by either epileptic or nonepileptic mechanisms. The suggestion that some events are epileptic in origin is based upon their precise and consistent relationship to electric seizure activity on EEG which was simultaneously recorded with the videotaped clinical seizures. The suggestion that some events were generated by nonepileptic mechanisms is based upon both EEG and clinical data. First, these clinical events were not consistently accompanied by EEG seizure activity and most often occurred in the absence of any electric seizure activity. Second, the spontaneously occurring clinical events could be suppressed by restraint or repositioning of the infant. For example, generalized tonic posturing could be controlled by repositioning of the infant's head and neck. In addition, clinical events identical to the spontaneously occurring events, could be provoked by tactile stimulation. For example, stroking the infant's back or rubbing the infant's limb could provoke posturing or motor automatisms. Finally, increasing intensity or sites of tactile stimulus would result in increasing the degree of paroxysmal movements, and stimulation at one site could provoke paroxysmal movements at another site. These clinical features of suppression of movement, evocation of clinical events, temporal and spatial summation and irradiation of the response are not suggestive of an epileptic process, but, rather, are characteristic of reflex physiology (Sherrington *et al.*, 1932; Starzl, Taylor and Magoun, 1951).

EPILEPTIC MECHANISMS

The concepts of epileptogenesis in the immature brain are complex and are rapidly evolving (Moshé, 1993; Shinnar, Moshé and Swann, 1994). However, some basic concepts still hold and are thought responsible for the predominantly focal features of epileptic neonatal seizures. The epileptic discharge is defined by the hypersynchronous firing of an aggregate of cortical neurons. Discharges may be confined to specific regions or spread rapidly to other regions. Thus, epileptic seizures tend to be manifested as unifocal or multifocal events, with irregular rather than sequential spread over cortical regions.

NONEPILEPTIC MECHANISMS

Animal models of reflex physiology demonstrate specific features which are characteristic of both the nonepileptic neonatal seizures and the interictal state of the infants who experience them (Table 9.2). Normally, brainstem structures facilitate the primitive movements of progression (such as stepping, pedalling, or swimming) and posture (such as truncal and limb extension or flexion). In the immature animal, these primitive movements may occur reflexly. Eventually, however, the forebrain develops and extends inhibitory influences on brainstem facilitatory centres. This, in essence, allows the cortex to 'override' primitive reflex behaviors in order for more voluntary movements to become manifest. If the forebrain is either depressed, removed, or disconnected, the facilitatory brainstem centres are allowed to mediate reflex behaviors without rostral inhibition. These unchecked reflex behaviors can be characterized by suppression and evocation of clinical events, spatial and temporal summation, and irradiation of the response, and may occur because of rich extrapyramidal sensory input to the brainstem (Sherrington *et al.*, 1932; Starzl, Taylor and Magoun, 1951; Sprague and Chambers, 1954).

All of these features are also characteristic of generalized tonic posturing and motor automatisms. In addition, these events most

Table 9.2 Comparison of findings in animal models demonstrating reflex physiology and in neonates with clinical seizures which have no consistent electrocortical signature

Animal models*	Neonate†
Decortication	Functional decortication (cortical depression)
	Coma or lethargy
	EEG: depressed and undifferentiated or isoelectric
Reflex movements	Spontaneous or provoked movements
Progression	Motor automatisms
Posturing	Tonic posturing
Response to stimulation	Response to stimulation
Temporal summation	Temporal summation
Spatial summation	Spatial summation
Irradiation of response	Irradiation of response
Response to restraint	Response to restraint
Arrest of movements	Arrest of movements

*Sherrington *et al.*, 1932; Lindsley Schreiner and Magoun, 1949; Sprague and Chambers, 1954; Mori, Shik and Yagodnitsyn, 1977.
†Mizrahi and Kellaway, 1987.

typically occur in infants with evidence of forebrain depression. The infants are comatose or lethargic and the background of their EEGs is typically characterized as depressed and undifferentiated. Because of this putative pathophysiologic mechanism of disinhibition of brainstem facilitatory centres, these clinical events in infants have been referred to as 'brainstem release phenomena' (Kellaway and Hrachovy, 1983; Mizrahi and Kellaway, 1984, 1987).

CLINICAL IDENTIFICATION OF PATHOPHYSIOLOGY

Because of their distinctive clinical features, it is possible, in many instances, to identify and classify seizures at the bedside according to their presumed pathophysiology. Epileptic seizures cannot be suppressed by restraint and, typically, cannot be provoked. On the other hand, clinical events which can be suppressed and evoked most likely can be classified as nonepileptic in origin. In addition to these characteristics, epileptic and nonepileptic neonatal seizures may have other constellations of clinical characteristics.

ETIOLOGY

REVIEW OF ETIOLOGIC FACTORS

Most of the previous discussion of neonatal seizures has emphasized seizure type and pathophysiology. However, this initial discussion of etiology will apply to all seizures regardless of pathophysiology. The occurrence of neonatal seizures indicates the presence of CNS dysfunction and should prompt an orderly and thorough clinical and laboratory investigation of the underlying etiology. A complete list of possible etiologies can be extensive (Goddard, Glaze and Fishman, 1982). Major etiologic factors are: hypoxic-ischemic encephalopathy, meningitis, encephalitis, intracranial hemorrhage (intraventricular, intracerebral, subarachnoid), cerebral infarction, congenital anomalies of the brain, metabolic disorders (hypoglycemia, hypomagnesemia, hypocalcemia), inborn errors of metabolism (Chapter 4c), and genetic disorders (Chapter 8). It should be noted that, for some infants, despite a thorough evaluation, no specific etiology of the seizures or associated risk factor will be identified.

The relative importance of various aetiologic factors has changed over the past few decades as neonatal care practices have changed and some etiologic factors became more completely understood. For example, prior to the mid 1970s hypocalcemia was an important factor associated with neonatal seizures, but this is now rare (Holden, Mellits and Freeman, 1982; Kellaway and Mizrahi, 1987). In addition, new technology has allowed for a greater appreciation of the importance of intracranial hemorrhage, cerebral infarction and congenital brain malformations, viral infections, and genetic disorders. These changes in the relative importance of various etiologic factors will have further significance in the discussions, below, of prognosis of neonatal seizures.

SELECTED ETIOLOGIC FACTORS

Attention has recently been focused on some specific etiologic factors, because of a re-examination of diagnostic criteria or because of development of new technology which has allowed their precise definition. The clinical signs and laboratory findings associated with the diagnosis of hypoxic-ischemic encephalopathy are currently considered, by some investigators, to lack specificity and to not consistently predict long-term neurologic outcome (Nelson and Leviton, 1991; Paneth, 1993). Thus, specific criteria for this diagnosis are currently being reevaluated. The eventual refinement may provide the basis for a clearer understanding of the relationships between perinatal hypoxia-ischemia, neonatal seizures, and brain injury. New criteria may also require a review of conclusions drawn from investigations utilizing less precise diagnostic criteria.

There has also been increased interest in two syndromes of benign neonatal convulsions: benign familial neonatal convulsions and benign neonatal convulsions. Benign familial neonatal convulsions are thought to have a pattern of autosomal transmission based upon a locus on chromosome 20 (Quattelbaum, 1979; Leppert *et al.*, 1989), although recent reports suggest some genetic heterogeneity (Lewis *et al.*, 1993) (Chapter 8). The disorder is considered to be benign because initial clinical descriptions reported no neurologic sequelae in affected infants. However, more recent studies suggest that not all infants with benign familial neonatal convulsions experience normal long-term outcome (Ronen *et al.*, 1993).

Benign neonatal convulsions occur in infants with no family history of neonatal seizures. The infants are typically full term and the produce of a normal pregnancy and delivery. The seizures are usually brief, often clonic and typically occur between the 4th and 6th day of life. No etiology can be identified. The infants are neurologically normal before, between and following the seizures (Plouin, 1990).

There has also been recent interest in the seizures which may follow cardiac surgery which requires periods of imposed circulatory arrest and extracorporeal membrane oxygenation (ECMO) procedures. These procedures are being performed with increased frequency – seizures may represent important short-term sequelae. Because the timing of the interruption of cerebral blood flow is known, new neuroprotective therapies are being tested which may prevent acute seizures as well as diffuse brain injury.

RELATIONSHIP BETWEEN ETIOLOGY AND SEIZURE TYPE

The previous discussion of etiology referred to all seizure types as if they were a homogeneous group. However, there is evidence to suggest that specific seizure types may be associated with various etiologic factors and their resulting degree and severity of brain injury (Kellaway and Mizrahi, 1987; Mizrahi and Kellaway, 1987). The presumed nonepileptic seizures of generalized tonic posturing and motor automatisms have been most often associated with etiologic factors responsible for diffuse brain injury: hypoxia-ischemia, severe meningitis or encephalitis, and infarction or hemorrhage which may involve both cerebral hemispheres. Seizures considered to be of epileptic origin, such as focal clonic or focal tonic seizures, have been most often associated with etiologic factors such as localized infarction or hemorrhage which tend to produce focal brain injury with relative sparing of other brain regions. In addition, focal epileptic seizures have been associated with some metabolic disorders such as hypocalcemia, hypoglycemia, and hypomagnesemia. It should also be noted that some infants with diffuse brain injury can experience epileptic seizures with or without nonepileptic events. In addition, although these generalizations may be helpful in initial bedside clinical assessment, they cannot be utilized to exclude specific etiologies.

PROGNOSIS

DETERMINANTS OF PROGNOSIS

Despite considerable clinical and animal-based investigations of the effect of seizures on the developing brain, there is still no clear consensus as to whether there are long-term neurologic or cognitive sequelae of neonatal seizures (Holmes, 1991). Clinical studies represent an important resource in understanding the prognosis of neonatal seizures. Reported sequelae include death, abnormal neurologic examination, mental retardation, and the development of postnatal epilepsy.

Early investigations of the sequelae of neonatal seizures reported mortality ranging from 20 to 42% and morbidity from 3 to 27% (Burke, 1954; Cadilhac, Passonant and Ribstein, 1959; Craig, 1960; Harris and Tizard, 1960). In later studies, outcome was analyzed in relation to etiology, demonstrating that certain risk factors were associated with different severities of sequelae. Normal outcomes occurred with increasing frequency in

association with each of the following etiologic factors: hypoxia-ischemia, CNS infection, cerebral hemorrhage, hypoglycemia, and hypocalcemia (McInerny and Schubert, 1969; Rose and Lombroso, 1970; Bergman *et al.*, 1983; Lombroso, 1983; Mannino and Trauner, 1983; Clancy *et al.*, 1985; Kellaway and Mizrahi, 1987).

Overall, it appears that the most important determinant of outcome is the degree of brain injury associated with seizure occurrence. The factors which caused the seizures and concomitant brain disturbance are the most likely factors which determine long-term outcome, rather than the seizures themselves (Holden, Mellits and Freeman 1982; Bergman *et al.*, 1983; Kellaway and Mizrahi, 1987).

POSTNATAL EPILEPSY

Few studies have specifically examined the relationship between neonatal seizures and the eventual development of epilepsy later in life. Clancy and colleagues (Clancy and Legido, 1991) indicated the incidence of epilepsy to be as high as 56% in children who had seizures in the newborn period. Risk factors which increased the probability of neonates with seizures developing postnatal epilepsy included: coma and significant background EEG abnormalities during the neonatal period; eventual development of cerebral palsy or mental retardation; spikes and sharp and slow wave activity on postnatal follow-up EEGs.

THERAPY

OVERVIEW OF THERAPY

The main objectives in the therapy of neonatal seizures are treatment of etiologic factors underlying the seizures and cessation of seizures with AEDs. Although these goals can be achieved for some infants, success may prove more difficult in others: etiologic factors may not be readily apparent, the precise relationship to the seizures of associated etiologic factors may not be known, features of the clinical seizures may suggest that AEDs may not be warranted, and AED administration may not be completely effective in control of seizures.

Treatment of neonatal seizures, ideally, is based upon the consideration of several interrelated factors. These include: etiology of the seizure or its associated risk factors, characterization and classification of seizure type, determination of pathophysiology, assessment of duration and severity of the seizures, understanding the natural history of the seizure disorder, and assessment of the expected effects of the seizures and the AEDs on the developing brain. Unfortunately, information concerning all of these factors may not be complete. However, efforts to consider each may provide the basis for rational management decisions at the bedside.

Overall, there are three phases of therapy for neonates with seizures. These phases, which should be individualized to each infant, include: initial medical management, etiology-specific therapy and AED therapy.

Initial medical management and etiology-specific therapy

The usual principles of general medical management also apply to the neonate with seizures. Adequate ventilation and circulatory perfusion are ensured, since changes in respirations, heart rate and blood pressure may occur in association with seizures, as a consequence of etiologic factors, or in association with AED therapy.

A major goal of the evaluation of neonates with seizures is the identification of treatable causes of the seizures. The therapy of identified specific etiologic factors is critical. Therapies can be directed toward CNS and systemic infections. Treatable metabolic factors include: hypocalcemia, hypomag-

nesemia and hypoglycemia. Pyridoxine dependency is a treatable cause of medically refractory neonatal seizures, although it is exceedingly rare.

Antiepileptic drug therapy

The AEDs traditionally utilized in controlling neonatal seizures are phenobarbitone, phenytoin and diazepam. In the USA, the dosages utilized are: phenobarbitone, 20 mg/kg as a loading dose, followed by additional dosages of 10 mg/kg to achieve serum levels between 20 and 40 µg/ml; phenytoin, 20 mg/kg as a loading dose to achieve serum levels between 15 and 20 µg/ml; diazepam, 0.1–0.3 mg/kg in repeated dosages. Reports of the use of other traditional AEDs cite carbamazepine, primidone, and paraldehyde (now unavailable in the USA) (Painter and Alvin, 1990). These AED have been utilized as additional therapy when first-line AEDs have failed to control seizures. Other AEDs have been the topic of clinical reports and have received considerable interest. Both lorazepam (Painter and Alvin, 1990; Maytal, Novak and King, 1991) and lidocaine (Painter and Alvin, 1990; Hellström-Westas *et al.*, 1992) have been reported to be safe and efficacious.

There have been few controlled studies of the relative efficacy of various AEDs in neonatal seizures. However, Painter and colleagues have recently reported no significant difference between acute administration of phenobarbitone and phenytoin in seizure control (Painter *et al.*, 1994).

FACTORS IN CONSIDERING INSTITUTION OF THERAPY

The decision to initiate AED therapy requires the consideration of seizure type, pathophysiology, duration and severity, natural history of the seizure disorder, and anticipated effects of both the seizures and the selected AED on the infant. Most often, clinicians consider instituting AED therapy without benefit of EEG or EEG/video monitoring. Under these circumstances, the clinician must first decide if the clinical seizures are of epileptic or nonepileptic origin. If the seizures are of epileptic origin, then they must be assessed for duration and severity.

Initiation of AED therapy based upon features of the clinical seizure

Four situations, described below, may be encountered in which AED use may be considered based solely upon the clinical features of the seizures.

Focal clonic or focal tonic seizures – prolonged and recurrent

The clinical features of focal clonic or focal tonic seizures help to designate them as epileptic in origin. Focal clonic seizures are repetitive and rhythmic muscle contractions which cannot be arrested by restraint or repositioning. Similarly, focal tonic seizures, such as sustained posturing of a limb cannot be altered by these maneuvers. The focal tonic seizures characterized by eye deviation can be differentiated from the random eye movements of nonepileptic motor automatisms, since the epileptic tonic eye deviation is sustained and cannot be evoked by stimulation. Once the clinical seizures are considered epileptic in origin, duration and severity must be considered. When they are thought to be sustained and prolonged, they are treated vigorously with AEDS.

Focal clonic or focal tonic seizures – brief and infrequent

The specific features of these seizures are the same as those described above, and provide the basis for their designation as epileptic in origin. As such, AEDS may be utilized in attempts to control the seizures. However, because these seizures may be brief, occur infrequently, and have a short natural history with relatively rapid spontaneous resolution, the use of AEDS for these seizures is being reevaluated. This is based upon the following concepts: epileptic seizures are reactive to an underlying brain disorder; for some infants following an initial injury, seizures may resolve spontaneously, and potential adverse effects of AEDS may outweigh the potential risk of brief and infrequent seizures on the developing brain (Moshé, 1987). Unfortunately, specific criteria for what constitutes brief and infrequent seizures have not been established, and issues of whether AEDs and seizures adversely effect the immature brain have not yet been completely resolved.

Generalized tonic posturing and motor automatism – responsive to stimulation and restraint

Generalized tonic posturing and motor automatisms (including ocular signs, oral-buccal-lingual movements, and movements of progression) may be presumed to be of nonepileptic origin. This determination can be made at the bedside based upon the characterization of the events and their response to clinical maneuvers: the spontaneous events can be suppressed by restraint or repositioning of the limbs or trunk and events similar to spontaneous events can be evoked by tactile stimulation. Traditionally, these clinical events have been treated with AEDs and in some instances, their frequency and severity have diminished. This finding has been utilized to support the notion that the events may be epileptic seizures. However, this effect is most likely not the result of specific antiepileptic properties, but rather because some of these drugs are also CNS depressants. Overall, if generalized tonic posturing and motor automatisms demonstrate characteristic clinical features, they can be presumed to be of nonepileptic origin and do not require AED therapy (Mizrahi and Kellaway, 1987; Mizrahi, 1989). Although the clinical events may be initially quite dramatic, their natural course is one of gradual spontaneous resolution without AED therapy.

Generalized tonic posturing and motor automatisms – not responsive to stimulation and restraint

For some infants, the clinical features of generalized tonic posturing and motor automatisms, are typical of nonepileptic events, but clinical maneuvres of restraint, repositioning or stimulation do not result in characteristic responses. In these instances, the infants are treated with AEDs with the understanding that clinical observation and maneuvers alone cannot provide data to indicate underlying pathophysiology.

Initiation of AED therapy based upon EEG or EEG/video monitoring

At some medical facilities, bedside EEG or EEG/video monitoring is available to complement clinical assessment. In these settings, in addition to the four clinical situations just described, two other clinical circumstances may be encountered which determine whether AED therapy should be initiated.

Clinical seizures present in the absence of EEG seizure activity

These clinical seizure types include generalized tonic posturing and motor automatisms. The clinical features suggest they are nonepileptic in origin. The lack of EEG seizure activity at the time of the clinical seizures provides further to the support of this determination. These clinical events are not treated with AEDs when they occur in the absence of electrical seizure activity.

EEG seizure activity in absence of any clinical seizures

Electrical seizure activity occurring in the absence of any clinical seizure activity is treated with AEDs. However, these electric seizures may be highly resistant to therapy despite high dosages of several AEDs.

GOALS OF AED THERAPY

The goals of AED therapy are to stop neonatal seizures, prevent their recurrence, and minimize any sequelae. However, specific issues must be addressed when considered these objectives.

Goals of acute therapy

Clinical seizures of epileptic origin may be controlled with AED therapy, but the electrical seizure activity accompanying the clinical seizures may persist (Mizrahi and Kellaway, 1987). What then is the end-point of AED therapy – cessation of clinical seizures or cessation of electrical seizure activity?

The response of epileptic seizures to AEDs has been described in studies utilizing EEG/video monitoring. Untreated, clinical epileptic seizures occur in a time-locked relationship to EEG seizure activity. The initial response to AEDs is cessation of clinical seizures, although the EEG seizure activity may continue to be present. This phenomena has been referred to as 'decoupling' of the clinical from the electric seizure (Mizrahi and Kellaway, 1987, 1992) (Figs 9.1, 9.2). Further AED therapy may eliminate electrical seizure activity. However, this may be difficult or, more often, may not be accomplished (Painter *et al.*, 1994). Attempts to eliminate electrical seizure activity may lead to high dosages of multiple AEDs. This strategy may not successfully control EEG seizure activity, and may also be associated with the clinical problems of CNS depression, systemic hypotension, and respiratory depression. Here, the clinician is faced with weighing the potential risks of vigorous AEDs against the potential benefits, and likelihood of success, of therapy. In these situations, therapeutic strategies may be devised to strike an even

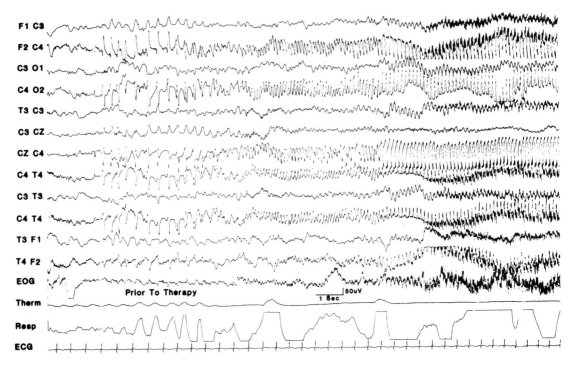

Fig. 9.1   Prior to AED therapy, an electrical seizure is recorded arising from the right central region. It is accompanied by a clinical seizure characterized by rhythmic clonic jerking of the left arm. (Reproduced with permission from Kellaway and Mizrahi, 1990.)

balance. One scheme is to attain high therapeutic levels of phenobarbital and phenytoin, and then utilize individual dosages of a benzodiazepine in attempts to reduce or eliminate electrical seizure discharges. Further AED therapy may not be attempted because of the systemic adverse effects which are frequently encountered.

Goals of chronic therapy

Once a desired therapeutic effect is obtained in the acute setting, infants are typically placed on regimens of maintenance AEDs. This is usually in the form of phenobarbitone alone or with phenytoin (maintenance dosages of each are 3–4 mg/kg/day). The decision to discontinue AEDs after a period of clinical seizure control is highly individualized, since no specific practice guidelines have been established. An important con-

sideration is the probable natural history of the treated disorder. Seizures may represent short-lived phenomena produced in reaction to acute injuries. If this is true, then long-term AED therapy may be maintained for a short-term clinical disorder. Reported maintenance schedules range from 1 week up to 12 months after the last seizure (Boer and Gal, 1983). Although specific clinical and EEG predictors of recurrent seizures following AED withdrawal have not been identified (Gal, Sharpless and Boer, 1984; Brod *et al.*, 1988), there has been increasing clinical interest in short-term therapy, with AED withdrawal 2 weeks following the infant's last clinical seizure.

RISK VERSUS BENEFIT OF AED THERAPY

As noted earlier, there is no clear consensus on whether epileptic seizures adversely effect

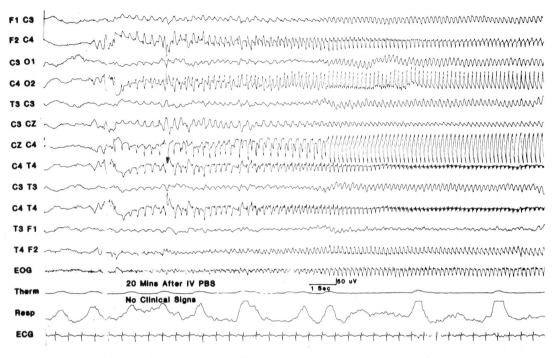

Fig. 9.2 EEG of the infant shown in Fig. 9.1 several minutes later after administration of phenobarbitone, demonstrates an electrical seizure arising from the same location, and with a similar character. However, no clinical seizure activity accompanied the electrical seizure activity – the electrical and clinical seizures have been 'decoupled'. (Reproduced with permission from Kellaway and Mizrahi, 1990.)

the developing brain (Holmes, 1991). Some investigators suggest that, in animals, there are important changes in the CNS at a cellular or molecular level, although changes may be transient and their impact on animal performance not detectable. No clinical studies have been able to effectively address this issue. In addition, there are no detailed clinical studies of the adverse systemic effects of seizures, although infants with prolonged seizures may experience changes in respiration, heart rate or blood pressure, and may have an increased level of energy utilization. These may be unwelcome clinical findings in an infant who may already be medically compromised.

On the other hand, there is an equal lack of consensus concerning the possible adverse effects of AEDs on the developing brain.

Experimental data suggest alteration in cell growth and energy substrate utilization (Diaz, Schain and Bailey, 1977; Diaz and Schain, 1978; Bergey *et al.*, 1981; Neale *et al.*, 1985), although the applicability of these findings to human neonates has been called into question. There have been few studies on adverse effects of acute AED therapy, although vigorous treatment may result in CNS depression, hypotension, bradycardia, and respiratory depression (Goldberg *et al.*, 1986). There are few studies of the effect of long-term therapy on neonates and young infants.

Overall, a regimen which may minimize perceived risk and maximize therapeutic benefit includes acute therapy to eliminate clinical seizures, maintenance therapy after seizure control is attained, and withdrawal of

AEDs 2 weeks following the last clinical seizure. However, much additional basic scientific and clinical investigation is needed in order to firmly establish the rational basis for this or other management schemes.

CLINICAL NEUROPHYSIOLOGY

This topic has been reserved for the end of this chapter for several reasons. The diagnosis and management of neonatal seizures are primarily based on clinical assessment of the infant. In addition, clinical neurophysiology services are not available at all medical facilities. However, when available, EEG can be a valuable adjunct to clinical assessment. This topic is discussed further in Chapter 19.

Considerations of analysis of neonatal EEG

Some principles of analysis of the background activity, interictal discharges and electrical seizures activity are helpful in understanding the role of EEG diagnosis and management of neonates suspected of seizures. The background activity may be useful in that it may provide some objective measure of degree and severity of CNS dysfunction which may be associated with seizures. Serial EEGs, with the initial recordings obtained in the acute period, are the most accurate in the characterization of the evolution of brain injury and in providing information concerning prognosis (Tharp, Scher and Clancy 1989; Hrachovy, Mizrahi and Kellaway 1990). Interictal discharges have limited utility in assessment, since interictal sharp waves in the neonate are considered epileptiform, as they are in older children or adults (Hrachovy, Mizrahi and Kellaway, 1990). The EEG recorded during a clinical or electrical seizure is certainly the most helpful in assessment. Ictal EEG will assist in identifying clinical episodes which are epileptic in origin. Conversely, the absence of electrical seizure activity during clinical seizures may suggest that they are not epileptic in origin. The critical factor in the analysis of ictal EEG recording is the precise documentation of the character, the beginning and the end of the clinical events in relation to the actual EEG tracing. This is best accomplished by a trained observer making notations directly on the EEG as it is being recorded.

EEG/polygraphic/video monitoring

Simultaneously recording at the infant's bedside of EEG; polygraphic measures such as electromyogram, electrooculogram, electrocardiogram, respiration, blood pressure, oxygen saturation and expiratory carbon dioxide; and video has been utilized for several years in research settings and in clinical management at only a few medical centers (Mizrahi and Kellaway, 1987; Mizrahi, 1989). Although there is much interest in the technique, instrumentation, personnel and logistic problems limit its widespread clinical applicability. However, the findings of clinical studies which have utilized EEG/polygraphic/video monitoring have, in part, formed the basis of some of the current principles of clinical practice.

ACKNOWLEDGMENTS

This chapter was supported, in part, by Grant NS11535 from the National Institutes of Neurological Disorders and Stroke and the Joseph P. Kennedy Jr Foundation for Mental Retardation. In addition, the assistance of the Michael Foundation (*Stiftung* Michael), Bonn, Germany, is gratefully acknowledged.

REFERENCES

Bergey, G.K., Swaiman, K.F., Schrier, B.K. *et al.* (1981) Adverse effects of phenobarbital on morphological and biochemical development of fetal mouse spinal cord neurons in culture. *Annals of Neurology*, **9**, 584–9.
Bergman, I., Painter, M.J., Hirsch, R.P. *et al.*

(1983) Outcome in neonates with convulsions treated in an intensive care unit. *Annals of Neurology*, **14**, 642–7.

Boer, H.R. and Gal, P. (1983) Neonatal seizures: a survey of current practice. *Clinical Pediatrics*, **21**, 453–7.

Brod, S.A., Ment, L.R., Ehrenkranz, R.A. and Bridgers, S. (1988) Predictors of success for drug discontinuation following neonatal seizures. *Pediatric Neurology*, **4**, 13–7.

Burke, J.B. (1954) Prognostic significance of neonatal convulsions. *Archives of Disease in Childhood*, **29**, 342–5.

Cadilhac, J., Passouant, P. and Ribstein, M. (1959) Convulsions in the newborn: EEG and clinical aspects. *Electroencephalography and Clinical Neurophysiology*, **11**, 604.

Clancy, R.R. and Legido, A. (1991) Postnatal epilepsy after EEG-confirmed neonatal seizures. *Epilepsia*, **32**, 69–76.

Clancy, R., Malin, S., Laraque, D. *et al.* (1985) Focal motor seizures heralding stroke in full-term neonates. *American Journal of Diseases of Children*, **139**, 601–6.

Craig, W.S. (1960) Convulsive movements occurring in the first ten days of life. *Archives of Disease in Childhood*, **35**, 336–44.

Diaz, J. and Schain, R.J. (1978) Phenobarbital: effects of long-term administration on behavior and brain of artificially reared rats. *Science*, **199**, 90.

Diaz, J., Schain, R.J. and Bailey, B.J. (1977) Phenobarbital: effects of long-term administration on behavior and brain of artificially reared rat pups. *Biology of the Neonate*, **32**, 77.

Dreyfus-Brisac, C. and Monod, N. (1964) Electro-clinical studies of status epilepticus and convulsions in the newborn, in *Neurological and Electroencephalographic Correlative Studies in Infancy* (eds P. Kellaway and I. Petersén), Grune and Stratton, New York, pp. 250–72.

Eriksson, M. and Zetterström, R. (1979) Neonatal convulsions. Incidence and causes in the Stockholm area. *Acta Paediatrica Scandinavica* **68**, 807–11.

Fenichel, G.M., Olson, B.J. and Fitzpatrick, J.E. (1980) Heart rate changes in convulsive and nonconvulsive neonatal apnea. *Annals of Neurology*, **7**, 577–82.

Gal, P., Sharpless, M.K. and Boer, H.R. (1984) Outcome in neonates with seizures: are chronic anticonvulsants necessary? *Annals of Neurology*, **15**, 610–1.

Goddard, J., Glaze, D.G. and Fishman, M.A. (1982) Neurological disorders of the neonate. *Current Neurology*, **4**, 241–61.

Goldberg, R.N., Goldman, S.L., Ramsay, R.E. *et al.* (1982) Detection of seizure activity in the paralyzed neonate using continuous monitoring. *Pediatrics*, **69**, 583–6.

Goldberg, R.N., Moscoso, P., Bauer, C.R. *et al.* (1986) Use of barbiturate therapy in severe perinatal asphyxia: a randomized controlled trial. *Journal of Pediatrics*, **109**, 851.

Harris, R. and Tizard, J.P.M. (1960) The electroencephalogram in neonatal convulsions. *Journal of Pediatrics*, **57**, 501–20.

Hellström-Westas, L., Svenningse, N.W., Westgren, U. *et al.* (1992) Lidocaine for treatment of severe seizures in newborn infants. II. Blood concentrations of lidocaine and metabolites during intravenous infusion. *Acta Paediatrica Scandinavica*, **81**, 35–9.

Holden, K.R., Mellits, E.D. and Freeman, J.M. (1982) Neonatal seizures. I. Correlation of prenatal and perinatal events with outcomes. *Pediatrics*, **70**, 165–76.

Holmes, G.L. (1991) Do seizures cause brain damage? *Epilepsia*, **32** (suppl. 5), S14–S28.

Hrachovy, R.A., Mizrahi, E.M. and Kellaway, P. (1990) Electroencephalography of the newborn, in *Current Practice of Clinical Electroencephalography*, 2nd edn (eds D. Daly and T.A. Pedley), Raven Press, New York, pp. 201–42.

Kellaway, P. and Hrachovy, R.A. (1983) Status epilepticus in newborns: a perspective on neonatal seizures, in *Advances in Neurology*, Vol. 34: *Status Epilepticus* (eds A.V. Delgado-Escueta, C.G. Wasterlain, D.M. Treiman and R.J. Porter), Raven Press, New York, pp. 93–9.

Kellaway, P. and Mizrahi, E.M. (1987) Neonatal seizures, in *Epilepsy: Electroclinical Syndromes* (eds H. Luders and R.P. Lesser), Springer-Verlag, New York, pp. 13–47.

Kellaway, P. and Mizrahi, E.M. (1990) Clinical, electroencephalographic, therapeutic, and pathophysiologic studies of neonatal seizures, in *Neonatal Seizures: Pathophysiology and Pharmacologic Management* (eds C.G. Wasterlain and P. Vert), Raven Press, New York, pp. 1–13.

Leppert, M., Anderson, V.E., Quattlebaum, T.G. *et al.* (1989) Benign familial neonatal convulsions linked to genetic markers on chromosome 20. *Nature*, **337**, 647–8.

Lewis, T.B., Leach, R.J., Ward, K. *et al.* (1993) Genetic heterogeneity in benign familial neonatal convulsions: identification of a new locus on chromosome-8q. *American Journal of Human Genetics*, **53**, 670–5.

Lindsley, D.B., Schreiner, L.H. and Magoun, H.W. (1949) An electromyographic study of spasticity. *Neurophysiology*, **12**, 197–205.

Lombroso, C.T. (1974) Seizures in the newborn, in *Handbook of Clinical Neurophysiology*, vol 15 (eds P.J. Vinken and G.W. Bruyn), North-Holland, Amsterdam, pp. 189–218.

Lombroso, C.T. (1983) Prognosis in neonatal seizures. *Advances in Neurology*, **34**, 101–13.

Lou, H.C. and Friis-Hansen, B. (1979) Arterial blood pressure elevations during motor activity and epileptic seizures in the newborn. *Acta Paediatrica Scandinavica*, **68**, 803–6.

Mannino, F.L. and Trauner, D.A. (1983) Stroke in neonates. *Journal of Pediatrics*, **102,**, 605–10.

Maytal, J., Novak, G.P. and King, K. (1991) Lorazepam in the treatment of refractory neonatal seizures. *Journal of Child Neurology*, **6**, 319–23.

McInerny, T.K. and Schubert, W.K. (1969) Prognosis of neonatal seizures. *American Journal of Diseases of Children*, **117**, 261–4.

Minkowski, A. and Sainte-Anne-Dargassies, S. (1956) Les convulsions du nouveau-nè. *Evolut Psychiatr*, **1**, 279–89.

Minkowski, A., Sainte-Anne-Dargassies, S., Dreyfus-Brisac, C. *et al.* (1955) L'état du mal convulsif du nouveau-né. *Archives Francaises de Pediatrie*, **12**, 271–84.

Mizrahi, E.M. (1987) Neonatal seizures: problems in diagnosis and classification. *Epilepsia*, **28** (**suppl. 1**), S46–55.

Mizrahi, E.M. (1989) Consensus and controversy in the clinical management of neonatal seizures. *Clinics in Perinatology*, **16**, 485–500.

Mizrahi, E.M. (1994) Neonatal seizures, in *Pediatric and Adolescent Medicine* (ed S. Shinnar) (in press).

Mizrahi, E.M. and Kellaway, P. (1984) Characterization of seizures in neonates and young infants by time-synchronized electroencephalographic/polygraphic/video monitoring. *Annals of Neurology*, **16**, 383.

Mizrahi, E.M. and Kellaway, P. (1987) Characterization and classification of neonatal seizures. *Neurology*, **37**, 1837.

Mizrahi, E.M. and Kellaway, P. (1992) The response of electroclinical neonatal seizures to antiepileptic drug therapy. *Epilepsia*, **33**, (**suppl. 3**), S114.

Mori, S., Shik, M.L. and Yagodnitsyn, A.S. (1977) Role of pontine tegmentum for locomotor control in mesencephalic cat. *Journal of Neurophysiology*, **40**, 284–95.

Moshé, S.L. (1987) Epileptogenesis and the immature brain. *Epilepsia*, **28** (**suppl. 1**), S3–15.

Moshé, S.L. (1993) Seizures in the developing brain. *Neurology*, **43**, (**suppl. 5**), S3–7.

Neale, E.A., Sher, P.K., Graubard, B.I. *et al.* (1985) Differential toxicity of chronic exposure to phenytoin, phenobarbital, or carbamazepine in cerebral cortical cell cultures. *Pediatric Neurology*, **1**, 143–50.

Nelson, K.B. and Leviton, A. (1991) How much of neonatal encephalopathy is due to birth asphyxia? *American Journal of Diseases of Children*, **145**, 1325–31.

Painter, M.J. and Alvin, J. (1990) Choice of anticonvulsants in the treatment of neonatal seizures, in *Neonatal Seizures* (eds C.G. Wasterlain and P. Vert), Raven Press, New York, pp. 243–56.

Painter, M.J., Scher, M.S., Paneth, N.S. *et al.* (1994) Randomized trial of phenobarbital v. phenytoin treatment of neonatal seizures. *Pediatric Research* (in press).

Paneth, N. (1993) The causes of cerebral palsy. Recent evidence. *Clinical and Investigative Medicine,* **16**, 95–102.

Plouin, P. (1990) Benign neonatal convulsions, in *Neonatal Seizures* (eds C.G. Wasterlain and P. Vert), Raven Press, New York, pp. 51–9.

Quattlebaum, T.G. (1979) Benign familial convulsions in the neonatal period and early infancy. *Journal of Pediatrics*, **95**, 257–9.

Ronen, G.M., Rosales, T.O., Connolly, M. *et al.* (1993) Seizure characteristics in chromosome 20 benign familial neonatal convulsions. *Neurology*, **43**, 1355–60.

Rose, A.L. and Lombroso, C.T. (1970) Neonatal seizure states. *Pediatrics*, **45**, 404–25.

Scher, M.S., Aso, K., Beggarly, M.E. *et al.* (1993) Electrographic seizures in pre-term and full-term neonates: clinical correlates, associated brain lesions, and risk for neurologic sequelae. *Pediatrics*, **91**, 128–34.

Schulte, F.J. (1966) Neonatal convulsions and their relation to epilepsy in early childhood. *Developmental Medicine and Child Neurology*, **8**, 381–92.

Sherrington, C.S., Creed, R.S., Denny-Brown, D.E. *et al.* (1932) *Reflex Activity of the Spinal Cord*, Oxford University Press, London.

Shinnar, S., Moshé, S. and Swann, J.W. (1994)

Focal seizures in developing brain, in *Brain Development and Epilepsy* (eds S. Moshé, J. Noebels, P. Schwartzkroin and J. Swann), Oxford University Press, London (in press).

Spellacy, W.N., Peterson, P.Q., Winegar, A. *et al.* (1987) Neonatal seizures after cesarean delivery: higher risk with labor. *American Journal of Obstetrics and Gynecology*, **157**, 377–9.

Sprague, J.M. and Chambers, W.W. (1954) Control of posture by reticular formation and cerebellum in intact, anesthetized and unanesthetized and in decerebrated cat. *American Journal of Physiology*, **176**, 52–64.

Starzl, T.E., Taylor, C.W. and Magoun, H.W. (1951) Collateral afferent excitation of reticular formation of the brain stem. *Journal of Neurophysiology*, **14**, 479–96.

Tharp, B.R., Scher, M.S. and Clancy, R.R. (1989) Serial EEGs in normal and abnormal infants with birthweights less than 1200 grams – a prospective study with long term follow-up. *Neuropediatrics*, **20**, 64–72.

Volpe, J.J. (1973) Neonatal seizures. *New England Journal of Medicine*, **289**, 413–5.

Volpe, J.J. (1989) Neonatal seizures. *Pediatrics*, **84**, 422–8.

FEBRILE SEIZURES 10

Sheila J. Wallace

INTRODUCTION

Seizures precipitated by febrile illnesses are much commoner than any other form of clinical epileptic manifestation. For the most part they are only passing, age-related responses to a noxious stimulus. Nevertheless, in some children such seizures are acute indications of life-long, underlying neurologic states which are less than optimal. The skill in the management of children who present with seizures in response to febrile illnesses lies in recognition of individual children in whom long-term neurologic, educational, and behavior dysfunctions persist; and in whom there is a high risk of subsequent epilepsy. A recent monograph has explored the natural history of febrile seizures in considerable detail (Wallace, 1988). Further information and a more extensive review of the literature is available therein.

DEFINITION

A seizure occurring in association with a fever is the inevitable starting point. Only later may an underlying intracranial infection or a deviation from normal neurodevelopmental progress be identified. There is no evidence that the actual seizure is different with respect to the underlying illness; and, now, considerable data to show that the long-term outlook relates more to the nature of the febrile illness or to the premorbid state than to the seizure, unless the latter is particularly severe.

It is usual to define the height of the body temperature necessary for the term 'febrile' to be applied as 38°C. The main area for contention relates to seizures which are part of the presentation of intracranial infections, particularly if these are bacterial. Many authors, for example, Nelson and Ellenberg (1976) and Verity, Butler and Golding (1985a), exclude children with meningitis and/or encephalitis from their studies; whereas others, for example, Wallace (1976), Lewis *et al.* (1979) and Frantzen, Lennox-Buchthal and Nygaard (1968), acknowledge that the actual seizure is no different, but that the importance of the underlying illness should be emphasised. There are particular difficulties in drawing firm guidelines when a viral infection causes only a minor rise in the CSF cell count.

Since many children with febrile seizures have very minor, and previously unrecognized, neurodevelopmental problems (Wallace, 1976, 1988), it is difficult to draw a firm dividing line between those considered normal or abnormal. Some children with frank cerebral palsy only ever have seizures when febrile. Therefore, most series include children with prior neurologic problems.

It is important to differentiate febrile seizures from nonepileptic attacks which occur in early childhood. These are considered in detail in Chapter 2.

Epilepsy in Children. Edited by Sheila Wallace. Published in 1996 by Chapman & Hall, London. ISBN 0 412 56860 8

In conclusion, the most satisfactory definition is that a febrile seizure itself is any seizure of cerebral origin which occurs in association with any febrile illness. Further qualifications of this definition may later be necessary. In particular, febrile seizures are considered simple if they are generalized, single within a defined illness, and of less than 15 minutes' duration. The terms complex, complicated or severe are used for seizures which have partial features, are repeated within the same illness, and/or are prolonged.

HISTORIC PERSPECTIVE

Hippocrates described febrile seizures, clearly differentiating them from rigors and breath-holding attacks. He noted that both generalized and partial seizures might occur. The strong association with age was recognized by Hippocrates and emphasized later by the seventeenth century pediatrician, Thomas Willis. Both noted that attacks were most frequent around about the time of teething. The importance of genetic factors was also emphasized from very early times; but, other predisposing events, reported in the Greek, Arabian, and early European literature, tend to reflect prevailing beliefs rather than scientific observations. Intervention by the gods; cold phlegm discharged into warm blood; plumpness and a hard belly; poor nutrition; vapors rising from the lower parts to the head; abnormal motility of body fluids; irritation or 'vellification'; and the predominance of the spinal over the cerebral system were all considered possible explanations. High fever and intracranial infection were recognized precipitants from the time of Hippocrates. From the beginning of the nineteenth century, emphasis on the symptomatic nature of febrile seizures can be found. Mortality was reported by the early Greeks, but the possibility of a benign outcome was also recognized. The importance to prognosis of the state of the child prior to a febrile seizure was noted early in the nineteenth century. The first monograph on febrile seizures was published in 1941.

EPIDEMIOLOGY

Much of the information on febrile seizures has been obtained from hospital or other special populations. In addition, criteria for inclusion in various reports has varied. Nevertheless, there is a fair measure of agreement that, overall, from 2 to 4% of all children are likely to have at least one febrile seizure before the age of 5 years. A recent study conducted in the Swedish county of Vasterbotten, where there were 21 544 children aged up to 6 years, found that 115 cases were newly diagnosed over a period of 20 months (Forsgren *et al.*, 1990a). In the same period 128 children were identified by district nurses, physicians and the neurophysiological laboratory as having febrile seizures (Forsgren *et al.*, 1990b). The annual first attendance rate in the age group up to 4 years was 500/100 000 and the annual incidence rate 460/100 000. The cumulative incidence was 4.1%.

Reports on prevalence according to various criteria have been reviewed by Wallace (1988). For the first febrile seizures, social class and race are irrelevant. Children of parents who themselves have had febrile seizures have a risk four times that in the general population, and this is greatest for male children of female probands. Children of parents with epilepsy have a slightly raised prevalence at 5%. Siblings of probands have a risk of febrile seizures 3.5 times that in the general population and an actual prevalence of 8%. Males are more likely to be affected than females: Forsgren *et al.* (1990b) found a ratio of 1.72 : 1. The type of precipitating event can be relevant. Viral, rather than bacterial, infections are prominent. However, both shigellosis and bacterial meningitis are well-recognized precipitants. Of routine vaccines, only measles has been associated with an increased incidence of febrile seizures, and even this is low at 0.93 : 1000 doses. Even when suffering from apparently provocative illnesses, only a minority of children convulse, emphasizing the need to acknowledge the importance of predisposing factors.

AGE

Age is the most critical of all the factors predisposing to febrile seizures. The biological evidence for this statement is emphasized by the tendency for all young mammals to have periods in early life when seizures are particularly likely to be precipitated by fever. In humans the critical age extends from 6 to 36 months, with particular vulnerability during the second year. Analysis of age of onset by sex suggests that males and females may have slightly different ages of peak incidence, but different study groups do not always agree (Forsgren *et al.*, 1990a, 1990b: Wallace 1988). For patients who later develop mesial temporal sclerosis, the initial prolonged lateralized seizure occurs earlier in girls than boys. Most studies find that complex febrile seizures are commoner before the age of 1 year than later, and that children with negative family histories for seizures are likely to present earlier (Wallace, 1988; Maytal and Shinnar 1990; Offringa *et al.*, 1992). Social class factors and pre- and perinatal histories do not influence age at onset.

Although previous studies (Wallace, 1988) have suggested that the subsequent seizure history and intellectual development are critically related to the age at the first seizure, Madge *et al.* (1993), who reported on children with severe febrile seizures only, were unable to find a significant association between age at presentation and dysfunction at follow-up. Nevertheless, as befits an age-related disorder, recurrence of febrile seizures is significantly associated with onset before 12–18 months. The age at each recurrence also has predictive value for subsequent episodes (Offringa *et al.* 1992).

GENETIC FACTORS

The percentages of probands with positive family histories for any seizure disorder or specifically for febrile seizures vary enormously from study to study (Wallace, 1988), but there is general agreement that genetic factors are important. Forsgren *et al.* (1990a) compared patients with controls and found significant increases of febrile seizures in mothers ($P < 0.001$) and fathers ($P < 0.002$), but not in siblings ($P < 0.49$): 24% of children with febrile seizures but only 5% of controls had parents or siblings with febrile seizures ($P < 0.001$). On the other hand, figures for nonfebrile seizures were comparable in cases and controls. In a twin study, Tsuboi (1987) found intrapair similarity to be much greater in monozygotic than dizygotic pairs. His study supported a multifactorial mode of inheritance. However Rich *et al.* (1987) consider a polygenic model appropriate only for families of probands with single febrile seizures. Those with probands with multiple febrile seizures fitted better with a single-major-locus model with nearly dominant seizure susceptibility.

Genetic factors have influences on age at onset and characteristics of the initial febrile seizure. These are variably advantageous or otherwise. There seems no doubt that a positive family history is associated with an increased risk of recurrence of febrile seizures. The influence on the development later of unprovoked seizures or epilepsy is less clear. The height of the fever at presentation and subsequently psychologic and social development are unrelated to the family history.

PREDISPOSING FACTORS IN THE PRE- AND PERINATAL PERIODS

A number of adverse factors occur more frequently than expected in children with febrile seizures. Chronic maternal ill-health, often secondary to illnesses recognized as likely to reduce fertility, which itself is a risk factor for febrile seizures in males, is found in approximately 16% of mothers of probands. Chronic pyelonephritis, glomerular nephritis, thyrotoxicosis, chronic mental disorders, epilepsy, hypertension, and autoimmune diseases have been reported (Wallace, 1988; Nelson and Ellenberg, 1990). Smoking is pregnancy can double the risk of simple febrile seizures, and alcohol doubles the likelihood of complex attacks (Cascano Koepsell and Farwell 1990; Nelson and Ellenberg, 1990). Early, repeated, slight vaginal bleeding, toxemia, maternal therapeutic drug use and seizures are further risk factors (Wallace, 1988; Nelson and Ellenberg, 1990).

Duration of gestation, birth order, duration of labor, prolonged rupture of the membranes, and fetal distress are not related to the occurrence of febrile seizures, but, delivery other than by the vertex (Verity, Butler and Golding, 1985a; Wallace, 1988; Madge *et al.*, 1993) and relative reduction in birth weight for gestation (Wallace, 1988) have been identified as risk factors. Sepsis and errors of metabolism significantly increase the risk, but present in extremely small numbers (Nelson and Ellenberg, 1990).

The perinatal history is considered independent of genetic factors, but there are several studies which suggest that children with adverse pre- or perinatal events have an increased risk of complex initial febrile seizures, and of later nonfebrile seizures.

POSTNATAL DEVELOPMENT BEFORE THE INITIAL SEIZURE

Social circumstances are unimportant in relation to the initial seizure. On the whole, affected children are normally healthy, but upper and lower respiratory infections and otitis media are significantly commoner than expected (Verity, Butler and Golding, 1985b). Congenital malformations are not unduly frequent, but abnormal dermatoglyphic patterns occur more often than in the general population.

Most affected children have unremarkable neurodevelopmental histories. However, the possibility that minor, as well as major, deviations from normal can reduce the threshold for seizures during febrile illnesses receives support from animal work, and from studies where 'soft' signs have been specifically sought. Occipitofrontal circumferences are comparable in range to those of unaffected children, though excesses of children with over-large and smaller than expected heads are found in most cohorts. In studies where those with frank cerebral palsy are not excluded, fewer than 5% have serious disabling conditions. A further 20–25% suffer from less obvious neurologic problems (Nelson and Ellenberg, 1976; Wallace, 1988). Minor delays in both age at walking (Wallace, 1976; Forsgren *et al.*, 1990a, 1990b) and age at talking (Wallace, 1976; Verity, Butler and Golding, 1985b) have been reported. Frank mental retardation is rare before the onset of febrile seizures, but occurs more frequently than in the general population.

Children who are later mentally retarded are likely to have an earlier onset, but it is not always clear whether slow development preceded the initial seizure. Prior neurologic abnormality predisposes to complicated, complex or severe febrile seizures (Wallace, 1988; Madge *et al.*, 1993), and to febrile status epilepticus (Maytal and Shinnar, 1990); to recurrence of febrile seizures; development of nonfebrile seizures and epilepsy; cognitive delay; and later EEG abnormalities. Death is an extremely rare complication, and is commoner with prior neurodevelopmental abnormalities.

PRECIPITATING FACTORS

Two main factors deserve attention: the fever and the underlying illness.

There are age-related metabolic responses to fever associated with upper respiratory tract infections (Fleming *et al.*, 1994), but their relevance to febrile seizures is doubtful. Most authors consider a temperature of at least 38°C necessary for inclusion within the term febrile seizure. Often the body temperature, usually taken in close proximity to the seizure rather than during it, is much higher than this. There is much debate about whether the rate of rise or the ultimate height of the fever is the factor determining the occurrence of a seizure in a susceptible individual. A review of previous studies suggests that the latter is the more important (Wallace, 1988). It is probable that a minor pyrexia precedes recognized illness (Jackson, Peterson and Wailoo, 1994). Differentiation between high fever and hyperthermia is not possible on the basis of body temperature alone, but is important for managment (Simon 1993). Since status epilepticus can cause hyperthermia, a vicious circle may arise.

Clinically the commonest underlying illnesses are upper respiratory tract infections, but otitis media, bronchopneumonia, pertussis, gastrointestinal infection, pyuria, measles, exanthem subitum, scarlet fever, meningitis, encephalitis, and malaria also feature in lists of associated disorders. Since the manifestations of fever are largely dependent on the causative agent (Saper and Breder, 1994), it is not surprising that a wide range of infections is involved. However, viruses are responsible for the precipitating illness in almost 90% of cases: viral invasion of the central nervous system can be implied from CSF immunoglobulin estimations (Lewis *et al.*, 1979; Wallace, 1988; Suga *et al.*, 1993; Hall, Long and Schnabel, 1994). The immunologic defense mechanisms are different in different viral infections (Isaacs, 1989), therefore responses of children aged 6–36 months could well be more dramatic than older subjects who have had prior exposure. Unexpected bacteremia with *Streptococcus pneumoniae* has been reported (Chamberlain and Gorman, 1988). A specific search for urinary tract infection is important (Lee and Verrier Jones, 1991). Bacterial meningitis must always be considered: more than a quarter of cases of meningitis present with seizures as well as other symptoms (Green *et al.*, 1993). Shigellosis also features prominently amongst bacterial causes. Vaccination is the cause of the precipitating fever in only 1.4% of children (Hirtz, Nelson and Ellenberg, 1983)

THE INITIAL SEIZURE

Complete characterization of the initial seizure is the most important historic information needed.

It is generally agreed that brief, generalized, and single seizures should be termed 'simple'. However the maximum duration accepted as brief varies widely, some authors choosing 10 minutes, and others 15, 30, or 60 minutes. Biochemical evidence suggests 30 minutes is critical, but in line with the National Childhood Perinatal Project (NCPP) (Nelson and Ellenberg, 1976) 15 minutes is now usual. Those seizures other than 'simple', i.e. those of longer duration, with partial features and/or repeated in the same illness are variously referred to as severe, complicated, complex, nonsimple, or prolonged. It would be helpful if 'complex' could become the accepted term.

Recording of the characterization of seizures depends on the assiduity of the observer: much higher percentages with partial features are recorded when these are specifically sought (Wallace, 1988). Overall, approximately 70% are reported to be generalized. In a study of interobserver agreement on classification of complex features of 100 febrile seizures, Berg *et al.* (1992a) found good agreement on whether the seizure was repeated or prolonged, but only fair to good agreement on focality. Problems arose mainly with interpretation of lateral eye deviation, staring episodes and motor asymmetries in the context of bilateral seizures. The observers agreed that 60 of the 100 seizures were completely generalized. Lateralized seizures suggest prior neurologic dysfunction

(Wallace, 1988; Al-Eissa *et al.*, 1992), but have also been correlated with asymmetry of hemispheric maturation (Taylor and Ounsted, 1971). They tend to occur at younger ages, particularly in females; in family history-negative children; and in those with adverse perinatal events and later suboptimal neuro-developmental histories: subsequent partial epilepsy and neurologic and cognitive problems occur in one-third of affected children.

ACUTE NEUROLOGIC FINDINGS

Considering that seizures of any nature are symptoms of acute cerebral dysfunction, it is surprising how infrequently early neurologic findings are reported. Prolonged disturbance of consciousness, which occurs in 31%, can be secondary to the underlying infection, related to the pyrexia (Simon, 1993), or consequent on prolonged seizures. Asymmetric features are of most significance. These are usually reported in up to 12% of patients, but where particularly careful examination is conducted and minor asymmetries are included, about a third of children are affected (Wallace, 1988). Asymmetries in pyramidal tract functions are most usual. Other early signs include cerebellar ataxia and upper motor neuron facial weakness. When an acute, usually transient, hemiparesis (Todd's paresis) follows a prolonged, lateralized febrile seizure, there is a high risk, possibly 50%, of subsequent complex partial seizures.

INVESTIGATION AT PRESENTATION

Investigation should aim to identify the underlying illness and highlight features which might lower the seizure threshold. Findings which have long-term implications should be noted. Appropriate tests are further reviewed in Chapter 21.

Blood counts, blood, urine and stool cultures for bacteria, and viral studies are relevant to the underlying infection. Examination of CSF is the most controversial issue.

Even though Green *et al.* (1993), have suggested that signs other than seizures are always present, when attempts have been made to establish absolute criteria for lumbar puncture, difficulties with exclusion of bacterial meningitis on clinical examination alone have been encountered in the younger children (Wallace, 1988). Therefore, it is concluded that lumbar puncture is essential when there is meningism or when the child is less than 18 months of age at presentation.

In some children low levels of serum IgA may be important, but further information is needed.

Secondary effects of the infection leading to alterations in: electrolytes and urea; acid–base status; blood glucose; calcium, phosphorus and magnesium; and liver enzymes are rarely found. Such tests should only be done if the underlying illness suggests they may be deranged.

Studies of chemical constituents of the CSF have shown some alterations in relation to both fever and seizures (Wallace, 1988). Complex, rather than simple, seizures are associated with raised lactate levels. CSF gamma-aminobutyric acid (GABA) levels are reduced but they tend, in any case, to be lower in younger children and in febrile children. GABA levels are, however, significantly lower in association with prolonged seizures (Schmieglow *et al.*, 1990). A transient decrease in 5-hydroxyvaleric acid is considered a secondary phenomenon (Giroud *et al.*, 1990). Raised prostaglandin E-2 levels are related to fever rather than to seizures (Loscher and Siemes, 1988). Brief febrile seizures do not alter CSF values of purine metabolites and pyrimidine bases (Livingston *et al.*, 1989; Rodriguez-Nunes *et al.*, 1991). Findings on free amino acids are equivocal (Cremades *et al.*, 1989) and on CSF arginine vasopressin of doubtful significance (Sharples *et al.*, 1992).

Plain skull X-rays are unhelpful and should not be requested. The roles of CT scans and

MRI have yet to be explored in the acute situation. MRI could well be relevant in prolonged lateralized seizures.

EEGs reflect the underlying illness and prior neurologic abnormalities (Wallace, 1988). A generalized increase in slow frequencies is the most usual finding, and is usually a nonspecific response to viral infection. Asymmetries and focal abnormalities are relatively common and almost certainly reflect prior brain abnormality (virtually always minor) rather than an acquired problem. Paroxysmal abnormalities tend to be, to some extent, age related. In 148 children with spike-wave complexes, spikes or sharp waves, the paroxysmal abnormalities occurred in 14% of those aged less than 1 year and 31% of those over 32 months, and were focal in just over one-third (Sofijanov *et al.*, 1992). Acute EEGs are not helpful in prognosis and should be requested only when considered useful for immediate management.

ACUTE THERAPY

Control of the seizure is paramount, but treatment of the fever and of the underlying illness are also important.

Seizures are self-limiting in 90%. Since there is biochemical and pathologic evidence that cerebral damage occurs after 30 minutes, control within this period is vital. Management of a continuing seizure starts with placement of the child in the recovery position. Drug therapy is identical to that suggested for status epilepticus (Chapter 18), with benzodiazepines, usually diazepam given intravenously 0.1 mg/kg or rectally in solution 0.5 mg/kg, the first choice. Intravenous lorazepam finds some favor in North America, where intravenous phenobarbitone is also still used acutely (Millichap and Colliver, 1991). Although numbers are small, comparison of rectal diazepam, followed by oral diazepam 8 hourly during the fever, with intramuscular and later oral phenobarbitone, suggests that the latter is more effective in

preventing repeated attacks during the same illness (Sopo *et al.*, 1991).

John Milton (1641, quoted by Simon, 1993) stated 'the Feaver is to the Physitians, the eternal Reproach'. However, comprehensive reviews of fever (Hull, 1989; Simon, 1993) recommend antipyretic medication, preferably with paracetamol, rather than physical cooling for the control of fever; but Simon (1993) points out that in hyperthermia, present when thermoregulatory measures fail, there is no benefit from antipyretics and external cooling is important.

Underlying infections should receive appropriate treatment.

PATHOLOGIC AND PATHOPHYSIOLOGIC FEATURES

Since the seizures themselves are, in essence, no different to others of cerebral origin, only features specific to febrile attacks will be considered. General points on pathology can be found in Chapter 5 and on pathophysiology in Chapter 6.

Modern imaging techniques have added considerably to the pool of information available, and are likely to continue to do so. Following investigation of a child with electrolyte imbalance using short-echo-time proton nuclear magnetic resonance (NMR) to obtain a biochemical spectrum of the cortical gray matter (Lee, Arcinue and Ross, 1994), it is clear that there is a potential for detailed investigation of metabolic and biochemical changes in the brain during fever and of their relevance to febrile seizures.

There is a well-recognized association between prolonged, particularly lateralized, febrile seizures and later temporal lobe pathology, particularly that involving the mesial temporal structures (Cendes *et al.*, 1993a, 1993b; Kuks *et al.*, 1994; Sloviter, 1994). In the past, it has been assumed that mesial temporal sclerosis is a consequence of the prolonged lateralized seizure, but Cendes *et al.*

(1993a) rightly question whether preexisting anomalies predispose to the final pathology. The lateralization of the initial seizure in response to a generalized stimulus, fever, is in keeping with this suggestion. NMR imaging confirms loss of volume in the mesial temporal structures when complex partial seizures of temporal lobe origin follow febrile seizures (Chapters 20, 23d).

RECURRENCE OF FEBRILE SEIZURES: PROPHYLACTIC THERAPY

Overall, the recurrence risk is in the region of 30–40% (Wallace, 1988; Berg *et al.*, 1990; Daugbjerg *et al.*, 1990; Forsgren *et al.*, 1990b; Maytal and Shinnar, 1990; Al-Eissa *et al.*, 1992; Berg *et al.*, 1992b; Offringa *et al.*, 1992; Rosman *et al.*, 1993; Van Esch *et al.*, 1994). However, the presence or absence of defined risk factors make overall figures irrelevant for the individual. Children at risk of further febrile seizures have the following characteristics: low social class; young age, particularly if less than 1 year at onset, family history positive for seizure disorders; continuing neurologic abnormality; and/or complex initial seizure (Wallace, 1988). A fever of more than 40°C is associated with a reduced recurrence risk (El-Radhi and Banajeh, 1989; Offringa *et al.*, 1992). EEG findings and the presence or absence of proven viral infections appear irrelevant (Rantala, Unari and Tuokho, 1990). Using a multivariate analysis, Offringa *et al.* (1992) found children at most risk of recurrence (48% risk) had temperatures of less than 40°C, a positive family history and multiple initial seizures: those with least recurrence risk (15%) had fevers of more than 40°C, negative family histories, and simple initial seizures. A meta-analysis (Berg *et al.*, 1990) found age at onset 12 months or less and family history of febrile seizures (not unprovoked seizures) distinguished between high- and low-risk groups. The recurrence risk rises with the number of first degree relatives affected (Van Esch *et al.*, 1994), and

with the total number of risk factors present (Kundsen, 1985).

Drug therapy may aim to prevent recurrences or ensure that they are brief when they occur. Prophylaxis can be short term, given at the onset of fever, or long term with daily long-acting antiepileptic drugs. Although there is no evidence that prevention of recurrences reduces the risk of later epilepsy, those with many recurring simple febrile seizures are at greater risk of having generalized epilepsy later (Annegers *et al.*, 1987). Antipyretic measures, alone, are not effective prophylaxis. Intermittent therapy has been reported to be effective by some authors: diazepam rectally in solution or as suppositories, or orally; clonazepam orally or rectally in solution; clobazam orally; nitrazepam orally; valproate as suppositories or, chloral hydrate as suppositories (Wallace, 1988; Tondi *et al.*, 1987; Rosman *et al.*, 1993; Rosman, Colton and Labazzo, 1993). Others have been unable to confirm a reduction in recurrence rates using intermittent therapy (Autret *et al.*, 1990; Daugbjerg *et al.*, 1990). Practical difficulties with intermittent therapy – failure to recognize a pyrexia, problems with administration and the likelihood of causing sedation and thus masking signs in a child who might have an intracranial infection – make intermittent prophylaxis a somewhat unattractive option.

Although initial studies with long-term prophylaxis using phenobarbitone or valproate were promising, more recent analyses using intention-to-treat methodology and pooled data have shown no benefit (Maytal and Shinnar, 1990; Daugbjerg *et al.*, 1990; Farwell *et al.*, 1990; Newton, 1988). Nevertheless, at the beginning of this decade, almost 90% of North American pediatric neurologists still gave prophylactic long-term phenobarbitone after a complex initial febrile seizure (Millichap and Colliver, 1991).

The current preferred drug management of febrile seizures is rectal diazepam in solution 2.5 mg for children aged less than 1 year and

5 mg for those aged 1 year or more given when the seizure starts. Parents are advised to place the child in the recovery position and avoid both overheating and excessive cooling during illnesses.

DEVELOPMENT OF NONFEBRILE SEIZURES AND EPILEPSY

Children who have febrile seizures have a significantly increased risk of subsequent epilepsy (recurrent unprovoked seizures). The NCPP found that by age 7 years 3% of children with febrile seizures had had non-febrile attacks, and 2% had epilepsy (Nelson and Ellenberg, 1976). Another population study (Annegers *et al.*, 1987), using life-table cumulative methods, estimated the risks of unprovoked seizures to be 2% at 5 years, 4.5% by age 10, 5.5% by 15 years and 7% at 25 years. Children with prior febrile seizures probably make up about one-third of the childhood population with epilepsy (Ross *et al.*, 1980).

Unprovoked seizures may present between 1 month and 28 years after the initial febrile attack, but 85% start within 4 years. Almost any seizure type may occur, but generalized tonic-clonic, absence and partial with auto-matisms or other motor symptomatology are those most often reported (Wallace, 1988; Pavone *et al.*, 1989; Wolf and Forsythe, 1989; Verity and Golding, 1991; Wallace, 1991; Al-Eissa *et al.*, 1992; Verity, Ross and Golding, 1993). A review of epileptic syndromes and their relationship to febrile seizures found some evidence of associations with: child-hood absence epilepsy (Chapter 13a); myo-clonic absences (Chapter 13b); severe myo-clonic epilepsy in infancy (Chapter 11e); benign partial epilepsies (Chapter 13c; Kajatani *et al.*, 1981, 1992); and juvenile myoclonic epilepsy (Chapter 14b; Wallace, 1991). How-ever, progression to an epileptic syndrome is very rare. Annegers *et al.* (1987) clarified the risks for generalized and partial epilepsies, demonstrating that generalized epilepsies

tend to occur when there is a positive family history of nonfebrile seizures and a large number of brief generalized febrile seizures have occurred. Partial epilepsies follow pro-longed lateralized febrile seizures in approx-imately 20% of cases. The pathologic findings associated with this sequence of events are explored in detail in Chapter 5. Early age at onset of seizures with fever and persisting neurologic dysfunction are further contrib-utory factors, particularly for later partial epilepsy. The type of infection and the EEG findings within 7 days of onset are irrelevant.

LONG-TERM NEUROLOGIC OUTLOOK

The neurologic status after a febrile seizure closely reflects that prior to the attack. Only in a maximum of 5% of cases selected by hospital admission has a definite persisting alteration in neurologic status been identi-fied. Even if febrile status epilepticus occurs, neurologic findings are unlikely to change (Maytal and Shinnar, 1990). The actual signs are very variable and range from severe disability secondary to cerebral palsy in 3–4%, to mild, hardly discernible deviations from normal in a minimum of 25–30%. When new abnormalities occur, they are usually hemipareses. In the children with previous severe febrile seizures examined during the follow-up of the National Childhood Ence-phalopathy Study (Madge *et al.*, 1993), 5.5% had cerebral palsy, 17% involuntary move-ments, 21% difficulties with gross motor coordination, 25% problems with fine motor coordination, 8% motor impersistence, 6% muscle weakness or spasticity, and 12% pathologic increase or decrease in tendon reflexes. Clearly this was a group selected for severity of the initial seizure, but cohorts who are more representative of the general popu-lation also contain many children with mild or minimal pyramidal tract abnormalities, cerebellar ataxia, dyspraxia, and general clumsiness (see Wallace, 1988). Such children have difficulties with the routine motor tasks of self-care. Speech delay has also been reported to occur more often than expected (Wallace, 1976; Verity, Butler and Golding, 1985b). Continuing neurologic abnormalities are closely associated with a persisting tendency to seizures.

LONG-TERM EEG CHANGES

EEGs are somewhat disappointing investigations in children with febrile seizures. Any abnormalities found initially are more likely to be secondary to the prior neurologic status and the acute illness than to the seizure. Later, generalized abnormalities, particularly paroxysmal discharges, are age dependent rather than indicative of clinical epilepsy. Between one-fifth and one-half of those who have EEGs 2 or more years after the initial seizure have spikes or spike-and-wave recorded (see Wallace, 1988). Sixty per cent of children who have had single febrile seizures between 8 and 10 years earlier have runs of theta activity, asymmetries and intermittent focal slow waves, but only 5% have spikes or spike-and-wave on their EEGs. For children with prolonged lateralized febrile seizures, asymmetric or focal slow waves, with or without spikes, seen on early records are likely to persist, with evolution to frankly epileptic foci in some cases. Centrotemporal spikes are seen much more frequently than expected in children who have had febrile seizures and do not necessarily imply that clinical attacks will appear (Kajitani *et al.*, 1981, 1992; Wallace, 1991). Genetically determined changes – abnormal theta activity, 3 Hz spike-wave and photosensitivity are found more often than would be expected in a random population.

Interpretation of the changes on EEGs of children who have had febrile seizures can be very difficult.

COGNITIVE ABILITIES

The cognitive abilities of children with febrile seizures identified in the general population are generally comparable with those of unaffected children but, when identified by hospital admission, the febrile seizure children are retarded in 5–15% of cases. In addition, specific learning difficulties are much commoner than expected. Discordant twin studies have always found the siblings with febrile seizures to be disadvantaged. Poor speech and language abilities, problems with short-term memory and failure to maintain developmental quotients occur more often than in the general population. Many affected children have difficulties with copying shapes and/or with drawing pictures of people. Between 12 and 19 per cent of children identified by hospital admission have specific difficulties with reading accuracy and/or reading comprehension when tested 8–10 years later. Attentional deficits, when corrected for mental age, are significantly commoner than in controls. For most children with later cognitive difficulties, there is evidence of developmental delay prior to the first febrile seizure; but, particularly when the seizure is severe, acquired difficulties can arise, and some children who progress to epilepsy fail to make adequate progress once a chronic seizure disorder becomes established. Poor cognitive abilities are associated with low social class, repeated febrile seizures, continuing neurologic handicap, and the later occurrence of nonfebrile seizures (Wallace, 1988). Wolf and Forsythe (1989) found that four of 400 children who had brief generalized febrile seizures had intelligence quotients (IQ) of 70 or less; whereas Verity, Ross and Golding (1993) and Madge *et al.* (1993) reported one-third and 21%, respectively, of children with lengthy or severe febrile seizures to have low ability later. In the series of Madge *et al.* (1993), 59% of those with severe attacks later had global ability scores of less than 95. Clearly individual assessment is necessary in many cases.

BEHAVIORAL PROBLEMS

Difficulties in behavior are commoner than in the general childhood population. Aggressive outbursts, temper tantrums, overactivity, sleeping problems, unsociability, enuresis, and encopresis are reported (Verity, Butler and Golding, 1985b; Madge *et al.*, 1993). Such difficulties seem, on the whole, to relate more to the overall developmental status than to the seizures.

SOCIAL ASPECTS

Childhood febrile seizures occur unexpectedly at a young age when the parents are likely to be relatively young and inexperienced. It is not surprising that many parents think that their child has died. This can lead to overprotectiveness, overindulgence, and disruption of the parent–child relationship. Balslev (1991) has reviewed parental reactions to an initial febrile seizure. Seventy-seven per cent thought the child dead or dying, and 15% thought their child was suffocating or had meningitis. Only 21% positioned the child correctly. Afterwards, parental behavior altered, with the commencement of overnight watching in 6%, watching when feverish in 8%, restless sleep (parents) in 60%, and dyspepsia in 29%. The rate of parental behavioral symptoms was not correlated with the child's sex, age, duration, or other characteristics of the seizure, the presence of cyanosis, previous parental knowledge of febrile seizures, the parents' thoughts during the seizure nor with the appropriateness of their management. However, there was a significant rise in parental behavioral symptoms if a further seizure occurred ($P < 0.02$).

CONCLUSIONS

For the majority of children with febrile seizures the outlook for further seizures, epilepsy, continuing neurologic, cognitive, educational and/or behavior problems is very good. However there is an important minority for whom the febrile seizure acts as an alerting mechanism to neurologic and other problems which are likely to continue. The febrile seizure should be recognized as a significant event in these cases.

REFERENCES

Al-Eissa, Y.A., Al-Omair, A.O., Al-Herbish, A.S. *et al.* (1992) Antecedents and outcome of simple and complex febrile convulsions among Saudi children. *Developmental Medicine and Child Neurology* **34**, 1085–90.

Annegers, J.F., Hauser, W.A., Shirts, S.B. *et al.* (1987) Factors prognostic of unprovoked seizures after febrile convulsions. *New England Journal of Medicine*, **316**, 493–8.

Autret, E., Billard, C., Bertrand, P. *et al.* (1990) Double-blind, randomized trial of diazepam versus placebo for prevention of recurrence of febrile seizures. *Journal of Pediatrics*, **117**, 490–4.

Balslev, T. (1991) Parental reactions to a child's first febrile convulsion. A follow-up investigation. *Acta Paediatrica Scandinavica*, **80**, 466–9.

Berg, A.T., Shinnar, S., Hauser, W.A. and Leventhal, J.M. (1990) Predictors of recurrent febrile seizures: a meta-analytic review. *Journal of Pediatrics*, **116**, 329–37.

Berg, A.T., Steinschneider, M., Kang, H. and Shinnar, S. (1992a) Classification of complex features of febrile seizures: inter-rater agreement. *Epilepsia*, **33**, 661–6.

Berg, A.T., Shinnar, S., Hauser, W.A. *et al.* (1992b) A prospective study of recurrent febrile seizures. *New England Journal of Medicine* **327**, 1122–7.

Cassano, P.A., Koepsell, T.D. and Farwell, J.R. (1990) Risk of febrile seizures in childhood in relation to prenatal maternal cigarette smoking and alcohol intake. *American Journal of Epidemiology*, **132**, 462–73.

Cendes, F., Andermann, F. and Gloor, P. *et al.* (1993a) Atrophy of mesial structures in patients with temporal lobe epilepsy: cause or consequence of repeated seizures? *Annals of Neurology*, **34**, 795–801.

Cendes, F., Andermann, F., Dubeau, F. *et al.* (1993b) Early childhood prolonged febrile convulsions, atrophy and sclerosis of mesial structures, and temporal lobe epilepsy: an MRI volumetric study. *Neurology*, **43**, 1083–7.

Chamberlain, J.M. and Gorman, R.L. (1988) Occult bacteremia in children with febrile seizures. *American Journal of Diseases in Children*, **142**, 1073–6.

Cremades, A., Penafiel, R., Monserrat, F. *et al.* (1989) Free amino acids in the cerebrospinal fluid of children with febrile seizures. *Neuropediatrics*, **20**, 129–31.

Daugbjerg, P., Brems, M., Mai, J. *et al.* (1990) Intermittent prophylaxis in febrile convulsions: diazepam or valproic acid? *Acta Neurologica Scandinavica*, **81**, 17–20.

El-Radhi, A.S. and Banajeh, S. (1989) Effect of fever on recurrence rate of febrile convulsions. *Archives of Disease in Childhood*, **64**, 869–70.

Farwell, J.R., Lee, Y.J., Hirtz, D.G. *et al.* (1992) Phenobarbital for febrile seizures – effects on intelligence and on seizure recurrence. *New England Journal of Medicine*, **326**, 144.

Fleming, P.J., Howell, T., Clements, M. and Lucas, J. (1994) Thermal balance and metabolic rate during upper respiratory tract infection in infants. *Archives of Disease in Childhood*, **70**, 187–91.

Forsgren, L., Sidenvall, R., Blomquist, H. K. *et al.* (1990a) An incident case-referrent study of febrile convulsions in children: genetical and social aspects. *Neuropediatrics*, **21**, 153–9.

Forsgren, L., Sidenvall, R., Blomquist, H.K. and Heijbel, J. (1990b) A prospective incidence study of febrile convulsions. *Acta Paediatrica Scandinavica*, **79**, 550–7.

Frantzen, E., Lennox-Buchthal, M. and Nygaard, A. (1968) Longitudinal EEG and clinical study of children with febrile convulsions. *Electroencephalography and Clinical Neurophysiology*, **24**, 197–212.

Giroud, M., Dumas, R., Dauvergne, M., *et al.* (1990) 5-Hydroxyindoleacetic acid and homovallinic acid in cerebrospinal fluid of children with febrile convulsions. *Epilepsia*, **31**, 178–81.

Green, S.M., Rothrock, S.G., Clem, K.J. *et al.* (1993) Can seizures be the sole manifestation of meningitis in febrile children? *Pediatrics*, **92**, 527–34.

Hall, C.B., Long, C.E. and Schnabel, K.C. (1994). Human herpesvirus-6 infection in children. A prospective study of complications and reactivation. *New England Journal of Medicine*, **331**, 432–3.

Hirtz, D.G., Nelson, K.B., and Ellenberg, J.H. (1983) Seizures following childhood immunizations. *Journal of Pediatrics*, **102**, 14–18.

Hull, D. (1989) Fever – the fire of life. *Archives of Disease in Childhood*, **64**, 1741–7.

Isaacs, D. (1989) Immunity to viruses. *Archives of Disease in Childhood*, **64**, 1649–52.

Jackson, J.A., Petersen, S.A. and Wailoo, M.P. (1994). Body temperature changes before minor illness in infants. *Archives of Disease in Childhood*, **71**, 80–3.

Kajitani, T., Ueoka, K., Nakamura, M. and Kumanomidu, Y. (1981) Febrile convulsions and rolandic discharges. *Brain and Development*, **3**, 351–9.

Kajitani, T., Kimura, T., Sumita, M. and Kaneko M. (1992) Relationship between benign epilepsy of children with centro-temporal EEG foci and febrile convulsions. *Brain and Development*, **14**, 230–4.

Knudsen, F.U. (1985) Recurrence risk after first febrile seizure and effect of short term diazepam prophylaxis. *Archives of Disease in Childhood*, **60**, 1045–9.

Kuks, J., Cook, M.J., Fish, D.R. *et al.* (1993) Hippocampal sclerosis in epilepsy and childhood febrile seizures. *Lancet*, **342**, 1391–4.

Lee, J.H., Arcinue, E. and Ross, B.D. (1994) Brief report: organic osmolytes in the brain of an infant with hypernatraemia. *New England Journal of Medicine*, **331**, 439–42.

Lee, P. and Verrier Jones, K. (1991) Urinary tract infection in febrile convulsions. *Archives of Disease in Childhood*, **66**, 1287–90.

Lewis, H.M., Parry, J.V., Parry, R.P. *et al.* (1979) Role of viruses in febrile convulsions. *Archives of Disease in Childhood*, **54**, 869–76.

Livingston, J.H., Brown, J.K., Harkness, R.A. *et al.* (1989) Cerebrospinal fluid nucleotide metabolites following short febrile convulsions. *Developmental Medicine and Child Neurology*, **31**, 161–7.

Loscher, W. and Siemes, H. (1988) Increased concentration of prostaglandin E-2 in cerebrospinal fluid of children with febrile convulsions. *Epilepsia*, **29**, 307–10.

Madge, N., Diamond, J., Miller, D. *et al.* (1993) The National Childhood Encephalopathy Study: a 10 year follow-up. *Developmental Medicine and Child Neurology*, **35** (Suppl. 68).

Maytal, J. and Shinnar, S. (1990) Febrile status epilepticus. *Pediatrics*, **86**, 611–16.

Millichap, J.G. and Colliver, J.A. (1991) Management of febrile seizures: survey of current practice and phenobarbital usage. *Pediatric Neurology*, **7**, 243–8.

Nelson, K.B. and Ellenberg, J.H. (1976) Predictors of epilepsy in children who have experienced febrile seizures. *New England Journal of Medicine*, **295**, 1029–33.

Nelson, K.B. and Ellenberg, J.H. (1990) Prenatal and perinatal antecedents of febrile seizures. *Annals of Neurology*, **27**, 127–31.

Newton, R. W. (1988) Randomised controlled trials of phenobarbitone and valproate in febrile convulsions. *Archives of Disease in Childhood*, **63**, 1189–91.

Offringa, M., Derksen-Lubsen, G., Bossuyi, P.M. and Lubsen, J. (1992) Seizure recurrence after a first febrile seizure: a multivariate approach. *Developmental Medicine and Child Neurology*, **34**, 15–24.

Pavone, L., Cavazzuti, G.B., Incorpora, G. *et al.* (1989) Late febrile convulsions: a clinical follow up. *Brain and Development*, **11**, 183–5.

Rantala, H., Uhari, M. and Tuokko, H. (1990) Viral infections and recurrences of febrile convulsions. *Journal of Pediatrics*, **116**, 195–9.

Rich, S.S., Annegers, J.F., Hauser, W.A. and Anderson, V.E. (1987) Complex segregation analysis of febrile convulsions. *American Journal of Human Genetics*, **41**, 249–57.

Rodriguez-Nunez, A., Camina, F., Lojo, S. *et al.* (1991) Purine metabolites and pyrimidine bases in cerebrospinal fluid of children with simple febrile seizures. *Developmental Medicine and Child Neurology*, **33**, 908–11.

Rosman, N.P., Colton, T. and Labazzo, J. (1993) Diazepam to prevent febrile seizures. *New England Journal of Medicine*, **329**, 2034.

Rosman, N.P., Colton, T., Labazzo, J. *et al.* (1993) A controlled trial of diazepam administered during febrile illnesses to prevent recurrence of febrile seizures. *New England Journal of Medicine*, **329**, 79–84.

Ross, E.M., Peckham, C.S., West, P.B. *et al.* (1980) Epilepsy in children: findings from The National Child Development Study. *British Medical Journal*, **1**, 207–10.

Saper, C.B. and Breder, C.D. (1994) The neurologic basis of fever. *New England Journal of Medicine*, **330**, 1880–6.

Schmieglow, K., Johnsen, A.H., Ebbesen, F. *et al.* (1990). Gamma-aminobutyric acid concentration in lumbar cerebrospinal fluid from patients with febrile convulsions and controls. *Acta Paediatrica Scandinavica*, **79**, 1092–8.

Sharples, P.M., Seckl, J.R., Human, D. *et al.* (1992) Plasma and cerebrospinal fluid arginine vasopressin in patients with and without fever. *Archives of Disease in Childhood*, **67**, 998–1002.

Simon, H.B. (1993) Hyperthermia. *New England Journal of Medicine*, **329**, 483–7.

Sloviter, R.S. (1994) The functional organization of the hippocampal dentate gyrus and its relevance to the pathogenesis of temporal lobe epilepsy. *Annals of Neurology*, **35**, 640–54.

Sofijanov, N., Emoto, S., Kuturec, M. *et al.* (1992) Febrile seizures: clinical characteristics and initial EEG. *Epilepsia*, **33**, 52–7.

Sopo, S.M., Pesarei, M.A., Celestini, E. and Stabile, A. (1991) Short-term prophylaxis of febrile convulsions. *Acta Paediatrica Scandinavica*, **80**, 248–9.

Suga, S., Yoshikawa, T., Asano, Y. *et al.* (1993) Clinical and virological analyses of 21 infants with exanthem subitum (roseola infantum) and central nervous system complications. *Annals of Neurology*, **33**, 597–603.

Taylor, D.C. and Ounsted, C. (1971) Biological mechanisms influencing the outcome of seizures in response to fever. *Epilepsia*, **12**, 33–45.

Tondi, M., Carboni, F., Deriu, A. *et al.* (1987) Intermittent therapy with clobazam for simple febrile convulsions. *Developmental Medicine and Child Neurology*, **29**, 830–1.

Tsuboi, T. (1987) Genetic analysis of febrile convulsions: twin and family studies. *Human Genetics*, **75**, 7–14.

Van Esch, A., Steyerberg, E.W., Berger, M.Y. *et al.* (1994) Family history and recurrence of febrile seizures. *Archives of Disease in Childhood*, **70**, 395–9.

Verity, C.M. and Golding, J. (1991) Risk of epilepsy after febrile convulsions: a national cohort study. *British Medical Journal*, **303**, 1373–6.

Verity, C.M., Butler, N.R. and Golding, J. (1985a) Febrile convulsions in a national cohort followed up from birth. I – Prevalence and recurrence in the first five years of life. *British Medical Journal*, **290**, 1307–10.

Verity, C.M., Butler, N.R. and Golding, J. (1985b) Febrile convulsions in a national cohort followed up from birth. II – Medical history and intellectual ability at five years of age. *British Medical Journal*, **290**, 1307–10.

Verity, C.M., Ross, E.M. and Golding, G. (1993) Outcome of childhood status epilepticus and lengthy febrile convulsions: findings of a national cohort study. *British Medical Journal*, **307**, 225–8.

Wallace, S.J. (1976) Neurological and intellectual deficits: convulsions with fever viewed as acute indications of life-long developmental defects, in *Brain Dysfunction in Infantile Febrile Convulsions* (eds M.A.B. Brazier and F. Coceani), Raven Press, New York: pp. 259–77.

Wallace, S.J. (1988) *The Child with Febrile Seizures*, Butterworth, London.

Wallace, S.J. (1991) Epileptic syndromes linked with previous history of febrile seizures, in *Modern Perspectives of Child Neurology* (eds Y. Fukuyama, S. Kamoshita, C. Ohtsuka and Y. Suzuki), The Japanese Society of Child Neurology: Tokyo, pp. 175–81.

Wolf, S.M. and Forsythe, A. (1989) Epilepsy and mental retardation following febrile seizures in childhood. *Acta Paediatrica Scandinavica*, **78**, 291–5.

EPILEPSIES WITH ONSET IN THE FIRST YEAR

EARLY EPILEPTIC ENCEPHALOPATHIES 11a

Shunsuke Ohtahara and Yoko Ohtsuka

In keeping with the morphologic and biochemical immaturity of the CNS, when compared with other times in childhood, seizures in the neonatal and early infantile periods are rare. There are only a few epileptic syndromes which begin in early infancy (Commission on Classification and Terminology of the International League Against Epilepsy, 1989), and most of them are refractory. Of these, early-infantile epileptic encephalopathy with suppression-burst – Ohtahara's syndrome (OS) and early myoclonic encephalopathy (EME) – are described in this chapter.

EARLY-INFANTILE EPILEPTIC ENCEPHALOPATHY WITH SUPPRESSION BURST: OHTAHARA'S SYNDROME

OS is the earliest type of age-dependent epileptic encephalopathy.

Overall, age-dependent epileptic encephalopathy comprises OS, West's syndrome, and Lennox–Gastaut syndrome. Although they are independent clinicoelectric entities, having their own clinical and electroencephalographic characteristics, they have the following characteristics in common:

1. Predominance in a certain age group.
2. A peculiar type of frequent, minor generalized seizures.
3. Severe and continuous epileptic EEG abnormality.
4. Heterogeneous etiology.
5. Frequent association with mental defect.
6. Resistance to treatment and grave prognosis (Ohtahara, 1977, 1978).

Furthermore, transition with age is often observed among these syndromes. Considerable numbers of OS cases evolve into West's syndrome, and further from West's syndrome to Lennox–Gastaut syndrome during their clinical course (Yamatogi and Ohtahara, 1981; Ohtsuka *et al.*, 1986; Ohtahara and Yamatogi, 1990). The common characteristics and transition with age led Ohtahara (1977, 1978) to apply the term 'age-dependent epileptic encephalopathy' to this group of disorders.

Although the etiology of these syndromes is heterogeneous, each occurs predominantly in a certain age range and has clinical and EEG characteristics in common. Since these clinical and electrical features characteristic of each type of syndrome are secondary to multiple etiologies, the age factor should be considered as the common denominator responsible for the manifestation of the specific features. Thus, these epileptic syndromes may be the age-specific epileptic reaction to various nonspecific exogenous brain insults, acting at the age-specific development stage.

OS was first described as an independent epileptic syndrome by Ohtahara *et al.* in 1976. Several tens of cases have been reported since then (Martin *et al.*, 1981; Konno *et al.*, 1982; Clark *et al.*, 1987; Bermejo

Epilepsy in Children. Edited by Sheila Wallace. Published in 1996 by Chapman & Hall, London. ISBN 0 412 56860 8

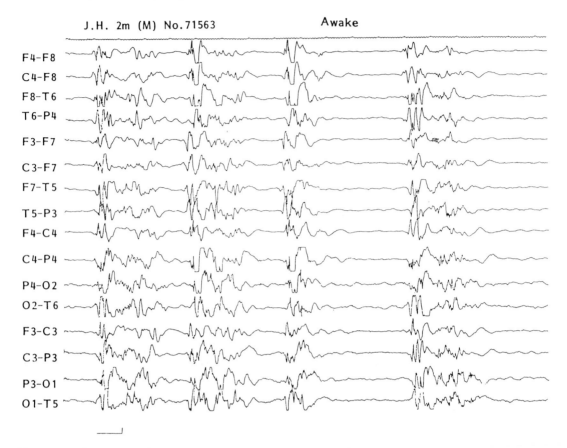

J.H. 2m (M) No.71563   Awake

F4–F8
C4–F8
F8–T6
T6–P4
F3–F7
C3–F7
F7–T5
T5–P3
F4–C4
C4–P4
P4–O2
O2–T6
F3–C3
C3–P3
P3–O1
O1–T5

Fig. 11a.1 Suppression-burst pattern in a 2-month-old boy with Ohtahara's syndrome. (a) Awake.

et al., 1992; Robain and Dulac, 1992), but compared with West's and Lennox–Gastaut syndromes their occurrence has been rare. No obvious sex difference in incidence has been observed.

CLINICAL FINDINGS

The onset of seizures is early, that is confined to within the first 2 or 3 months after birth, and mainly within 1 month. The main seizure type is tonic spasms which occur with or without clustering. They present not only while awake, but in most cases during sleep also. In addition, partial seizures, such as erratic focal motor seizures and hemiconvulsions, are observed in some cases. Myoclonic seizures are rare.

EEG FINDINGS

The most characteristic feature is the suppression-burst (S-B) pattern, which is consistently seen both while awake and asleep (Fig. 11a.1). The S-B pattern is characterized by high voltage bursts alternating with nearly flat patterns at an approximately regular rate. Bursts last 1–3 seconds and comprise 150–350 μV slow waves intermixed with spikes. The duration of the suppression phase is 3–4 seconds. The burst–burst interval measured from the beginning–beginning of bursts ranges from 5 to 10 seconds.

OTHER INVESTIGATIONS

CT scans and MRI reveal abnormal findings, particularly asymmetric lesions, even at an

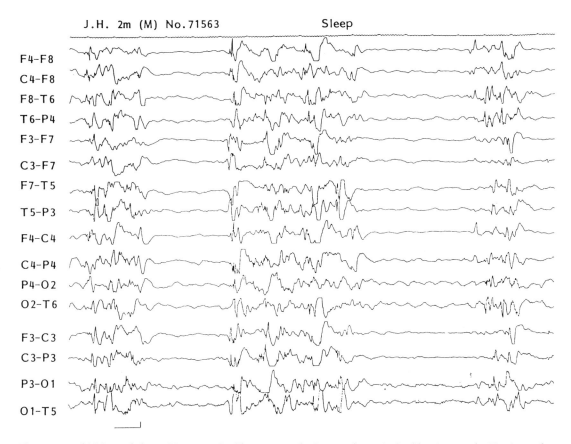

Fig. 11a.1 (b) Natural sleep. Horizontal calibration mark, 1 second, vertical calibration mark, 50 microvolts.

early stage, in most cases. Abnormalities are often found in auditory brainstem responses and visual evoked potentials (Ohtahara *et al.*, 1992).

No abnormalities are found in analyses of serum and urinary amino acids, cerebrospinal fluid, bone marrow, enzyme assay of white blood cells, serum pyruvate and lactate, ammonia, liver function, serum immunoglobulin, or TORCH screen.

UNDERLYING PATHOLOGIES AND PRESUMPTIVE CAUSES

Although the etiology of OS is heterogeneous, obvious brain lesions such as malformations are often found. Porencephaly,

Aicardi's syndrome, cerebral dysgenesis (Ohtahara *et al.*, 1992), olivary-dentate dysplasia (Harding and Boyd, 1991; Robain and Dulac, 1992), hemimegalencephaly (Bermejo *et al.*, 1992), linear sebaceous nevus (Hirata, Ishikawa and Somiya, 1985), Leigh's encephalopathy (Tatsuno *et al.*, 1984), and subacute diffuse encephalopathy (Ohtahara *et al.*, 1992) have been reported. There are also a few cryptogenic cases (Clark, Gill and Noronha, 1987; Ohtahara *et al.*, 1992).

TREATMENT AND PROGNOSIS

Seizures are very intractable. Synthetic ACTH therapy has shown a partial effect in only a few cases. All cases are severely handicapped, both mentally and physically, at final follow-up. Many cases die, especially in the early stages of the disease.

EVOLUTION OF THE CLINICAL AND EEG FEATURES

Characteristically a specific pattern of evolution develops. In mid-infancy, namely during 3–6 months of age, OS evolves to West's syndrome in many cases; and in early childhood, i.e. 1–3 years of age, in some cases further from West syndrome to Lennox–Gastaut syndrome.

In the EEG, the S-B pattern evolves to hypsarrhythmia in many, and further from hypsarrhythmia to diffuse slow spike-waves in some cases.

DIFFERENTIAL DIAGNOSIS FROM WEST'S SYNDROME (Chapter 11b)

The age at onset is different being from neonatal to early infancy in OS and from the middle to late infancy in West's syndrome. Although the main seizure type is tonic spasms in both syndromes, in OS tonic spasms appear not only while awake but also during sleep, and also in many cases with and without clustering. Partial seizures are also observed in some OS cases. Most cases with OS show severe cortical pathology, often with asymmetric lesions on neuroimaging.

With reference to the EEG findings, the S-B pattern is seen in OS, in contrast to hypsarrhythmia in West's syndrome. The S-B pattern differs from the periodic type of hypsarrhythmia in which periodicity becomes distinct only during sleep. In OS seizures are more intractable and ACTH therapy is not effective in most cases. The prognosis is less favourable in OS than in West's syndrome.

EARLY MYOCLONIC ENCEPHALOPATHY

Early myoclonic encephalopathy (EME) is a rare epileptic syndrome, first reported by Aicardi and Goutières in 1978. Males and females are equally affected.

CLINICAL FEATURES

The onset of seizures is confined to the first 3 months of age, and most commence within 1 month of birth.

Fragmentary myoclonias predominate. In addition, frequent erratic partial seizures, massive myoclonias, and tonic spasms are seen, but fragmentary myoclonias are the essential symptom in EME and, in most cases, the earliest type of seizure (Aicardi, 1992). Dalla Bernardina *et al.* (1982, 1983) claim that partial seizures, associated with erratic myoclonias, are particularly characteristic. Massive myoclonias and tonic spasms are not necessarily observed in all cases. Some cases have tonic spasms at 3–4 months of age and have been considered to have atypical West's syndrome. However, the period of atypical West's syndrome is transient and the EME state persists for a prolonged period thereafter.

EEG FINDINGS

The EEG shows the S-B pattern, consisting of alternating bursts lasting 1–5 seconds and almost flat periods of suppression of 3–10 seconds duration. The S-B pattern of EME becomes more distinct during sleep, in many cases especially during deep sleep (Dalla Bernardina *et al.*, 1983; Murakami, Ohtsuka and Ohtahara, 1993) (Fig. 11a.2).

S-B tends to be replaced by atypical hypsarrhythmia or by multifocal paroxysms after 3–5 months of age. However, in most cases, the appearance of atypical hypsarrhythmia is transient and a subsequent return to S-B is observed; thereafter, S-B characteristically persists for a prolonged period (Dalla Bernardina *et al.*, 1983; Murakami, Ohtsuka and Ohtahara, 1993).

NEUROIMAGING

Imaging is normal at the beginning in most cases, but in some cases, progressive cortical

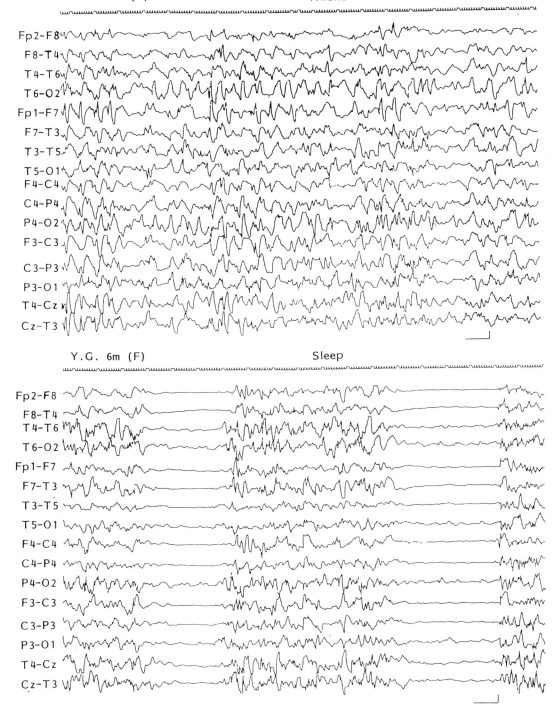

Fig. 11a.2 Suppression-burst pattern in a 6-month-old girl with early myoclonic encephalopathy. (a) Awake. (b) Natural sleep. Horizontal calibration mark, 1 second; vertical calibration mark, 50 microvolts.

and periventricular atrophy are observed later (Aicardi, 1992; Murakami, Ohtsuka and Ohtahara, 1993).

UNDERLYING PATHOLOGIES AND PRESUMPTIVE CAUSES

The most striking feature is the frequency of familial cases (four of 12 families reported by Aicardi (1992) and two of eight in the series of Dalla Bernardina *et al.* (1982, 1983)). This suggests that an inborn error of metabolism is likely to be responsible (see Chapter 4c). Nonketotic hyperglycinemia (Dalla Bernardina *et al.*, 1979; Terasaki *et al.*, 1988), propionic aciduria and D-glycine acidemia have been reported so far (Lombroso, 1990), but there are many cases with as yet unidentified causes.

TREATMENT AND PROGNOSIS

Neither the conventional antiepileptic drugs nor ACTH, corticosteroids, or pyridoxine have been effective. Many cases die early, mostly before 2 years of age. All surviving cases show progressive deterioration and finally reach a vegetative state.

DIFFERENTIAL DIAGNOSIS BETWEEN OHTAHARA'S SYNDROME AND EARLY MYOCLONIC ENCEPHALOPATHY

OS and EME have common clinical and electrical characteristics, i.e. onset in the neonatal and early infantile periods, and the S-B pattern on the EEG. Therefore differential diagnosis between these syndromes requires consideration.

CLINICAL FEATURES

With regard to the clinical seizure types; the main seizure type is tonic spasms in OS, but myoclonias, especially erratic myoclonias, and frequent partial seizures predominate in EME. In contrast, myoclonias are rarely seen in OS.

EEG FINDINGS

The S-B pattern is a feature common to both syndromes, but the form, time of appearance, and duration of appearance differ considerably. S-B in OS is characterized by periodic and consistent appearances during both the awake and sleeping states, whereas in EME, it is enhanced by sleep and often not manifest in the awake state. In OS, S-B is present at the onset and disappears within the first 6 months, whereas in EME, it appears at 1–5 months of age in some cases and characteristically persists for a prolonged period (Dalla Bernardina *et al.*, 1983; Murakami, Ohtsuka and Ohtahara, 1993).

EVOLUTION DURING THE CLINICAL COURSE

A characteristic feature of OS is the evolution of the EEG during the clinical course: from the S-B pattern to hypsarrhythmia in many cases and further from hypsarrhythmia to diffuse slow spike-waves in some cases (Ohtahara *et al.*, 1992). In contrast, in EME, although a transient appearance of atypical hypsarrhythmia is observable during the clinical course in some cases (Murakami, Ohtsuka and Ohtahara, 1993), S-B reappears and persists for a prolonged period. Thus, the pattern of evolution with age differs considerably in the two syndromes.

In relation to evolution in epileptic syndromes, OS shows a specific pattern of evolution as an age-dependent epileptic encephalopathy, while EME has no specific evolution with age.

ETIOLOGY

In OS, obvious brain lesions, such as brain malformations, are often seen, and CT scans and MRI show abnormal findings even at an early stage. No familial cases have been reported in OS. In contrast, the frequent occurrence of familial cases suggests that a congenital familial metabolic disorder is causative in EME.

These features emphasize definite differences between OS and EME, and strongly suggest that they belong to different clinico-electrical entities. They also support the results of the research in which Schlumberger, Dulac and Plouin (1992) demonstrated characteristic clinical and symptomatologic features in these two syndromes with no overlap.

REFERENCES

Aicardi, J. (1992) Early myoclonic encephalopathy (neonatal myoclonic encephalopathy), in *Epileptic Syndromes in Infancy, Childhood and Adolescence*, 2nd edn, (eds J. Roger, M. Bureau, C. Dravet *et al.*), John Libbey, London, pp. 13–23.

Aicardi, J. and Goutières, F. (1978) Encephalopathie myoclonique neonatale. *Revue d'Electroencephalographie et de Neurophysiologie Clinique*, **8**, 99–101.

Bermejo, A.M., Martin, V.L., Arcas, J. *et al.* (1992) Early infantile epileptic encephalopathy: a case associated with hemimegalencephaly. *Brain and Development*, **14**, 425–8.

Clark, M., Gill, J., Noronha, M. *et al.* (1987) Early infantile epileptic encephalopathy with suppression burst: Ohtahara syndrome. *Developmental Medicine and Child Neurology*, **29**, 520–8.

Commission on Classification and Terminology of the International League Against Epilepsy (1989) Proposal for revised classification of epilepsies and epileptic syndromes. *Epilepsia*, **30**, 389–99.

Dalla Bernardina, B., Aicardi, J., Goutières, F. *et al.* (1979) Glycine encephalopathy. *Neuropaediatrie*, **10**, 209–25.

Dalla Bernardina, B., Dulac, O., Bureau, M. *et al.* (1982) Encephalopathie myoclonique précoce avec epilepsie. *Revue d'Electroencephalographie et de Neurophysiologie Clinique*, **12**, 8–14.

Dalla Bernardina, B., Dulac, O., Fejerman, N. *et al.* (1983) Early myoclonic epileptic encephalopathy (EMEE). *European Journal of Pediatrics*, **140**, 248–52.

Harding, B.N. and Boyd, S.G. (1991) Intractable seizures from infancy can be associated with dentato-olivary dysplasia. *Journal of the Neurological Sciences*, **104**, 157–65.

Hirata, Y., Ishikawa, A. and Somiya, K. (1985) A case of linear nevus sebaceous syndrome associated with early-infantile epileptic encephalopathy with suppression burst (EIEE). *No To Hattatsu*, **17**, 577–82.

Konno, K., Miura, Y., Suzuki, H. *et al.* (1982) A study on clinical features of the early infantile epileptic encephalopathy with suppression burst or Ohtahara syndrome. *No To Hattatsu*, **14**, 395–404.

Lombroso, C.T. (1990) Early myoclonic encephalopathy, early infantile epileptic encephalopathy, and benign and severe infantile myoclonic epilepsies: a critical review and personal contributions, *Journal of Clinical Neurophysiology*, **7**, 380–408.

Martin, H.-J., Deroubaix-Tella, P. and Thelliez Ph. (1981) Encephalopathie epileptique neo-natale à bouffées periodiques. *Revue d'Electroencephalographie et de Neurophysiologie Clinique*, **11**, 397–403.

Murakami, N., Ohtsuka, Y. and Ohtahara, S. (1993) Early infantile epileptic syndromes with suppression-bursts: early myoclonic encephalopathy vs. Ohtahara syndrome. *Japanese Journal of Psychiatry and Neurology*, **47**, 197–200.

Ohtahara, S. (1977) A study on the age-dependent epileptic encephalopathy. *No To Hattatsu*, **9**, 2–21.

Ohtahara, S. (1978) Clinico-electrical delineation of epileptic encephalopathies in childhood. *Asian Medical Journal*, **21**, 499–509.

Ohtahara, S. and Yamatogi, Y. (1990) Evolution of seizures and EEG abnormalities in childhood onset epilepsy, in *Clinical Neurophysiology of Epilepsy, Handbook of Electroencephalography and Clinical Neurophysiology*, Revised Series, vol. 4, (eds J.A. Wada and R.J. Ellingson), Elsevier, Amsterdam, pp. 457–77.

Ohtahara, S., Ishida, T., Oka, E. *et al.* (1976) On the specific age dependent epileptic syndrome: the early-infantile epileptic encephalopathy with suppression-burst. *No To Hattatsu*, **8**, 270–80.

Ohtahara, S., Ohtsuka, Y., Yamatogi, Y. *et al.* (1992) Early-infantile epileptic encephalopathy with suppression-bursts, in *Epileptic Syndromes, in Infancy, Childhood and Adolescence*, 2nd edn, (eds J. Roger, M. Bureau, C. Dravet *et al.*), John Libbey, London, pp. 25–34.

Ohtsuka, Y., Ogino, T., Murakami, N. *et al.* (1986) Developmental aspects of epilepsy with special reference to age-dependent epileptic encephalopathy. *Japanese Journal of Psychiatry and Neurology*, **40**, 307–13.

Robain, O. and Dulac, O. (1992) Early epileptic encephalopathy with suppression bursts and olivary-dentate dysplasia. *Neuropediatrics*, **23**, 162–4.

Schlumberger, E., Dulac, O. and Plouin, P. (1992) Early infantile epileptic syndrome(s) with suppression-burst: nosological considerations, in *Epileptic Syndromes in Infancy, Childhood and Adolescence*, 2nd edn, (eds J. Roger, M. Bureau, C. Dravet, *et al.*), John Libbey, London, pp. 35–42.

Tatsuno, M., Hayashi, M., Iwamoto, H., *et al.* (1984) Leigh's encephalopathy with wide lesions and early infantile epileptic encephalopathy with burst-suppression: an autopsy case. *No To Hattatsu*, **16**, 68–75.

Terasaki, T., Yamatogi, Y., Ohtahara, S. *et al.* (1988) A long-term follow-up study on a case with glycine encephalopathy. *No To Hattatsu*, **20**, 15–22.

Yamatogi, Y. and Ohtahara S. (1981) Age-dependent epileptic encephalopathy: a longitudinal study. *Folia Psychiatrica et Neurologica Japanica*, **35**, 321–31.

Raili Riikonen

West's syndrome consists of infantile spasms, hypsarrhythmia, and mental retardation. The spasms are usually resistant to conventional antiepileptic drugs. Typically, the onset is between 3 and 7 months of age and virtually never after the age of 1 year. The incidence has been estimated to vary between 1.6 and 4.3 per 10 000 live births (Nelson, 1972; Riikonen and Donner, 1979), and has not changed during the past 30 years (Riikonen, 1995).

INFANTILE SPASMS AND HYPSARRHYTHMIA

In his letter to *The Lancet*, West (1841) described the characteristic spasms and noted an association with development retardation. Gibbs and Gibbs (1952) first described the EEG pattern commonly seen in infants with infantile spasms, and gave the pattern of hypsarrhythmia its name. Infantile spasms are classified as generalized epilepsies in the International Classification (Commission on Classification and Terminology of the International League Against Epilepsy, 1989).

SPASMS

The spasms usually involve the muscles of the neck, trunk, and extremities. A cry frequently follows an attack. The spasms may be flexor, extensor or, most commonly, mixed (Hrachovy and Frost 1989). The individual child can have various types of the spasms. The presence of asymmetric spasms and focal signs suggests a symptomatic etiology. Spasms occur in series. They are common during drowsiness and occur especially on arousal or soon thereafter. Motor components can be minimal. A vast number of spasms are missed by parents when compared to those seen in polygraphic and video recordings. The diagnosis of the spasms is easy when they are typical. However, they are often misinterpreted, (in as many as 88% of cases by primary care physicians, Bellman, Ross and Miller, 1983), and considered to be colic, startle responses or normal infant behavior. The spasms may be infrequent or atypical at the onset. Repetitive, stereotyped characterization of any movements in infancy should arouse the suspicion of infantile spasms and lead to an immediate EEG examination.

EEG

Hypsarrhythmia consists of a pattern of irregular, diffuse, asymmetric, high-voltage slow waves interspersed with sharp waves and spikes, distributed randomly throughout scalp recordings (a total, chaotic disorganization of cortical electrogenesis, Fig. 11b.1). The term 'modified hypsarrhythmia' is used if there is some preservation of background rhythms, synchronous bursts of generalized spike-wave activity, significant asymmetry, or burst-suppression on the tracing. A constant focus of abnormal discharges may also

Epilepsy in Children. Edited by Sheila Wallace. Published in 1996 by Chapman & Hall, London. ISBN 0 412 56860 8

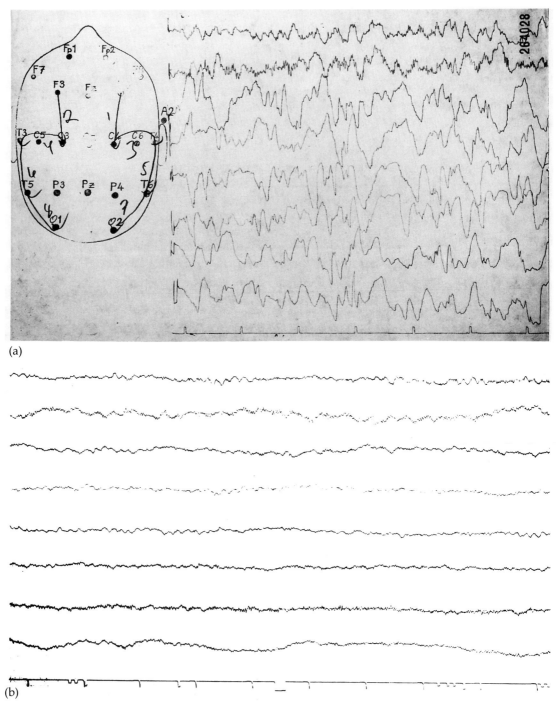

(a)

(b)

Fig. 11b.1 (a) Hypsarrhythmia in a patient with cryptogenic infantile spasms. Irregular, diffuse, asymmetric, high-voltage slow waves interspersed with sharp waves and spikes arising multifocally (waking EEG before therapy). (b) Effect of corticotrophin therapy over 2 weeks.

precede, accompany, and/or follow hypsar-rhythmia. Such atypical patterns can be observed in up to 40% of patients (Jeavons and Bower, 1973). Extremely rarely, infantile spasms may occur when the EEG does not show a hypsarrhythmic pattern. However, this pattern is usually present at some time in the course of the disorder, if only in slow-wave sleep. 'Hypsarrhythmic pattern is a highly variable and dynamic EEG pattern from minute to minute, from hour to hour' (Hrachovy, Frost and Kellaway, 1984). Imme-diately following a clinical seizure and during rapid eye movement (REM) sleep, EEG trac-ings tend to be closer to normal, showing a marked decrease in abnormal activity (Kel-laway *et al.*, 1979). Persisting hypsarrhythmia during a cluster of spasms appeared to be an EEG pattern that correlated with a favorable outcome (Fusco and Vivevagno, 1993). A constantly normal tracing, including sleep-recording, effectively rules out the diagnosis of infantile spasms. Sometimes the infant ceases to take interest in his surroundings, and blindness is suspected. This functional amaurosis is seen in association with missing or grossly abnormal patterns of visual evoked potentials (Wenzel, 1987) and probably cor-responds to perfusion defects involving the parieto-occipital areas (Chugani *et al.*, 1993; Jambaqué *et al.* 1993). In addition, behavioral regression of an infant under 1 year of age should lead to an EEG examination, when hypsarrhythmia may reveal the cause of the regression. Some brain malformations such as Aicardi's syndrome (Fariello *et al.*, 1977), lissencephaly syndrome (Hakamada *et al.*, 1979), or hemimegalencephaly (Paladin *et al.*, 1989), have characteristic EEG patterns.

DIFFERENTIAL DIAGNOSIS

Benign myoclonus of early infancy may closely mimic infantile spasms, but the EEG is normal (Lombroso and Fejerman, 1977). Benign myoclonic epilepsy (Chapter 11d), with a favorable outcome, is also often misdiagnosed as infantile spasms, but the EEG shows generalized spike-waves occur-ring in brief bursts during the early stages of sleep (Dravet, Bureau and Roger, 1985). Syndromes closely related to West's syn-drome include early myoclonic encephalo-pathy (Aicardi, 1985) (Chapter 11a), early infantile epileptic encephalopathy (Ohtahara *et al.* 1987, Chapter 11a), and the syndrome of periodic, lateralized spasms (Gobbi *et al.*, 1987). The two former syndromes both have a burst-suppression pattern in EEG. The three syndromes include patients with very serious brain pathology and outcome. Early infantile encephalopathy will often evolve to West's syndrome. West's syndrome evolves in about one-quarter of the patients to Lennox–Gastaut syndrome, which is an important differential diagnosis for patients more than 1 year of age.

ETIOLOGY

Many different disorders which cause abnor-malities of the brain seem to be etiologic in West's syndrome (Table 11b.1). Since the study of Zellweger (1948) infantile spasms have been divided into two groups on the basis of the identified or presumed cause of the seizures: symptomatic and cryptogenic. The symptomatic group comprises infants who have a definite history suggesting a prenatal, perinatal or postnatal insult, when the predisposing etiologic factor can usually be identified. Children with cryptogenic spasms are those who have been healthy and developed normally prior to the spasms and for which no cause can be identified. The sizes of the groups has varied amongst reports. Classification depends heavily on the extent of the investigations performed. In modern series, the proportion of cryptogenic cases has decreased to about 15%, following careful neuroradiologic, virologic, and meta-bolic studies (Matsumoto *et al.*, 1981; Riiko-nen, 1982; Glaze *et al.*, 1988).

Various pre- and perinatal insults are

Table 11b.1   Presumed etiologic factors in West's syndrome

---

1. Prenatal

Placental dysfunction:
Maternal toxemia
Abruptio placentae (Crichton 1968, Riikonen and Donner 1979)

Intrauterine hypoxia-ischemia:
Multicystic encephalomalacia (Jeavons and Bower 1973)
Porencephaly
Hydrancephaly (Neville 1972)
Ulegyria
Cortical dysplasia (Palm, Blennow and Brun, 1986)

Congenital malformations:
Dysgenetic
Tuberous sclerosis (Riikonen and Simell 1990)
Aicardi's syndrome
Other types of agenesis of corpus callosum
Lissencephaly
Miller–Dieker syndrome (Dobyns, Stratton and Greenberg, 1984)
Holoprosencephaly (Watanabe, Hara and Iwase, 1976)
Megalencephaly (Lombroso 1983)
Heterotopias
PEHO syndrome (Salonen *et al.*, 1991)
Incontinentia pigmenti (Esquivel, Pitt and Boyd, 1991)
Linear nevus syndrome (Vivegano *et al.*, 1984)
Chromosomal – trisomy 21 (Cassidy *et al.*, 1983), fragile X chromosome (Rugtveit, 1986)

Infections:
Cytomegalovirus
Rubella
Toxoplasma (Riikonen, 1993)

Genetic:
Metabolic defect:
Phenylketonuria
Lipid storge disease
Tuberous sclerosis etc. (Bignami *et al.*, 1966)
Pyridoxine-dependency seizures (Bankier, Turner and Hopkins, 1983)
Nonketotic hyperglycinemia (Dalla Bernardina *et al.*, 1979)
Hyperornithinemia, hypercitrullinemia and homocitrullinemia (HHH) syndrome (Shih, Efron and Moser, 1963)
Histidinuria (Duffner and Cohen, 1975)

Degenerative diseases:
Leigh's necrotizing encephalomyelopathy (Kamoshita, Mizurani and Fukuyama, 1970)
Sudanophilic leukodystrophy

Endogenous/exogenous toxic factors:
Lead and lithium (Lombroso, 1983)

2. Perinatal

Hypoxia-ischemia
Hypoglycemia (Riikonen and Donner, 1979)
Infections

3. Postnatal

Intracranial hemorrhage, sepsis, CNS infections:
Herpes simplex virus
Purulent meningitis (Riikonen, 1995)
Hypoxia-ischemia (Hrachovy *et al.*, 1987)
Secondary metabolic derangements
Exogenous toxins
Cerebral infarcts (Alvarez, Shinnar and Moshé, 1987)
Brain tumors (Ruggieri, Carabello and Fejerman, 1989)

---

responsible for the majority of cases in the symptomatic group (Table 11b.1). In one population-based cohort including 209 children with West's syndrome, the actual incidence of identified etiologic factors was as follows: 22% of the children had brain malformations or malformation syndromes and tuberous sclerosis; insults at birth were the cause in 7.1%; unknown pre- and/or perinatal factors in 17.7%; early infections in 4.3%; symptomatic neonatal hypoglycemia in 14.8%, and familial or metabolic diseases in 8.6%; and 18.2% were cryptogenic (Riikonen, 1995). From 1960 to 1991 the proportion of brain malformations and malformation syndromes, as well as metabolic diseases identified, increased, secondary to greater refinement in neuroradiologic and metabolic diagnostic methods. Conversely, the number attributed to birth insults, infections and neonatal hypoglycemia decreased. Small-for-gestational age infants seem to be more liable to develop infantile spasms than approriate-for age preterm infants (Crichton, 1968; Riikonen, 1995). Increased survival of infants with very low birth weight does not seem to increase the number with West's syndrome.

Tuberous sclerosis is an important etiologic factor, accounting for up to 25% of patients. A variety of other syndromes have been reported: Aicardi's syndrome (corpus callosum agenesis or hypoplasia, chorioretinal lacunae, other anomalies; Aicardi, Lefébure and Lerique-Koechlin, 1965), Miller–Dieker syndrome (type I lissencephaly, specific facial dysmorphic features, chromosomal anomaly 17 p-; Dobyns, Stratton and Greenberg, 1984), PEHO syndrome (Progressive Encephalopathy, Hypsarrhythmia, Optic atrophy, Salonen *et al.*, 1991). Metabolic diseases have also rarely been connected with West syndrome (Table 11b.1). The empiric recurrence risk among siblings is estimated to be 1.5% and for all first-degree relatives 0.7% (Fleiszar, Daniel and Imrey, 1977), but certain families may have a high recurrence risk, due to still unidentified autosomal recessive disorders. Familial cases, i.e. more than one patient in a family, may occur in 4.4–4.8% of the patients (Riikonen, 1987; Dulac *et al.*, 1993).

At autopsy, two-thirds of the patients are considered to have epilepsy of embryofetal origin (Meencke and Gerhard, 1985; Jellinger, 1987). At epilepsy surgery, too, patients are often found to have microdysgenesis (Vinters *et al.*, 1992; Chugani *et al.*, 1993). However, these series consist of selected cases, since autopsy material usually comes from patients who die at an early age; thus severe malformations are, presumably, overrepresented. On the other hand, patients selected for surgery usually have focal structural anomalies. In clinical and radiologic series, 18–20% are found to have malformations.

PATHOPHYSIOLOGY

The pathophysiologic mechanism of West's syndrome is unknown. There are at least four main theories, which are detailed below.

DISTURBANCE OF CORTICAL SYNAPTOGENESIS

It is believed that there is a problem in the modulation of neurotransmitters at a specific period of brain maturation. The age when infantile spasms usually appear corresponds to the critical period of maximal cerebral development (Riikonen, 1983). The discrepancy between brain development and age is supported by the following: West's syndrome and hypsarrhythmia have a tendency to disappear spontaneously with age; defective dendritic development has been demonstrated at autopsies of children with West's syndrome, suggesting the possibility of arrested development; glucocorticoids have an accelerating effect on some physiologic events (enzymes, myelination, neuroblast growth); positron emission tomography (PET) has shown that subcortical, phylogenetically old structures, where the maturation of the brain starts, are hypermetabolic in these patients, compared to age-matched controls (Chugani, Phelps and Mazziotta *et al.*, 1987; Chugani *et al.*, 1992).

DYSFUNCTION OF THE BRAINSTEM

More localized lesions, especially of the brainstem, are also thought to be responsible for infantile spasms (biochemical or anatomic imbalance between neurons in the giganto-cellular area, raphe (Hrachovy and Frost, 1989)). This theory is supported by some neuropathologic findings (Satoh *et al.*, 1986) and studies of brainstem-evoked potentials or magnetic resonance imaging (MRI) of lesions in this area (Miyazahi *et al.*, 1993); brain serotonin neurons are concentrated in or near the midline of brain, and altered serotonin metabolism may play some role in the pathophysiology of infantile spasms (Silverstein and Johnston, 1984); and the spasms are related to awakening.

ABNORMAL CORTICAL–SUBCORTICAL INTERACTION

According to Chugani *et al.*, 1992, cortical abnormality exerts a noxious influence over the brainstem, from where discharges spread rostrally to the lenticular nuclei and caudally to the spinal cord, accounting for the relative symmetry of the spasms. This cortical trigger-ing mechanism is supported by the observa-tions that: initially, partial seizures may evolve to infantile spasms with a bilateral hypsarrhythmic pattern (Yamamato *et al.*, 1988); and partial seizures can precede, co-exist with, or follow infantile spasms, and resections of focal abnormalities seen on EEG and PET scans can stop infantile spasms (Chugani *et al.*, 1993).

ABNORMAL BRAIN–ADRENAL AXIS

More recently, Baram (1993) has suggested that corticotrophin releasing hormone (CRH) synthesis and activity is increased, secondary

to early stress during a critical perinatal period (high CRH receptor abundance), which can result in long-term effects. How-ever, CSF CRH has been normal (Baram *et al.*, 1992), as are tests on the hypophyseal–adrenal (HPA) axis of patients prior to ther-apy (Perheentupa, Riikonen and Dunkel, 1986). Further, studies of neurotransmitter metabolism in CSF, including ACTH and serotonin metabolites, have yielded conflict-ing results (Nalin *et al.*, 1985; Riikonen and Gupta, 1988; Airaksinen, Tuomisto and Riikonen, 1992; Baram *et al.*, 1992).

It appears that heterogeneous pathophysio-logic mechanisms may be operative in the genesis of infantile spasms. In some cases a focal cortical lesion probably produces in-fantile spasms; in others, lesions might exist elsewhere.

ETIOLOGIC INVESTIGATIONS

A careful search for etiologic factors should be undertaken in every case to formulate a more accurate prognosis, and establish whether there is a need for genetic counsel-ing. When carefully sought, etiologic factors can be detected in up to two-thirds of the cases. A comprehensive history, especially with regard to heritable disorders and pre-natal and perinatal events, as well as a careful clinical examination, e.g. to check for signs of tuberous sclerosis (TS), should always be undertaken. The importance of neuro-ophthalmologic, neuroimaging, virologic, and neurometabolic studies is further stressed.

Neuroophthamologic evaluation can identify the ocular hallmarks of a variety of diseases including structural malformations, meta-bolic disorders, early infections and TS. CT may reveal pathology in two-thirds of cases: malformations, calcifications and/or brain atrophies (Cusmai, Dulac and Diebler, 1988). The calcifications of TS can be detected under the age of 1 year (Riikonen and Simell, 1990). It is important that CT is done before ACTH therapy, since the latter leads to reversible dilatation of the ventricles and appearances suggestive of atrophy. The cause of this change is unknown (Glaze, Hrachovy and Frost, 1986); MRI can detect disturbances of myelination and focal abnormalities which cannot be seen on CT (van Bogaert *et al.*, 1993).

CSF (cells, protein, IgG index, viral antibody index) should be studied if the etiology is still unclear. Immunoglobulin production in the CNS can be active for a long time, even years after a primary infection. Therefore estimation of the IgG index can provide important clues to past herpes simplex virus (HSV), cytomegalovirus (CMV) or rubella infection at the age when spasms appear. Infections may represent 10% of etiology (Riikonen, 1993).

Screening of serum and urine for inborn errors of metabolism including amino acids is justified, even though it is uncommon to discover an abnormality. In some infants chromosomal analysis will be indicated because of dysmorphic features or structural anomalies of the brain.

When considering surgical treatment single photon emission cerebral tomography (SPECT) and PET studies can be valuable (Chapter 20). They may reveal abnormalities in patients though CT and MRI have been normal (Chiron *et al.*, 1993; Chugani *et al.*, 1993). However, despite significant correlations with lesional foci, or with EEG foci, in the absence of neuroradiologically detectable lesions, PET and SPECT have no absolute localizing value, and cannot be used alone for preoperative assessment (Chiron *et al.*, 1989; Shields *et al.*, 1992). At present, the precise value of these techniques remains to be defined. The significance of focal abnormalities is also a problem worthy of future study.

TREATMENT

STEROIDS

Infantile spasms are usually resistant to antiepileptic drugs. Since the first results were reported with ACTH (Sorel and Dusaucy-Bauloye, 1958), corticoids have remained the therapy of choice. A good response occurs to ACTH in about 60–80% of children with infantile spasms and to oral steroid therapy in 50% (Singer, Rabe and Haller, 1980; Snead, Benton and Hosey, 1983). Most examiners find ACTH more effective than corticosteroids but opinions vary. In the only prospective double-blind study, which included 24 children with infantile spasms, there was no significant difference between corticotropin and oral steroids but some minor differences may have been overlooked because the number of patients was small (Hrachovy *et al.*, 1984). Since the response may be favorable, even for patients with symptomatic etiology, short-term treatment with ACTH is probably advisable for this group also. However, because side-effects of ACTH are frequent, some authors prefer to use steroid therapy only for patients with cryptogenic spasms, for whom it may improve the long-term outcome.

Dose and duration of therapy

The optimal dose and optimal duration of ACTH therapy is still unknown. The modalities of treatment have been extremely variable and comparisons between studies are almost impossible. The daily intramuscular dosage of ACTH administered either alone or combined with glucocorticoids, has varied from 5 to 180 units, and the duration of treatment from 3 weeks to 6 months or longer. The daily oral corticosteroid usually used is hydrocortisone 5–25 mg/kg or prednisolone 2–10 mg/kg. Some authors favor prolonged high-dose treatments using ACTH (Singer, Robe and Haller, 1980; Lerman and Kivity, 1982; Snead *et al.*, 1989) or hydrocortisone (Pinsard, 1981), while others prefer short treatments with lower doses of ACTH (Riikonen, 1982; Hrachovy and Frost, 1989; Hrachovy, Frost and Glaze, 1994) or hydrocortisone (Aicardi 1992). In one study children treated with lower doses of ACTH had a better long-term mental outcome than those treated with higher doses (Riikonen and Donner, 1980). Large doses and synthetic derivatives seem to have more side-effects, probably due to their overprolonged effect (Riikonen and Donner, 1980; Perheentupa, Riikonen and Dunkel, 1986).

The relapse rate is about 30% with treatment schedules of 6 weeks. The relapses sometimes occur during corticosteroid treatment, perhaps due to downregulation of the receptors (Tornello *et al.*, 1982), but are more usual within 2 months of cessation of treatment. A lower relapse rate has been found in studies with longer treatment. However, it is difficult to be sure whether longer treatment or spontaneous remission accounts for the cessation of the spasms. West's syndrome may disappear within 1 year in 25% of the patients (Hrachovy, Glaze and Frost, 1991). Further, the following are good reasons for short-term treatment:

1. The rapid response with regard to both spasms and hypsarrhythmia (within 2 weeks from the start of therapy).
2. Frequent side-effects (which can be deleterious for the growing brain).
3. A second course leads to a further remission in up to two-thirds of the cases.

My own recommendation is as follows: Treatment is started by giving oral pyridoxine 150 mg daily for 3–4 days. If there is no response, corticotrophin (Acton prolongatum) is started, and the dose adjusted for individuals in a step-wise manner on the basis of etiology and response to therapy. Initially Acton prolongatum 3 IU/kg is given daily and any concomitant anticonvulsants are tapered down. The first evaluation for cessation of the spasms and hypsarrhythmia is arranged after 2 weeks' treatment. In patients with a cryptogenic etiology who respond, the dose is tapered in the sequence 1.5, 0.75 IU/kg/daily, each given for a week. In symptomatic patients the initial dose is continued for a total of 4 weeks and then similarly tapered. If the response is not good (reassessing at 2-week intervals), the dose will be doubled twice at 2-week intervals up to 12 IU/kg both for cryptogenic and symptomatic patients. If there is still no response the dose will be tapered stepwise at 1-week intervals halving the dose each times; and, therapy with anticonvulsants, preferably nitrazepam, will be started. If there is a relapse, the highest preceding dose will be resumed. The children are treated as inpatients because daily evaluation of the spasms and daily injections and observation of the side-effects of the therapy are important.

With this regimen all the cryptogenic patients have had a good long-lasting effect with the short treatment period and with low doses (4 weeks, beginning with 3 IU/kg/day) (Heiskala *et al.*, in press). No other drugs during the steroid therapy are recommended, since there is no evidence that addition of anticonvulsants to steroid therapy improves the control rate. In contrast, they may shorten the half-life of steroids, and valproate may have antagonistic effects on the HPA axis (Kritzler, Vining and Plotnick, 1983; Gambertoglio *et al.*, 1984).

Side-effects of steroid therapy

Severe side-effects and fatal results from ACTH treatment have been reported (Riikonen and Donner, 1980). Since steroids suppress each stage of the immune response, infections are common. Atypical infections may even occur. Other side-effects of the therapy are arterial hypertension, intracranial hemorrhages, osteoporosis, renal calcifications (Rausch, Hanefeld and Kaufman, 1984; Riikonen *et al.*, 1986), electrolyte and fluid disturbances (Riikonen *et al.*, 1989), subdural haematoma, severe neurological symptoms such as apathy, hypotonia and irritability, transient brain atrophy (Glaze *et al.*, 1986), and hypertrophic cardiomyopathy with cardiac insufficiency (Lang *et al.*, 1984). One of the most dangerous side-effects of steroid therapy seems to be adrenocortical hyporesponsiveness following discontinuance of treatment (Perheentupa, Riikonen and Dunkel, 1986; Rao and Willis, 1987). This probably explains why most deaths occur within 2 weeks of cessation of therapy. Dramatic endocrine-related changes in fluid balance with hypoadrenalism occur at the same time (Riikonen *et al.*, 1989).

Nevertheless, most side-effects may be prevented or treated, if the following recommendations are needed.

1. Infections should be excluded and treated before the start of treatment. Concomitant prophylactic treatment with trimethoprim sulfamethaxazole has been efficacious for children with a history of frequent infections and in immunosuppressed patients.
2. Steroid therapy should be avoided for children with congenital CMV infection (the signs of which are retardation, brain calcifications, and microcephaly) or symptomatic acquired CMV infection (encephalitis, pneumonitis), since steroids may activate a latent infection, render a child susceptible to a new infection; or, an infection may be aggravated and even persist.
3. The blood pressure and electrolyte levels must be measured regularly. Hypertension and electrolyte disturbances should be corrected. If there is acute weight gain or renal failure, the kidneys and heart should be studied by ultrasound. Brain CT should be repeated if severe focal neurologic symptoms present, since hemorrhages and tumors occur rarely.
4. The dose of ACTH should be tapered slowly. If cortisol levels are low, stressful situations should be covered by hydrocortisone. It is advisable to monitor HPA function until it has normalized. Therapy

should be given at the minimal effective dosage and for the minimal effective time.

Action of steroids

ACTH can have its effect either by stimulation of corticosteroids; by stimulation of other adrenal steroids (Riikonen and Perheentupa, 1986); or, by a direct effect on the brain. Direct actions of ACTH/corticosteroids on the brain could cause: acceleration of physiologic events over a critical stage of brain maturation (balance between excitatory and inhibitory mechanisms); a cell membrane stabilizing effect (hyperpolarization and thereby decreasing the probability of firing of neurons); neuroregulation (neurotransmitter, neuromodulator, or as a trophic hormone), or amelioration of CRH overactivity (Baram, 1993).

ALTERNATIVES TO STEROID THERAPY

Alternative treatments are seen in Table 11b.2. In general, these drugs have not been shown to be as effective as steroids, the response rate being up to 50% (valproate 58%). Further, the studies of the efficacy of these drugs have not included evaluation of

Table 11b.2 Alternative therapy in the treatment of infantile spasms

Therapy	Patients (no.)	% Response in 4 weeks
ACTH fragments	9*	22
Immunoglobulin	49*	31
TRH	13	54
Large doses of valproate	82*†‡	58
Nitrazepam	27‡	52
Vigabatrin	68‡§‖	43
Pyridoxine	118	13
Surgery	29*‖	72

*Patients summarized from different series.
†Only cessation of hypsarrhythmia given (no data on spasms).
‡Only cessation of spasms reported (none or insufficient data on EEG).
§Response in 22–150 days.
‖Of children given vigabatrin 69%, and, of those undergoing surgery, 100%, had refractory epilepsy.

both the spasms and EEG and assessment has always been in relation to their short-term rather than long-term effects.

Large doses of **valproate** (up to 100 mg/kg) have been used as a first drug for treatment of infantile spasms (Pavone *et al.*, 1981; Siemens *et al.*, 1988; Prats *et al.*, 1991). The response rate has been up to 58%. Because of a high risk of hepatotoxicity in this group of young, often brain-abnormal patients, this therapy carries a high risk (Dreifuss *et al.*, 1987). **Nitrazepam** is also efficacious in about 50% (Dreifuss *et al.*, 1986). High doses of **pyridoxine** have been reported in Japan to have good results (Ohtsuka *et al.*, 1987), especially in idiopathic cases. However, ACTH therapy has been more efficient.

Vigabatrin

In a single uncontrolled study vigabatrin (an irreversible inhibitor of GABA transaminase) has been reported to have excellent effects on intractable spasms, especially symptomatic spasms, and, particularly in patients with tuberous sclerosis (Chiron *et al.*, 1991). Since this report, the use of vigabatrin for infantile spasms has increased dramatically, so Chiron's study is reviewed in detail. Sixty-one per cent (43) of the 68 patients had received steroid therapy. Vigabatrin was used as add-on therapy to steroids or conventional anticonvulsant treatment. The doses ranged from 50 to 200 mg/kg/day, administered in two daily doses. The ages of the patients ranged from 2 months to 13 years; the onset of the spasms was before the age of 1 year. All the children were retarded. All subjects were evaluated after 5 months of treatment and then again after at least 12 months of therapy. Forty-three per cent of the patients (29/68 patients) showed a complete suppression of the spasms by the end of the evaluation phase of 5 months. The symptomatic patients showed a better response (16/32 patients) than the cryptogenic group (13/36 patients); this was contrary to the usual reports on therapeutic

responses in infantile spasms. The best result was observed in tuberous sclerosis (10/14 patients). Relapse occurred in almost half the patients with cryptogenic spasms, whereas all patients with tuberous sclerosis remained free of the spasms after a mean of 3 years on vigabatrin. The results of this study are difficult to compare with those from others, since the latter include infants under 1 year of age; and response to therapy is followed closely both clinically and by EEG recording. Disappearance of hypsarrhythmia is generally considered to be an important criterion of therapeutic response, but in the study by Chiron *et al.* (1991) evaluation of the spasms was made by the parents and EEGs were recorded for only 41 of 68 patients. Therefore the transition to partial seizures which occurred in nine patients after cessation of the spasms might have been difficult to interpret.

A good sustained effect on seizures was achieved for 20 of 68 patients (29%). This treatment, like any other, is difficult to assess because infantile spasms usually disappear spontaneously (25% were in remission 11 months after onset, Hrachovy, Glaze and Frost, 1991).

In other studies, Appleton (1993) has given vigabatrin as the drug of first choice to 11 children with infantile spasms. Spasms ceased in four of 11 children (36%) within 3–5 days. Smitt, Wohtrab and Boltshauser (1994) gave vigabatrin as monotherapy to seven children and as add-on therapy to 10 children with infantile spasm, and concluded that although vigabatrin has an impressive clinical effect in some patients, the effect on the EEG is disappointing in most infants; hypsarrhythmia was unchanged in 13 of 17 children (76%). In a multicentre study of 135 children, including 13 children with West's syndrome, it was concluded that dosages in excess of 100 mg do not give any additional effect (Livingston *et al.*, 1989).

Vigabatrin is usually well tolerated but side-effects are seen in 25% of children

(Chiron *et al.*, 1991; Dulac *et al.*, 1991). The commonest are hyperexcitability and hypotonia. Vigabatrin may also cause an increase in seizure frequency, relapse, and appearance of new seizure types. Seizures are most likely to increase in nonprogressive myoclonic epilepsy and Lennox–Gastaut syndrome, but infantile spasms may also become more frequent (Lortie *et al.*, 1993). On the other hand no change in myelination has been seen in neuropathologic examination of adults (Cannon *et al.*, 1991) or in MRI studies in children (Chiron *et al.*, 1991). In adults vigabatrin did not cause any cognitive impairment either acutely or in the long term. In contrast, the responders have shown a significant improvement in cognitive functions (Gillham *et al.*, 1993).

Although vigabatrin awaits controlled studies and studies on evaluation of long-term effects in children with infantile spasms, it seems to be worth trying as an add-on drug after failure of steroid treatment for symptomatic infantile spasms, in partial epilepsy developing after infantile spasms, and as a first-line treatment in tuberous sclerosis. An increasing number of doctors use vigabatrin as their initial choice for symptomatic infantile spasms. My personal approach to management of the spasms will remain with steroids as first-line treatment, until other drugs have been shown to be more effective.

Immunoglobulins

Immunoglobulins have been used in a small number of children with infantile spasms (Ariizumi *et al.*, 1987; Echenne *et al.*, 1991). The immunologic basis for this therapy is unknown.

SURGERY

Some children with medically refractory infantile spasms have a localized brain defect. The association of hypsarrhythmia with a constant focus of abnormal discharge on EEG has been long recognized (Druckman and Chao, 1955; Jeavons and Bower, 1964). Local abnormalities are seen in the EEG in up to 57% of the patients (Riikonen, 1982), and in 65% when studied by EEG and neuroimaging (Shields *et al.*, 1992). Whether the cortical lesions are significant for the development of the spasms or merely coincidental, remains unknown. However, control of spasms following removal of **structural** abnormalities found on CT or MRI, such as tumors, porencephaly, or hemimegalencephalic changes, has been reported (Branch and Dyken, 1979; Mimaki, Ono and Yabuuchi, 1983; Palm, Brandt and Korinthenberg, 1988; Ruggieri, Carabello and Fejerman, 1989; Uthman *et al.*, 1991). Surgical removal of cortical **hypometabolic** lesions identified by PET was initiated at The University of California, Los Angeles. In 23 patients with intractable spasms, PET was, in 14 patients, the only neuroimaging modality to identify abnormal areas of cortex which were presumably also epileptogenic areas. The parietal-occipital-temporal region was the most common site. Fifteen of the 23 patients (most still on medication) remained seizure free at follow-up 4–47 months after surgery (Chugani *et al.*, 1993). Carrazana *et al.* (1993) have reported six more patients with surgical resections, all with good outcome. The authors recommend that surgical intervention should be considered early in the medically refractory cases, prior to the onset of epileptic encephalopathy. However, there remain some unresolved questions: the term intractability is difficult to define in a very young child; epileptic focal abnormalities tend to disappear spontaneously or migrate (posteroanterior migration of epileptic foci, Gibbs and Gibbs, 1952); prolonged barbiturate anesthesia may stop the spasms (Riikonen *et al.*, 1988); and the long-term effects of the surgery on cognitive functions have not yet been evaluated. Good results following the removal of hypometabolic areas await confirmation.

Other treatments which have been tried and have been reported to have some effect

Table 11b.3 Long-term outcome for children with West's syndrome

'Normal' mental outcome	Jeavons and Bower (1973) n=105	Matsumoto et al. (1981) n=139	Riikonen (1982) n=162	Snead et al. (1983) n=46	Lombroso (1983) n=90	Glaze et al. (1988) n=64
All cases (%)	17	23	24			9
Cryptogenic (%)	37	44	44		40	38
Seizure-free (%)	37	44	36	52		50
Duration of follow-up (yr)	2–12	5	3–19		6	0.75–9

Table 11b.4 Long-term outcome in relation to time-lag between onset of spasms and start of ACTH

'Normal' development	Glaze et al. (1988) n=64	Riikonen (1982) n=162	Lombroso (1983) n=72*	Koo et al. (1993) n=32
In early treated	3/22 (14%)	28/87 (32%)	11/21 (52%)	3/6 (50%)
In late treated	3/42 (7%)	11/75 (15%)	13/51 (27%)	6/26 (23%)

*Etiology in all patients cryptogenic.

are as follows: thyrotropin releasing hormone (Matsumoto *et al.*, 1987), ACTH fragments (Pentella, Bachman and Sandman, 1982), barbiturate anesthesia (Riikonen *et al.* 1988), ketogenic diet (De Vivo, 1983), tetrabenazine (Hrachovy, Frost and Glaze, 1988), methysergide, and methylparatyrosine (Hrachovy *et al.*, 1989).

PROGNOSIS

The long-term outcome of children from different series is very similar in many respects (Table 11b.3). The overall figures for normal development are 12–25%, but for cryptogenic cases 40–44%. Other seizures, after cessation of infantile spasms, are seen in 60%. The most common later epilepsies are Lennox–Gastaut epilepsy (Chapter 12a) and partial epilepsy (Chapter 16). The temporal lobes are the most common sites of abnormality. Psychiatric disorders such as infantile autism and hyperkinetic behavior occur in about 25% of cases; hyperkinetic behavior and autism being equally represented (Riikonen and Amnell, 1981). In patients with tuberous sclerosis infantile autism occurred in 26–58% of patients in the series of Hunt and Dennis (1987) and Jambaqué *et al.* (1991),

whereas it was seen in only 13% of the whole series of children with West's syndrome of Riikonen and Amnell (1981). The prognosis is strongly influenced by the structural abnormality underlying the syndrome. In a recent study the long-term outcome was not influenced by whether treatment was early or late or by response to therapy (Glaze *et al.*, 1988). However, in two series with larger numbers of patients and longer follow-up time, a short time between onset and treatment correlated with a more favorable outcome than a long lag in institution of ACTH (Table 11b.4). Since steroids bring cessation of the spasms more rapidly than other regimens, early treatment of infantile spasms seems to be important. A good response to therapy is also important in predicting a more favorable outcome (Riikonen, 1991).

CONCLUSIONS

There are many crucial problems still unresolved in West's syndrome. However, much has been achieved: the identification of this syndrome is nowadays more precise, using time-synchronized video and polygraphic recordings; and, more accurate etiologic diagnoses can be made by clinical, neuroimaging, virologic, biochemical, and pathologic methods. Various genetic patterns are recognized (e.g. tuberous sclerosis, some metabolic diseases). There is better clinical experience of drugs such as steroids, vigabatrin and other anticonvulsants, pyridoxine, thyrotropin releasing hormone, and immuno-globulins. A better knowledge of the prevention and treatment of side-effects of steroid therapy exists. In some patients a surgical approach seems to be of benefit: PET has proven to be useful in assisting selection of such patients.

The only consistent factor in West's syndrome seems to be age specificity. Therefore, the understanding of brain maturation will be the focus of all studies concerned with the unclear metabolic and pathophysiologic mechanism of West's syndrome, and its treatment by drugs and surgery.

REFERENCES

Aicardi, J. (1992) Diseases of the nervous system in childhood, in *Clinics in Developmental Medicine*, No 115/118, (eds M. Bax, C. Gillberg and H. Ogier), MacKeith Press, Oxford, p. 937.

Aicardi, J. (1985) Early myoclonic encephalopathy, in *Epileptic Syndromes in Infancy, Childhood and Adolescence*, (eds J. Roger, C. Dravet, M. Bureau, F.E. Dreifuss and P. Wolf), John Libbey, Euro-text, London, pp. 12–22.

Aicardi, J., Lefébure, J. and Lerique-Koechlin, A. (1965) A new syndrome: spasms in flexion, callosal agenesis, ocular abnormalities. *Electro-encephalography and Clinical Neurophysiology*, **19**, 609–10.

Airaksinen, E., Tuomisto, L. and Riikonen, R. (1992) The concentrations of GABA, 5-HIAA and HVA in the cerebrospinal fluid of children with infantile spasms and the effects of ACTH treatment. *Brain and Development*, **14**, 386–90.

Alvarez, L.A., Shinnar, S. and Moshé, S.L. (1987) Infantile spasms due to unilateral cerebral infarcts. *Pediatrics*, **79**, 1024–6.

Appleton, R. (1993) The role of vigabatrin in the management of infantile epileptic syndromes. *Neurology*, **43**, (suppl. 5), S21–3.

Ariizumi, M., Baba, K., Hibio, S. *et al.* (1987) Immunoglobulin therapy in the West syndrome. *Brain and Development*, **9**, 422–5.

Bankier, A., Turner, M. and Hopkins, I.J. (1983) Pyridoxine-dependent seizures. A wider clinical spectrum. *Archives of Disease in Childhood*, **58**, 415–8.

Baram, T.Z. (1993) Pathophysiology of massive infantile spasms: perspective on the putative role of the brain adrenal axis. *Annals of Neurology*, **33**, 231–6.

Baram, T.Z., Mitchell, W.G., Snead, O.C. *et al.* (1992) Brain–adrenal axis hormones are altered in the CSF of infants with massive infantile spasms. *Neurology*, **42**, 1171–5.

Bellman, M., Ross, E. and Miller, D. (1983) Infantile spasms and pertussis immunisation. *Lancet*, **i**, 1031–4.

Bignami, A., Maccagnami, F., Zapella, M. and Tingey, A. (1966) Familial infantile spasms and hypsarrhythmia associated with leucodystrophy. *Journal of Neurology Neurosurgery and Psychiatry*, **29**, 129–34.

Branch, C.E. and Dyken, P.R. (1979) Choroid plexus papilloma and infantile spasms. *Annals of Neurology*, **5**, 302–4.

Cannon, D., Butler, W., Mumford, J. and Lewis, P. (1991) Neuropathologic findings in patients receiving long-term vigabatrin therapy for chronic intractable epilepsy. *Journal of Child Neurology*, **6** (suppl.2), S17–24.

Carrazana, E.J., Lombraso, C., Mikati, M. *et al.* (1993) Facilitation of infantile spasms by partial seizures. *Epilepsia*, **34**, 97–109.

Cassidy, S., Gainey, A., Holmes, G. *et al.* (1983) Infantile spasms in Down syndrome: an unappreciated association. *American Journal of Human Genetics*, **35**, 82A (abstr. 244).

Chiron, C., Raynaud, C., Dulac, O. *et al.* (1989) Study of cerebral blood flow in partial epilepsy of childhood using SPECT method. *Journal of Neuroradiology*, **16**, 317–24.

Chiron, C., Dulac, O., Beaumont, D. *et al.* (1991) Therapeutic trial of vigabatrin in refractory infantile spasms. *Journal of Child Neurology*, **6** (suppl.2), S52–9.

Chiron, C., Dulac, O., Bulteau, C. *et al.* (1993) Study of regional cerebral blood flow in West Syndrome. *Epilepsia*, **34**, 707–15.

Crichton, J. (1968) Infantile spasms in children with low birthweight. *Developmental Medicine and Child Neurology*, **10**, 36–41.

Chugani, H.T., Phelps, M.E. and Mazziotta, J.C.

(1987) Positron emission tomography study of human brain functional development. *Annals of Neurology*, **22**, 487–97.

Chugani, H.T., Shewmon, D.A., Sankar, R. *et al.* (1992) Infantile spasms: II. Lenticular nuclei and brain stem activation on positron emission tomography. *Annals of Neurology*, **131**, 212–9.

Chugani, H., Shewmon, A., Shields, D. *et al.* (1993) Surgery for intractable spasms: neuro-imaging perspectives. *Epilepsia*, **34**, 764–71.

Commission on Classification and Terminology of the International League Against Epilepsy (1989) Proposal for revised classification of epilepsies and epileptic syndromes. *Epilepsia*, **30**, 389–99.

Cusmai, R., Dulac, O. and Diebler, C. (1988) Lesions focales dans les spasmes infantiles. *Neurophysiological Clinics*, **18**, 235–41.

Dalla Bernardina, B., Aicardi, J., Goutiéres, F. and Plouin, P. (1979) Glycine encephalopathy. *Neuropediatrics*, **10**, 209–25.

De Vivo, D. (1983) How to use drugs (steroids) and the ketogenic diet, in *Antiepileptic Drug Therapy in Pediatrics*, (eds P.L. Morselli, C.E. Pippenger and J.K. Penry), Raven Press, New York, pp. 283–95.

Dobyns, W.B., Stratton, R.F. and Greenberg, F. (1984) Syndromes with lissencephaly. I: Miller–Dieker and Norman–Roberts syndromes and isolated lissencephaly. *American Journal of Medical Genetics*, **18**, 509–26.

Dravet, C., Bureau, M. and Roger, J. (1985) Benign myoclonic epilepsy in infants, in *Epileptic Syndromes in Infancy, Childhood and Adolescence*, (eds J. Roger, C. Dravet, M. Bureau, F. Dreifuss and P. Wolf), John Libbey, London, pp. 51–7.

Dreifuss, F., Farwell, J., Holmes, G. *et al.* (1986) Infantile spasms, comparative trial of nitrazepam and corticotropin. *Archives of Neurology*, **43**, 1107–10.

Dreifuss, F.E., Santilli, N., Langer, D.H. *et al.* (1987) Valproic acid hepatic fatalities – a retrospective review. *Neurology*, **37**, 379–85.

Druckman, R. and Chao, D. (1955) Massive spasms in infancy and childhood. *Epilepsia*, **4**, 61–72.

Duffner, P. and Cohen, M. (1975) Infantile spasms associated with histidinemia. *Neurology (Minneapolis)*, **25**, 195–7.

Dulac, O., Chiron, C., Luna, D., Cusmai, R. *et al.* (1991) Vigabatrin in childhood epilepsy. *Journal of Child Neurology*, **6** (suppl. 2), S30–37.

Dulac, O., Feingold, J., Plouin, P. *et al.* (1993) Genetic predisposition to West syndrome. *Epilepsia*, **34**, 732–7.

Echenne, B., Parayre-Chanez, M.J., Taillebois, L. *et al.* (1991) Treatment of infantile spasms with intravenous gamma-globulins. *Brain and Development*, **13**, 313–9.

Esquivel, E.E., Pitt, M.C. and Boyd, S.G. (1991) EEG findings in hypomelanosis of Ito. *Neuropediatrics*, **27**, 216–9.

Fariello, R.G., Chun, R.W., Doro, J.M. *et al.* (1977) EEG recognition of Aicardi's syndrome. *Archives of Neurology*, **34**, 563–6.

Fleiszar, K., Daniel, W. and Imrey, P. (1977) Genetic study of infantile spasms with hypsarrhythmia. *Epilepsia*, **18**, 55–62.

Fusco, L and Vigevano, F. (1993) Ictal clinical electroencephalographic findings of spasms in West syndrome. *Epilepsia*, **34**, 671–8.

Gambertoglio, J.G., Holford, N.G., Kapusnik, J.E. *et al.* (1984) Disposition of total and unbound prednisolone in renal transplant patients. *Kidney International*, **25**, 119–23.

Gibbs, F.A. and Gibbs, E.L. (eds) (1952) *Atlas of Electroencephalography, Epilepsy*, vol. II, Addison-Wesley, Cambridge, Massachussets.

Gillham, R., Blacklaw, J., McKee, P. and Brodie, M. (1993) Effect of vigabatrin on sedation and cognitive function in patients with refractory epilepsy. *Journal of Neurology, Neurosurgery and Psychiatry*, **56**, 1271–5.

Glaze, D., Hrachovy, R., Frost, J. *et al.* (1986) Computed tomography in infantile spasms: effects of hormonal therapy. *Pediatric Neurology*, **2**, 23–7.

Glaze, D.J., Hrachovy, R.A., Frost, J.D. *et al.* (1988) Prospective study of outcome of infants with infantile spasms treated during controlled studies of ACTH and prednisone. *Journal of Pediatrics*, **112**, 389–96.

Gobbi, G., Bruno, L., Pini, A. *et al.* (1987) Periodic spasms: an unclassified type of epileptic seizure in childhood. *Developmental Medicine and Child Neurology*, **27**, 766–75.

Hakamada, S., Watanabe, K., Hara, K. and Miyazaki, S. (1979) The evolution of electroencephalographic features in lissencephaly syndrome. *Brain and Development*, **1**, 277–83.

Heiskala, H., Riikonen, R., Santavuori, P. *et al.* (1995) Infantile spasms: individualized ACTH therapy. *Acta Pediatr.*, in press.

Hrachovy, R.A. and Frost, J.D. (1989) Infantile spasms. *Pediatric Clinics of North America*, **36**, 311–29.

Hrachovy, R.A., Frost, J.D. and Kellaway, P. (1984) Hypsarrhthmia: variations on the theme. *Epilepsia*, **28**, 317–25.

Hrachovy, R., Frost, J. and Glaze, D. (1988) Treatment of infantile spasms with tetrabenazine. *Epilepsia*, **29**, 561–3.

Hrachovy, R., Frost, J., Glaze, D. and Rose, D. (1989) Treatment of infantile spasms with methysergide and α-methylparatyrosine. *Epilepsia*, **30**, 607–10.

Hrachovy, R., Frost, J. and Glaze, D. (1994) High-dose, long-duration versus low-dose, short-duration corticotrophin therapy for infantile spasms. *Journal of Paediatrics*, **124**, 803–6.

Hrachovy, R., Glaze, D. and Frost, J. (1991) A retrospective study of spontaneous remission and long-term outcome in patients with infantile spasms. *Epilepsia* **32**, 212–4.

Hrachovy, R., Frost, J., Kellaway, P. and Zion, T. (1984) Double-blind study of ACTH vs prednisone therapy in infantile spasms. *Journal of Pediatrics*, **103**, 641–5.

Hrachovy, R., Frost, J., Gospe, S. and Glaze D. (1987) Infantile spasms following near-drowning: a report of two cases. *Epilepsia*, **28**, 45–6.

Hunt, A. and Dennis, J. (1987) Psychiatric disorder among children with tuberous sclerosis. *Developmental Medicine and Child Neurology*, **29**, 190–8.

Jambaqué, I., Chiron, C., Dulac, O. *et al.* (1993) Visual inattention in West syndrome: a neuropsychological and neurofunctional imaging study. *Epilepsia*, **34**, 692–700.

Jambaqué, I., Cusmai, R., Curatolo, P. *et al.* (1991) Neuropsychological aspects of tuberous sclerosis in relation to epilepsy and MRI findings. *Developmental Medicine and Child Neurology*, **33**, 698–705.

Jeavons, P.M. and Bower, B.D. (1964) Infantile spasms: a review of the literature and a study of 112 cases, in *Clinics of Developmental Medicine*, no. 15, Spastics Society and W. Heinemann Medical Books, London.

Jeavons, P. and Bower, B. (1973) Long-term prognosis of 150 cases of West syndrome. *Epilepsia*, **14**, 153–64.

Jellinger, K. (1987) Neuropathological aspects of infantile spasms. *Brain and Development*, **9**, 349–57.

Kamoshita, S., Mizutani, I. and Fukuyama, Y. (1970) Leigh's subacute necrotizing encephalomyelopathy in a child with infantile spasms and hypsarrhythmia. *Developmental Medicine and Child Neurology*, **12**, 430–5.

Kellaway, P., Hrachovy, R.A., Frost, J.D. Jr and Zion, T. (1979) Precise characterization and quantification of infantile spasms. *Annals of Neurology*, **6**, 214–8.

Koo, B., Hwang, P. and Logan, W. (1993) Infantile spasms: outcome and prognostic factors of cryptogenic and symptomatic groups. *Neurology*, **43**, 2322–7.

Kritzler, R.K., Vining, E.P.G. and Plotnick, L.P. (1983) Clinical and laboratory observations. Sodium valproate and corticotrophin suppression in the child treated for seizures. *Journal of Pediatrics*, **102**, 142–3.

Lang, D., Muhler, E., Kupferschmid, C.H. *et al.* (1984) Cardiac hypertrophy secondary to ACTH treatment in children. *European Journal of Pediatrics*, **142**, 121–5.

Lerman, P. and Kivity, S. (1982) The efficacy of corticotrophin in primary infantile spasms. *Journal of Pediatrics*, **101**, 294–6.

Livingston, J., Beamont, D., Arzimanglou, A. and Aicardi, J. (1989) Vigabatrin in the treatment of epilepsy in children. *British Journal of Clinical Pharmacology*, **27**, 109S–12S.

Lombroso, C.T. (1983) A prospective study of infantile spasms: clinical and therapeutic correlates. *Epilepsia*, **24**, 135–58.

Lombroso, C.T. and Fejerman, N. (1977) Benign myoclonus of early infancy. *Annals of Neurology*, **1**, 38–148.

Lortie, A., Chiron, C., Mumford, J. and Dulac, O. (1993) The potential for increasing seizure frequency, relapse, and appearance of new seizure types with vigabatrin. *Neurology*, **43** (suppl. 5), S24–7

Matsumoto, A., Watanabe, K., Negoro, T. *et al.* (1981) Long-term prognosis after infantile spasms: a statistical study of prognostic factors in 200 cases. *Developmental Medicine and Child Neurology*, **23**, 51–65.

Matsumoto, A., Kumagai, T., Takeuchi, T. *et al.* (1987) Clinical effects of thyrotropin-releasing hormone for severe epilepsy in childhood: a comparative study with ACTH therapy. *Epilepsia*, **28**, 49–55.

Meencke, H.J. and Gerhard, C. (1985) Morphological aspects of aetiology and the course of infantile spasms (West-Syndrome). *Neuropediatrics*, **16**, 58–66.

Mimaki, T., Ono, J. and Yabuuchi, H. (1983)

Temporal lobe astrocytoma with infantile spasms. *Annals of Neurology*, **14**, 695–6.

Miyazaki, B., Hashimoto, T., Tayama, M. and Kuroda, Y. (1993) Brainstem involvement in infantile spasms: a study employing brainstem evoked potentials and magnetic resonance imaging. *Neuropediatrics*, **24**, 126–30.

Nalin, A., Facchinetti, F., Galli, V. *et al.* (1985) Reduced ACTH content in cerebrospinal fluid of children affected by cryptogenic infantile spasms with hypsarrhythmia. *Epilepsia*, **26**, 446–9.

Nelson, K. (1972) Discussion, in *The Epidemiology of Epilepsy: A Workshop NINSDS*, monograph no 14, (eds M. Alter and W.A. Hauser), US Government Printing Office, Washington, p. 78.

Neville, B. (1972) The origin of infantile spasms: evidence from a case of hydrancephaly. *Developmental Medicine and Child Neurology*, **14**, 644–56.

Ohtahara, S., Ohtsuka, Y., Yamatogi, Y. and Oka, E. (1987) The early-infantile epileptic encephalopathy with suppression-burst: developmental aspects. *Brain and Development*, **9**, 418–21.

Ohtsuka, Y., Matsuda, M., Ogino, T. *et al.* (1987) Treatment of the West syndrome with high-dose pyridoxal phosphate. *Brain Development*, **9**, 418–21.

Paladin, F., Chiron, C., Dulac, O. *et al.* (1989) Electroencephalographic aspects of hemimegalencephaly. *Developmental Medicine and Child Neurology*, **31**, 377–83.

Palm, L., Blennow, G. and Brun, A. (1986) Infantile spasms and neuronal heterotopias. *Acta Paediatrica Scandinavica*, **75**, 855–9.

Palm, D. G., Brandt, M. and Korinthenberg, R. (1988) West syndrome and Lennox–Gastaut syndrome in children with porencephalic cysts: long-term follow-up after neurosurgical treatment, in *The Lennox–Gastaut syndrome*, (eds E. Niedermeyer and R. Degen), Alan R. Liss, New York, pp. 491–526.

Pavone, L., Incorpora, G., La Rosa, M. *et al.* (1981) Treatment of infantile spasms with sodium dipropylacetic acid. *Developmental Medicine and Child Neurology*, **23**, 454–61.

Pentella, K., Bachman, D. and Sandman, C. (1982) Trial on ACTH 4–9 analogue (ORG 2766) in children with intractable seizures. *Neuropediatrics*, **13**, 59–62.

Perheentupa, J., Riikonen, R. and Dunkel, L. (1986) Adrenocortical hyporesponsiveness after ACTH therapy of infantile spasms. *Archives of Disease in Childhood*, **61**, 750–3.

Pinsard, N. (1981) Encéphalopathies épileptiques évolutives du nourrisson (syndrome de West et syndrome de Lennox-Gastaut). *Revue de Electroencephalographie et de Neurophysiologie Clinique*, **11**, 419–24.

Prats, J., Garaizar, C., Rua, M. *et al.* (1991) Infantile spasms treated with high doses of sodium valproate: initial response and follow-up. *Developmental Medicine and Child Neurology*, **33**, 617–25.

Rao, J. and Willis, J. (1987) Hypothalamo-pituitary-adrenal function in infantile spasms: effects of ACTH therapy. *Journal of Child Neurology*, **2**, 220–3.

Rausch, H., Hanefeld, F. and Kaufman, H. (1984) Medullary nephrocalcinosis and pancreatic calcifications demonstrated by ultrasound and CT in infants after treatment with ACTH. *Radiology*, **153**, 105–7.

Riikonen, R. (1982) A long-term follow-up study of 214 children with the syndrome of infantile spasms. *Neuropediatrics*, **13**, 14–23.

Riikonen, R. (1983) Infantile spasms: some new theoretical aspects. *Epilepsia*, **24**, 159–68.

Riikonen, R. (1987) Infantile spasms in siblings. *Journal of Pediatric Neurosciences*, **34**, 235–44.

Riikonen, R. (1991) Modern trends in the treatment of infantile spasms, in *Proceedings of the International Symposium, New Trends in Pediatric Epileptology*, (eds S. Ohtahara and J. Roger), Okayama Japan, pp. 149–54.

Riikonen, R. (1993) Infantile spasms: infectious disorders. *Neuropediatrics*, **24**, 274–280.

Riikonen, R. (1995) Decreasing perinatal mortality – unchanged infantile spasms morbidity. *Developmental Medicine and Child Neurology*, **37**, 232–8.

Riikonen, R. and Amnell, G. (1981) Psychiatric disorders in children with earlier infantile spasms. *Developmental Medicine and Child Neurology*, **23**, 747–60.

Riikonen, R. and Donner, M. (1979) Incidence and aetiology of infantile spasms from 1960 to 1976: a population study in Finland. *Developmental Medicine and Child Neurology*, **21**, 333–43.

Riikonen, R. and Donner, M. (1980) ACTH therapy in infantile spasms: side-effects. *Archives of Disease in Childhood*, **55**, 664–72.

Riikonen, R. and Gupta, D. (1988) Effect of ACTH treatment on CSF ACTH, IgG index and CSF albumin ratio in children with infantile spasms: preliminary observations. *Neuroendocrinology*, **10**, 355–62.

Riikonen, R. and Perheentupa, J. (1986) Serum

steroids and success of corticotropin therapy in infantile spasms. *Acta Paediatrica Scandinavica*, **75**, 598–600.

Riikonen, R. and Simell, O. (1990) Tuberous sclerosis and infantile spasms. *Developmental Medicine and Child Neurology*, **32**, 203–9.

Riikonen, R., Simell, O., Jääskeläinen, J. *et al.* (1986) Disturbed calcium and phosphate homeostasis during treatment with ACTH of infantile spasms. *Archives of Disease in Childhood*, **61**, 671–6.

Riikonen, R., Santavuori, P., Sainio, K. *et al.* (1988) Can barbiturate anesthesia cure infantile spasms? *Brain and Development*, **10**, 300–4.

Riikonen, R., Perheentupa, J., Simell, O. *et al.* (1989) Hormonal background of hypertension and fluid derangements associated with ACTH treatment of infants. *European Journal of Pediatrics*, **148**, 737–41.

Ruggieri, V., Caraballo, R. and Fejerman, N. (1989) Intracranial tumors and West syndrome. *Pediatric Neurology*, **5**, 327–9.

Rugtveit, J. (1986) X-linked mental retardation and infantile spasms in two brothers. *Developmental Medicine and Child Neurology*, **28**, 543–9.

Salonen, R., Somer, M., Haltia, M. *et al.* (1991) Progressive encephalopathy with edema, hypsarrhythmia, and optic atrophy (PEHO syndrome). *Clinical Genetics*, **39**, 287–93.

Satoh, J., Mizutani, T., Horimatsu, Y. *et al.* (1986) Neuropathology of the brain-stem in age-dependent epileptic encephalopathy – especially in cases with infantile spasms. *Brain and Development*, **8**, 443–9.

Shields, D., Shewmon, A., Chugani, H.T. *et al.* (1992) Treatment of infantile spasms: medical or surgical? *Epilepsia*, **33** (suppl. 4), S26–31.

Shih, V., Efron, M., and Moser, H. (1969) Hyperornithinemia, hyperammonemia and homociatrullinuria: a new disorder of amino acid metabolism associated with myoclonic seizures and mental retardation. *American Journal of Diseases in Childhood*, **117**, 83–92.

Siemens, H., Spohr, H., Michael, T. *et al.* (1988) Therapy of infantile spasms with valproate: results of a prospective study. *Epilepsia*, **29**, 553–60.

Singer, W.D., Rabe, E.F. and Haller, J.S. (1980) The effect of ACTH therapy upon infantile spasms. *Journal of Pediatrics*, **96**, 485–98.

Silverstein, F. and Johnston, M.V. (1984) Cerebro-spinal fluid monoamine metabolites in patients with infantile spasms. *Neurology*, **34**, 102–5.

Smitt, B., Wohlrab, G. and Boltshauser, E. (1994) Vigabatrin in newly diagnosied infantile spasms. *Neuropediatrics*, **25**, 54.

Snead, O.C., Benton, J.W., Hosey, B.S.N. *et al.* (1989) Treatment of infantile spasms with high dose ACTH: efficacy and plasma levels of ACTH and cortisol. *Neurology*, **39**, 1027–31.

Snead, O.C., Benton, J.W., Hosey, L.C. *et al.* (1983) ACTH and prednisone in childhood seizure disorders. *Neurology*, **33**, 966–70.

Sorel, L. and Dusaucy-Bauloye, A. (1958) À propos de 21 cas d'hypsarrhythmia de Gibbs – son traitement spectaculaire par l'ACTH. *Acta Neurologica Psychiatrica Belgica*, **58**, 130–41.

Tornello, S., Orti, E., Alejandro, F. *et al.* (1982) Regulation of glucocorticoid receptors in brain by corticosterone treatment of adrenalectomized rats. *Neuroendocrinology*, **35**, 411–7.

Uthman, B., Reid, S., Wilder, B. *et al.* (1991) Outcome for West syndrome following surgical treatment. *Epilepsia*, **32**, 668–71.

van Bogaert, P., Chiron, C., Adamsbaum, C. *et al.* (1993) Value of magnetic resonance imaging in West syndrome of unknown etiology. *Epilepsia*, **34**, 701–6.

Vigevano, F., Aicardi, J., Lini, M. and Pasquinelli, A. (1984) La sindrome del nevo sebaceo lineare: presentazione di una casistica multicentrica. *Bolletin Lega Italiana contra la Epilepsia*, **45/46**, 59–63.

Vinters, H.V., Fisher, R.S., Cornford, M.E. *et al.* (1992) Morphological substrates of infantile spasms: studies based on surgically resected cerebral tissue. *Child's Nervous System*, **8**, 8–17.

Watanabe, K., Hara, K. and Iwase, K. (1976) The evolution of neurophysiological features in holoprosencephaly. *Neuropediatrics*, **7**, 19–41.

Wenzel, D. (1987) Evoked potentials in infantile spasms. *Brain and Development*, **9**, 365–86.

West, W. J. (1841) On a peculiar form of infantile convulsions. *Lancet*, **i**, 724–5.

Yamamoto, N., Watanabe, K., Negoro, T. *et al.* (1988) Partial seizures evolving to infantile spasms. *Epilepsia*, **29**, 34–40.

Zellweger, H. (1948) Blitz-Nick- und Salaam-Krämpfe (Grusskrämpfe). In: Krampfe in Kindesalter. *Helvetica Paediatrica Acta*, **3** (Suppl. 5), 4–11.

PARTIAL EPILEPSIES IN INFANCY

11c

Olivier Dulac

When referring to infants, pediatricians are often reluctant to use the term 'epilepsy'. They prefer 'convulsion', thus highlighting the high frequency of occasional, symptomatic seizures in this age range. However, even in infancy, epileptic seizures may be nonconvulsive, i.e. restricted to vegetative or staring episodes. A major reference work concerning seizures in the first year of life classified them as 'infantile spasms', 'status epilepticus', 'febrile convulsions', and 'others' (Chevrie and Aicardi, 1977). The latter probably included partial seizures, but there is no clear reference to these types of attack. Most textbooks of pediatric neurology, including those especially devoted to pediatric epileptology, do not mention the occurrence of partial epilepsies in infancy. With reference to infancy, the term 'partial epilepsy' has benefited only from a very short existence, though it seems from now to be promised a long period of recognition. The first reports date back to 1978 (Di Cagno *et al.*, 1978), and literature has appeared consistently since then, including the proceedings of a symposium on partial epilepsies held in Marseilles (Roger, 1989). These studies will be reviewed in this chapter.

INCIDENCE

Very few data are available. Indeed, the incidence is very difficult to assess since children, in particular infants, often exhibit several types of seizures (Luna *et al.*, 1988) and generalized epilepsies may include or be preceded by partial seizures. The only epidemiologic study involving incidence in the first year of life according to seizure types reported an incidence of partial seizures of 15/100 000 (Luna *et al.*, 1988).

SEMIOLOGY

ICTAL CLINICAL MANIFESTATIONS

Motor and vegetative features are the most frequent ictal manifestations. Tonic or clonic movements may involve the face, one or both arms, or one side of the body. The involved arm is typically elevated, with abduction of the shoulder and flexion of the elbow, wrist, and fingers (Luna, Dulac and Plouin, 1989). Bilateral eyelid jerking and lateral deviation of the mouth are frequent. Lateral deviation of the head and/or eyes is usually tonic. Lateral jerks of the eyes, otherwise called 'epileptic nystagmus', occasionally occur.

Vegetative manifestations include apnea. It may be difficult to determine whether this consists of a respiratory pause or a tonic contraction of the respiratory muscles. Flushing or pallor may involve the whole body, the face or only the lips. Tachypnea and mydriasis have also been reported.

Automatisms have been reported (Luna, Dulac and Plouin, 1989). These consist of swallowing, chewing and tongue smacking or licking of the lips and, purposeless hand movements. Generally, gestural automatisms

Epilepsy in Children. Edited by Sheila Wallace. Published in 1996 by Chapman & Hall, London. ISBN 0 412 56860 8

are simple, localized, and nonpurposeful (extension and/or flexion of limbs, head shaking) (Yamamoto *et al.*, 1987). In other instances, seizures only consist of motion arrest, decreased responsiveness, staring, and blank eyes (Watanabe, Negoro and Aso, 1993).

Usually, it is not possible to determine whether consciousness is altered, although lack of reaction to stimulation is reported in over three-quarters of the cases in one series (Luna, Dulac and Plouin, 1989). An aura of fear, the patient approaching his parents with a terrified expression before the occurrence of other ictal manifestations, is occasionally reported in the second year of life (Luna, Dulac and Plouin, 1989). Tonic-clonic secondary generalization is mentioned in 25% (Luna, Dulac and Plouin, 1989) to 100% (Watanabe, Negoro and Aso, 1993) of cases. Postictal symptoms of confusion, disorientation, lethargy, or focal motor defect are frequent (Luna, Dulac and Plouin, 1989).

The sequence of events is variable. Vegetative manifestations usually precede motor activity, whereas alimentary automatisms tend to be seen more often after, than before, convulsive movements (Luna, Dulac and Plouin, 1989). A very unusual and previously not reported sequence was mentioned in two patients (Luna, Dulac and Plouin, 1989): generalized tonic seizures evolving to partial clonic manifestations.

The ictal sequence may vary according to age: one-quarter of the patients reported by Luna, Dulac and Plouin (1989) had changes in ictal patterns in the course of the disorder: generalized seizures became partial or new focal features appeared during the second year of life. There is a trend toward more focal manifestations as the patient grows older.

The duration of each seizure ranges from 30 seconds to 4 minutes, with secondary generalization lasting 1–2 minutes (Luna, Dulac and Plouin, 1989; Watanabe, Negoro and Aso, 1993). Yamamoto *et al.* (1987) found

seizures to be significantly longer in infants than in older children.

Seizure classification according to the International League Against Epilepsy (ILAE) criteria (Commission on Classification and Terminology of the International League Against Epilepsy, 1981) shows that there are three types of seizures, simple partial seizures, complex partial seizures (CPS) with striking motor manifestations, and CPS with impairment of consciousness at onset (Luna, Dulac and Plouin, 1989).

Another combination of generalized and focal features is the occurrence of a partial seizure intermingled with a cluster of spasms. Although focal features usually precede the first spasms, as if the focal discharge 'triggered' the cluster of spasms and they indicated secondary generalization (Dalla Bernardina *et al.*, 1984; Bour *et al.*, 1986), other patterns have been reported including the occurrence of focal features at the end of the cluster or during the course of the cluster (Carrazzana *et al.*, 1993). In these cases, the clinical expression of the focal seizure consists mainly of arrest of activity, staring or lateral deviation of head or eyes, complex nystagmus (Shewmon, 1994), or hemitonia. It may even be entirely subclinical.

ICTAL EEG MANIFESTATIONS

Ictal discharges consist of low-voltage fast waves, or rhythmic sharp waves or spikes, in the theta or beta ranges with decreasing frequency and increasing amplitude, thus resembling recruiting rhythms (Yamamoto *et al.*, 1987; Luna, Dulac and Plouin, 1989; Watanabe, Negoro and Aso, 1993). Later in the discharge, because of additional slow waves, a pattern of spikes and sharp waves can be produced (Yamamoto *et al.*, 1987). In most instances, the discharge is focal and spreads to adjacent or contralateral areas, and then becomes generalized. Less often, it remains in the same area throughout. In some instances, the discharge involves a whole hemisphere or is generalized from the onset, and it is only later in the course of the disease that a clear focal onset emerges (Luna, Dulac and Plouin, 1989).

CLINICAL EEG CORRELATIONS OF ICTAL FEATURES

Conflicting patterns have been reported, but few studies were based on video EEG recording. The ictal discharge may involve any area of the cerebral cortex (Yamamoto *et al.*, 1987; Chiron *et al.*, 1988; Luna, Dulac and Plouin, 1989). One study found no correlation between topography of the ictal discharge and clinical manifestations (Yamamoto *et al.*, 1987), but elsewhere tonic or clonic movements were found to be contralateral to the EEG discharge (Luna, Dulac and Plouin, 1989), and ocular clonus contralateral to the occipital discharge (Chiron *et al.*, 1988). Versive phenomena could be ipsilateral or contralateral (Luna, Dulac and Plouin, 1989), and chewing movements resulted from a temporal discharge.

STATUS EPILEPTICUS AND HH SYNDROME

Long-lasting or repeated seizures without interictal recovery of consciousness are frequent in infancy. Prolonged hemiclonic seizures followed by hemiplegia defines the HH syndrome that mainly relates to seizures occurring in infancy (Gastaut *et al.*, 1960; Aicardi *et al.*, 1969).

INTERCITAL EEG ACTIVITY

Interictal EEG is normal in 12–50% of patients. Focal spikes are recorded in one-quarter (Dravet *et al.*, 1989) to one-half (Luna, Dulac and Plouin, 1989) the cases. In most instances, only the background activity is abnormal.

ETIOLOGY

IDENTIFIABLE CAUSES

Various neurocutaneous disorders may be involved. Sturge–Weber disease often produces status epilepticus (SE), i.e. HH syndrome, when seizures begin in the first year of life, particularly between 3 and 6 months of age (Dulac *et al.*, 1982). In incontinentia pigmenti, also, the first seizure often consists of an episode of focal SE (Avrahami *et al.*, 1985). In both instances, focal ischemia causes SE.

In tuberous sclerosis, partial seizures may precede the occurrence of infantile spasms (IS), from the very first weeks of life. They may emerge after IS have been controlled (Chiron *et al.*, 1991). They may also start after 6 months of life without previous IS (Dulac, Plouin and Motte, 1984). Cases with HH syndrome have been reported.

Major malformations, i.e. Aicardi's syndrome (Bour *et al.*, 1986), agyria (Dulac, Plouin and Motte, 1984), and hemimegalencephaly (Vigevano *et al.*, 1989) often produce focal seizures at onset, before the age of 3 months and the occurrence of IS. The incidence of epilepsy in focal dysplasia is more problematic given the difficulty in identifying the lesion radiologically in the first year of life, before myelination is completed (Van Bogaert *et al.*, 1993). In prepeduncular hamartoma, focal motor seizures may occur very early in life, before gelastic seizures become the characteristic ictal hallmark (Plouin *et al.*, 1983). Various chromosomal aberrations may be associated with partial epilepsy (Chapter 4b).

Due to bleeding in infancy, both arteriovenous and cavernous angiomas may produce occasional seizures before chronic epilepsy develops.

Hamartomas and tumors underlie 1–2% of epilepsies beginning in infancy. The latter usually have the histologic characteristics of benign tumors, astrocytomata, gangliogliomata, or dysembryoplastic neuroepithelial tumors (DNT), but it may be difficult to distinguish some benign tumors from dysplasia, and both are occasionally found together in a single patient (Prayson, Estes and Morris, 1993). DNT is claimed to combine characteristics of both conditions (Daumas-Duport *et al.*, 1988).

Sequelae of pre-, peri- or postnatal acute circulatory failure, including porencephaly or ulegyria, may be involved. Like other focal lesions, the latter often produce IS before focal epilepsy develops (Diebler and Dulac, 1987). The same applies to neonatal bacterial meningitis, and to neo- or postnatal herpetic encephalitis. The latter may be overlooked in the newborn and be recognized later, based on the characteristics of the epilepsy and the neuroradiologic findings.

Partial epilepsy is rarely the only ictal expression in metabolic diseases. Alper's disease is a notable exception, producing epilepsia partialis continua (Egger *et al.*, 1987). The combination with hepatic failure causes confusion with valproate toxicity.

Although hippocampal gliosis has been reported histologically in severe infantile epilepsy, affected patients did not suffer from 'temporal lobe' epilepsy, and the lesions were definitely a consequence of severe seizure activity (Coppola *et al.*, 1995).

CRYPTOGENIC PARTIAL EPILEPSY

Cryptogenic partial epilepsy in infancy (in the sense that clinical and EEG characteristics suggest a lesion, but it is not demonstrable clinically or radiologically) has been recognized recently. Luna, Dulac and Plouin (1989) found it began mainly before 4 months or after 8 months, thus before or after the age when IS present, and noted clinical/EEG correlation. The age of onset may be determined in part by the topography of the epileptogenic focus. No case was found to involve the leg in the first year of life. In addition, cryptogenic epilepsy involving the occipital areas seems to begin mostly in the first 2 months of life (Lortie *et al.*, 1995). This unique condition combines very frequent seizures that remain intractable for several months, and major and prolonged disorders of vision and interpersonal contact.

The correlation between age of onset and topography of the epileptogenic zone is probably related to the time scale of maturation of the cerebral cortex, as shown by development milestones and functional imaging (Chugani, Phelps and Mazziotta, 1987; Chiron *et al.*, 1992; Chapters 4a, 20). Indeed, occipital areas undergo early and rapid maturation, within the first 2 months; whereas maturation in the prefrontal and temporopolar areas occurs later and is slower, and poor motor development suggests delayed maturation of paracentral areas.

The cause of cryptogenic partial epilepsy in infancy does not seem to be homogeneous, since the outcome may be very variable. Some patients suffer a chronic disease and the discharges involve a single cortical area throughout, as though a radiologically undetectable focal lesion was involved. In other instances, a stormy onset with very frequent daily seizures and deterioration of the neurologic condition is followed by a decrease in seizure frequency or cessation of seizures after a few months. In these cases, a kind of maturational disorder at a specific stage of cortical development seems to be involved.

MIGRATING PARTIAL SEIZURES

This very peculiar pattern is characterized by onset before six, and mainly between two and four, months, in previously normal infants with normal neuroradiologic investigations (Coppola *et al.*, 1995). During a mean of 5 weeks, the patients suffer a few focal seizures, before the second phase of the disorder appears. This consists of more or less continuous focal seizures with random topography of onset, involving both hemispheres. The EEG pattern of the ictal discharge is homogeneous, although its site of onset varies from one seizure to the next in a given patient. It consists of rhythmic activity of decreasing frequency and increasing amplitude, involving an increasing area, as if there was progressive recruitment of an increasingly wide area of the cortex. Each discharge lasts 1–4 minutes. Discharges involving different areas may overlap. Occipital, temporal, and rolandic areas are involved from the onset, whereas frontal involvement is delayed until after the age of 6 months. Video/EEG studies show clear clinical and EEG correlation of ictal events relating to the topography of the discharge (Chiron *et al.*, 1988).

During this period of very frequent seizures, patients lose all previously acquired skills. The head circumference stops growing and the patient becomes very hypotonic between the seizures. After a few months of evolution, the seizures become less frequent, occurring in clusters of a few days, more or less regularly. Of the series of 14 reported patients, three died and two were studied neuropathologically. Gliosis of the hippocampus was seen in both cases (Coppola *et al.*, 1995).

BENIGN INFANTILE PARTIAL EPILEPSY

Benign convulsions begin between 1 and 6 weeks of age and the patients exhibit the clinical and EEG characteristics of benign neonatal convulsions: partial seizures with random origin and high frequency contrast with a normal interictal clinical condition, normal sleep and wake interictal EEG, and a favorable outcome after a few days or weeks (Dulac, Cusmai and de Oliveira, 1989).

Although a hospital-based study failed to disclose cases of benign partial epilepsy in infancy (Dulac, Cusmai and de Oliveira 1989), the existence of such a syndrome has been demonstrated by Japanese authors (Watanabe *et al.* 1987, 1990; Watanabe,

Negoro and Aso, 1993). In benign partial epilepsy of infancy, seizures often occur in clusters, between 3 and 20 months of age. They consist of motor arrest, staring eyes, and eventually secondary generalization. The EEG at onset shows a pattern of focal recruiting rhythm, later mixed with slow waves of decreasing frequency, and ending in spikes, polyspikes and sharp wave complexes, involving rolandic, occipital, temporal, or parietal areas of both hemispheres.

Radiology and laboratory investigations are normal. Seizures are easily controlled and psychomotor outcome is excellent. Four of seven patients in one series had a first degree relative with benign infantile convulsions or febrile convulsions (Watanabe *et al.*, 1990).

BENIGN FAMILIAL INFANTILE CONVULSIONS

Benign familial infantile convulsions (BFIC) begin between 4 and 6 months of age with partial seizures with secondary generalization, occurring in clusters of four to 10 a day, for 2 to 4 days and involving both hemispheres (Vigevano *et al.*, 1992). The seizures consist of arrest of activity, slow lateral deviation of the head and eyes, loss of consciousness, diffuse hypertonia, unilateral clonic jerks becoming secondarily generalized. The side of lateral deviation may vary from one seizure to the next. Seizures last a few minutes. The ictal EEG pattern is similar to that of the previous group. It shows rhythmic spikes and spike-waves of increasing amplitude starting in the centroposterior areas of one hemisphere, involving progressively the whole hemisphere, and then the contralateral one. The side of onset may vary from one seizure to the next, as do the clinical manifestations. The interictal EEG is normal. The seizures are easily controlled by antiepileptic drugs and did not recur during 6–9 years of follow-up. BFIC have been shown not to be genetically related to benign familial neonatal convulsions (Malafosse *et al.*, 1995).

Some cases of the previous series may belong to BFIC.

CONCLUSIONS

As occurs in older children, infants may suffer from idiopathic, cryptogenic, or symptomatic partial epilepsy. However, partial seizures may be the only expression of a diffuse involvement of the cortex, probably as a consequence of immature pathways. Indeed, migrating partial seizures, and familial and nonfamilial benign infantile convulsions may be considered as generalized epilepsies, although seizures are only focal. From the therapeutic point of view, the distinction is very important, since the drugs effective in partial epilepsy may worsen some patients with generalized epilepsy, i.e. severe myoclonic epilepsy in infancy, which often begins with focal seizures in the first year of life.

REFERENCES

Aicardi, J., Amsili, J. and Chevrie, J.J. (1969) Acute hemiplegia in infancy and childhood. *Developmental Medicine and Child Neurology*, **11**, 162–73.

Avrahami, E., Harel, S., Jurgehson, U. *et al.* (1985) Computed tomographic demonstration of brain changes in incontinentia pigmenti. *American Journal of Diseases of Children*, **139**, 372–4.

Bour, F., Chiron, C., Dulac, O. and Plouin, P. (1986) Caractères électrocliniques des crises dans le syndrome d'Aicardi. *Revue d'Electroencephalographie et de Neurophysiologie Clinique*, **16**, 341–53.

Carrazzana, E.J., Lombroso, C.T., Mikati, M. *et al.* (1993) Facilitation of infantile spasms by partial seizures. *Epilepsia*, **34**, 97–109.

Chevrie, J.J. and Aicardi, J. (1977) Convulsive disorders in the first year of life: etiologic factors. *Epilepsia*, **18**, 489–98.

Chiron, C., Soufflet, C., Pollack, C. and Cusmai, R. (1988) Semiology of cryptogenic multifocal partial seizures in infancy. *Electroencephalography and Clinical Neurophysiology*, **70**, 9P–16P.

Chiron, C., Dulac, O., Beaumont, D. *et al.* (1991) Therapeutic trial of vigabatrin in refractory infantile spasms. *Journal of Child Neurology*, **6** (suppl. 2), S52–9.

Chiron, C., Raynaud, C., Maziere, B. *et al.* (1991) Changes in regional cerebral blood flow during brain maturation in children and adolescents. *Journal of Nuclear Medicine*, **33**, 696–703.

Chugani, H.T., Phelps, M.E. and Mazziotta, J.C. (1987) Positron emission tomography study of human brain functional development. *Annals of Neurology*, **22**, 487–497.

Commission on Classification and Terminology of the International League Against Epilepsy (1981) Proposal for revised clinical and electroencephalographic classification of epileptic seizures. *Epilepsia*, **22**, 489–501.

Coppola, G., Plouin, P., Chiron, C. *et al.* (1995) Migrating partial seizures in infancy: a malignant disorder with developmental arrest. *Epilepsia* (in press).

Dalla Bernardina, B., Colamaria, V., Capovilla, G. *et al.* (1984) Sindromi epilettiche precoci e malformazion bi cerebrali: studio multicentrico. *Boll Lega It Epil*, **45/46**, 65–7.

Daumas-Duport, C, Scheithauer, B.W., Chodkiewicz, J.P. *et al.* (1988) Dysembryoplastic neuroepithelial tumor: a surgically curable tumor of young patients with intractable partial seizures. Report of 39 cases. *Neurosurgery*, **23**, 454–6.

Di Cagno, L., Ravetto, F., Rigardetto, R. and Capizzi, G. (1978) Aspetti clinici ed evolutivi a medio termine delle crisi partiali dei primi due anni. *Boll Lega It*, **22/23**, 145–52.

Diebler, C. and Dulac, O. (1987) *Pediatric Neurology and Neuroradiology. Cerebral and Cranial Diseases*, Springer-Verlag, Berlin, pp. 408.

Dravet, C., Catani, C., Bureau, M. and Roger, J. (1989) Partial epilepsies in infancy: a study of 40 cases. *Epilepsia*, **30**, 807–12.

Dulac, O., Plouin, P. and Motte, J. (1984) L'épilepsie dans l'agyrie-pachygyrie type Bielchowsky. *Boll Lega It Epi*, **45/46**, 29–32.

Dulac, O., Cusmai, R. and De Oliveira, K. (1989) Is there a partial benign epilepsy in infancy? *Epilepsia*, **30**, 798–801.

Dulac, O., Larrègue, M., Roger, J. and Arthuis, M. (1982) Maladie de Sturge–Weber. Intérêt de l'analyse topographique de l'angiome cutané dans le diagnostic d'angiome pial associé. *Archives Françaises de Pediatrie*, **39**, 155–8.

Egger, J., Harding, B.N., Boyd, S.G. *et al.* (1987) Progressive neuronal degeneration of childhood (PNDC) with liver disease. *Clinical Pediatrics*, **26**, 167–73.

Gastaut, H., Poirier, F., Payan, H. *et al.* (1960)

HHE syndrome: hemiconvulsions-hemiplegia-epilepsy. *Epilepsia*, **1**, 418–47.

Lortie, A., Plouin, P., Pinard, J.M. and Dulac, O. (1995) *Occipital Epilepsy in Neonates and Infants* (eds A. Beaumanoir *et al.*),

Luna, D., Dulac, O. and Plouin, P. (1989) Ictal characteristics of cryptogenic partial epilepsies in infancy. *Epilepsia*, **30**, 827–32.

Luna, D., Chiron, C., Pajot, N. *et al.* (1988) *Epidémiologie des épilepsies de l'enfant dans le département de l'Oise (France). Epidémiologie des Epilepsies*, J. Libbey, Eurotext, London, Paris, pp. 41–53.

Malafosse, A., Beck, C., Bellet, H. *et al.* (1995) Benign familial convulsions is not an allelic form of the benign familial neonatal convulsions gene. *Annals of Neurology* (in press).

Plouin, P., Ponsot, G., Dulac, O. *et al.* (1983) Hamartomes hypothalamiques et crises de rire. *Rev EEG Neurophysiol clin*, **13**, 312–6.

Prayson, R.A., Estes, M.L. and Morris, H.H. (1993) Coexistence of neoplasia and cortical dysplasia in patients presenting with seizures. *Epilepsia*, **34**, 609–15.

Roger, J. (1989) Introduction: partial epilepsies symposium. *Epilepsia*, **30**, 797.

Shewmon, D.A. (1995) Ictal aspects, with emphasis on unusual variants, in *Infantile Spasms and West syndrome*, (eds O. Dulac, H. Chugani, B. Dalla Bernardina), Saunders, London, pp. 36–57.

Van Bogaert, P., Chiron, C., Andamsbaum, C. *et al.* (1993) Value of magnetic resonance imaging in West syndrome of unknown etiology. *Epilepsia*, **34**, 701–6.

Vigevano, F., Bertini, E., Boldrini, R. *et al.* (1989) Hemimegalencephaly and intractable epilepsy: benefits of hemispherectomy. *Epilepsia*, **30**, 833–43.

Vigevano, F., Fusco, L., di Capua, M. *et al.* (1992) Benign infantile familial convulsions. *European Journal of Pediatrics*, **151**, 608–12.

Watanabe, K., Negoro, T. and Aso, K. (1993) Benign partial epilepsy with secondary generalized seizures in infancy. *Epilepsia*, **34**, 635–8.

Watanabe, K., Yamamoto, N., Negoro, T. *et al.* (1990) Benign infantile epilepsy with complex partial seizures. *Journal of Clinical Neurophysiology*, **7**, 409–16.

Watanabe, K., Yamamoto, N., Negoro, T. *et al.* (1987) Benign complex partial epilepsies in infancy. *Pediatric Neurology*, **3**, 208–11.

Yamamoto, N., Watanabe, K., Negoro, T. *et al.* (1987) Complex partial seizures in children: ictal manifestations and their relation to clinical course. *Neurology*, **37**, 1379–82.

Natalio Fejerman

INTRODUCTION

The nosological delineation of true myoclonic epilepsies (ME) in infancy and childhood has been and is still a controversial subject (Harper, 1968; Loiseau *et al.*, 1974; Jeavons, 1977; Aicardi, 1981; Dalla Bernardina *et al.*, 1983; Dravet, Bureau and Roger, 1985; Aicardi and Levy-Gomes, 1989; Lombroso, 1990; Fejerman, 1991). The accepted Classification of the International League Against Epilepsy (Commission on Classification and Terminology of the International League Against Epilepsy, 1989) includes benign myoclonic epilepsy in infancy (BMEI) among idiopathic generalized epilepsies, whereas severe myoclonic epilepsy in infancy (SMEI) is placed as a syndrome with generalized and partial seizures without specifying whether it is idiopathic, cryptogenic, or symptomatic. Despite some persisting controversies, BMEI is now fully recognized as the early presentation of an idiopathic myoclonic epilepsy, even though the term 'benign' should only be accepted for a condition associated neither with the need for long-lasting treatment, nor with the slightest deficit in neuropsychologic development. Following its first description in 1981, 37 cases of BMEI had been reported by 1992 (Dravet and Bureau, 1981; Dravet, Bureau and Roger, 1985, 1992). The neurodevelopment history prior to the onset of seizures was usually normal. There were family members with epilepsy in 25% and

febrile seizures (FS) occurred in four of the 37 affected children. An important point is that in BMEI, FS preceding myoclonic seizures are always brief and infrequent (Dravet, Bureau and Roger, 1992).

CLINICAL AND EEG FEATURES

The usual sequence is the onset of brief bilateral myoclonic seizures (MS) in a neurologically normal infant aged between 6 months and 2 years. Jerks are more prominent in the upper part of the body causing a head-drop and upwards and outwards extension of upper limbs. The jerks may be single and very brief or repetitive with a pseudorhythmic pattern, lasting several seconds. Even if the eyes roll up, consciousness is never completely lost; and, only very rarely, when the lower limbs are more involved, does the child fall.

Even when closely observing an attack, it is difficult to be sure whether a head-drop is due to a myoclonic jerk, a brief tonic contraction, or an atonic seizure. Polygraphic recordings have shown that in BMEI the jerks are myoclonic and that absences or tonic seizures are never detected (Dravet, Bureau and Roger, 1992).

MS occur at any time of the day. Every seizure is associated with a discharge of generalized spike-waves or polyspike-waves. It is rare to find subclinical discharges in the

Epilepsy in Children. Edited by Sheila Wallace. Published in 1996 by Chapman & Hall, London. ISBN 0 412 56860 8

waking EEG. On the other hand, drowsiness and the early stages of sleep activate the discharges, some of which are unaccompanied by a clinical expression. A photosensitive response is seen in the EEG in about 20% of the cases. In a personal case, occasional daytime MS started in infancy. Interictal EEGs were normal during waking and sleep. Around 3 years of age clinical myoclonia occurred only in the early stages of sleep, when there were concomitant spike-wave discharges. This case serves to stress the point that the interictal EEG is usually normal in the waking state. The EEG may also be normal when the child is pharmacologically sedated and the recording omits the drowsy state and the early stages of sleep.

Valproate has been found to be the drug of choice and gives excellent control of seizures. In some cases generalized tonic-clonic seizures have appeared later in childhood or adolescence upon stopping medication (Dravet, Bureau and Roger, 1992).

The major concern about the evolution of BMEI is that 21–41% of the cases do not achieve normal school performance. The claim that early treatment might prevent occurrence of this nonbenign evolution (Aicardi and Levy-Gomes, 1989; Dravet *et al.*, 1992; Todt and Müller, 1992) is not yet substantiated. The following case histories exemplify the problems.

Patient 1
Seizures started at 6–7 months of age with loss of awareness and elevation of the eyes, slight trunk flexion, and occasional loss of posture. They were particularly noticeable just after awakening and when overtired. At 15 months there were jerks with backward falls. Although these had resolved spontaneously by 18 months they recurred at 19 months. At 2 years, following many single myoclonic jerks, a generalized clonic seizure occurred in association with a fever. Subsequently infrequent episodes associated with interruption in activities and staring have occurred, particularly during systemic

illnesses. An EEG at age 18 months while awake recorded a dominant rhythm of high-amplitude theta rhythms with infrequent bursts of high-amplitude 3-Hz waves, at times associated with spikes. Photic stimulation at a wide range of frequencies from 2 to 50 Hz evoked bursts of high-amplitude spikes and/or polyspikes and waves. Treatment with valproate led to an initial improvement, and at times when seizures have become more prominent, an increase in valproate dosage has been effective. Investigations for metabolic, postinfective and structural lesions have been negative.

General status at age 5 years: *After a slightly slow start, speech and language development are commensurate with age. There are movement difficulties, particularly in the fine and gross motor planning areas. Problems with dressing, pencil skills and use of feeding utensils have been identified. Discrete finger movements, imitation of gestures and balancing skills are all less well developed than expected. There is no gross cognitive problem, but the parents have not agreed to a full psychologic assessment. At 20 months, all skills were appropriate for age.*

Patient 2
Seizures were first noted at 15 months. They were characterized by sudden cessation of activity, an upward roll of the eyes, a glazed look, and a sway of the body. Soon after, falls were noted during the attacks; and while crawling there would be suddenly loss of power in the upper limbs with a fall on to the head. Valproate was started within 3 months of the onset of seizures, but control was variable over the next 6 months. Valproate was discontinued at 5 years, after 3 years of freedom from seizures. There has been no recurrence in the subsequent 2 years. An EEG at 17 months showed a background of theta rhythms. During a seizure lasting 2.5 seconds, stillness and rolling-up of the eyes were noted in association with a high-amplitude generalized spike and wave discharge. Photic stimulation did not produce any epileptic discharges. A further EEG

when aged 4 years and 9 months, while still receiving valproate, was normal.

At 20 months of age, a formal development assessment produced evidence of age-appropriate skills except for speech and language development, which was at a 15.5-month level. At 29 months, speech development continued to lag and eye-hand coordination was also poor. By 4 years, it was clear that there were severe problems with communication: both comprehension and expression were affected. Physically, there were difficulties with fine movement, imitation of gestures, tests of balance, and pursuit movements of the eyes. Education in a unit for children with communication and other specific difficulties was arranged.

It is clear that children who have had BMEI require detailed assessment, followed by assistance with their individual difficulties, and that the term 'benign' is not always appropriate.

DIFFERENTIAL DIAGNOSIS

Table 11d.1 lists the main nonepileptic and epileptic conditions which should be considered when diagnosing BMEI. More detailed analyses of these nonepileptic and epileptic paroxysmal disorders or episodic symptoms with onset during the first year of life are given in Chapters 2, 11b, 12a, 12b and 15 and also elsewhere (Fejerman, 1994).

Table 11d.1 Differential diagnosis of benign myoclonic epilepsy in infancy

---

Nonepileptic conditions
  Physiologic myoclonus (sleep jerks)
  Hyperekplexia
  Shuddering attacks
  Benign myoclonus of early infancy

Epileptic syndromes
  West's syndrome
  Severe myoclonic epilepsy in infancy
  Early-onset Lennox–Gastaut syndrome
  Cryptogenic or symptomatic myoclonic or
    myoclonic-astatic epilepsies

Nevertheless, it is important to stress the differentiation of BMEI from a nonepileptic condition which has the same abbreviation in initial letters: Benign Myoclonus of Early Infancy (Fejerman 1977, 1984; Lombroso and Fejerman, 1977; Fejerman and Medina 1986; Fejerman, 1991). In both syndromes, at comparable ages, in babies with prior normal development, myoclonia appear, mostly in the awake state, and predominantly in the head and upper limbs. Brief jerks tend to be repeated for some seconds, without loss of consciousness. In a proportion of cases of benign nonepileptic myoclonus the jerks resemble shuddering attacks (Vanasse, Bedard and Andermann, 1976), or may simulate infantile spasms, leading to the proposal of the term 'benign nonepileptic infantile spasms' (Dravet *et al.*, 1986). The clinical evolution is different, since in all cases, the nonepileptic benign myoclonia tend to disappear during the second and third year of life. In addition, antiepileptic drugs have no clear effect on them.

In view of the clinical similarities the differential diagnosis rests on the EEG. Either an ictal record or one capturing drowsiness and the early stages of sleep will confirm the diagnosis of BMEI. Waking, nonictal EEGs are not sufficient.

West's syndrome is undoubtedly the main condition to consider when a baby has brief repetitive seizures affecting axial and upper limb musculature. Again, the EEG will clearly be helpful in differentiating spike-wave or polyspike-wave discharges on a normal background rhythm from hypsarrhythmia. The differential diagnosis between BMEI and another epileptic syndrome described by the Marseilles School (Dravet, 1978; Dravet and Bureau, 1985), namely severe myoclonic epilepsy of infancy (SMEI), has provoked some controversies. It has been suggested that these syndromes may only reflect different degrees of severity in a single condition described as infantile myoclonic epilepsy following febrile convulsions (Lombroso,

1990). However, clinical and EEG differences seem to be clear: FS are always prolonged in SMEI and brief in BMEI; in any case, only 10–20% of the cases of BMEI in other series had previous FS; MS are very rare during the first year of life in SMEI and are the unique seizures in BMEI; the EEG is usually normal during the first year of life in SMEI; and arrest of neurodevelopment progress appears earlier and is invariable in SMEI, whereas in BMEI only 20–40% of cases are affected and cognitive problems become evident later, rather than in the early stages.

Early-onset Lennox–Gastaut syndrome (LGS) may show MS, but most frequently the seizures will be myoclonic-atonic or atonic, causing falls. On the other hand, LGS, by definition, is a combination of different types of seizures, mainly atonic, tonic and atypical absences. In most of the cases an EEG during drowsiness shows the classic slow spike-wave interictal discharges, and particularly the recruiting rhythm associated with brief tonic seizures (Beaumanoir, 1985; Aicardi, 1986).

Finally, epilepsy with myoclonic-astatic seizures (MAE) may start in early childhood and pose difficulties for nosologic identification. In this syndrome, the course and outcome are recognized as quite variable (Commission on Classification and Terminology of the International League Against Epilepsy, 1989; Doose 1985) and it probably encompasses syndromes that many authors might consider as separate, ranging from BMEI to the myoclonic variant of LGS (Aicardi and Levy-Gomes, 1989; Delgado-Escueta *et al.*, 1990; Fejerman, 1991; Chapter 12c). Nevertheless, the main features of MAE are the association of myoclonic-astatic seizures leading to drop attacks with absences and tonic-clonic seizures; the frequent occurrence of absence status; and, the presence of 4–7 Hz rhythms in the EEG, in addition to numerous spike-wave and polyspike-wave discharges. These features are not shared by BMEI.

REFERENCES

Aicardi, J. (1981) Myoclonic epilepsies. *Research and Clinical Forums*, **2**(2), 47–59.

Aicardi, J. (1986) *Epilepsy in Children: International Review of Child Neurology Series*, Raven Press, New York.

Aicardi, J. and Levy-Gomes, A.L. (1989) The myoclonic epilepsies of childhood. *Cleveland Clinic Journal of Medicine*, **56** (suppl.1), 534–9.

Beaumanoir, A. (1985) The Lennox–Gastaut syndrome, in *Epileptic Syndromes in Infancy, Childhood and Adolescence* (eds J. Roger *et al.*), John Libbey Eurotext, London, pp. 89–99.

Commission on Classification and Terminology of the International League Against Epilepsy (1989) Proposal for revised classification of epilepsies and epileptic syndromes. *Epilepsia*, **30**, 389–99.

Dalla Bernardina, B., Colamaria, V., Capovilla, G. and Bondavalli, S. (1983) Nosological classification of epilepsies in the first three years of life, in *Epilepsy: An Update in Research and Therapy* (eds G. Nistico *et al.*) Alan Liss, New York, pp. 165–83.

Delgado-Escueta, A.V., Greenberg, D., Weissbecker, K. *et al.* (1990) Gene mapping in the idiopathic generalized epilepsies: juvenile myoclonic epilepsy, childhood absence epilepsy, epilepsy with grand mal seizures, and early childhood myoclonic epilepsy. *Epilepsia*, **31**(suppl.3), S19–29.

Doose, H. (1985) Myoclonic astatic epilepsy of early childhood, in *Epileptic Syndromes in Infancy, Childhood and Adolescence* (eds J. Roger *et al.*), John Libbey Eurotext, London, Paris, pp. 78–88.

Dravet, C. (1978) Les epilepsies graves de l'enfance. *Vie Méd*, **8**, 543–8.

Dravet, C. and Bureau, M. (1981) L'epilepsie myoclonique benigne du nourrisson. *Revue d'Electroencephalographie Neurophysiologie*, **11**, 438–44.

Dravet, C. and Bureau, M. (1985) Severe myoclonic epilepsy in infants, in *Epileptic Syndromes in Infancy, Childhood and Adolescence* (eds J. Roger *et al.*), John Libbey Eurotext, London, Paris, pp. 58–67.

Dravet, C., Bureau, M. and Roger, J. (1985) Benign myoclonic epilepsy in infants, in *Epileptic Syndromes in Infancy, Childhood and Adolescence* (eds J. Roger *et al.*), John Libbey Eurotext, London, Paris, pp. 51–57.

Dravet, C., Bureau, M. and Roger, J. (1992) Benign myoclonic epilepsy in infants, in *Epileptic Syndromes in Infancy, Childhood and Adolescence*, 2nd edn (eds J. Roger *et al.*), John Libbey, London, pp. 67–74.

Dravet, C., Giraud, N., Bureau, M. *et al.* (1986) Benign myoclonus of early infancy or benign non epileptic infantile spasms. *Neuropediatrics*, 1;17, 33–8.

Fejerman, N. (1977) Mioclonías benignas de la infancia temprana. Comunicación preliminar in, *Actas IV Jornadas Rioplatenses de Neurología Infantil. 1976. Neuropediatría Latinoamericana*, Delta, Montevideo, pp. 131–4.

Fejerman, N. (1984) Mioclonías benignas de la infancia temprana. *Annales Espanoles de Pediatria*, **21**, 725–31.

Fejerman, N. (1991) Myoclonies et epilepsies chez l'enfant. *Revue Neurologique (Paris)*, **147**, 782–97.

Fejerman, N. (1994) Differential diagnosis, in *Infantile Spasms and West Syndrome* (eds O. Dulac *et al.*), W.B. Saunders, London, pp. 88–98.

Fejerman, N. and Medina, C.S. (1986) *Convulsiones en la infancia*, 2nd edn, El Ateneo, Buenos Aires.

Harper, J.R. (1968) True myoclonic epilepsy in childhood. *Archives of Disease in Childhood*, **43**, 28–35.

Jeavons, P.M. (1977) Nosological problems of myoclonic epilepsies in childhood and adolescence. *Developmental Medicine and Child Neurology*, **19**, 3–8.

Loiseau, P., Legroux, H.M., Grimond, P. *et al.* (1974) Taxometric classification of myoclonic epilepsies. *Epilepsia*, **15**, 1–11.

Lombroso, C.T. (1990) Early myoclonic encephalopathy, early infantile epileptic encephalopathy, and benign and severe infantile myoclonic epilepsies: a critical review and personal contributions. *Journal of Clinical Neurophysiology*, **7**, 380–408.

Lombroso, C.T. and Fejerman, N. (1977) Benign myoclonus of early infancy. *Annals of Neurology* **1**, 138–48.

Todt, H. and Müller, D. (1992) The therapy of benign myoclonic epilepsy in infants, in *Benign Localized and Generalized Epilepsies in Early Childhood, Epilepsy Research* (eds. R. Degen and F. Dreifuss), Elsevier, Amsterdam.

Vanasse, M., Bedard, P. and Andermann, F. (1976) Shuddering attacks in children: an early clinical manifestation of essential tremor. *Neurology*, **26**, 1027–30.

SEVERE MYOCLONIC EPILEPSY IN INFANCY

Natalio Fejerman

INTRODUCTION

Severe myoclonic epilepsy in infancy (SMEI) is, without doubt, a recognizable epileptic syndrome even though the term 'myoclonic' has been questioned (Aicardi and Levy-Gomes, 1989). Since the first description in 1978, details of 172 cases had been published by 1992 (Dravet, 1978; Dravet *et al.*, 1992). The prevalence has been estimated around one in 20 000 to one in 40 000 infants (Hurst, 1990; Yakoub *et al.*, 1992). The nosologic placement of SMEI is still debatable, not only in terms of seizure types, but particularly in relation to whether SMEI should be considered as an idiopathic, cryptogenic, or symptomatic syndrome (See Chapter 7). Genetic influences seem to be strong. In most of the published series, positive family histories of epilepsy and/or febrile seizures (FS) were found, ranging from to 20% to 64% of cases (Table 11e.1) (Dulac and Arthuis, 1982; Ogino, 1986; Dalla Bernardina *et al.*, 1987; Giovanardi Rossi *et al.*, 1991; Dravet *et al.*, 1992). In the largest reported series, 18% had family histories of epilepsy and 14% of FS (Dravet *et al.*, 1992). Isolated cases of SMEI have been seen in siblings and only one pair of affected monozygotic twins has been reported (Fujiwara *et al.*, 1990). However, the significance of these genetic data should be contrasted with the finding that seizures are almost always intractable in SMEI and all patients show mental retardation at follow-

Table 11e.1 SMEI: family history of epilepsy and/or febrile seizures

	Cases of SMEI (no.)	Positive family history (%)
Dulac and Arthuis (1982)	20	20
Ogino (1986)	14	64.3
Dalla Bernardina *et al.* (1987)	40	30
Hurst (1987)	7	57
Aicardi and Levy-Gomes (1989)	11	9
Giovanardi Rossi *et al.* (1991)	15	33
Dravet *et al.* (1992)	63	32

up. Such characteristic are more typical of an epileptic encephalopathy than of an idiopathic condition (Fejerman, 1991). In one autopsied case, microdysgenetic lesions were found in the spinal cord and cerebellum (Renier and Renkawek, 1990), but the vast majority of cases seem to be cryptogenic, at least with current knowledge since it is unusual to find personal pathologic antecedents and extensive investigation, including metabolic and neuroimaging studies, is always negative.

CLINICAL AND EEG FEATURES

The most common sequence of events in SMEI is: normal initial development; a first seizure at around 5–6 months (range 2–9 months), usually associated with fever (when

Epilepsy in Children. Edited by Sheila Wallace. Published in 1996 by Chapman & Hall, London. ISBN 0 412 56860 8

afebrile, a recent history of vaccination or infectious disease is present); a prolonged clonic or tonic-clonic attack, either generalized or unilateral; after an interval of weeks or a few months, second and further seizures occur with or without fever; antiepileptic drugs (AED) do not prevent recurrence of the seizures; by 1 year of age the children usually start walking and using the first isolated words; from the second year of life onwards, myoclonic seizures (MS) appear; they may vary from segmentary, mild and occasional, causing only jerks of a limb, facial muscles or axial muscles, to generalized, massive and frequent seizures progressing to drop attacks or rarely to status (Yakoub *et al.*, 1992); myoclonia occur mainly on awakening and can be triggered by variations in light intensity, closure of the eyes, or hot baths (Ogino, 1986; Fujiwara *et al.*, 1990; Dravet *et al.*, 1992); a clear increase in their frequency often precedes generalized seizures (Yakoub *et al.*, 1992); other types of afebrile seizures also appear from 1 to 4 years of age in most of the patients; these can be partial clonic seizures, versive seizures and complex partial seizures.

Absences are less frequent, very rarely typical, and consist of brief isolated loss of consciousness or an arrest of activity with a myoclonic component. There are disagreements in the literature as to whether absences form part of repeated myoclonic attacks (Dalla Bernardina *et al.*, 1982; Dravet *et al.*, 1992; Dulac and Arthuis, 1982; Yakoub *et al.*, 1992). Tonic seizures are not usually seen in SMEI. When present, they suggest a different diagnosis.

As the seizures start, the child slows up in neuropsychological development: language acquisition is poor, intellectual quotients become low, some degree of hyperactivity (which may also be influenced by AEDs) is present, and mild cerebellar and pyramidal signs cause clumsiness and ataxia of gait.

EEGs have been extensively studied with standard and polygraphic recordings (Dalla Bernardina *et al.*, 1987; Dravet *et al.*, 1992;

Yakoub *et al.*, 1992). They are usually normal during the first year. However, spontaneous or photically induced spike-wave discharges have been described at this age in four of 63 cases (Dravet *et al.*, 1992) and in 13 of another 40 patients (Dalla Bernardina *et al.*, 1987).

In parallel with the clinical deterioration, EEG abnormalities appear between the second and third years of life. Short bursts of generalized polyspikes, polyspikes and waves, or spikes and waves are found, either interictally or associated with myoclonic jerks. The background rhythms probably remain normal in a significant proportion of the patients, although data about this aspect of the EEG are scarce. A particular theta (4–5 Hz) monomorphic activity has been described in awake traces from the frontocentral and lateral regions (Dalla Bernardina *et al.*, 1982; Dravet and Bureau, 1985; Giovanardi Rossi *et al.* 1991).

TREATMENT AND OUTCOME

Long-term follow-up has been reported in several series and is summarized in Table 11e.2. Over the course of time, the frequency of myoclonia decreases progressively (Ogino, 1986; Dalla Bernardina *et al.*, 1987; Aicardi and Levy-Gomes, 1989; Giovanardi Rossi *et al.*, 1991; Dravet *et al.*, 1992; Yakoub *et al.*, 1992). Complex partial seizures seem to disappear after a few years (Fujiwara *et al.*, 1990; Dravet *et al.*, 1992), but generalized or secondary generalized tonic-clonic seizures tend to persist.

The seizures in SMEI are highly intractable, and in only a small series has a good response been reported with high doses of valproate (Hurst, 1987). The numbers of patients treated with the newer AEDs is not known. Perhaps lamotrigine might be worth a trial, since it has been useful in atypical absences, atonic and myoclonic seizures (Richens and Yuen, 1991; Yuen, 1994). Felbamate might have been used following reports of responses in the Lennox–Gastaut syn-

Table 11e.2 SMEI: series of patients with long-term follow-up

Author	Patients (no.)	Time of follow-up (yr)	Seizures	EEG	Mental status
Ogino (1986)	14	Range: 4–17	AA and MS stopped at 4–17 years, in 5 patients GTCS remained intractable	BGR deteriorated. Diffuse and focal discharges persisted	MR in 100%
Dalla Bernardina et al. (1987)	40	Mean: 8 Range: 3–20	Brief GTCS persisted in series. Other types of seizures disappeared		38%: Lack of speech 31%: MR with LDD 31%: Lear.D
Aicardi and Levy-Gomes (1989)	11	Mean: 5 Range: 1.5–20	Seizures intractable in 100%		91%: MR 91%: LDD and Lear.D
Giovanardi Rossi et al. (1991)	15	Mean: 14 Range: 8–23	Secondary GTCS and PS persisted in 100%	Slowing in BGR. MfD in 100%	IQ>50:26.7% IQ<50:73.3% BD in most of patients
Dravet et al. (1992)	63	Mean: 11 Range: 3–27	Active epilepsy up to 11–12 years. Less dramatic GTCS during sleep persist longer	BGR remained normal in 20 patients. Generalized SW and PSW disappeared in 19%. MfD in 82.5%	MR in all patients over 10 years of age IQ<50:50%

AA = Atypical absences; GTCS = generalized tonic-clonic seizures; PS = simple and complex partial seizures; MS = myoclonic seizures; SW = spike and waves; PSW = polyspike and waves; BGR = background rhythm; MfD = multifocal discharges; MR = mental retardation; LDD = language development disorder; Lear.D = learning disorders; BD = behavioral disorders.

drome (Ritter *et al.*, 1993), but it has been withdrawn due to bone marrow and liver failure. Fairly good control of seizures with vigabatrin has been attained, personally, in four SMEI patients treated from the second year of life, but follow-up is still too short. Probably the best initial therapeutic measure would be to teach the parents to use rectal diazepam at the onset of new febrile or afebrile seizures occurring after the first attack.

Some secondary cerebral lesions found in one autopsied case have been interpreted as probable sequelae to the prolonged clonic or tonic-clonic febrile or afebrile seizures which take place during the first years of life (Renier and Renkawek, 1990). The final outcome is always poor in terms of intellectual abilities and in the largest series presented all the patients aged more than 10 years are dependent and institutionalized (Dravet *et al.*, 1992). It is noteworthy that three of 40 patients in one series died (Dalla Bernardina *et al.*, 1987), as did 10 of 63 in another report (Dravet *et al.*, 1992).

DIFFERENTIAL DIAGNOSIS

The sequence of clinical events and EEG features characteristic of SMEI is such that a positive diagnosis is possible only when enough time has elapsed to allow the full picture to evolve (Commission on Classification and Terminology of the International League Against Epilepsy 1989; Dalla Bernardina *et al.*, 1982; Dravet *et al.*, 1985; Fejerman and Medina, 1986; Fejerman, 1991). Nevertheless, stricter criteria for the early diagnosis of SMEI have recently been presented (Yakoub *et al.*, 1992). These authors state: 'the occurrence of afebrile generalized clonic seizures in the first year of life in previously normal children with normal CT scanning and EEG is the major clue for an early diagnosis'. Their criteria for selecting cases included at least one afebrile seizure, but afebrile was defined as associated with a temperature under 38.5°C. Therefore, these

Table 11e.3 Epileptic syndromes to be considered in differential diagnosis of SMEI

Benign myoclonic epilepsy in infancy
Epilepsy with myoclonic-astatic seizures
Lennox–Gastaut syndrome
Intermediate forms
Temporal lobe epilepsy linked with previous history of febrile seizures

criteria are not really contrary to the general experience which dates the onset to prolonged seizures, either febrile or associated with vaccinations or infectious diseases (Dravet *et al.*, 1992). Furthermore, the term myoclonic can be retained only if attainment of the second or third years of life are awaited before the diagnosis is made. It is noted that some cases with similar features and evolution, but without myoclonic seizures, have been reported (Ogino *et al.*, 1989; Yakoub *et al.*, 1992). The differential diagnosis of SMEI includes several early-onset epileptic syndromes (Table 11e.3). Some of them are considered in the preceding section of this chapter, namely benign myoclonic epilepsy in infancy (Chapter 11d), and the next chapter, epilepsy with myoclonic-astatic seizures (MAE) (Chapter 12b) and Lennox–Gastaut syndrome (LGS) (Chapter 12a). SMEI shares with some cases of MAE and LGS the presence of different types of seizures, their intractability, and the association of mental retardation with the course of time (Beaumanoir, 1985). In fact some of the patients reported as having MAE might have been cases of SMEI, since the boundaries allowed for its definition are somewhat loose (Doose, 1985).

If one considers that cryptogenic LGS (Boniver *et al.*, 1987) may start in infancy, may include myoclonic seizures, and may even not show its typical EEG pattern at the beginning, the differential diagnosis with SMEI would be difficult, especially when, in some series, up of 10% of the LGS cases have had previous FS. However this is not usual, in that in 369 children with FS followed for at least 2 years, only one case of LGS was reported (Wallace, 1991).

Intermediate or borderline cases straddling the boundaries between MAE, LGS, and SMEI probably exist (Aicardi, 1986; Fejerman, 1991; Yakoub *et al.*, 1992). Finally, the differential diagnosis with temporal lobe epilepsy secondary to prolonged FS must be considered in the early stages of SMEI (Wallace, 1988). The antecedent of FS, and the appearance of complex partial seizures and secondary generalized clonic or tonic-clonic seizures with normal interictal EEGs, are similar at the beginning, but the later clinical-EEG evolution emphasizes the differences.

In summary, nosologic recognition of SMEI as a distinct epileptic syndrome is being achieved with more certainty as new and larger series of cases are presented. In fact, most pediatric neurologists now consider SMEI with the appearance of new seizures, despite preventive treatment, after a first prolonged unilateral or generalized clonic seizure associated with fever, particularly if the temperature was not very high at the time.

REFERENCES

Aicardi, J. (1986) *Epilepsy in Children: International Review of Child Neurology Series*, Raven Press, New York.

Aicardi, J. and Levy-Gomes, A.L. (1989) The myoclonic epilepsies of childhood. *Cleveland Clinic Journal of Medicine*, **56**(suppl.1), 534–9.

Beaumanoir, A. (1985) The Lennox–Gastaut syndrome, in *Epileptic Syndromes in Infancy, Childhood and Adolescence* (eds J. Roger *et al.*), John Libbey Eurotext, London, Paris, pp. 89–99.

Boniver, C., Dravet, C., Bureau, M. and Roger J. (1987) Idiopathic Lennox–Gastaut syndrome, in *Advances in Epileptology*, vol. 16 (eds P. Wolf *et al.*), Raven, New York. pp. 195–200.

Commission on Classification and Terminology of the International League Against Epilepsy (1989) Proposal for revised classification of epilepsies and epileptic syndromes. *Epilepsia*, **30**, 389–99.

Dalla Bernardina, B., Capovilla, G., Gattoni, M.B. *et al.* (1982) Epilepsie myoclonique grave de la première année. *Revue d'Electroencéphalographie et de Neurophysiologie Clinique*, **12**, 21–5.

Dalla Bernardina, B., Capovilla, G., Chiamenti, C. *et al.* (1987) Cryptogenetic myoclonic epilepsies of infancy and early childhood: nosological and prognostic approach, in *Advances in Epileptology* (eds P. Wolf *et al.*), Raven, New York, vol. 16, pp. 175–9.

Doose, H. (1985) Myoclonic astatic epilepsy of early childhood, in *Epileptic Syndromes in Infancy, Childhood and Adolescence* (eds J. Roger *et al.*), John Libbey Eurotext, London, Paris, pp. 78–88.

Dravet, C. (1978) Les epilepsies graves de l'enfance. *Vie Méd*, **8**, 543–8.

Dravet, C. and Bureau, M. (1985) Severe myoclonic epilepsy in infants, in *Epileptic Syndromes in Infancy, Childhood and Adolescence* (eds J. Roger *et al.*), John Libbey Eurotext, London, Paris, pp. 58–67.

Dravet, C., Bureau, M., Guerrini, R. *et al.* (1992) Severe myoclonic epilepsy in infancy, in *Epileptic Syndromes in Infancy, Childhood and Adolescence*, 2nd edn (eds J. Roger *et al.*), John Libbey, London, pp. 75–88.

Dulac, O. and Arthuis, M. (1982) Epilepsie Myoclonique Sévère de l'Enfant, *Journées Parisiennes de Pédiatrie*, Flammarion, Paris, pp. 259–68.

Fejerman, N. (1991) Myoclonies et epilepsies chez l'enfant. *Revue Neurologique* (*Paris*), **147**, 782–97.

Fejerman, N. and Medina, C.S. (1986) *Convulsiones en la Infancia*, 2nd edn, El Ateneo, Buenos Aires.

Fujiwara, T., Nakamura, H., Watanabe, M. *et al.* (1990) Clinicoelectrographic concordance between monozygotic twins with severe myoclonic epilepsy in infancy. *Epilepsia*, **31**, 281–6.

Giovanardi Rossi, P., Santucci, M., Gobbi, G. *et al.* (1991) Long-term follow-up of severe myoclonic epilepsy in infancy, in *Modern Perspectives of Child Neurology* (eds Y. Fukuyama *et al.*), The Japanese Society of Child Neurology, Asahi Daily News Co., Tokyo, pp. 205–13.

Hurst, D.L. (1987) Severe myoclonic epilepsy in infancy. *Pediatric Neurology*, **3**, 269–72.

Hurst, D.L. (1990) Epidemiology of severe myoclonic epilepsy in infancy. *Epilepsia*, **31**, 297–400.

Ogino, T. (1986) Severe myoclonic epilepsy in infancy – a clinical and electroencephalographic study. (Summary in English.) *Journal of the Japanese Epileptic Society*, **4**, 114–26.

Ogino, T., Ohtsuka, Y., Yamatogi, Y. *et al.* (1989) The epileptic syndromes sharing common characteristics during early childhood with severe myoclonic epilepsy in infancy. *Japanese Journal of Psychiatric Neurology (Tokyo)*, **43**, 479–81.

Renier, W. O and, Renkawek, K. (1990) Clinical and neuropathological findings in a case of severe myoclonic epilepsy in infancy. *Epilepsia*, **31**, 287–91.

Richens, A. and Yuen, A.W.C. (1991) Overview of the clinical efficacy of lamotrigine. *Epilepsia*, **32** (suppl. 2), S13–60.

Ritter, F. J. *et al.* The Felbamate Study Group in Lennox–Gastaut Syndrome (1993) Efficacy of felbamate in childhood epileptic encephalo-pathy (Lennox–Gastaut syndrome). *New England Journal of Medicine*, **328**, 29–33.

Wallace, S.J. (1988) *The Child with Febrile Seizures*, John Wright, London.

Wallace, S.J. (1991) Epileptic syndromes linked with previous history of febrile seizures, in *Modern Perspectives of Child Neurology* (eds Y. Fukuyama *et al.*), The Japanese Society of Child Neurology, Asahi Daily News Co., Tokyo, pp. 175–81.

Yakoub, M., Dulac, O., Jambaqué, I. *et al.* (1992) Early diagnosis of severe myoclonic epilepsy in infancy. *Brain and Development*, **14**, 209–303.

Yuen, A.W.C. (1994) Lamotrigine: a review of antiepileptic efficacy. *Epilepsia*, **35** (suppl. 5), S33–6.

EPILEPTIC SYNDROMES WITH ONSET IN EARLY CHILDHOOD 12

INTRODUCTION

The epilepsies that have their onset in early childhood are often severe and difficult to treat. Their clinical presentation can be extremely varied, with multiple seizure types and associated features. As a result of their variable expressions, they are difficult to include within well-defined epilepsy syndromes (Chevrie and Aicardi, 1977).

Among the currently recognized syndromes in children aged 1–5 years, some, such as severe and benign myoclonic epilepsies, or some epilepsies with partial seizures, often begin in the first year of life and are described elsewhere (Chapter 11).

The Lennox–Gastaut syndrome (LGS) and some types of epilepsy with prominent myoclonic or atonic seizures are the subject of this chapter, which deals with recognizable epilepsy syndromes with onset after the age of 1 year. Age limits, however, are arbitrary as some cases of severe or benign myoclonic epilepsy and some syndromes with benign infantile partial seizures (Dravet *et al.*, 1989; Dulac, Cusmai and De Oliveira, 1989; Watanabe *et al.*, 1990) can appear or develop characteristic features after the first birthday. Conversely, the LGS and some cases of myoclonic-astatic epilepsy may begin before the age of 1 year.

The LGS and several types of myoclonic epilepsy share a number of features, notably frequent brief seizures with falls, mental retardation or deterioration, occurrence of minor status epilepticus, and resistance to conventional drug treatment, so their nosologic classification is difficult and variably understood (Aicardi 1986, 1994).

Currently, reasonable, if not universal, agreement has been reached with regard to characterization of the LGS (Aicardi and Levy Gomes, 1988; Roger, Dravet and Bureau, 1989; Zifkin, 1990; Beaumanoir and Dravet, 1992), but the nosologic situation of the various forms of myoclonic or myo-astatic epilepsy remains confused.

This chapter will consider in succcessive sections: Lennox–Gastaut syndrome; the concept of myoclonic-astatic epilepsy; and other epilepsies with tonic, atonic, or astatic seizures that are difficult to classify in any well-defined syndrome.

REFERENCES

Aicardi, J. (1986) *Epilepsy in Children*, Raven Press, New York.
Aicardi, J. (1994) *Epilepsy in Children*. 2nd edn, Raven Press, New York.
Aicardi, J. and Levy Gomes, A. (1988) The Lennox–Gastaut syndrome: clinical and electroencephalographic features, in *The Lennox–Gastaut Syndrome* (eds E. Niedermeyer and R. Degan), Alan Liss, New York, pp. 25–46.

Beaumanoir, A. and Dravet, C. (1992) The Lennox–Gastaut syndrome, in *Epileptic Syndromes in Infancy, Childhood and Adolescence*, 2nd edn, John Libbey, London, pp. 115–32.

Chevrie, J.J. and Aicardi, J. (1972) Childhood epileptic encephalopathy with slow spike-wave: a statistical study of 80 cases. *Epilepsia*, **13**, 259–71.

Dulac, O., Cusmai, R. and De Oliveira, K. (1989) Is there a partial benign epilepsy in infancy? *Epilepsia*, **30**, 798–801.

Roger, J., Dravet, C. and Bureau, M. (1989) The Lennox–Gastaut syndrome. *Cleveland Clinical Journal of Medicine*, **56**(suppl.), S172–80.

Watanabe, K., Yamamoto, N., Negoro, T. *et al.* (1990) Benign infantile epilepsy with complex partial seizures. *Journal of Clinical Neurophysiology*, **7**, 409–16.

Zifkin, B.G. (1990) The Lennox–Gastaut syndrome, in *Comprehensive Epileptology* (eds M. Dam and L. Gram), Raven Press, New York, pp. 123–31.

Jean Aicardi

The Lennox–Gastaut syndrome (LGS) is currently defined as an epilepsy syndrome characterized by multiple types of seizure including a nucleus of brief tonic, atonic and myoclonic attacks and atypical absences associated with an interictal EEG pattern of diffuse, slow spike-wave complexes. Mental retardation or deterioration is a very frequent but not constant feature (Aicardi and Levy Gomes, 1988). Some authors (Beaumanoir, 1985; Beaumanoir and Dravet, 1992; Roger, Dravet and Bureau, 1989) find this definition too inclusive and consider that the mere presence of multiple seizure types and an interictal slow spike-wave pattern is not diagnostic. They propose two additional criteria:

1. The occurrence of generalized tonic seizures.
2. The presence of runs of fast (10 Hz) EEG rhythms during slow sleep that may be ictal or interictal.

However, these features are not found in every case. In recent series, tonic seizures were present in 80–92% of patients (Gastaut *et al.*, 1973; Beaumanoir and Dravet, 1992) and fast EEG rhythms during slow sleep in only 55% of those patients who had whole-night EEG sleep recordings (Baldy-Moulinier *et al.* 1988). Nevertheless, they are of considerable value and make a diagnosis of LGS much more likely, even though they are not pathognomonic.

INCIDENCE AND ETIOLOGY

The incidence of the LGS is poorly known. Its frequency has been variously estimated to be 1–10% of childhood epilepsies (Gastaut *et al.*, 1973; Luna *et al.*, 1988), the former figure being probably closer to reality. Males are affected more often than females (54 to 63%). Onset is between 1 and 7 years in the vast majority. The peak age of onset is between 3 and 5 years of age. Up to 20% of cases have their onset before 2 years, but late cases with onset in late childhood, adolescence, or even adulthood are known to occur (Roger *et al.*, 1987).

Between 25 and 30% of cases occur in children without previous development or neurologic abnormality or epilepsy, and without imaging evidence of brain damage. Such cases are now termed cryptogenic in the ILAE Classification of Epilepsies and Epileptic Syndromes (Commission on Classification and Terminology of the International League Against Epilepsy, 1989) where LGS is considered to be a cryptogenic or symptomatic syndrome. However, the term 'cryptogenic' as defined by the ILAE implies the presence of an underlying, if undefined, brain disease that has not been demonstrated in such cases. Mental deterioration is usually the only evidence of brain dysfunction and it may well be a consequence of the epileptic activity itself, rather than of any previous brain damage. If so, the term idiopathic epilepsy would apply, the more so since a

Epilepsy in Children. Edited by Sheila Wallace. Published in 1996 by Chapman & Hall, London. ISBN 0 412 56860 8

family history of epilepsy has been found in a high proportion of cases by some investigators who have isolated an 'idiopathic' form of LGS (Boniver *et al.*, 1987; Ohtahara *et al.*, 1988), not currently included in the ILAE classification. However, the frequency of a family history of epilepsy in LGS patients varies considerably from 2.5% (Chevrie and Aicardi, 1972) to 47.8% (Dravet and Roger, 1988).

Approximately 70–75% of cases result from demonstrable brain abnormality or occur in patients with previous development delay or epilepsy (Chevrie and Aicardi, 1972; Gastaut *et al.*, 1973; Ohtahara *et al.*, 1988). These are often termed symptomatic cases, by analogy with infantile spasms. However, the correct term, according to the ILAE scheme, should be 'cryptogenic' when the nature of the underlying condition is undetermined, as is often the case. Thus, the same term is used with two different meanings, illustrating the difficulties inherent in a comprehensive classification of the epilepsies.

Some symptomatic cases are due to known brain diseases or lesions, most of which are of developmental origin. Tuberous sclerosis is a relatively common cause of LGS. Abnormal cortical development may also be a cause. In 16 of 30 autopsy cases, cortical dysplasia was present and was extensive in nine (Roger and Gambarelli-Dubois, 1988). Bilateral perisylvian and central dysplasia (Guerrini *et al.* 1992a, 1992b; Ricci *et al.*, 1992; Kuzniecky *et al.*, 1993) and diffuse subcortical laminar heterotopias (Palmini, Andermann and Tampieri, 1991; Palmini *et al.*, 1991) can cause a fully-fledged LGS, and even focal areas of dysplastic cortex (Palmini *et al.*, 1991; Guerrini *et al.*, 1992a, 1992b) may be responsible. Rare cases are due to hamartomas of the floor of the third ventricle (Berkovic *et al.*, 1988), Sturge–Weber syndrome (Chevrie, Specola and Aicardi, 1988; Roger and Gambarelli-Dubois, 1988), or tumors, especially in the frontal lobes (Angelini *et al.*, 1979).

Very little is known of the pathologic basis

of the 'cryptogenic' cases of the LGS. Biopsy studies (Renier, 1988; Renier, Gabreëls and Jaspar, 1988) have shown only relatively minor changes, such as poor dendritic arborizations and disturbed synaptic development of pyramidal cells in the inner layers of the cortex.

PET studies (Chugani *et al.*, 1987; Theodore *et al.*, 1987 – in five and 10 cases respectively) have also given variable results confirming the etiologic heterogeneity of the LGS. In some cases, a focal area of hypometabolism was found, while in others multiple abnormal areas or diffuse hypometabolism were demonstrated. It seems likely that LGS is also heterogeneous from a physiopathologic point of view, some cases representing diffusion on a bisynchronous mode from a focal lesion and others being due to multifocal or diffuse epileptogenic activity.

Acquired destructive lesions are less common but hypoxic brain damage is mentioned in most series (Ohtahara, 1988; Roger and Gambarelli-Dubois, 1988). Large porencephalic defects can also result in a picture of LGS (Ohtahara *et al.*, 1988; Palm, Brandt and Korithenberg, 1988).

The LGS often follows other epileptic syndromes, most commonly West's syndrome, which is found to have preceded the LGS in 17.5–41% of cases (Aicardi and Levy Gomes, 1988; Ohtahara *et al.*, 1988; Weinman, 1988). Cases following infantile spasms may represent a special subgroup of the LGS, with early onset, predominance of tonic seizures with a repetitive character and a particularly poor prognosis (Aicardi and Levy Gomes, 1988; Ohtahara *et al.*, 1988). LGS is included by Ohtahara (1988) among the age-dependent epileptic encephalopathies together with West and early infantile epileptic encephalopathy (Ohtahara's syndrome). However, many cases are not preceded by other epileptic encephalopathies and the causes of the different syndromes may not be the same. Major brain malformations are less commonly a cause of LGS than of infantile spasms (Aicardi, 1986, 1994). Other types of epileptic seizures preceding the appearance of LGS include unilateral seizures, generalized tonic-clonic seizures, and episodes of convulsive status epilepticus. Partial seizures are relatively common (Chevrie and Aicardi, 1972; Gastaut *et al.*, 1973; Roger, Dravet and Bureau, 1989; Zifkin, 1990). Primary generalized seizures, including typical absences, have been observed only rarely (Roger, Dravet and Bureau, 1989; Beaumanoir and Dravet, 1992).

ICTAL MANIFESTATIONS

The seizures of the LGS are, in most cases, frequently repeated and usually occur many times, or even several dozen times, daily. They are especially frequent during sleep.

TONIC SEIZURES

Tonic seizures are present in 74–92% of cases (Chevrie and Aicardi, 1972; Gastaut *et al.*, 1973; Roger, Dravet and Bureau, 1989). The axial type produces a flexor movement of the head and trunk as a result of the brief, but sustained, bilateral symmetric contraction of axial muscles, and is usually associated with clouding of consciousness and autonomic manifestations. In axo-rhizomelic seizures, there is associated abduction and elevation of the arms, while global tonic attacks result in falls if the child is standing. Tonic seizures may be quite mild, especially in sleep, when they are often limited to a brief apnea and/or an upwards deviation of the eyes. Axial spasms (Egli *et al.*, 1985; Ikeno *et al.*, 1985) are very brief tonic seizures of 1–3 seconds' duration that are the most common cause of falls in LGS patients. In infants, tonic seizures tend to occur in clusters and to be followed by atonia so they may be difficult to distinguish from infantile spasms (Roger, Dravet and Bureau, 1989; Donat and Wright, 1991). In older patients, episodes of automatic behavior may follow the tonic phase or alternate with tonic contractions (Oller

Daurella, 1970). Such tonic-automatic seizures were found in 16% of cases (Roger, Dravet and Bureau, 1989).

ATYPICAL ABSENCE SEIZURES

These are the second most common type of seizure in the LGS. They are observed in 13–100% of patients (Gastaut *et al.*, 1973; Aicardi and Levy Gomes, 1988). They may resemble closely typical absence attacks, although their onset and termination are said to be less abrupt, or be mild and hardly detectable clinically, since loss of consciousness can be incomplete, allowing the child to continue ongoing activities, albeit at a slower pace, and in an imperfect manner. Decreased consciousness may be associated with loss of muscle tone, erratic myoclonic jerks, sialorrhea or mild hypertonia of neck and back muscles.

MYOCLONIC AND ATONIC SEIZURES

Myoclonic and atonic seizures are less common and less characteristic of the LGS than tonic seizures or absences. They are difficult to distinguish from one another by clinical observation alone and require polygraphic recording for precise qualification. Myoclonic seizures are associated with spike-wave or polyspike-wave discharges whereas atonic seizures paradoxically are associated with the same EEG discharges as tonic seizures. Myoclonic seizures occur in 4–22.5% of LGS patients (Gastaut *et al.*, 1973). Atonic seizures are seen in 14–36% of patients (Gastaut *et al.*, 1973).

These four major types of seizures are usually associated in variable proportions and all can be responsible for falls. The noncommittal terms of astatic seizures (Gastaut *et al.*, 1973) or drop-attacks are clinically useful, as the mechanism of falls is often impossible to determine without polygraphic studies (Oguni *et al.*, 1992).

EPISODES OF NONCONVULSIVE STATUS EPILEPTICUS

These episodes occur in 50–75% of patients. The most common type consists of sub-continuous atypical absences interrupted periodically by recurring tonic seizures (Dravet *et al.*, 1985; Beaumanoir *et al.*, 1988). Other episodes may feature obtundation of variable degree associated with erratic myoclonus, or purely tonic seizures that often tend to become attenuated when the episodes are long-lasting. Tonic status can be accompanied by considerable autonomic disturbances and may be life-threatening (Dravet *et al.*, 1985; Beaumanoir *et al.*, 1988) and resistant to drugs. The duration exceeds 1 week in up to half the cases (Dravet *et al.*, 1985). Nonconvulsive status may be difficult to distinguish from the 'bad periods' that are common in the course of LGS. Indeed, all transitions can be observed and the distinction can be to some extent arbitrary (Shorvon, 1994).

In addition to the nucleus of tonic, atonic and myoclonic seizures and of nonconvulsive status, a variety of less suggestive attacks are often observed; these may precede, accompany or follow the 'core' seizures and include generalized or partial clonic or tonic-clonic seizures, complex partial seizures, and unilateral clonic seizures.

EEG FEATURES

INTERICTAL PATTERNS

The classic interictal EEG feature of LGS is the slow spike-wave (SSW) pattern, originally reported as 'petit mal variant' pattern because it was erroneously thought to be related to the 3-Hz spike-wave pattern of 'true petit mal' (absence epilepsy) (Fig. 12a.1). The SSW complexes consist of a spike (<70 ms) or sharp wave (70–200 ms) followed by a sinusoidal electronegative slow wave of 350–400 ms duration. A prominent positive trough is present between the fast and the slow components (Blume, David and Gomez, 1973; Blume, 1988). The SSW complexes may appear singly or in runs, with a repetition rate of 1–2.5 Hz. They are bilateral and roughly symmetric, though shifting asymmetries are often evident. They are diffuse but usually predominate over the frontocentral part of the scalp (Niedermeyer, 1969), though they may be more obvious over the occipitotemporal areas in a few patients (Blume, 1988). The SSWs are usually abundant, appearing in long sequences but, in a few cases, they are rare and may be only visible during slow wave sleep which in all cases increases their frequency (Baldy-Moulinier *et al.*, 1988; Roger, Dravet and Bureau, 1989). The SSWs are not responsive to photic stimulation and very little, if at all, to hyperventilation.

Bursts of diffuse or bilateral fast (10 Hz) rhythms (or polyspikes), originally termed 'grand mal pattern', are frequently recorded during slow wave sleep. They usually last a few seconds but tend to recur at relatively brief intervals. Some are associated with mild tonic attacks but many are subclinical even when polygraphic recording of electromyograms and respiration is performed simultaneously (Baldy-Moulinier *et al.*, 1988, Beaumanoir, 1985; Beaumanoir and Dravet, 1992). Such discharges are highly suggestive of the LGS. However, they are not pathognomonic of the syndrome as they have been recorded in cases of focal epilepsy (Pazzaglia *et al.*, 1985; Roger *et al.*, 1991) and they are not present in all cases. Baldy-Moulinier *et al.* (1988) found them in 44 (55%) of 80 patients diagnosed with LGS who had all-night recording. Fast bursts disappear during REM sleep.

Other sleep discharges include polyspike-wave complexes (Degen and Degen, 1984; Roger, Dravet and Bureau, 1989) that are also very frequent in slow wave sleep, possibly more than the 10-Hz bursts.

Slowing of background rhythms is present in over half the cases but not necessarily

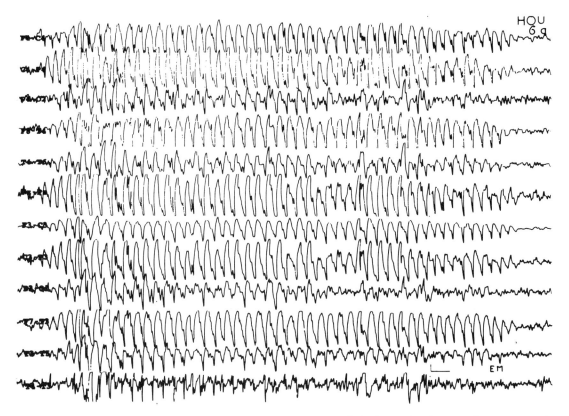

Fig. 12a.1 Atypical absence seizure. Regular succession of high-amplitude, synchronous, and symmetric slow spike-wave complexes at 2 Hz. Calibration: 100 μv, 1 second.

on every record. Focal paroxysmal activity (sharp waves) or slow activity are seen in some cases.

ICTAL PATTERNS

Ictal patterns include, in addition to 10 Hz discharges (Fig. 12a.2), sudden voltage attenuation, sometimes with superimposed 20-Hz, low-amplitude activity which may accompany some tonic seizures or be associated with atypical absences and, rarely, with myoclonic attacks (Gastaut *et al.*, 1974). The EEG concomitants of most myoclonic-atonic seizures are polyspike-wave complexes although SSW or fast rhythms can occur with atonic attacks. Atypical absences may be accompanied by high-voltage slow spike-waves, but other ictal patterns such as fast rhythms and paroxysmal decrement may be more common.

MENTAL RETARDATION OR DETERIORATION

Mental retardation is the third component of the classical LGS triad. However, 7–10% of children with LGS remain mentally unaffected (Chevrie and Aicardi, 1972, Beaumanoir, 1985; Aicardi and Levy Gomes, 1988; Ohtahara *et al.*, 1988; Roger, Dravet and Bureau, 1989; Beaumanoir and Dravet, 1992) even after long follow-up periods. A majority of patients are already delayed at onset of the syndrome, but 25–30% seemed to develop normally before the first seizures. The declining IQ

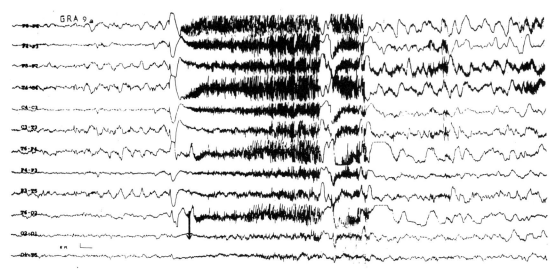

Fig. 12a.2 Tonic seizure in a child with Lennox–Gastaut syndrome. Discharge of fast rhythms of increasing amplitude followed by postictal slow waves. Calibration: 50 μv, 1 second.

may be due to slow progress resulting in increasing discrepancy between development and chronologic ages (Gastaut *et al.*, 1973), but true regression with loss of previously acquired skills undoubtedly occurs in some children (Aicardi, 1986). Even in cases with progressive deterioration, however, the process is self-limited, does not lead to complete dementia, is not associated with neurologic signs and may be partially reversible. It is therefore different from that seen in neurodegenerative diseases.

The degree of mental retardation is often severe: 48 of 89 patients in one series had an IQ of less than 25 (Ohtsuka *et al.* 1990), and 21 of 40 children in another series had an IQ of less than 50 (Aicardi and Levy Gomes, 1988). Many children have, in addition, severe psychiatric problems, frequently with autistic components (Gastaut *et al.*, 1973). Some children are also hyperactive, insecure, and aggressive (Oller-Daurella 1973).

The resulting overall disability precludes normal school attendance and learning, and later social integration, even when the cognitive deficit is of a relatively mild degree.

COURSE AND PROGNOSIS

The course of most cases of LGS is fluctuating with 'good' and 'bad' periods that appear to be related, at least in part, to the epileptic activity as indicated by the frequency of seizures and/or the intensity of paroxysmal EEG abnormalities.

Seizures persist into adolescence and early adulthood in most patients. Reported remission rates range from nil (Beaumanoir and Dravet, 1992) to 4% (Roger, Dravet and Bureau, 1989) or 6.7% (Gastaut *et al.*, 1973). In one series (Ohtsuka *et al.*, 1990), a rate of 24% was found. The characteristic types of LGS seizures continue to occur in the majority of patients, especially those who initially present with a complete clinical and EEG picture including tonic seizures, episodes of nonconvulsive status and runs of 10-Hz rhythms during slow sleep (Beaumanoir, 1985; Beaumanoir and Dravet, 1992). In patients with a less typical syndrome, with mainly atonic and/or myoclonic attacks, the characteristic LGS seizures often tend to be replaced by others, mostly simple or complex partial in type. In such patients, the LGS may be only a transient phase in the course of a focal or multifocal epilepsy (Beaumanoir, 1985; Roger, Dravet and Bureau, 1989; Beaumanoir and Dravet, 1992), possibly representing secondary bilateral synchrony (Gastaut and Zifkin, 1988).

The EEG abnormalities also tend to persist. Ohtsuka *et al.* (1990), however, found that the SSW pattern was replaced by multifocal independent spike foci in 31% of their 89 cases. These tended to run an especially severe course and were often associated with clinical or imaging evidence of cortical damage. In contrast, the SSW pattern persisted in almost all the cases of Beaumanoir and Dravet (1992) and of Roger, Dravet and Bureau (1989), even though focal or multifocal spikes were superimposed in 75% of cases. These differences might reflect different selection criteria.

Several studies have looked for more precise predictors of prognosis. Roger, Dravet and Bureau (1989) isolated four factors of poor prognosis: a symptomatic etiology, an early age of onset (even in cryptogenic cases), a high frequency of seizures with repeated episodes of nonconvulsive status, and a constantly slow EEG background. Aicardi and Levy Gomes (1988) found that a late onset of seizures, a normal CT scan, a paroxysmal response to hyperventilation, and a relatively high proportion of fast SW complexes, were associated with a better outcome; on the contrary, a history of infantile spasms was of ominous significance. In this study, as in those of Beaumanoir *et al.* (1988) and of Dravet and Roger (1988), the occurrence of episodes of status had no prognostic significance. This is at variance with the findings of Doose and Völtzke (1979) who found that such a history was strongly correlated with ultimate dementia.

DIAGNOSTIC AND NOSOLOGIC ISSUES

Even with the relatively exclusive criteria used in this chapter, the clinical presentation of the LGS is not entirely homogeneous and there is clearly room for many different clinical patterns variably overlapping with one another and with other syndromes, depending on any individual combination of seizure types and EEG anomalies. Beaumanoir (1985) found that 63% of 103 patients presented with a typical picture including tonic seizures, 10-Hz EEG bursts and episodes of status, and that 37% of them exhibited only some classic features but also had other seizure types including partial seizures or, rarely, generalized tonic-clonic seizures or even absences suggestive of primary generalized epilepsy. Gastaut and Zifkin (1988) have also proposed to exclude from typical LGS cases characterized by the predominance of atonic drop-attacks, commonly in association with partial seizures and with focal EEG abnormalities. They regarded such cases as secondary bilateral synchrony due to diffusion from focal epileptigenic lesions and emphasized the frequent asymmetry of EEG abnormalities and sometimes the presence of unilateral neurologic signs. It is difficult, however, to reject, on hypothetical physiopathologic bases, cases that otherwise satisfy all the criteria for LGS. Asymmetry of the EEG and focal neurologic signs can be found in typical LGS (Gastaut and Zifkin, 1988), so the exclusion of such cases is motivated only by the theoretical reason that they represent a form of localization-related epilepsy, whereas the LGS is classified as a secondary generalized epilepsy. In the absence of pathologic and pathophysiologic data, such a position is not tenable and it may well be that many cases of classic LGS are due to diffusion of epileptic discharges from currently undetectable localized lesions.

It is likely that the cases of post-traumatic epilepsy with diffuse slow spike-wave complexes reported by Niedermeyer (1972) belong in the same or a similar category.

Patients with SSW and only one type of seizure (usually tonic) do not meet the criteria of LGS. However, some have a course quite similar to complete cases and can probably be regarded simply as variants of LGS, while others may belong to different syndromes. The so-called 'intermediate petit mal', as described by Lugaresi *et al.* (1973), differs from typical LGS by the presence of relatively typical absence seizures during the initial course associated with, or preceding, more characteristic LGS seizures, and, by the occurrence of a high proportion of fast SW complexes in addition to the SSW of LGS. Lugaresi *et al.* regarded it as intermediate between the primary and the secondary generalized epilepsies, which is a physio-pathologic concept. From a clinical point of view, such cases fulfil the criteria for LGS and cannot be clearly separated from typical LGS by any single feature or combination of features (Aicardi and Levy Gomes, 1988) and should therefore be regarded as an integral part of the syndrome.

Several investigators (Aicardi and Chevrie, 1971; Dravet *et al.*, 1982) have set apart a **myoclonic variant of the LGS**, characterized by the prominence of myoclonic or myoclonic-atonic attacks, the rarity of tonic seizures that are exclusively nocturnal and by episodes of absence status, often with marked erratic myoclonus. The onset is usually later than in tonic-atonic cases (average four years) and the outcome may be less unfavorable (Aicardi, 1982). The situation of these cases *vis-à-vis* the myoclonic epilepsies is discussed in Chapter 12c.

Other epileptic syndromes with myo-atonic attacks may raise diagnostic problems, as myoclonic attacks are relatively frequent in typical LGS.

Severe myoclonic epilepsy (Dalla Bernardina *et al.*, 1982; Dravet *et al.*, 1992., Chapter 11d), also termed polymorphic epilepsy of early childhood (Aicardi 1991), also features re-peated brief seizures with falls and cognitive deterioration. However, the early history of affected children is quite different, since the onset is virtually always in the first year of life, with repeated and often long-lasting convulsive seizures commonly precipitated by mild fevers. At this stage, the differential diagnosis lies more with febrile convulsions than with LGS. The EEG never features SSW and there are no, or only rare and late, tonic seizures (Chapter 11e).

The less severe types in the spectrum of the myoclonic epilepsies do not feature tonic attacks and only uncommonly SSWs (Aicardi, 1991; Dravet, Bureau and Roger, 1992). Transitional forms between the myoclonic epilepsies and LGS are discussed in a later section.

Atypical partial benign epilepsy is the term coined by Aicardi and Chevrie (1982) to designate a rare epilepsy syndrome also called pseudo-Lennox syndrome by Doose and Baier (1989). It is characterized by rare focal, often nocturnal, seizures and by periods, usually of a few weeks' duration, during which intense clinical and EEG epileptic activity is evident. During these periods, the seizures are characteristically atonic attacks that can be focal or generalized and can result in multiple daily falls. The EEG abnormalities are extremely intense in slow sleep, amount-ing to continuous spike-wave of slow sleep (or 'electrical status epilepticus') but persist in the waking state in the form of bursts of fast or slow SW that often accompany atonic seizures. The active periods are separated by intervals of several months and only two to five such episodes occur before apparently complete recovery (Aicardi, 1986; Deonna, Ziegler and Despland, 1986; Aicardi and Levy Gomes, 1992).

Atypical benign partial epilepsy is probably an intermittent form of the syndrome of electrical status epilepticus of slow sleep (Chapter 13d), now renamed 'syndrome of continuous spike-waves of slow sleep (CSWSS), whose cognitive outcome is un-favorable, possibly because of the persistence of intense epileptic activity for prolonged periods in contrast to that which occurs in atypical partial benign epilepsy. The syn-drome is frequently mistaken for LGS because of the gross clinical and EEG abnormalities, but its prognosis seems to be completely different as patients followed up so far have all remitted and none is retarded. Minor learning/cognitive difficulties are not excluded, however, as follow-up data on these children are incomplete. Atypical benign partial epilepsy differs from LGS by the absence of tonic seizures, the frequent history of partial nocturnal attacks, and the absence of polyspike-wave complexes during sleep. The same differences exist between the syndrome of continuous spike-waves of slow sleep and the LGS, but the outcome is rather poor in both.

Isolated sleep dystonia (Lugaresi, Cirignotta and Montagna, 1986) does not raise major diagnostic problems as the attacks are mainly dystonic with violent writhing movements rather than tonic seizures. Vigilance-dependent tonic seizures (Rajna, Kundra and Halasz, 1983) may be a variant of sleep dystonia but are more likely to represent an epileptic manifestation of possible frontal origin. Similar cases have been recently reported by Vigevano and Fusco (1993). In their patients, the frequent repetition of tonic attacks might initially suggest the possibility of LGS. However, awareness remained normal during the seizures, the interictal EEG was normal, and ictal EEGs showed rhythmic theta activity quite different from LGS seizures. Such cases probably represent partial epileptic seizures of frontal origin. Their course appears to be benign.

TREATMENT

LGS is notoriously resistant to therapy and represents a common type of intractable epilepsy of childhood. Drug treatment however can decrease the frequency of seizures in at least some patients. Sodium valproate, benzodiazepines, especially clobazam, and carbamazepine are probably most useful. Each drug should be used first in isolation, then in association. In my experience, the combination of sodium valproate with cloba-

zam has been relatively satisfactory. In some cases, carbamazepine, that may be more effective against tonic seizures, can be combined with valproate that may be more active against atypical absences and drop attacks (O'Donohoe, 1985).

As many cases are resistant to these drugs, other antiepileptic agents should be tried. However, care should be taken to avoid multiple drug associations and/or agents that depress the level of consciousness, which may result in a paradoxical increase in seizure frequency. Many patients are actually improved by a decrease in polypharmacy, even though this does not result in complete seizure control.

The new antiepileptic agents should certainly be tried in resistant cases. Vigabatrin is only rarely effective in the long run (Aicardi, 1994). Lamotrigine has shown an encouraging effect on drop attacks and may be especially effective when combined with sodium valproate (Pisani *et al.*, 1993). Controlled trials are needed before firm recommendations can be made, but preliminary results seem promising. Felbamate proved effective against LGS in a controlled trial (Felbamate Study, 1993), but has now been withdrawn as a result of unacceptable side-effects. The exact results and modalities of treatment remain to be worked out.

Nonconventional agents have been used. Corticosteroids or ACTH may be indicated to tide the patients over a particularly difficult period (Aicardi, 1986, 1994). Their prolonged use is proposed by some investigators but their value remains to be proved since major side-effects are unavoidable with long-term, high-dose therapy. The value of immunoglobulins is currently difficult to assess (Rapin, Astruc and Etienne, 1988), despite favorable uncontrolled trials. Some authors have used amantadine (Shields, Lake and Chugani, 1985) or thyroid-releasing hormone but the results remain to be confirmed in larger controlled studies. The ketogenic diet has been extensively used (O'Donohoe, 1985;

Schwartz *et al.*, 1983) and seems to be effective in the short run, but it is difficult to maintain for a long duration and has not been submitted to properly controlled trials.

Surgical treatment has been used in a few cases (Chapter 23d). Resection of a focal lesion can be indicated when a localized abnormality is present (Palmini, Andermann and Tampieri, 1991; Palmini *et al.*, 1991). In most cases the only surgical possibility is anterior or total callosotomy. This operation has been found effective in selected cases (Oguni *et al.*, 1991; Pinard, 1991), especially against the drop attacks that are the most incapacitating type of seizure; but, recurrences have been observed and the exact value and indications of this technique remain to be established.

REFERENCES

Aicardi, J. (1982) Childhood epilepsies with brief myoclonic, atonic or tonic seizures (eds J. Laidlaw and A. Richens), *A Textbook of Epilepsy*, Churchill Livingstone, Edinburgh.

Aicardi, J. (1986) *Epilepsy in Children*, Raven Press, New York.

Aicardi, J. (1991) Myoclonic epilepsies in childhood. *International Pediatrics*, **6**, 195–200.

Aicardi, J. (1994) *Epilepsy in Children*, 2nd edn. Raven Press, New York.

Aicardi, J. and Chevrie, J.J. (1971) Myoclonic epilepsies of childhood. *Neuropädiatrie*, **3**, 177–90.

Aicardi, J. and Chevrie, J.J. (1982) Atypical benign partial epilepsy of childhood. *Developmental Medicine and Child Neurology*, **24**, 281–92.

Aicardi, J. and Levy Gomes, A. (1988) The Lennox–Gastaut syndrome: clinical and electroencephalographic features, in *The Lennox–Gastaut Syndrome* (eds E. Niedermeyer and R. Degen), Allan Liss, New York, pp. 25–46.

Aicardi, J. and Levy Gomes, A. (1992) Clinical and EEG symptomatology of the 'genuine' Lennox–Gastaut syndrome and its differentiation from other forms of epilepsy of early childhood, in *The Benign Localized and Generalized Epilepsies of Early Childhood* (ed. R. Degen), Elsevier, Amsterdam, pp. 185–93.

Angelini, L., Broggi, G., Riva, D. and Solero, C.L. (1979). A case of Lennox–Gastaut syndrome successfully treated by removal of a parietotemporal astrocytoma. *Epilepsia*, **20**, 665–9.

Baldy-Moulinier, M., Touchon, J., Billiard, M. *et al.* (1988) Nocturnal sleep study in the Lennox–Gastaut syndrome, in *The Lennox–Gastaut Syndrome* (eds E. Niedermeyer and R. Degen), Allan Liss, New York, pp. 243–60.

Beaumanoir, A. (1985) The Lennox–Gastaut syndrome, in *Epileptic Syndromes in Infancy, Childhood and Adolescence* (eds J. Roger, C. Dravet, M. Bureau *et al.*), John Libbey, London, pp. 88–99.

Beaumanoir, A. and Dravet C. (1992) The Lennox–Gastaut syndrome, in *Epileptic Syndromes in Infancy. Childhood and Adolescence*, 2nd edn (eds. J. Roger, C. Dravet, M. Bureau, *et al.*) John Libbey, London, pp. 115–32.

Beaumanoir, A., Foletti, G., Magistris, M. and Volanschi, D. (1988). Status epilepticus in the Lennox–Gastaut syndrome, in *The Lennox–Gastaut Syndrome*, (eds E. Niedermeyer and R. Degen) Alan Liss, New York, pp. 283–99.

Berkovic, S.F., Andermann, F., Melanson, D. *et al.* (1988) Hypothalamic hamartoma and ictal laughter: evolution of a characteristic epileptic syndrome and diagnostic value of magnetic resonance imaging. *Annals of Neurology*, **23**, 429–39.

Blume, W.T. (1988) The EEG features of the Lennox–Gastaut syndrome, in, *The Lennox–Gastaut syndrome* (eds E. Neidermeyer and R. Degen), Alan Liss, New York, pp. 159–76.

Blume, W.T., David, R.B. and Gomez, M.R. (1973) Generalized sharp and slow wave complexes – associated clinical features and long-term follow-up. *Brain*, **96**, 289–306.

Boniver, C., Dravet, C., Bureau, M. and Roger, J. (1987) Idiopathic Lennox–Gastaut syndrome, in *Advances in Epileptology, 16th Epilepsy International Symposium* (eds P. Wolf, M. Dam, D. Janz and F. Dreifuss), Raven Press, New York, pp. 195–200.

Chevrie, J.J. and Aicardi, J. (1972) Childhood epileptic encephalopathy with slow spike-wave: a statistical study of 80 cases. *Epilepsia*, **13**, 259–71.

Chevrie, J.J. and Aicardi, J. (1977) Convulsive disorders in the first year of life. Etiologic factors. *Epilepsia*, **18**, 489–98.

Chevrie, J.J., Specola, N. and Aicardi, J. (1988) Secondary bilateral synchrony in unilateral pial angiomatosis: successful surgical treatment. *Journal of Neurology, Neurosurgery and Psychiatry*, **51**, 663–70.

Chugani, H.T., Mazziota, J.C., Engel, J. Jr and Phelps, M.E. (1987) The Lennox–Gastaut syndrome: metabolic subtypes determined by 2-dioxy-2^{18} fluoro-D-glucose positron emission tomography. *Annals of Neurology*, **21**, 4–13.

Commission on Classification and Terminology of the International League Against Epilepsy (1989) Proposal for revised classification of epilepsy and epileptic syndromes. *Epilepsia*, **30**, 389–99.

Dalla Bernardina, B., Capovilla, G., Gattoni, M.B. *et al.* (1982) Epilepsie myoclonique grave de la première année. *Revue d'Electroencéphalographie et de Neurophysiologie Clinique*, **12**, 21–5.

Degen, R. and Degen, H.E. (1984) Sleep and sleep deprivation in epileptology, in *Epilepsy, Sleep and Sleep Deprivation* (eds R. Degen and E. Niedermeyer), Elsevier, Amsterdam, pp. 273–86.

Delgado-Escueta, A.V., Greenberg, D., Weissbecker, K. *et al.* (1990) Gene mapping in the idiopathic generalized epilepsies: juvenile myoclonic epilepsy, childhood absence epilepsy, epilepsy with grand mal seizures, and early childhood myoclonic epilepsy. *Epilepsia*, **31** (suppl. 3) S19–29.

Deonna, T., Ziegler, A.L., and Despland, P.A. (1986) Combined myoclonic-astatic and 'benign' focal epilepsy of childhood ('atypical benign partial epilepsy of childhood'). A separate syndrome. *Neuropediatrics*, **17**, 144–51.

Donat, J.F. and Wright, F.S. (1991) Seizures in series: similarities between seizures of the West and Lennox–Gastaut syndromes. *Epilepsia*, **32**, 504–9.

Doose, H. and Baier, W.K. (1989) Benign partial epilepsies and related syndromes – multifactorial pathogenesis with hereditary impairment of brain maturation. *European Journal of Pediatrics*, **149**, 152–8.

Doose, H. and Völzke, E. (1979) Petit mal status in early childhood and dementia. *Neuropädiatrie*, **10**, 10–14.

Dravet, C. and Roger, J. (1988) The Lennox–Gastaut syndrome: historical aspects from 1966 to 1987, in *The Lennox–Gastaut Syndrome* (eds E. Niedermeyer and R. Degen), Alan Liss, New York, pp.9–23.

Dravet, C., Bureau, M., Guerrini, R. *et al.* (1992). Severe myoclonic epilepsy in infants, in *Epileptic Syndromes in Infancy, Childhood and Adolescence*, (eds J. Rogers *et al.*), Raven Press, New York, pp. 75–88.

Dravet, C., Bureau, M. and Roger, J. (1992). Benign myoclonic epilepsy in infants, in *Epileptic Syndromes in Infancy, Childhood and Adolescence*, (eds J. Rogers, M. Bureau, C. Dravet *et al.*), John Libbey, London, pp. 67–74.

Dravet, C., Catani, C., Bureau, M. and Roger, J. (1989) Partial epilepsies in infancy: a study of 40 cases. *Epilepsia*, **30**, 807–12.

Dravet, C., Natale, O., Magaudda, A. *et al.* (1985) Les états de mal dans le syndrome de Lennox–Gastaut. *Revue d'Electroencéphalographie et de Neurophysiologie Clinique*, **15**, 361–8.

Dravet, C., Roger, J., Bureau, M. and Dalla Bernardina, B. (1982) Myoclonic epilepsies in childhood, in *Advances in Epileptology; XIIIth Epilepsy Intenational Symposium*, (eds A. Akimoto, A. Kazamatsuri, M. Seino and A. Ward), Raven Press, New York, pp.135–40.

Egli, M., Mothersill, I., O'Kane, M. and O'Kane, F. (1985) The axial spasm – the predominant type of drop seizure in patients with secondary generalized epilepsy. *Epilepsia*, **26**, 401–15.

Felbamate Study in Lennox–Gastaut syndrome (1993) Efficacy of felbamate in childhood epileptic encephalopathy (Lennox–Gastaut syndrome). *New England Journal of Medicine*, **328**, 29–33.

Gastaut, H. and Zifkin, B.G. (1988) Secondary bilateral synchrony and Lennox–Gastaut syndrome, in *The Lennox–Gastaut Syndrome* (eds E. Niedermeyer and R. Degen), Alan Liss, New York, pp. 221–242.

Gastaut, H., Bughton, R., Roger, J. and Tassinari, C.A. (1974) Generalized convulsive seizures without local onset, in *Handbook of Clinical Neurology*, vol. 15. *The Epilepsies* (eds P.J. Vinken and G.W. Bruyn), Elsevier, Amsterdam, p. 107–29.

Gastaut, H., Dravet, C., Loubier, D. *et al.* (1973) Evolution clinique et pronostic du syndrome de Lennox–Gastaut, in *Evolution and Prognosis of Epilepsies* (eds E. Lugaresi, P. Pazzaglia and C.A. Tassinari), Aulo Gaggi, Bologna, pp. 133–54.

Guerrini, R., Dravet, C., Raybaud, C. *et al.* (1992a) Neurological findings and seizure outcome in children with bilateral opercular macrogyric-like changes detected by magnetic resonance imaging. *Developmental Medicine and Child Neurology*, **34**, 694–705.

Guerrini, R., Dravet, C., Raybaud, R. *et al.* (1992b) Epilepsy and focal gyral anomalies detected by MRI: electroclinicomorphological correlations and follow-up. *Developmental Medicine and Child Neurology*, **34**, 706–18.

Kuzniecky, R. *et al.* (1993) Congenital bilateral perisylvian syndrome. *Lancet*, **341**, 608–12.

Lugaresi, E., Cirignotta, F. and Montagna, P. (1986) Nocturnal paroxysmal dystonia. *Journal of Neurology, Neurosurgery and Psychiatry*, **49**, 375–80.

Lugaresi, E., Pazzaglia P., Franck, L. *et al.* (1973) Evolution and prognosis of primary generalized epilepsies of the petit mal absence type, in *Evolution and Prognosis of Epilepsies* (eds E. Lugaresi *et al.*), Aulo Gaggi, Bologna, pp. 3–22.

Luna, D., Chiron, C., Dulac, O. and Pajot, N. (1988) Epidémiologie des épilepsies de l'enfant dans le département de l'Oise (France), in *Epidémologie des Epilepsies, Journées d'Etudes de la Ligue Française contre l'Epilepsie* (ed. P. Jallon), J. Libbey, London, pp.41–53.

Niedermeyer, E. (1969) The Lennox–Gastaut syndrome. A severe type of childhood epilepsy. *Deutsche Zeitschrift für Nervenheilkunde*, **195**, 263–82.

Niedermeyer, E. (1972) *The Generalized Epilepsies*, C.C. Thomas, Springfield, IL.

O'Donohoe, N. (1985) *Epilepsies of Childhood*, 2nd edn. Butterworth, London.

Oguni, H., Fukuyama, Y., Imaizumi, Y. and Uehara, T. (1992) Video-EEG analysis of drop-seizures in myoclonic-astatic epilepsy of early childhood (Doose syndrome). *Epilepsia*, **33**, 805–13.

Oguni, H., Olivier, A., Andermann, F. and Comair, J. (1991) Anterior callosotomy in the treatment of medically intractable epilepsy: a study of 43 patients with a mean follow-up of 39 months. *Annals of Neurology*, **30**, 357–64.

Ohtahara, S. (1988) Lennox–Gastaut syndrome: considerations in its concept and categorization. *Japanese Journal of Psychiatry and Neurology*, **42**, 535–42.

Ohtahara, S., Ohtsuka, Y., Yoshinaga, H. *et al.* (1988). Lennox–Gastaut syndrome: etiological considerations, in *Lennox–Gastaut Syndrome* (eds E. Niedermeyer and R. Degen), Alan Liss, New York, pp.47–63.

Ohtsuka, Y, Amano, R, Mizukawa, M. and Ohtahara, S. (1990) Long-term prognosis of the Lennox–Gastaut syndrome. *Japanese Journal of Psychiatry and Neurology*, **44**, 257–64.

Oller-Daurella, L. (1970) A special type of attack observed in the Lennox–Gastaut syndrome in adults. *Electroencephalography and Clinical Neurophysiology*, **29**, 529.

Oller-Daurella, L. (1973) Evolution et pronostic du syndrome de Lennox–Gastaut, in *Evolution and Prognosis of Epilepsies*, (eds E. Lugaresi, P. Pazzaglia and C.A. Tassinari) Aulo Gaggi, Bologna, pp. 155–64.

Palm, D.G., Brandt, M. and Korithenberg, R. (1988) West syndrome and Lennox–Gastaut syndrome in children with porencephalic cysts, in *The Lennox–Gastaut Syndrome* (eds E. Niedermeyer and R. Degen), Alan Liss, New York, pp. 419–26.

Palmini, A., Andermann, F., Olivier, A. *et al.* (1991). Focal neuronal migration disorders and intractable partial epilepsy: results of surgical treatment. *Annals of Neurology*, **30**, 750–7.

Palmini, A., Andermann, F. and Tampieri, D. (1991) Neuronal migration disorders: a contribution of modern neuroimaging to the etiologic diagnosis of epilepsy. *Canadian Journal of Neurological Sciences*, **18**, 580–7.

Pazzaglia, R., d'Alessandro, R., Ambrosetto, G. and Lugaresi, E. (1985) Drop attacks: an ominous change in the evolution of partial epilepsy. *Neurology*, **33**, 1725–30.

Pinard, J.M. (1991) Anterior and total callosotomy in epileptic children: prospective one-year follow-up study. *Epilepsia*, **32** (suppl. 3) 54.

Pisani, F., Di Perri, Perucca, E. and Richens, A. (1993) Interaction of lamotrigine with sodium valproate. *Lancet*, **341**, 1224.

Rajna, P., Kundra, O. and Halasz, P. (1983) Vigilance level-dependent tonic seizures. Epilepsy or sleep disorder? *Epilepsia*, **24**, 725–33.

Rapin, F., Astruc, J. and Etienne, B. (1988) Utilisation pédiatrique des immunoglobulines intraveineuses en immuno-modulation. A propos de 34 observations. *Annales de Pédiatrie*, **35** 481–8.

Renier, W.O. (1988) Neuromorphological and biochemical analysis of a brain biopsy in a second case of idiopathic Lennox–Gastaut syndrome, in *The Lennox–Gastaut Syndrome* (eds E. Niedermeyer and R. Degen). Alan Liss, New York, pp. 427–32.

Renier W.O., Gabreëls, F.J.M. and Jaspar, H.H.J. (1988) Morphological and biochemical analysis of a brain biopsy in a case of idiopathic Lennox–Gastaut syndrome. *Epilepsia*, **29**, 644–9.

Ricci, B., Cusmai, R., Fariello, G. *et al.* (1992) Double cortex: a neuronal migration anomaly as a possible cause of Lennox–Gastaut syndrome. *Archives of Neurology*, **49**, 61–5.

Roger, J. and Gambarelli-Dubois, D. (1988) Neuro-pathological studies of the Lennox–Gastaut syndrome, in *The Lennox–Gastaut Syndrome* (eds E. Niedermeyer and R. Degen), Alan Liss, New York, pp. 73–93.

Roger, J., Gobbi, G., Bureau, M. *et al.* (1991) Severe partial epilepsies in childhood, in *Modern Perspectives of Child Neurology* (eds Y. Fukuyama, S. Kamoshita, C. Ohtsuka and Y. Suzuki), Japanese Society of Child Neurology, Tokyo, pp. 223–30.

Roger, J., Rémy, C., Bureau, M. *et al.* (1987) Le syndrome de Lennox–Gastaut chez l'adulte. *Revue Neurologique*, **143**, 401–5.

Schwartz, R.H., Eaton, J., Ainsley–Green, A. and Bower, B.D. (1983) Ketogenic diets in the management of childhood epilepsy, in *Research Progress in Epilepsy* (ed. F. Clifford-Rose), Pitman, London, pp. 326–32.

Shields, W.D., Lake, J.L. and Chugani, H.T. (1985) Amantadine in the treatment of refractory epilepsy: an open trial in 10 patients. *Neurology*, **35**, 579–81.

Shorvon, S. (1994) *Status Epilepticus*, Cambridge University Press, Cambridge.

Theodore, W.H., Rose, D., Patronas, W. *et al.* (1987) Cerebral glucose metabolism in the Lennox–Gastaut syndrome. *Annals of Neurology*, **21**, 14–21.

Vigevano, F. and Fusco, L. (1993) Hypnic tonic postural seizures in healthy children provide evidence for a partial epileptic syndrome of frontal origin. *Epilepsia*, **34**, 110–9.

Weinman, H.M. (1988) Lennox–Gastaut syndrome and its relationship to infantile spasms (West syndrome), in *The Lennox–Gastaut Syndrome* (eds E. Niedermeyer and R. Degen), Alan Liss, New York, pp. 301–17.

MYOCLONIC-ASTATIC EPILEPSY   12b

Jean Aicardi

The concept of myoclonic-astatic epilepsies (MAE) is difficult to circumscribe, so MAE is variably understood by different investigators.

Doose *et al.* (1970) first proposed the term myoclonic-astatic petit mal, later (Doose and Baier, 1987) changed to MAE, to designate the primary generalized epilepsies of childhood whose main clinical manifestations are myoclonic and/or astatic seizures, i.e. seizures characterized by repeated falls attributed to lapses in muscular tone. Doose and his colleagues did not report on the polygraphic features of the attacks that could have been due either to atonia or to myoclonic jerking. They emphasized the significance of biparietal theta waves in the EEG, the importance of genetic factors in the etiology, the absence of apparent organic brain damage, and the preponderance of fast spike-wave or polyspike-wave complexes (as opposed to hysparrhythmia): all features that are also found in the primary generalized epilepsies of later ages. In Doose's conception, these features separated MAE from the secondary generalized epilepsies due to diffuse brain damage, of which the LGS is the main representative in the same age range. Doose has made it clear that he did not intend to describe a limited 'rigidly defined syndrome', but rather to draw attention to a large group of patients with emphasis on 'the wide variability of the idiopathic, generalized epilepsies of early childhood . . . as a result of multifactorial background responsible for electroclinical differences in presentation' (Doose, 1992). His concept of MAE embraces all forms of primary myoclonic epilepsies, including both the benign and the severe types of the ILAE classification (Commission on Classification and Terminology of the International League Against Epilepsy, 1989; Dravet, 1992; Dravet *et al.*, 1992; Dravet, Bureau and Roger, 1992; Dalla Bernardina *et al.*, 1982), that do not apply to any specific subtype.

Despite Doose's writings, MAE has often been regarded as a clinical and electroencephalographic syndrome, notwithstanding the fact that the basis for its delineation was a pathophysiologic concept rather than the EEG and clinical criteria used in other classifications, especially that of the International League Against Epilepsy. MAE, also termed 'Doose syndrome', has thus been entered into the ILAE classification of epilepsies and epileptic syndromes, on the same level as, and in addition to 'benign' and 'severe' myoclonic epilepsies, although no precise criteria have been provided.

Other authors, more recently, have used the term MAE (Roger, Dravet and Bureau, 1989; Dravet, 1992) or that of nonprogressive myoclonic epilepsy of childhood (Dulac, 1992; O. Dulac, personal communication) in a much more restricted sense to designate a specific electroclinical syndrome. These investigators thought that this syndrome corresponded at least in part to the MAE of Doose. It seems, however, that there are some differences among authors as to the limits

Epilepsy in Children. Edited by Sheila Wallace. Published in 1996 by Chapman & Hall, London. ISBN 0 412 56860 8

and precise features of the syndrome. Roger, Dravet and Bureau (1989) stated that patients with MAE presented with a single type of seizure (myo-atonic drop attacks). Dravet (1992) accepted, in addition, the occurrence of 'major afebrile convulsive seizures and of status of minor seizures with stupor'. Dulac (Dulac, 1992; O. Dulac, personal communications) emphasized the occurrence of multiple seizure types and distinguished two subgroups: one with mainly massive or axial myoclonic attacks, the other with mainly erratic myoclonus and 'vibratory tonic seizures'. From the viewpoint of the EEG, all authors have reported the presence of fast ($\geq$3 Hz) spike-wave or polyspike-wave complexes, often grouped in long bilateral and symmetric bursts. Dravet (1992) mentioned the presence of monomorphic theta rhythms, often recorded over the centroparietal areas. The course of the syndrome is reported as somewhat variable and may depend on the frequency and duration of the episodes of nonconvulsive status, the longest and most frequent being associated with the worst outcome (Dulac 1992).

The cases of 'early childhood myoclonic epilepsy' mentioned by Delgado-Escueta *et al.* (1990) and those of 'childhood intermediate myoclonic epilepsy' described by Giovanardi Rossi *et al.* (1985) appear to be closely related to MAE (Dravet *et al.*, 1992). Intermediate myoclonic epilepsy was described as a syndrome of massive myoclonic seizures, sometimes responsible for multiple falls, accompanied in some cases by atypical absences and generalized tonic-clonic attacks, but not by tonic seizures. Such cases did not show evidence of brain damage and the EEG showed fast spike-waves or polyspike-waves. Photosensitivity was present in half the cases and the course was more favorable than that of LGS, although seizures persisted in one-third of the patients and mental retardation was common. The syndrome was thought to be 'intermediate' between the primary and the secondary generalized

myoclonic epilepsies, in the same manner as 'intermediate petit mal' was thought to feature characteristics of both the LGS and typical absence epilepsy (Lugaresi *et al.*, 1973).

Aicardi and Levy Gomes (1989) have proposed separation of myoclonic epilepsies of early childhood into three subgroups:

1. Polymorphic epilepsy of early childhood.
2. Myoclonic epilepsy with isolated myoclonic attacks or occasional generalized tonic-clonic seizures.
3. Myoclonic epilepsies with multiple types of brief seizures often including tonic seizures.

The first two subgroups correspond approximately to severe and benign myoclonic epilepsies as described by other investigators (Chapter 11c, 11d). The third subgroup is closely related to MAE. Approximate relationships between myoclonic epilepsy syndromes, as understood by various authors, are indicated in Table 12b.1, but some consensus on the various types, to improve the present 'nosological jungle', is badly needed.

ETIOLOGY

MAE belongs to the idiopathic or cryptogenic groups of the ILAE classification of epilepsies and epileptic syndromes (Commission on Classification and Terminology of the International League Against Epilepsy, 1989). Symptomatic cases are rare and genetic factors are often operative, as indicated by the frequency of a family history of seizures. The overall incidence of seizures of any type in first- and second-degree relatives of probands with myoclonic epilepsy varies from 26 to 38% (Giovanardi Rossi *et al.*, 1988; Aicardi and Levy Gomes, 1989; Dravet *et al.*, 1992), and similar figures seem to apply to individual forms, including MAE (Doose, 1992). A multifactorial mode of inheritance is favored by Doose and Baier (1987) and Doose (1992).

Imaging of the brain gives consistently

Table 12b.1 Approximate relationships between syndromes of myoclonic epilepsy according to various authors

Doose (1992)*	Dravet et al. (1992)	Giovanardi Rossi et al. (1988)	Present author
	Severe myoclonic epilepsy (FS, followed by myoclonic seizures, atypical absences, partial or GTCS, FSW)	Severe myoclonic epilepsy (same as Dravet)	Polymorphic epilepsy of infants (severe myoclonic epilepsy, but one-third of cases without myoclonic seizures)
Myoclonic-astatic epilepsy (primary generalized epilepsy with myoclonic, atonic and other types of seizure including nonconvulsive status, GTCS or FS, rare or absent tonic attacks. FSW)	Benign myoclonic epilepsy (myoclonic seizures only, occasional FS, FSW)	Benign myoclonic epilepsy (same as Dravet)	Cryptogenic myoclonic epilepsy with only myoclonic attacks and occasional GTCS, FSW
	Unclassified myoclonic epilepsy (myoclonic and various types of seizures, FSW)	Unclassified myoclonic epilepsy (same as Dravet)	
	Myoclonic-astatic epilepsy (myoclonic and atonic seizures, nonconvulsive status, FSW)	Childhood intermediate myoclonic epilepsy (intermediate between primary, generalized epilepsies)	Myoclonic epilepsy with other brief seizures (myo-atonic-tonic, atypical absences, FSW, rarely SSW)
	Myoclonic variant of LGS (as above + rare tonic seizure, SSW)		
Lennox–Gastaut syndrome (secondary generalized epilepsy, tonic seizures and other types, SSW)	LGS (tonic + atonic seizures nonconvulsive status, SSW)	LGS (same as Dravet)	LGS (same as Dravet)

*Doose's classification uses both electroclinical and etiologic criteria, while other classifications are essentially electroclinical.
FS = febrile seizures; FSW = fast spike-waves; SSW = slow spike-waves; LGS = Lennox–Gastaut syndrome; GTCS = generalized tonic-clonic seizures.

normal results. The pathologic basis, if any, of the genetic propensity is unknown.

CLINICAL AND EEG FEATURES

The age of onset of MAE is overwhelmingly during the first 5 years of life when 94% of cases begin (Doose, 1992). Myoclonic seizures are most frequent, in most series, at 3–4 years of age (Aicardi and Chevrie, 1971; Dravet et al., 1982; Doose, 1992).

Myoclonic seizures, mostly of the massive or axial variety (Aicardi and Chevrie, 1971; Gastaut et al., 1974; Dravet et al., 1982) and atonic seizures with sudden loss of postural tone, are the major ictal manifestations. Myoclonic attacks can be of more limited extent and involve only the eyelids and/or facial muscles, but the axial type is predominant, with either head-nods, often saccadic, or diffuse involvement of upper and lower limbs with resulting violent falls. Polygraphic records show an extremely brief muscle contraction that often affects simultaneously both agonist and antagonist muscles and is synchronous with the EEG spike (Tassinari *et al.*, 1971). The contraction can remain single or be repeated – usually at rhythms of about 3 Hz – producing saccadic jerking. Myoclonic attacks are generally repeated many times daily and often tend to be more frequent and intense shortly after awakening (Aicardi and Chevrie, 1971). They sometimes occur in prolonged series but seldom reach a true myoclonic status.

Atonic seizures often follow a myoclonic jerk, although this may be so slight and limited as to go unrecognized clinically, or even with polygraphic recording. They are characterized by abrupt loss of muscle tone resulting in a complete fall or a head-nod or sagging of the knees, with mild nodding in the least severe cases. Oguni *et al.* (1992) have studied 36 drop seizures in five patients with MAE with simultaneous split-screen video recording and polygraphy. The seizures lasted 0.3–1 seconds and resulted in a fall on 16 occasions. Nine seizures were purely myoclonic with predominant involvement of flexor muscles. Two were myoclonic-atonic, with brief myoclonic flexor spasms immediately followed by loss of tone and fall. The majority of the seizures, 25 in all, were purely atonic in type. However, a change in facial expression and/or a brief twitch of the extremities sometimes preceded atonic resolution, suggesting the probability of a brief positive phenomenon in a few muscles. Electromyographic tracings show that the muscle contraction responsible for myoclonic jerks is usually followed by a brief period of EMG silence during which tonic muscle activity disappears for a duration of up to 120 ms (Tassinari *et al.*, 1971). The silent period sometimes occurs without a preceding jerk, although it is difficult to exclude the possibility of a mild contraction in muscles that are not being sampled (Shewmon and Erwin, 1988; Oguni *et al.*, 1992). In some patients, however, loss of muscle tone is a primary phenomenon. In such cases, the silent period tends to be longer, lasting up to 400 ms (Guerrini *et al.*, 1993). The clinical result of atonic seizures, whether or not associated with a myoclonia, varies from a mild head-nod to a complete fall, depending on the location and duration of the tonic lapse. A saccadic appearance, known as epileptic negative myoclonus, may result from periodically repeated atonia (Guerrini *et al.*, 1993). Atonia is usually associated with the slow wave of a single or multiple spike-wave complex (Tassinari *et al.*, 1971; Shewmon and Erwin, 1988), although the relationship with the spike may be variable.

Atypical absences are a feature in some cases of MAE. They may be accompanied by: changes in muscle tone (hypertonia or hypotonia); myoclonus of the facial musculature: or, only with a change in facial expression.

Episodes of nonconvulsive status epilepticus are mentioned by all authors. Doose and Völzke (1979) regard them as especially characteristic of MAE. They are marked by variable blurring of consciousness (stupor, apathy or milder obtundation) often associated with serial head-nodding due to repeated lapses of axial muscle tone and irregular twitching of muscles of the face or extremities (Brett, 1966). Some investigators (Dulac, 1992) think that obtundation with erratic myoclonus is a hallmark of the severe type of MAE, whereas true myoclonic status is a feature of the more benign myoclonic epilepsies. All agree that the episodes of status in MAE differ from the mixed type, with obtundation periodically interrupted by tonic seizures that is most characteristic of the LGS.

Tonic seizures are rare or absent in MAE (Dravet *et al.*, 1985; Giovanardi Rossi *et al.*, 1988; Roger, Dravet and Bureau, 1989; Dravet, 1992). Dulac (1992) has stressed the occurrence of a special type of 'vibratory tonic seizure' with cyanosis. Generalized tonic-clonic seizures occur in many cases. Simple or complex partial seizures are not a feature.

The ictal EEG of both myoclonic and atonic

seizures is characterized by sporadic discharges of irregular spike-waves or polyspike-waves at a frequency of 3 Hz or more (Gastaut *et al.*, 1974; Aicardi 1986, 1994). Similar discharges are frequently seen interictally. The background rhythm is usually normal or mildly slowed. The presence of monomorphic biparietal theta rhythm in the fully awake patient is considered an essential feature by Doose and Baier (1988), and has also been observed by Dravet *et al.* (1992). Ictal and interictal spike-wave complexes are bilateral but may show shifting asymmetries. A photoparoxysmal response is frequent (Giovanardi Rossi *et al.*, 1988; Doose, 1992), but has not been found by all authors (Dulac, 1992). It is not observed in the first year of life, contrary to the findings in about one-quarter of cases of severe myoclonic epilepsy (polymorphic epilepsy of early childhood).

Neurologic examination is normal in most children. Some patients, however, may appear grossly ataxic for variable periods even in the absence of obvious decrease in awareness (Aicardi and Chevrie, 1971; Aicardi, 1986; Bennett *et al.*, 1982), a phenomenon probably related to subclinical non-convulsive status.

COURSE AND OUTCOME

The course of MAE is variable, as is to be expected in such a heterogeneous syndrome. Most affected children have normal development and no neurologic abnormalities before the appearance of the seizures, but some have had other types of seizures, especially generalized tonic-clonic ones (Doose, 1992; Dulac, 1992). A substantial proportion remains unscathed. In cases with a prolonged course, particularly when repeated and protracted episodes of status occur, variable degrees of mental retardation become apparent (Doose *et al.*, 1970; Doose and Völtzke, 1979). Tonic seizures are particularly apt to occur in such cases and often appear in clusters during the latter part of the night. Persistence of rhyth-

mic EEG slowing until adolescence, without development of a stable alpha rhythm, may be an indicator of an unfavorable course (Gundel, Baier and Doose, 1981). In a series of 115 patients, Doose (1992) found that 54% had been seizure-free for at least 2 years after 7 years of age. In rare cases, the seizures disappeared without therapy and the development of these children remained normal. Such cases correspond to the benign myoclonic epilepsy of infancy described by Dravet, Bureau and Roger (1992; Chapter 11c). Patients whose epilepsy started during the first year of life with febrile or afebrile tonic-clonic seizures often of long duration had a poor outcome, in Doose's series, especially when they suffered prolonged episodes of nonconvulsive status epilepticus. Such cases correspond mostly to the severe myoclonic epilepsy of other authors (Chapter 11d). Dulac (1992; personal communication) found that 17 of his 28 patients had a favorable course with ultimate disappearance of seizures and no major cognitive defect following epilepsy, whereas 11 children ran an unfavorable course with resistant seizures and cognitive deterioration. The latter patients differed from the former in having prolonged episodes of nonconvulsive status and erratic myoclonus. Aicardi and Levy Gomes (1989) divided their 29 patients with myoclonic epilepsy, excluding those with polymorphic epilepsy, into two groups: 19 patients had exclusively myoclonic attacks or a few generalized tonic-clonic seizures in a predominantly myoclonic epilepsy, while 10 had myoclonic seizures and other types of brief seizures (e.g. atypical absences and sometimes a few tonic attacks). Patients of the first group fared relatively well, two-thirds of them being seizure-free after 6 years and none being severely retarded, although about half had learning and/or behavioral difficulties. Patients of the second group had a more severe outcome, with mental retardation in half of them and control of seizures in only 20%.

The discrepancies between various studies

clearly result from different selection criteria. If cases of severe myoclonic epilepsy (or polymorphic epilepsy of infants) are excluded, the outcome of patients with myoclonic or myoclonic-astatic epilepsy remains variable, but a significant proportion of the children will eventually be seizure-free and have reasonably normal development, even though minor behavioral and/or cognitive problems are common. Occasional patients may develop typical absence epilepsy (Kruse 1968; Chapter 13a) or juvenile myoclonic epilepsy (Dulac 1992; Chapter 14b).

It is, however, difficult to predict the outcome, and even in cases of benign myoclonic epilepsy (Dravet, Bureau and Roger, 1992) mental retardation and behavioral anomalies are not rare. Seven of the 12 patients reported by Dravet *et al.* were mildly retarded or behaviorally disturbed at the end of follow-up. However, the overall prognosis of the myoclonic epilepsies is clearly better than that of the LGS.

DIAGNOSTIC AND NOSOLOGIC PROBLEMS

Some of the conditions discussed in the differential diagnosis of LGS may also be difficult to separate from MAE, for example atypical partial benign epilepsy or the myoclonic variant of the LGS.

The progressive myoclonic epilepsies (Berkovic *et al.*, 1993; Chapter 15a) such as MERRF (myoclonic epilepsy with ragged-red fibers, Lafora's disease or Unverricht–Lundborg disease) can be indistinguishable initially from MAE, but the later emergence of neurologic abnormalities will establish the diagnosis. Episodes of nonconvulsive status epilepticus observed in some cases of MAE can present as ataxia and cognitive deterioration and mimic a degenerative disorder (Aicardi and Chevrie, 1971; Bennett *et al.*, 1982). The grossly abnormal EEG tracings are diagnostic.

In a few children with various forms of epilepsy, the administration of carbamazepine may induce the appearance of myoclonic attacks which disappear on discontinuation of the drug (Snead and Hosey, 1985). A similar phenomenon may also be observed with the use of vigabatrin (Marciani *et al.*, 1995).

Nonepileptic myoclonus, i.e. myoclonus unassociated with any paroxysmal EEG abnormalities, can be observed in many neurologic disorders but rarely raises a diagnostic problem with MAE, unless it is a part of a degenerative disease with associated epileptic features.

Finally, myoclonus is a common phenomenon in many forms of epilepsy (e.g. in some cases of absences or in the LGS) and the proportion of myoclonias necessary to make a diagnosis of myoclonic epilepsy cannot be precisely defined. This problem is further discussed in Chapter 12c.

TREATMENT

Drug treatment of MAE is primarily with sodium valproate but some patients, probably corresponding more to the benign myoclonic epilepsy of Dravet, respond dramatically to either valproate or ethosuximide in regular doses.

In the majority of patients, treatment is more difficult and high doses of valproate (from 50 mg/kg up to 80 mg/kg) are sometimes necessary. A combination of sodium valproate and ethosuximide may prove effective in cases for which either drug in isolation has failed to control the seizures.

The benzodiazepines, especially clonazepam and clobazam, are often very effective. However, the side-effects of clonazepam are often difficult to tolerate, so clobazam may be preferred. In difficult cases, a combination of clobazam and sodium valproate is often helpful.

Second-line drugs include acetazolamide, primidone (Doose, 1992), methosuximide (Tennyson, Greenwood and Miles, 1991), and sulthiame. Lamotrigine seems to be effective against many types of generalized seizures and may well become a major drug in the treatment of resistant forms, but more experience is required.

The treatment of episodes of nonconvulsive status epilepticus poses special problems. Intravenous benzodiazepines (diazepam or clonazepam) are often efficacious, although in some cases they may precipitate tonic status (Tassinari *et al.*, 1972; Bittencourt and Richens, 1981). For long-lasting periods of intense paroxysmal activity, the use of ACTH or corticosteroids can be considered (Doose, 1992).

The duration of treatment needs to be long as recurrences are common. In my own series, discontinuation of treatment was successful in approximately one-third of patients after a 4–5-year period.

REFERENCES

Aicardi, J. (1986) *Epilepsy in Children*, Raven Press, New York.

Aicardi, J. (1994) *Epilepsy in Children*, 2nd edn. Raven Press, New York.

Aicardi, J. and Chevrie, J.J. (1971) Myoclonic epilepsies of childhood. *Neuropädiatrie*, **3**, 177–90.

Aicardi, J. and Levy Gomes, A. (1989) The myoclonic epilepsies of childhood. *Cleveland Clinic Journal of Medicine*, **59**, S9–34.

Bennett, H.M., Selman, J.E., Rapin, I. and Rose, A. (1982) Nonconvulsive epileptiform activity appearing as ataxia. *American Journal of Diseases of Children*, **136**, 30–2.

Berkovic, S.F., Cochins, J., Andermann, E. and Andermann, F. (1993) Progressive myoclonus epilepsies: clinical and genetic aspects. *Epilepsia*, **34** (suppl. 3), S19–30.

Bittencourt, P.R.M. and Richens, A. (1981) Anticonvulsant-induced status epilepticus in Lennox–Gastaut syndrome. *Epilepsia*, **22**, 129–34.

Brett, E. M. (1966) Minor epileptic status. *Journal of the Neurological Sciences*, **3**, 52–75.

Commission on Classification and Terminology of the International League Against Epilepsy (1989) Proposal for revised classification of epilepsy and epileptic syndromes. *Epilepsia*, **30**, 389–99.

Dalla Bernardina, B., Capovilla, G., Gattoni, M.B.

et al. (1982) Epilepsie myoclonique grave de la première année. *Revue d'Electroencéphalographie et de Neurophysiologie Clinique*, **12**, 21–5.

Doose, H., Gerken, H. and Leonhardt, R. *et al.* (1970). Centrencephalic myoclonic-atastic petit mal. *Neuropädiatrie*, **2**, 59–78.

Doose, H. (1992) Myoclonic-astatic epilepsy of early childhood, in *Epileptic Syndromes in Infancy, Childhood and Adolescence*, (eds J. Roger, M. Bureau, C. Dravet *et al.*), John Libbey, London, pp. 103–14.

Doose, H. and Baier, W.K. (1987) Epilepsy with primarily generalized myoclonic-astatic seizures: a genetically determined disease. *European Journal of Pediatrics*, **146**, 550–4.

Doose, H. and Baier, W.K. (1988) Theta rhythms in the EEG – a genetic trait. *Brain and Development*, **10**, 347–54.

Doose, H. and Völzke, E. (1979) Petit mal status in early childhood and dementia. *Neuropädiatrie*, **10**, 10–14.

Dravet, C. (1992) Myoclonic-astatic epilepsy, in *Marseille Meeting on Myoclonic Epilepsies*, Marseille, June 1992.

Dravet, C., Bureau, M., Guerrini, R. *et al.* (1992) Severe myoclonic epilepsy in infants, in *Epileptic Syndromes in Infancy, Childhood and Adolescence* (eds J. Roger *et al.*), Raven Press, New York, pp. 75–88.

Dravet, C., Bureau, M. and Roger, J. (1992). Benign myoclonic epilepsy in infants, in *Epileptic Syndromes in Infancy, Childhood and Adolescence*, (eds J. Roger, M. Bureau, C. Dravet *et al.*), John Libbey, London, pp. 67–74.

Dravet, C., Natale, O., Magaudda, A. *et al.* (1985) Les états de mal dans le syndrome de Lennox–Gastaut. *Revue d'Electroencéphalographie et de Neurophysiologie Clinique*, **15**, 361–8.

Dravet, C., Roger, J., Bureau, M. and Dalla Bernardina, B. (1982) Myoclonic epilepsies in childhood, in *Advances in Epileptology: XIIIth Epilepsy Intenational Symposium* (eds A. Akimoto, A. Kazamatsuri, M. Seino and A. Ward), Raven Press, New York, pp. 135–40.

Dulac, O. (1992) Myoclonic-astatic epilepsy, in *Marseilles Meeting on Myoclonic Epilepsies in Children*, Marseille, June 1992.

Gastaut, H., Bughton, R., Roger, J. and Tassinari, C.A. (1974) Generalized convulsive seizures without local onset, in *Handbook of Clinical Neurology*, vol. 15. *The Epilepsies* (eds P.J. Vinken and G.W. Bruyn), Elsevier, Amsterdam, p. 107–29.

Giovanardi Rossi, P., Gobbi, G., Melideo, A. *et al.* (1988) Myoclonic manifestations in the Lennox–Gastaut syndrome and other childhood epilepsies, in *The Lennox–Gastaut Syndrome* (eds E. Niedermeyer and R. Degen), Alan Liss, New York, pp. 137–58.

Guerrini, R., Dravet, C., Genton, P. *et al.* (1993) Epileptic negative myoclonus. *Neurology*, **43**, 1078–83.

Gundel, A., Baier, W. and Doose, H. (1981) Spectral analysis of EEG in the late course of primary generalized myoclonic-astatic epilepsy. II. Cluster analysis of the power spectrum. *Neuropediatrics*, **12**, 110–8.

Kruse, R. (1968) *Das Myoklonisch-astatische Petit Mal*, Springer, Berlin.

Lugaresi, E., Pazzaglia, P., Franck, L. *et al.* (1973) Evolution and prognosis of primary generalized epilepsies of the petit mal absence type, in *Evolution and Prognosis of Epilepsies* (eds E. Lugaresi *et al.*), Aulo Gaggi, Bologna, pp. 3–22.

Marciani, M.G., Maschio, M., Spaneda, F. *et al.* (1995) Development of myoclonus in patients with partial epilepsy during treatment with vigabatrin: an electroencephalographic study. *Acta neurologica Scandinavica*, **91**, 1–5.

Oguni, H., Fukuyama, Y., Imaizumi, Y. and Uehara, T. (1992) Video-EEG analysis of drop-seizures in myoclonic-astatic epilepsy of early childhood (Doose syndrome). *Epilepsia*, **33**, 805–13.

Roger, J., Dravet, C. and Bureau, M. (1989) The Lennox–Gastaut syndrome. *Cleveland Clinic Journal of Medicine*, **56** (suppl.), S172–80.

Shewmon, D.A. and Erwin, R.J. (1988) Focal spike-induced cerebral dysfunction is related to the after-coming slow wave. *Annals of Neurology*, **23**, 131–7.

Snead, O.C. and Hosey, L.C. (1985) Exacerbation of seizures in children by carbamazepine. *New England Journal of Medicine*, **313**, 916–21.

Tassinari, C.A., Dravet, C., Roger, J. *et al.* (1972) Tonic status epilepticus precipitated by intravenous benzodiazepines in five patients with Lennox–Gastaut syndrome. *Epilepsia*, **13**, 431–5.

Tassinari, C.A., Lyagoubi, S., Gambarelli, F. *et al.* (1971) Relationships between EEG discharges and neuromuscular phenomena. *Electroencephalography and Clinical Neurophysiology*, **31**, 176.

Tennyson, M.B., Greenwood, R.S. and Miles, M.V. (1991) Methosuximide for intractable childhood seizures. *Pediatrics*, **87**, 186–9.

MYOCLONIC EPILEPSIES DIFFICULT TO CLASSIFY AS EITHER LENNOX–GASTAUT SYNDROME OR MYOCLONIC-ASTATIC EPILEPSY

Jean Aicardi

Classification of the epilepsies with myoclonic attacks and other brief seizures is a very difficult task. Dravet *et al.* (1982) left 34 of their 142 cases unclassified. Lombroso (1990) did not even think it possible to isolate the syndrome of severe myoclonic epilepsy, a distinction accepted by most other authors.

The separation of such cases from the LGS is relatively easy in typical cases but may be difficult in atypical forms. Two main characteristics are generally thought to separate LGS from the myoclonic epilepsies proper:

1. The presence and prominence of tonic seizures.
2. The predominance of interictal slow spike-wave complexes.

However, these features are not pathognomonic. A few tonic seizures may be observed in children with severe myoclonic epilepsy (Dravet *et al.*, 1992) or MAE (Doose, 1992). The EEG of some LGS patients can include a significant proportion of fast (≥ 2.5 Hz) spike-wave complexes (Gastaut *et al.*, 1973; Aicardi 1986; Blume, 1988). Conversely slow spike-waves may occur in occasional children with myoclonic epilepsies (Aicardi, 1982; Roger, Dravet and Bureau, 1989), and the 'accept-able' proportions of atypical clinical and/or EEG features in an individual case are obviously arbitrary. Such a difficulty is apparent in the case of the so-called myoclonic variant of the LGS (see Chapter 12a) which, for all practical purposes, is impossible to distinguish from MAE. In both MAE and the myoclonic variant of LGS myoclonic seizures are a prominent feature whilst tonic seizures are few and occur only during sleep (Dravet, 1992). In both cases, spike-wave complexes may be of either the fast or the slow variety and most cases are of cryptogenic origin, with a similar outcome (Aicardi and Chevrie, 1971). Therefore, there is no reason to maintain the myoclonic variant of LGS as a separate category.

It seems also that the cases of myoclonic epilepsy with other types of brief seizures reported by Aicardi and Levy Gomes (1989) may represent one aspect of MAE. Among the 10 patients described, eight had fast and two had slow spike-wave complexes in their EEGs. The outcome was less favorable than that of cases with only myoclonic seizures. Ninety per cent had learning or behavioral difficulties, 50% were retarded, and only 20% became seizure-free. Such cases can be

Epilepsy in Children. Edited by Sheila Wallace. Published in 1996 by Chapman & Hall, London. ISBN 0 412 56860 8

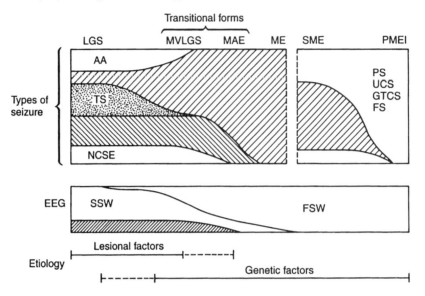

Fig. 12c.1 The spectrum of the Lennox–Gastaut syndrome and the myoclonic epilepsies. The left end of the spectrum is represented by the Lennox–Gastaut syndrome (LGS), with multiple seizure types including tonic and astatic seizures, slow spike-waves on EEG and predominantly lesional causes. The right end shows that the myoclonic epilepsies proper do not feature astatic or tonic seizures, are associated with fast spike-waves and are mainly genetically determined. Severe myoclonic epilepsy (or polymorphic epilepsy of infancy) is shown separated from the rest of the spectrum (vertical broken lines) to indicate that its clinical presentation is distinct, with onset by tonic-clonic usually febrile convulsions that may be the predominant type of attacks, even though it is closely related etiologically to other myoclonic epilepsies. ▨▨ = Myoclonic seizures; ▨▨ = continuous spike-waves of slow sleep; ◪◪ = astatic seizures; ▥▥ = tonic seizures. MVLGS = myoclonic variant of Lennox–Gastaut syndrome; MAE = myoclonic astatic epilepsy; ME = myoclonic epilepsy; SME = severe myoclonic epilepsy; PMEI = polymorphic epilepsy of infancy; AA = atypical absences; TS = tonic seizures; NCSE = nonconvulsive status epilepticus; PS = partial seizures; UCS = unclassified seizures; GTCS = generalized tonic-clonic seizures; FS = febrile seizures; SSW = slow spike-wave; FSW = fast spike-wave.

regarded as truly intermediate between LGS and the more benign cases of myoclonic epilepsy, but could also be attributed to the myoclonic variant of the LGS or to MAE and this may also be the case for the patients reported by Dulac (1992). Indeed, the proportion of various features among individual patients varies from case to case, creating a spectrum of conditions with all intermediary types between the LGS and the 'pure' myoclonic or myo-atonic epilepsies as illustrated in Fig. 12c.1. Only the more typical syndromes are reasonably well defined, but many patients are impossible to include in a definite category.

REFERENCES

Aicardi, J. (1982) Childhood epilepsies with brief myoclonic, atonic or clonic seizures, in *A Textbook of Epilepsy* (eds J. Laidlaw and A. Richens), Churchill Livingstone, Edinburgh.

Aicardi, J. (1986) *Epilepsy in Children*, Raven Press, New York.

Aicardi, J. and Chevrie, J.J. (1982) Myoclonic epilepsies of childhood. *Neuropädiatrie*, **3**, 177–90.

Aicardi, J. and Levy Gomes, A. (1989) The myoclonic epilepsies of childhood. *Cleveland Clinic Journal of Medicine*, **59**, S9–34.

Blume, W.T. (1988) Anticonvulsant-induced status epilepticus in Lennox–Gastaut syndrome. *Epilepsia*, **22**, 129–34.

Doose, H. (1992) Myoclonic-astatic epilepsy of

early childhood, in *Epileptic Syndromes in Infancy, Childhood and Adolescence* (eds J. Roger, M. Bureau, C. Dravet *et al.*), John Libbey, London, pp. 103–14.

Dravet, C. (1992) Myoclonic-astatic epilepsy, in *Marseille Meeting on Myoclonic Epilepsies*, Marseille, June 1992.

Dravet, C., Bureau, M., Guerrini, R. *et al.* (1992) Severe myoclonic epilepsy in infants, in *Epileptic Syndromes in Infancy, Childhood and Adolescence* (eds J. Roger *et al.*), Raven Press, New York, pp. 75–88.

Dravet, C., Roger, J., Bureau, M. *et al.* (1982) Myoclonic epilepsies in childhood, in *Advances in Epileptology: XIIIth Epilepsy International Symposium* (eds A. Akimoto, A. Kazamatsuri, M. Seino and A. Ward), Raven Press, New York, pp. 135–40.

Dulac. O. (1992) Myoclonic-astatic epilepsy, in *Marseilles Meeting on Myoclonic Epilepsies in Children*, Marseille, June 1992.

Gastaut, H., Dravet, C., Loubier, D. *et al.* (1973) Evolution clinique et pronostic du syndrome de Lennox–Gastaut, in *Evolution and Prognosis of Epilepsies* (eds E. Lugaresi, P. Pazzaglia and C.A. Tassinari), Aulo Gaggi, Bologna, pp. 133–54.

Lombroso, C.T. (1990) Early myoclonic encephalopathy, early infantile epileptic encephalopathy, and benign and severe infantile myoclonic epilepsies: a critical review and personal contribution. *Journal of Clinical Neurophysiology*, **7**, 380–408.

Roger, J., Dravet, C. and Bureau, M. (1989) The Lennox–Gastaut syndrome. *Cleveland Clinic Journal of Medicine*, **56**(suppl.), S172–80.

EPILEPTIC SYNDROMES WITH ONSET IN MIDDLE CHILDHOOD

13

CHILDHOOD ABSENCE EPILEPSY

Roberto Michelucci and Carlo Alberto Tassinari

INTRODUCTION

Childhood absence epilepsy (CAE), otherwise known as pyknolepsy (Sauer, 1916; Adie, 1924) or Friedmann's syndrome (Friedmann, 1906), is an age-dependent, idiopathic form of generalized epilepsy (Commission on Classification and Terminology of the International League Against Epilepsy, 1989), characterized by the following features (Dreifuss, 1990; Loiseau, 1992; Porter, 1993):

1. A strong family history of similar seizures.
2. Onset before puberty in previously normal children.
3. Female preponderance.
4. Absence seizures (AS) as the initial and predominant seizure type.
5. High recurrence of AS (several to many per day) of any kind except myoclonic absences.
6. Ictal EEG pattern with a bilateral, symmetric, and synchronous discharge of regular 3-Hz spike-waves (SW) on a normal background activity (Fig. 13a.1).
7. Frequent development of grand mal tonic-clonic seizures (GTCS) during adolescence.
8. Good response to treatment and good prognosis.

As defined above, CAE represents the paradigm of idiopathic generalized epilepsy. AS, however, may be the symptom of a variety of generalized epilepsies and a multiplicity of conditions have commonly been referred to as 'petit mal' in the past, leading to confusion and misunderstanding of their prognostic significance.

CLINICAL DATA

GENERAL

CAE represents 8% of epilepsy in school-age children (Cavazzuti, 1980), whereas its annual incidence has been estimated at 6.3/100 000 (Loiseau *et al.*, 1990) to 8.0/100 000 (Blom, Heijbel and Bergfors, 1978) children aged 0–15 years.

There is a female preponderance. Sixty to 76% of affected children are girls.

A positive family history of epilepsy is reported in 15 (Lugaresi *et al.*, 1973) to 44% (Currier, Kooi and Saidman, 1963) of children with AS. These seizures in parents and relatives are absences or tonic-clonic seizures, whereas febrile seizures are frequent in the siblings of children with CAE. On the other hand, the risk of epilepsy in the offspring of subjects having had CAE has been estimated at 6–8% (Beck Mannagetta *et al.*, 1989). Overall, there is a great deal of evidence for a genetic predisposition to CAE, but the nature of this genetic abnormality remains unknown (see Chapter 8). An autosomal dominant monogenic mode of inheritance (Metrakos and Metrakos, 1972), polygenic factors (Doose *et al.*, 1973), or a combination of both genetic and environmental factors (Berkovic *et al.*, 1987) have been suggested to explain the inheritance of CAE.

In recent years, the chromosomal localiza-

Epilepsy in Children. Edited by Sheila Wallace. Published in 1996 by Chapman & Hall, London. ISBN 0 412 56860 8

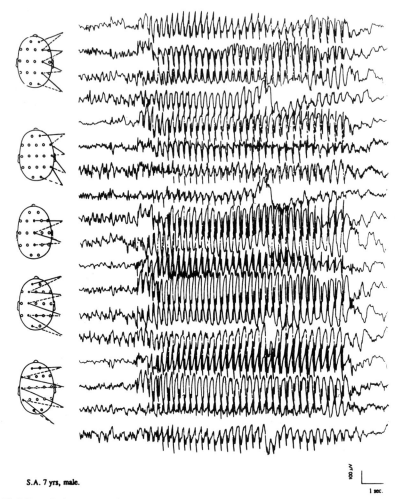

S.A. 7 yrs, male.

Fig. 13a.1   Childhood absence epilepsy: a typical simple absence seizure. The generalized SW have the highest amplitude under the frontocentral leads. The frequency of the discharge is faster, about 4 Hz, at the onset and slows to 2.5–3 c/s towards the end of the absence seizure.

tion of some genetic epilepsies has been identified with use of molecular genetics techniques: these entities include juvenile myoclonic epilepsy (Chapter 14b) (Greenberg *et al.*, 1988), benign familial neonatal convulsions (Chapter 9) (Leppert *et al.*, 1989) and progressive myoclonus epilepsy of the Unverricht–Lundborg type (Chapter 15a) (Lehesjoki *et al.*, 1991; Malafosse *et al.*, 1992; Tassinari *et al.*, 1992).

CAE is also likely to be successfully mapped in the near future (Delgado-Escueta *et al.*, 1990; Whitehouse, Curtis and Gardiner, 1990; Treiman, 1993), due to its relative frequency and inheritance pattern. The age of onset of CAE ranges between 3 and 12 years, with a peak around 6–7 years.

ABSENCE SEIZURES

The uncontested essence of an absence attack consists of a loss of awareness and responsive-

Table 13a.1 Classification of absence seizures in childhood absence epilepsy

Simple
Impairment of consciousness only
Complex
With mild clonic components (usually eyelids)
With 'tonic' components (usually arching of the back)
With 'atonic' components (usually head nodding)
With automatisms (perseverative or de novo)
With autonomic components
Absence continuing (absence status or spike wave stupor)

Modified from Commission on Classification and Terminology of the International League Against Epilepsy (1981), Dreifuss (1990) and Porter (1993).

ness with cessation of on-going activities. Different degrees of decrease in consciousness have been described, but a complete abolition of awareness, responsiveness and memory is usual in seizures of CAE.

Classic studies with intensive video-EEG monitoring (Penry, Porter and Dreifuss, 1975; Drury and Dreifuss, 1985; Holmes, McKeever and Adamson, 1987; Panayiotopoulos, Obeid and Waheed, 1989a) have demonstrated that loss of consciousness represents the only clinical finding (**simple** absence) in less than 10% of AS. More frequently, there is a variety of associated clinical features (clonic, tonic, atonic, vegetative components, or automatisms) (Table 13a.1). Mild **clonic** components exist in approximately one-half of the cases, and consist of eye blinking (at a rhythm of 3 Hz) or, less often, facial twitching. In some attacks there may be an increase in postural tone with **tonic** muscular contraction, usually limited to the eyes (which rotate upwards) or the head (which draws backwards). Decrease in postural tone may also occur, resulting in a gradual lowering of the head and/or arms. The **atonic** components rarely cause the patient to fall.

Automatisms are frequently seen during AS (60%): they may be either perseverative (the patient persists in what he is doing) or *de*

novo, with simple or complex movements. Automatisms are related to the duration of seizures, since their frequency increases with increasing seizure duration (Penry and Dreifuss, 1969). **Autonomic** or **vegetative** phenomena may be seen, including pupil dilatation, color change, piloerection, tachycardia, urinary incontinence, and salivation.

Interestingly, in many cases several components are noted during a given AS and several types of AS may be present in the same patient. AS are characterized by a short duration (5–30 seconds in most cases) and abrupt onset and termination. AS recur at a high frequency (10–100 per day), being often precipitated by emotional, intellectual, or metabolic (e.g. hyperventilation) factors, or occurring at particular times of day. However, the true frequency of AS is usually difficult to estimate because of the short duration of the attacks. Therefore, prolonged EEG recordings are sometimes needed to assess seizure frequency and to evaluate the efficacy of therapy.

Episodes of AS status (also known as spike-wave stupor or petit mal status) are relatively rare in CAE (10–16% of the cases) (Porter and Penry, 1983).

NEUROPHYSIOLOGIC DATA

INTERICTAL EEG

The interictal background EEG activity is usually normal. Interictal paroxysmal activity consists of single or brief discharges of generalized SW at 3 Hz, occurring either spontaneously or during hyperventilation. These paroxysms are found in almost all children with active CAE. If repeated EEG recordings with hyperventilation fail to show generalized discharges or clinical AS, the diagnosis of CAE must be questioned. The interictal SW discharges are also numerous during non REM sleep; however the bursts have a modified appearance in sleep, as they are briefer, irregular and slow to 1.5–2.5 Hz

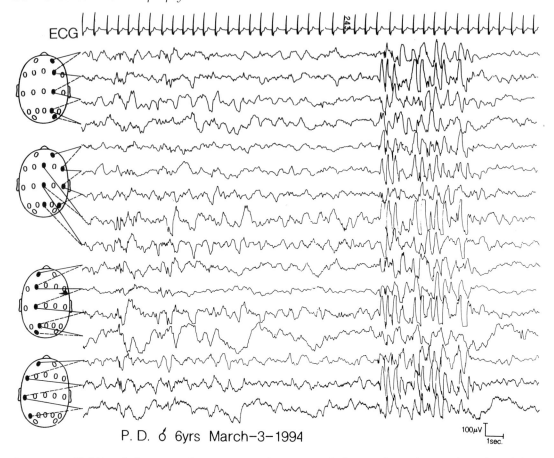

ECG

P. D. ♂ 6yrs March-3-1994

100μV
1sec.

Fig. 13a.2　Childhood absence epilepsy: interictal paroxysmal abnormalities during slow sleep (phase 3). The discharges are briefer, slower and more irregular when compared to wakefulness.

(Sato, Dreifuss and Penry, 1973) (Fig. 13a.2) Some children exhibit a particular posterior delta rhythm, i.e. long bursts of high sinusoidal activity at 3 Hz, symmetric or asymmetric from the occipito-parietal areas, blocked by eye opening and enhanced by hyperventilation (Cobb *et al.*, 1961) (Fig. 13a.3). The interictal paroxysmal abnormalities in CAE are 'generalized' by definition. However, because of the known link existing between CAE and benign epilepsy of childhood with centrotemporal (rolandic) spikes (Beaumanoir *et al.*, 1974, Chapter 13c), unilateral 'central' or 'midtemporal' SW may be observed (Fig. 13a.4). In some patients, isolated interictal fast spikes and waves either predominate

over or occasionally involve one or both frontal regions; this occurs particularly during sleep (Gastaut *et al.*, 1974; Gomez and Westmoreland, 1987).

ICTAL EEG

The ictal EEG consists of rhythmic SW discharge at 3 Hz, bilateral, synchronous and symmetric, with the highest amplitude under the frontocentral leads (Gomez and Westmoreland, 1987) (Figs 13a.1, 13a.3). The onset of the discharge is abrupt, whereas termination is less sudden. The frequency tends to be faster, about 4 Hz, at the onset and slows to 2.5–2 Hz towards the end of the discharge.

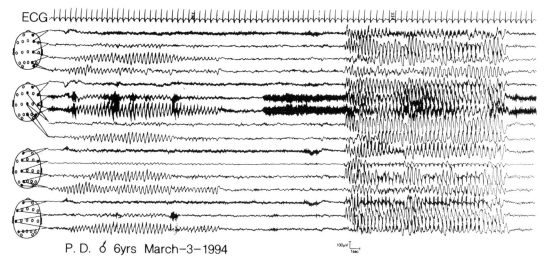

ECG

P. D. ♂ 6yrs March-3-1994

100µV ⌐
└ 1sec

Fig. 13a.3 Same patient as in Fig. 13a.2. On the left: long bursts of high sinusoidal activity at 3 Hz over both occipitoparietal areas. On the right: typical absence seizure.

More irregular SW discharges (polyspike-waves, changing rhythm within a discharge) are compatible with a diagnosis of CAE (Livingston *et al.*, 1965).

CT mapping of AS shows a maximum positivity as well as negativity of the individual SW complexes over both frontal areas (Rodin and Ancheta, 1987) (Fig. 13a.5).

In CAE, the distinction between 'ictal' and 'interictal' EEG paroxysms is sometimes difficult. Indeed, isolated SW discharges are usually interictal and subclinical phenomena. However they may also be ictal and give rise to a brief lapse of consciousness (micro-absence) or transient autonomic phenomena (pupillary hippus, an electrodermal response, etc.) (Gastaut *et al.*, 1974). Sophisticated testing in the form of both continuous performance tasks and response testing indicates impairment even with short paroxysms (less than 3 seconds in duration) (Dreifuss, 1990).

EVOLUTION

Once an adequate antiepileptic treatment is instituted, AS disappear in about 80% of patients. (Livingston *et al.*, 1965; Dalby, 1969;

Sato, Deifuss and Penry, 1976; Sato *et al.*, 1983). AS may cease soon after the onset of therapy or persist for a time, so that a complete resolution of CAE may occur at all ages, and not just at puberty. In a minority of patients (about 6%), AS are refractory to treatment and continue during adulthood, although at a lower frequency (Currier, Kooi and Saidman, 1963).

Whatever the evolution (disappearance or persistence) of AS, GTCS develop in about 40% of patients with CAE (Currier, Kooi and Saidman, 1963; Livingston *et al.*, 1965). GTCS usually begin between 10 and 15 years of age, occur at a low frequency and are easily controlled by treatment. Predisposing features for GTCS would be a late onset (after 8 years) of AS, male patients, a poor response of AS to initial treatment, incorrect therapy, abnormal background activity and photosensitivity (Loiseau, 1992).

Although CAE mostly occurs in neurologically and intellectually normal children, some degree of mental subnormality, mild IQ decrease and behavioral problems may develop during the evolution in about one-third

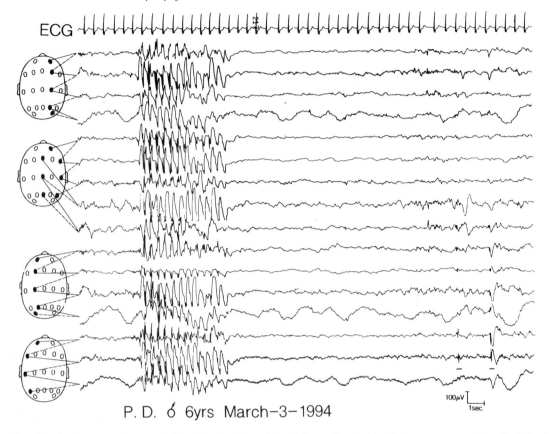

Fig. 13a.4 Same patient as in Fig. 13a.2. Slow sleep (phase 2). On the left: an apparently subclinical discharge of SW at 3 Hz. On the right: left focal 'temporal' spikes and SW.

of cases (Loiseau *et al.*, 1983). Such problems are likely to be due to a variety of reasons (antiepileptic therapy, frequency of AS, parents' attitude, etc.).

DIAGNOSIS

A great deal of confusion and misunderstanding arose in the past from the fact that all epilepsies with AS were called petit mal. Only in the past few years has progress been made in classifying the epileptic syndromes (Commission on Classification and Terminology of the International League Against Epilepsy, 1989), and a number of conditions, featuring AS as a prominent seizure type, have been recognized as distinct clinical

entities. Therefore, CAE should be differentiated from the following disorders:

Juvenile absence epilepsy (Wolf, 1992) (Chapter 14a), in which AS begin during adolescence and occur at a lower frequency.

Epilepsy with myoclonic absences (Tassinari, Bureau and Thomas, 1992; Manonmani and Wallace, 1994) (Chapter 13b), in which AS are accompanied by rhythmic jerks of the proximal muscles of the upper limbs and are usually resistant to treatment.

Juvenile myoclonic epilepsy (Chapter 14b), in which AS occur in 10–38% of cases and usually begin 1–9 years prior to the onset of myoclonic jerks and GTCS. AS heralding juvenile myoclonic epilepsy are less frequent and briefer than in CAE and are probably

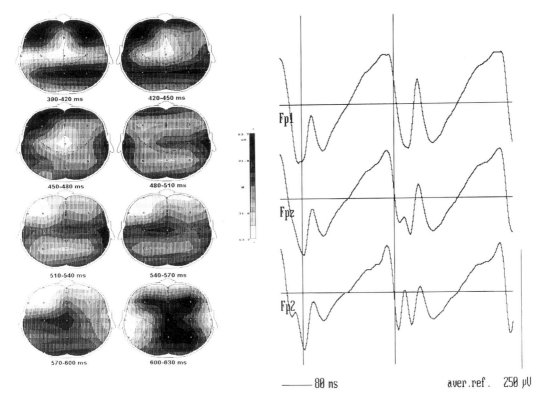

Fig. 13a.5 Same patient as in Fig. 13a.1. On the left, integrated maps, in 30-ms increments, of the spike-wave complex delineated by the vertical cursors, shown on the right of the figure. The positive transient (from 390 to 480 ms), preceding the spike, as well as the maximum negativity, represented by the slow wave (from 510 to 600 ms), are distributed over the frontopolar and frontal regions, with left predominance. (Courtesy of Dr G. Rubboli, Bologna.)

accompanied by a different EEG pattern (Panayiotopoulos, Obeid and Waheed, 1989b).

Other forms of idiopathic generalized epilepsy, in which AS show distinct features: eyelid myoclonia (Jeavons 1977; Appleton *et al.*, 1993), onset during the first year of life (Cavazzuti *et al.*, 1989), or occurrence after 'initial grand mal' (Dieterich *et al.*, 1985).

Symptomatic or cryptogenic generalized epilepsies (such as Lennox–Gastaut syndrome, Chapter 12a), in which AS are 'atypical' in that they are associated with slow (at 1.5–2.5 Hz), irregular or asymmetric SW discharges. Moreover, atypical AS are characterized by a less abrupt onset or cessation, more pronounced changes in tone, and longer duration than the typical AS occurring in CAE (Commission on Classification and Terminology of the International League Against Epilepsy, 1981). AS have been also reported in progressive encephalopathies, such as lipidosis (Andermann, 1967) and progressive myoclonus epilepsies (Roger *et al.*, 1992, Chapter 15a).

Partial epilepsies of frontal origin (Chapter 7) in which more or less regular bilateral SW discharges may arise from frontal foci. At least for a time frontal epilepsies may give rise to apparently similar 'AS', admittedly of a focal nature. In these cases, a focal motor component, asymmetric ictal discharges or an interictal focus may be the clue to a correct diagnosis. Head trauma and brain tumors (Loiseau and Cohadon, 1971) have been reported to be possible causes of AS of frontal origin.

TREATMENT

Traditionally, antiabsence drugs include valproic acid and ethosuximide. Although either drug alone may be used as the initial treatment, valproic acid is usually considered the drug of first choice. The rationale for preferring valproic acid is mainly due to the fact that this drug is also effective against GTCS, whereas ethosuximide is not.

When valproic acid does not control AS, ethosuximide alone is the drug of second choice. Sometimes a combination of valproic acid plus ethosuximide is needed to obtain seizure control. Clonazepam and clobazam are also effective against AS, but display frequent side-effects and tolerance develops in one-half of the cases. Lamotrigine, particularly in association with valproate, shows promise (Ferrie *et al.*, 1993). Benzodiazepines – either i.v. or orally – are the first-line drugs for the treatment of 'absence status' (Tassinari *et al.*, 1983).

REFERENCES

Adie, W.J. (1924) Pyknolepsy: a form of epilepsy occurring in children, with a good prognosis. *Brain*, **47**, 96–102.

Andermann, F. (1967) Absence attacks and diffuse neuronal disease. *Neurology*, **17**, 205–12.

Appleton, R.E., Panayiotopoulos, C.P., Acomb, B.A. and Beirne, M. (1993) Eyelid myoclonia with typical absences: an epilepsy syndrome. *Journal of Neurology, Neurosurgery and Psychiatry*, **56**, 1312–16.

Beaumanoir, A., Ballis, T., Warfis, G. and Ansari, K. (1974) Benign epilepsy of childhood with rolandic spikes. *Epilepsia*, **15**, 301–15.

Beck-Mannagetta, G., Janz, D., Hoffmeister, G. *et al.* (1989) Morbidity risk for seizures and epilepsy in offspring of patients with epilepsy, in *Genetics of the Epilepsies* (eds G. Beck-Mannagetta, V.E. Anderson, H. Doose and D. Janz), Springer-Verlag, Berlin, pp. 119–26.

Berkovic, S.F., Andermann, F., Andermann, E. and Gloor, P. (1987) Concepts of absence epilepsies: discrete syndromes or biological continuum? *Neurology*, **37**, 993–1000.

Blom, S., Heijbel, J. and Bergfors, P.G. (1978) Incidence of epilepsy in children: a follow-up study three years after the first seizure. *Epilepsia*, **19**, 343–50.

Cavazzuti, G.B. (1980) Epidemiology of different types of epilepsy in school-age children of Modena, Italy. *Epilepsia*, **21**, 57–62.

Cavazzuti, G.B., Ferrari, F., Galli, V. and Benatti, A. (1989) Epilepsy with typical absence seizures with onset during the first year of life. *Epilepsia*, **30**, 802–6.

Cobb, W.A., Gordon, N., Matthews, C. and Nieman, E.A. (1961) The occipital delta rhythm in petit mal. *Electroencephalography and Clinical Neurophysiology*, **13**, 142–3.

Commission on Classification and Terminology of the International League Against Epilepsy (1981) Proposal for revised clinical and electroencephalographic classification of epileptic seizures. *Epilepsia*, **22**, 489–501.

Commission on Classification and Terminology of the International League Against Epilepsy (1989) Proposal for revised classification of epilepsies and epileptic syndromes. *Epilepsia*, **30**, 389–99.

Currier, R.D., Kooi, K.A. and Saidman, L.J. (1963) Prognosis of pure petit mal: a follow-up study. *Neurology*, **13**, 959–67.

Dalby, M.A. (1969) Epilepsy and 3 per second spike and wave rhythms. A clinical, electroencephalographic and prognostic analysis of 346 patients. *Acta Neurologica Scandinavica*, **45**(suppl.), 1–83.

Delgado-Escueta, A.V., Greenberg, D., Weissbecker, K. *et al.* (1990) Gene mapping in the idiopathic generalized epilepsies: juvenile myoclonic epilepsy, childhood absence epilepsy, epilepsy with grand mal seizures, and early childhood absence epilepsy. *Epilepsia*, **31**(suppl.3), S19–29.

Dieterich, E., Doose, H., Baier, W.K. and Fichsel, H. (1985) Longterm follow-up of childhood epilepsy with absences. II: absence-epilepsy with initial grand mal. *Neuropediatrics*, **16**, 155–8.

Doose, H., Gerken, H., Horstmann, T. and Volzke, E. (1973) Genetic factors in spike wave absences. *Epilepsia*, **14**, 57–75.

Dreifuss, F.E. (1990) Absence epilepsies, in *Com-*

prehensive Epileptology (eds M. Dam and L. Gram), Raven Press, New York, pp. 145–53.

Drury, I. and Dreifuss, F.E. (1985) Pyknoleptic petit mal. *Acta Neurologica Scandinavica*, **72**, 353–62.

Ferrie, C.D., Robinson, R.O., Panayiotopoulos, C.P. and Knott, C. (1993) Lamotrigine in typical absence seizures. *Neuropediatrics*, **24**, 172.

Friedmann, M. (1906) Uber die nichtepileptischen absencen oder kurzen narkolepileptischen anfalle. *Dtsch. Z. Nervenheilk.*, **30**, 462–92.

Gastaut, H., Broughton, R., Roger, J. and Tassinari, C.A. (1974) Generalized non-convulsive seizures, in *The Epilepsies, Handbook of Clinical Neurology* (eds O. Magnus and A. M. Lorentz De Haas), North-Holland Publishing Company, Amsterdam, pp. 130–44.

Gomez, M.R. and Westmoreland, B.F. (1987) Absence seizures, in *Clinical Medicine and the Nervous System: Epilepsy: Electroclinical Syndromes* (eds H. Luders and R.P. Lesser), Springer-Verlag, New York, pp. 105–29.

Greenberg, D.A., Delgado-Escueta, A.V., Widlitz, H. *et al.* (1988) Juvenile myoclonic epilepsy may be linked to the BF and HLA loci on human chromosome 6. *American Journal of Medical Genetics*, **31**, 185–92.

Holmes, G.L., McKeever, M. and Adamson, M. (1987) Absence seizures in children: clinical and electroencephalographic features. *Annals of Neurology*, **21**, 268–73.

Jeavons, P.M. (1977) Nosological problems of myoclonic epilepsies in childhood and adolescence. *Developmental Medicine and Child Neurology*, **19**, 3–8.

Lehesjoki, A.E., Koskiniemi, M., Sistonen, P. *et al.* (1991) Localization of a gene for progressive myoclonus epilepsy to chromosome 21q22. *Proceedings of the National Academy of Sciences USA*, **88**, 3696–9.

Leppert, M., Anderson, V.E., Quattlebaum, T. *et al.* (1989) Benign familial neonatal convulsions linked to genetic markers on chromosome 20. *Nature*, **337**, 647–8.

Livingston, S., Torres, I., Pauli, L.L. and Rider, R.V. (1965) Petit mal epilepsy. Results of prolonged follow-up study of 117 patients. *Journal of the American Medical Association*, **194**, 113–8.

Loiseau, P. (1992) Childhood absence epilepsy, in *Epileptic Syndromes in Infancy, Childhood and Adolescence*, 2nd edn (eds J. Roger, M. Bureau, Ch. Dravet *et al.*), John Libbey, London, pp. 135–50.

Loiseau, P. and Cohadon, F. (1971) *Le petit mal et ses frontieres*, Masson, Paris.

Loiseau, P., Pestre, M., Dartigues, J.F. *et al.* (1983) Long-term prognosis in two forms of childhood epilepsy: typical absence seizures and epilepsy with rolandic (centrotemporal) EEG foci. *Annals of Neurology*, **13**, 642–8.

Loiseau, J., Loiseau, P., Guyot, M. *et al.* (1990) Survey of seizure disorders in the French Southwest. I: incidence of epileptic syndromes. *Epilepsia*, **31**, 391–6.

Lugaresi, E., Pazzaglia, P., Franck, L. *et al.* (1973) Evolution and prognosis of primary generalized epilepsy of the petit mal absence type, in *Evolution and Prognosis of Epilepsy* (eds E. Lugaresi, P. Pazzaglia and C.A. Tassinari), Aulo Gaggi, Bologna, pp. 2–22.

Malafosse, A., Lehesjoki, A.E., Genton, P. *et al.* (1992) Identical genetic locus for Baltic and Mediterranean myoclonus. *Lancet*, **339**, 1080–1.

Manonmani, V. and Wallace, S. (1994) Epilepsy with myoclonic absences. *Archives of Disease in Childhood*, **70**, 288–90.

Metrakos, J.D. and Metrakos, K. (1972) Genetic factors in epilepsy, in *The Epidemiology of Epilepsy: A Workshop*, NINDS monograph no. 14, (eds R. Alter and W.A. Hauser), US Government Printing Office, Washington DC, pp. 97–102.

Panayiotopoulos, C.P., Obeid, T. and Waheed, G. (1989a) Differentiation of typical absence seizures in epileptic syndromes: a video EEG study of 224 seizures in 20 patients. *Brain*, **112**, 1039–56.

Panayiotopoulos, C.P., Obeid, T. and Waheed, G. (1989b) Absences in juvenile myoclonic epilepsy: a clinical and video-electroencephalographic study. *Annals of Neurology*, **25**, 391–7.

Penry, J.K. and Dreifuss, F.E. (1969) Automatisms associated with the absence petit mal epilepsy. *Archives of Neurology*, **21**, 142–8.

Penry, J.K., Porter, R.J. and Dreifuss, F.E. (1975) Simultaneous recording of absence seizures with video tape and electroencephalography. *Brain*, **98**, 427–40.

Porter, R.J. (1993) The absence epilepsies. *Epilepsia*, **34**(suppl. 3), S42–8.

Porter, R.J. and Penry, J.K. (1983) Petit mal status, in *Status Epilepticus: Mechanisms of Brain Damage and Treatment* (eds A.V. Delgado-Escueta, C.G. Wasterlain, D.M. Treiman and R.J. Porter), Raven Press, New York, pp. 61–7.

Rodin, E. and Ancheta, O. (1987) Cerebral electrical fields during petit mal absences. *Electroencephalography and Clinical Neurophysiology*, **66**, 457–66.

Roger, J., Genton, P., Bureau, M. and Dravet, Ch. (1992) Progressive myoclonus epilepsies in childhood and adolescence, in *Epileptic Syndromes in Infancy, Childhood and Adolescence*, 2nd edn (eds J. Roger, M. Bureau, Ch. Dravet *et al.*), John Libbey, London, pp. 381–400.

Sato, S., Dreifuss, F.E. and Penry, J.K. (1973) The effect of sleep on spike-wave discharges in absence seizures. *Neurology*, **23**, 1335–45.

Sato, S., Dreifuss, F.E. and Penry, J.K. (1976) Prognostic factors in absence seizures. *Neurology*, **26**, 788–96.

Sato, S., Dreifuss, F.E., Penry, J.K. *et al.* (1983) Long-term follow-up of absence seizures. *Neurology*, **33**, 1590–5.

Sauer, H. (1916) Uber gehaufte kleine anfalle bei kindern (Piknolepsie). *Monatsschrift für Psychiatric Neurology*, **40**, 276–300.

Tassinari, C.A., Daniele, O., Michelucci, R. *et al.* (1983) Benzodiazepines: efficacy in status epilepticus, in *Advances in Neurology: Status Epilepticus* (eds A.V. Delgado-Escueta, C.G. Wasterlain, D.M. Treiman and R.J. Porter), Raven Press, New York, pp. 465–75.

Tassinari, C.A., Bureau, M. and Thomas, P. (1992) Epilepsy with myoclonic absences, in *Epileptic Syndromes in Infancy, Childhood and Adolescence*, 2nd edn (eds J. Roger, M. Bureau, Ch. Dravet *et al.*), John Libbey, London, pp. 151–60.

Tassinari, C.A., Michelucci, R., Lehesjoki, A.E. *et al.* (1992) Ramsay Hunt syndrome (mediterranean myoclonus) and Unverricht–Lundborg syndrome (baltic myoclonus) map to the same genetic locus. *Italian Journal of Neurological Sciences* (suppl. 1), 117–9.

Treiman, L.J. (1993) Genetics of epilepsy: an overview. *Epilepsia*, **34** (Suppl. 3), S1–11.

Whitehouse, W.P., Curtis, D. and Gardiner, R.M. (1990) Linkage analysis with HLA-DQ A_1 and A_2 in juvenile myoclonic epilepsy and childhood absence epilepsy. *Acta Neurologica Scandinavica*, **133**, 12.

Wolf, P. (1992) Juvenile absence epilepsy, in *Epileptic Syndromes in Infancy, Childhood and Adolescence*, 2nd edn (eds J. Roger, M. Bureau, Ch. Dravet *et al.*), John Libbey, London, pp. 307–12.

EPILEPSY WITH MYOCLONIC ABSENCES

Carlo Alberto Tassinari, Guido Rubboli and Roberto Michelucci

INTRODUCTION

Epilepsy with myoclonic absences (MA) is characterized clinically by absences accompanied by rhythmic and bilateral myoclonic jerks of severe intensity. On polygraphic recording (EEG+ EMG of deltoid muscles), MA correspond to a rhythmic spike and wave (SW) discharge at 3 Hz, which is bilateral, synchronous and symmetric (as observed in typical absences) and associated with an EMG discharge of myoclonias at 3 Hz and an increasing tonic contraction (Fig. 13b.1).

Since the early description of MAs (Tassinari *et al.*, 1969; Lugaresi *et al.*, 1973; Tassinari and Bureau, 1985), it has been believed that an epileptic syndrome characterized by the presence of MA as the only or predominant seizure type could be identified and separated from other forms of generalized epilepsy, such as childhood absence epilepsy. Indeed MA were shown to be often associated with some degree of mental retardation and a clear-cut resistance to medical treatment, so that the prognosis was more severe than in idiopathic generalized epilepsy. This view was accepted by the Commission on Classification and Terminology of the International League against Epilepsy (ILAE) (1989), and epilepsy with MA was classified as a separate entity in the group of cryptogenic or symptomatic generalized epilepsies.

CLINICAL DATA

GENERAL

MA is a rare seizure type, accounting for 0.5–1% of the epilepsies observed in a selected population with epilepsy who attend the Centre St Paul, Marseilles.

There is a male preponderance (69%), at variance with the female preponderance in childhood absence epilepsy. Etiologic factors are absent, except for a genetic susceptibility, as demonstrated by a positive family history of epilepsies in about 20% of cases.

The mean age of onset of MA is 7 years, with a range between 11 months and 12.2 years.

MYOCLONIC ABSENCES

MA are characterized by:

Impairment of consciousness, which is quite variable in intensity, ranging from a mild disruption of contact to a complete loss of consciousness. Sometimes the patients are aware of the jerks and may recall the words pronounced by the examiner during the seizures.

Motor manifestations, which consist of bilateral myoclonic jerks, often associated with a discrete tonic contraction. The myoclonias mainly involve the muscles of shoulders, arms and legs. When facial myoclonias

Epilepsy in Children. Edited by Sheila Wallace. Published in 1996 by Chapman & Hall, London. ISBN 0 412 56860 8

occur, they are more evident around the chin and the mouth (Fig. 13b.2), whereas eyelid twitching is typically absent or rare. Due to concomitant tonic contraction, the jerking of the arms is accompanied by a progressive elevation of the upper extremities, giving rise to a quite constant and recognizable pattern. When the patient is standing, falling is uncommon. Head and body deviation can be a feature present in some patients.

Autonomic manifestations, which consist of an arrest of respiration and inconstant loss of urine.

MA last for 10–60 seconds, and recur at a high frequency (many seizures per day), being often precipitated by hyperventilation or awakening. MA may be also observed during the early stages of sleep.

Episodes of MA status are distinctly rare.

SEIZURES OTHER THAN MYOCLONIC ABSENCES

In about one-third of cases MA represent the only seizure type. In the remaining patients, other seizures occur either before the onset of MA or in association with MA. They consist

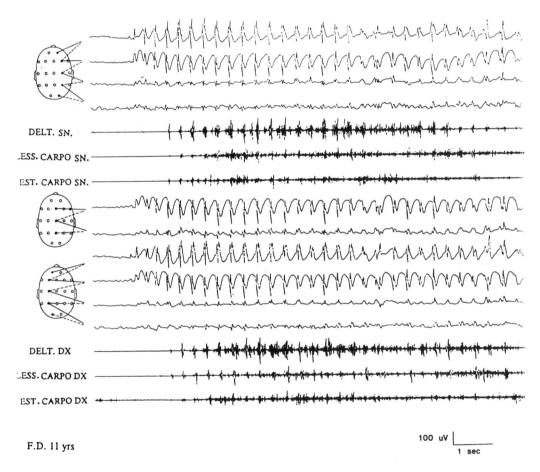

DELT. SN.

‑ESS. CARPO SN.

EST. CARPO SN.

DELT. DX

‑ESS. CARPO DX

EST. CARPO DX

F.D. 11 yrs

100 uV

1 sec

Fig. 13b.1 Spontaneous myoclonic absence. **EEG**: rhythmic SW discharge at 3 Hz, bilateral, synchronous and symmetrical, as observed in typical absences. **EMG**: rhythmic myoclonias, at the same frequency as the SW, which involve the upper extremities, begin 1 second after the onset of the EEG paroxysmal discharge and are progressively associated with a tonic contraction.

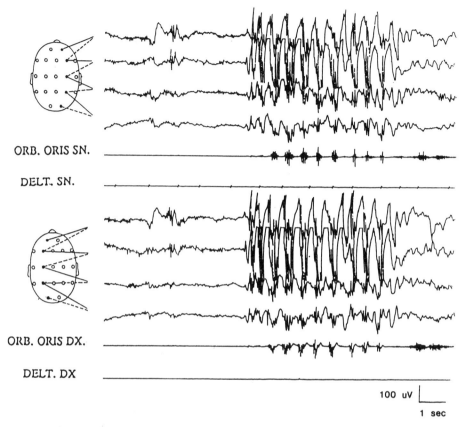

ORB. ORIS SN.

DELT. SN.

ORB. ORIS DX.

DELT. DX

100 uV

1 sec

B.D. 14 yrs

Fig. 13b.2 This patient had a past history of myoclonic absences in which myoclonias involved the upper extremities. At the time of our observation, he had only frequent and brief 'absences' associated with rhythmic twitching of the mouth and chin.

of rare generalized tonic-clonic seizures, absences, or epileptic falls.

NEUROLOGIC AND NEUROPSYCHOLOGIC EXAMINATION

Neurologic examination is normal in all cases. Mental retardation is present in about 45% of cases before the onset of MA. During the course of MA, mental retardation becomes apparent in a further 25% of cases, so that a total of 70% of patients present mental impairment at some time in the evolution of MA. These data constitute a very significant difference when compared with

the cognitive status observed in childhood absence epilepsy.

NEUROPHYSIOLOGIC DATA

INTERICTAL EEG

The interictal EEG shows a normal background activity in all cases, with superimposed generalized SW (in one-third of cases) or, more rarely, focal or multifocal SW.

ICTAL EEG

The ictal EEG consists of rhythmic SW discharges at 3 Hz, which are bilateral, synchronous, and symmetric, as observed in typical absences (Figs 13b.1, 13b.2). The onset and the end of SW are abrupt. Polygraphic (EMG) recording discloses the appearance of bilateral myoclonias, at the same frequency as the SW, which begin 1 second after the onset of EEG paroxysmal discharges and are followed by a tonic contraction, maximal in the shoulder and deltoid muscles (Fig. 13b.1). Tassinari *et al.* (1969, 1971) provided a detailed analysis of the relationships between the EEG SW and motor events by means of high-speed oscilloscopic recording. They found that there is a strict and constant relation between the spike of the SW discharge and the myoclonia. In the spike there is a component, a positive transient (Weir, 1965) of high amplitude, which is followed on the EMG by a myoclonia with a latency of 15–40 ms for the more proximal muscles and of 50–70 ms for the more distal muscles. This myoclonia is itself followed by a brief silent period (60–120 ms) which breaks the tonic contraction.

SLEEP EEG

Sleep organization is constantly normal and physiologic patterns are symmetrically present. During sleep the evolution of the SW discharges is similar, on the whole, to that observed in childhood absence epilepsy (Tassinari *et al.*, 1974).

MA may occur during stage I of sleep awakening the subject. During stage II, SW discharges, of brief or long duration, are also observed, sometimes associated with bursts of myoclonias.

EVOLUTION

Classical data on the evolution of MA indicate that these are still present in one half of the cases followed up for a mean period of 10 years, whereas they disappear in the remaining patients after a mean period of 5.5 years from the onset (Tassinari, Bureau and Thomas, 1992). The two groups of patients differ in the frequency and type of associated seizures: in fact patients with 'refractory' MA have a high incidence (85%) of associated seizures, mainly of generalized tonic-clonic and atonic types. On the contrary, patients with remitting MA have a lower incidence (50%) of associated seizures, mainly of the absence type. Another factor which seems to influence the evolution is medical therapy. Indeed recent observations indicate that a combination of valproic acid and ethosuximide at high doses with appropriate control of plasma levels leads to rapid remission of MA in most cases (Tassinari and Michelucci, 1994). On the other hand, the therapeutic history of patients with 'refractory' MA often discloses that the above drugs have been given at lower doses or that different medical therapies have been used. The long duration of MA is likely to be an important factor for the appearance of mental retardation, since intellectual functions are always preserved in children with rapid remission of MA. In rare cases, the disappearance of MA has been followed by the onset of other seizure types, namely absences with atypical SW discharges, clinical and subclinical tonic seizures, giving rise to a clinical picture similar to the Lennox–Gastaut syndrome (Tassinari, Bureau and Thomas, 1992; Tassinari *et al.*, 1995).

DIAGNOSIS

The diagnosis of MA mainly rests on the polygraphic demonstration of SW discharges at 3 Hz (as in typical absences) accompanied by rhythmic myoclonias. Therefore, polygraphic recording is mandatory when the clinical suspicion of MA is raised. Since the anamnestic data may be sometimes misleading (asymmetric MA may be misdiagnosed as partial motor seizures, MA with mild myoclonias may be misdiagnosed as typical petit mal absences,etc.), we suggest polygraphic recording should be performed also in patients with 'drug-resistant' absence seizures and in cases with refractory 'myoclonic' or 'partial motor' seizures.

TREATMENT

Data on outcome suggest that the correct medical therapy for MA consists of the associated use of valproic acid and ethosuximide at high doses, with serum plasma levels ranging from 80 to 130 μg/ml and 70 to 110 μg/ml, respectively.

In individual cases, good seizure control was achieved by using a combination of phenobarbitone, valproic acid and benzodiazepines. A recent study found lamotrigine, particularly in combination with valproate, or in one case ethosuximide, to be useful when other measures had failed (Manonmani and Wallace, 1994).

ACKNOWLEDGMENTS

We thank Professor G. Avanzini and Dr S. Franceschetti from the Neurological Institute C. Besta of Milan for providing a case of MA (see Fig. 13b.1). The financial support of Telethon (grant no. E109) is gratefully acknowledged.

REFERENCES

Commission on Classification and Terminology of the International League Against Epilepsy (1989) Proposal for revised classification of epilepsies and epileptic syndromes. *Epilepsia*, **30**, 389–99.

Lugaresi, E., Pazzaglia, P., Franck, L. *et al.* (1973) Evolution and prognosis of primary generalized epilepsies of the petit mal absence type, in *Evolution and Prognosis of Epilepsy* (eds E. Lugaresi, P. Pazzaglia and C.A. Tassinari), Aulo Gaggi, Bologna, pp. 2–22.

Manonmani, V. and Wallace, S. (1994) Epilepsy with myoclonic absences. *Archives of Disease in Childhood*, **70**, 288–90.

Tassinari, C.A. and Bureau, M. (1985) Epilepsy with myoclonic absences, in *Epileptic Syndromes in Infancy, Childhood and Adolescence* (eds J. Roger, C. Dravet, M. Bureau, F.E. Dreifuss and P. Wolf), John Libbey, London, pp. 123–31.

Tassinari, C.A. and Michelucci, R. (1994) Epilepsy with myoclonic absences: a reappraisal, in *Epileptic Seizures and Syndromes* (ed. P. Wolf), John Libbey, London, pp. 137–41.

Tassinari, C.A., Bureau, M. and Thomas, P. (1992) Epilepsy with myoclonic absences, in *Epileptic Syndromes in Infancy, Childhood and Adolescence*, 2nd edn (eds J. Roger, M. Bureau, C. Dravet *et al.*), John Libbey, London, pp. 151–60.

Tassinari, C.A., Lyagoubi, S., Santos, V. *et al.* (1969) Etude des décharges de pointes ondes chez l'homme. II. Les aspects cliniques et electroencephalographiques des absences myocloniques. *Revue Neurologique*, **121**, 379–83.

Tassinari, C.A., Lyagoubi, S., Gambarelli, F. *et al.* (1971) Relationships between EEG discharge and neuromuscular phenomena. *Electroencephalography and Clinical Neurophysiology*, **31**, 176.

Tassinari, C.A., Bureau-Paillas, M., Dalla Bernardina, B. *et al.* (1974) Generalized epilepsies and seizures during sleep: a polygraphic study, in *Brain and Sleep* (eds H.M. Van Praag and H. Meinardi), De Erven Bhon, Amsterdam, pp. 154–66.

Tassinari, C.A., Michelucci, R., Rubboli, G. *et al.* (1995) Myoclonic absence epilepsy in *Typical Absences and Related Epileptic Syndromes* (eds J.S. Duncan and C.P. Panayiotopoulos), Churchill Livingstone, London, pp. 187–95.

Weir, B. (1965) The morphology of the spike-wave complex. *Electroencephalography and Clinical Neurophysiology*, **19**, 284–90.

Kazuyoshi Watanabe

BENIGN CHILDHOOD EPILEPSY WITH CENTROTEMPORAL SPIKES

DEFINITION

In the International Classification (Commission on Classification and Terminology of the International League Against Epilepsy, 1989), benign childhood epilepsy with centrotemporal spikes (BCECT) is defined as a syndrome of brief, simple, partial, hemifacial motor seizures, frequently having associated somatosensory symptoms, which have a tendency to evolve into generalized tonic-clonic seizures. Both seizure types are often related to sleep. The EEG has blunt high-voltage centrotemporal spikes, often followed by slow waves that are activated by sleep and tend to spread or shift from side to side. If this definition is strictly adhered to, a patient with typical centrotemporal spikes and a benign course in whom only a history of nocturnal generalized convulsions is elicited might be placed in the category of unclassified epilepsy, because of an absence of hemifacial motor seizures. Such a case should be classified as BCECT, because initial hemifacial seizures are often missed during nocturnal sleep. Oropharyngeal symptoms and arrest of speech are also frequent (Loiseau and Beaussart, 1973) and should be incorporated into the definition, in addition to hemifacial seizures.

CLINICAL FEATURES

This syndrome represents about 16% of all epileptic seizures in children aged 0–15 years, being four times more frequent than typical absence seizures (Heijbel, Blom and Bergfors, 1975). Benign focal sharp waves frequently occur without clinical seizures; only 9% of children with such sharp waves have clinical seizures (Lüders *et al.*, 1987). The ratio of boys to girls is 6:4.

The age of onset ranges from 2 to 12 years, but is mostly between 4 and 10 years with a peak at 7–9 years (Lüders *et al.*, 1987).

There is a high incidence of a positive family history of epilepsy and of sharp waves on EEG (Blom, Heijbel and Bergfors, 1972; Blom and Heijbel, 1975, Lüders *et al.*, 1987; Degen and Degen, 1990; Roger *et al.*, 1990; Degen and Degen, 1992; Holmes, 1993), suggesting that genetic factors are important in this disorder. This is also supported by the study of monozygotic twins (Kajitani *et al.*, 1980). Most authors postulate an autosomal dominant inheritance with age-dependent penetrance. Eeg-Olofsson (1992) also suggested dominant inheritance on the basis of his study on HLA antigens and haplotypes. Another interesting finding was a statistically significant low incidence of the haplotype A1,B8 in both probands and parents. Some 7–10% of patients also have a past history of febrile seizures. This may indicate a genetic link between the two conditions, or a genetic

Epilepsy in Children. Edited by Sheila Wallace. Published in 1996 by Chapman & Hall, London. ISBN 0 412 56860 8

predisposition to febrile seizures at a younger age in patients with BCECT (Chapter 10). Some differences in the clinical manifestations of patients with a past history of febrile seizures may suggest that these conditions may be independent but with closely linked genes (Haga *et al.*, 1992).

As a rule, the patients show normal development and are neurologically normal. However, considering its prevalence, this syndrome may occur in developmentally or neurologically abnormal childen (Blom, Heijbel and Bergfors, 1972; Santanelli *et al.*, 1989). Therefore, the presence of development retardation or neurologic deficits does not preclude its diagnosis.

Higher cerebral functions such as language may be affected by focal sharp waves even in these benign partial epileptic syndromes (Piccirilli *et al.*, 1988).

Transitory cognitive impairment occurs in association with rolandic spikes (D'Alessandro *et al.*, 1990; Binnie, de Silva and Hurst, 1992), and in some patients interferes with scholastic performance (Kasteleijn-Nolst Trenité *et al.*, 1988; Chapter 24) or with general psychosocial functioning (Aarts *et al.*, 1984).

Recurrent headaches or migraine are frequent symptoms in BCECT (Bladin, 1987; Giroud *et al.*, 1990), but may not be significantly more frequent than in control children (Santucci *et al.*, 1985; Giovanardi Rossi *et al.*, 1987). Septien *et al.* (1991) found migraine in 63% of patients with a history of this disorder, on the basis of a long-term controlled study, and have concluded that the association of the two conditions is not fortuitous.

SEIZURE MANIFESTATIONS

Seizure manifestations are related to the somatosensory and motor area in the lower rolandic region just above the sylvian fissure, and consist of unilateral paresthesiae involving the tongue, lips, gums and inner cheeks, and unilateral motor phenomena involving the face, lips, tongue, pharyngeal and laryn-geal muscles (Lombroso, 1967; Loiseau and Beaussart, 1973). Difficulty with speech and vocalization is caused by a peripheral type of motor disturbance or dysarthria and occurs irrespective of the laterality of the epileptogenic focus. Sialorrhea, drooling, gurgling sounds from the throat, and a feeling of suffocation are also common. These orofacial symptoms should not be mistaken for oral automatisms. Speech and oromotor deficits may be an initial or a sole symptom of the disorder (Kellerman, 1978; Boulloche *et al.*, 1990; Deonna *et al.*, 1993). Consciousness is usually preserved unless seizures become secondarily generalized. Failure to respond secondary to arrest of speech should not be mistaken for impaired consciousness. Hemifacial seizures may spread to the upper arm but rarely to the lower limb. Secondary generalization of seizures is rare during wakefulness, but frequent during sleep. In diurnal seizures, somatosensory symptoms may be the only manifestation. The initial focal manifestations of the nocturnal seizures are usually missed, and these seizures although in fact, secondarily generalized, tend to be diagnosed as generalized tonic-clonic attacks. According to Loiseau and Beaussart (1973), 70% of generalized seizures were apparently primarily generalized. Three types of nocturnal seizures occur (Lerman, 1992):

1. Hemifacial seizures associated with speech arrest and drooling.
2. Seizures similar to the above but with loss of consciousness, usually with gurgling-grunting noises.
3. Generalized convulsions.

However, the presence or absence of consciousness is often difficult to determine in nocturnal seizures in children with speech arrest and uncertain memory. In older children, hemifacial seizures are commoner, whereas in younger ones hemiconvulsive or generalized nocturnal seizures are more frequent in some series (Beaussart, 1972);

Ishikawa *et al.* (1988) did not observe any difference in seizure type according to age. Haga *et al.* (1992) reported that those who had a family and/or a past history of febrile seizures tended to have generalized seizures.

The duration of seizures is usually brief, lasting several seconds to a few minutes, although status epilepticus has been reported rarely (Fejerman and Di Blasi, 1987; Roulet, Deonna and Despland, 1989; Colamaria *et al.*, 1991). Diurnal seizures, especially those showing somatosensory symptoms, are usually of short duration.

The frequency of seizures is usually low (Lerman and Kivity, 1975; Ambrosetto, Giovanardi Rossi and Tassinari, 1987). Some 50–60% of the patients have sporadic seizures infrequently at intervals of 2–12 months and 10–20% experience only a single seizure. In 20%, seizures occur frequently and usually in clusters.

Seizures occur only during sleep in 51–80% of the patients, both during sleep and wakefulness in 13–40%, and only during wakefulness in 0–32% (Lüders *et al.*, 1987).

EEG FEATURES

The background activity is generally normal. A power spectral analysis has shown slower occipital basic rhythms (Hongo *et al.*, 1990), but contamination of slow waves from the reference electrode near the midtemporal region cannot be ignored.

The interictal EEG shows characteristic focal spikes in the left or right central and/or midtemporal region (Fig. 13c.1). These spikes are typically a negative sharp wave with a blunted peak, preceded by a small positive wave and followed by a prominent positive wave with an amplitude frequently up to 50% that of the preceding negative sharp wave. This may be followed by an inconspicuous negative slow wave of lower amplitude than the preceding negative sharp wave (Lüders *et al.*, 1987). Frost, Hrachovy and Glaze (1992) analyzed spike morphology of

different childhood partial epilepsies more precisely and found the spikes of this syndrome to be higher in amplitude, longer in duration, and less sharp in comparison with those of patients with other syndromes. When these sharp waves occur unilaterally, they are always synchronous in the central and midtemporal regions (Lerman, 1992), and when bilateral they may be bilaterally asynchronous, and occur with different frequencies and amplitudes in the left and the right hemispheres. In about 60% of patients, the spike focus is unilateral and in 40%, bilateral. When bilateral, the spike foci tend to shift from side to side. During sleep, rolandic spikes occur maximally in slow wave sleep and minimally in REM sleep (Clemens and Majoros, 1987).

Centrotemporal sharp waves have a typical field of distribution forming a dipole with a negative pole at the midtemporal-central region and a positive pole at the superior frontal area (Lüders *et al.*, 1987). This has been confirmed by topographic mapping analysis (Gregory and Wong, 1984; Graf, Lischka and Gremel, 1990), and further supported by more recent investigations using a dipole localization method, a dipole tracing method, or a dipole source analysis. The dipoles of children with BCECT were found to be more concentrated in the rolandic region compared with those with features similar to BCECT but with signs of brain damage (Wong, 1989; Weinberg *et al.*, 1990; Yoshinaga *et al.*, 1992). However, van der Meij, Wieneke and van Huffelen (1993) did not find clear differences between various clinical groups in the localization of the sources describing the activity around the maximal amplitudes of the spike, the trough and the wave of the rolandic spike-wave complex.

The centrotemporal regions are not exclusive locations of the sharp waves. Drury and Beydoun (1991) found a focus outside the centrotemporal area in one-fifth of patients with histories and clinical courses completely

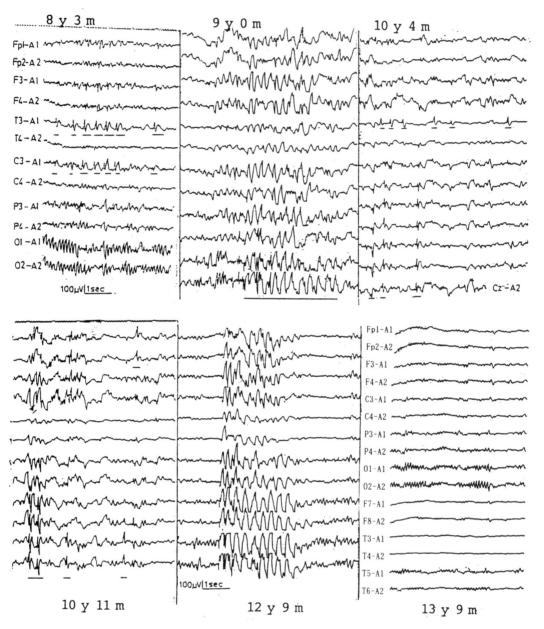

Fig. 13c.1   This neurologically and developmentally normal 15-year-old girl with a past history of febrile convulsions had typical nocturnal sylvian seizures at the age of 8 years. The EEG at 8 years 3 months disclosed typical sharp and slow wave discharges in the left midtemporal and central regions. The EEG at 9 years showed spike and wave complexes in both occipital regions on eye closure. The EEG at 10 years 4 months also displayed sporadic sharp waves in the left midtemporal area and spike and waves in the occipitoparietal regions independently. The EEG at 10 years 11 months demonstrated sporadic sharp waves independently in both frontal and occipital regions. She complained of blurred vision and headache occasionally. The EEG at 12 years 9 months revealed parieto-occipital dominant diffuse spike and wave bursts. EEGs at 13 years 9 months and thereafter were normal. She has been seizure free without treatment.

compatible with BCECT. A number of authors have mentioned the coexistence of other foci, multiple independent sharp wave foci, shifting of the location of sharp waves from a posterior to a centrotemporal location, and vice versa (Beaussart, 1972; Lerman and Kivity, 1975; Dalla Bernardina and Beghini, 1976; Amit, 1987; Lüders *et al.*, 1987; Watanabe, 1989; Beydoun, Garofalo and Drury, 1992. Holmes 1992 (Figs. 13c.1, 13c.4). Generalized spike-waves are also observed in some cases (Beaussart, 1972; Lerman and Kivity, 1975; Dalla Bernardina and Beghini, 1976; Petersen, Nielsen and Gulmann, 1983; Degen and Degen, 1990; Beydoun, Garofalo and Drury, 1992). Degen and Degen (1990) observed generalized spike-wave complexes in 32% of the siblings of patients with BCECT but focal discharges in various locations in only 6%.

There have been a few documentations of ictal recordings (Dalla Bernardina and Tassinari, 1975; Roger *et al.*, 1990). They usually show frequent rhythmic spikes or low voltage fast activity beginning in the centrotemporal region on one side (Fig. 13c.2). The paroxysmal discharges increase in amplitude and decrease in frequency, spreading to the adjacent regions and then to the whole hemisphere, evolving to high amplitude rhythmic spikes, and then to spike and waves when secondary generalization occurs. Lerman (1992) recorded a diurnal seizure beginning with focal decremental activity followed by dense spikes in the centrotemporal area during the tonic phase and spike-waves in the clonic phase with no spread and no postictal slowing. One of our patients showed frequent discharges of sharp waves in the right midtemporal, central, and the left central areas during a diurnal simple partial seizure (Fig. 13c.3). Guiterrez, Brick and Bodensteiner (1990) recorded a subclinical seizure with paroxysmal discharges showing a dipole reversal relative to the interictal discharges, and postulated the origin of the seizure discharge to be deep in the sylvian fissure in areas within cortical folds.

PATHOPHYSIOLOGY

Both clinical seizure manifestations and the location of EEG foci suggest that the epileptogenic focus is in the part of the lower rolandic cortex representing the face and the oropharynx. The bluntness of the spikes and the frequent association with slow waves may suggest a true focus, deep in the sylvian fissure (Lombroso, 1967).

Only a fraction of patients with typical rolandic sharp waves have clinical seizures. Factors which contribute to the expression of clinical epilepsy have not been elucidated. Heijbel, Blom and Rasmuson (1975) postulated the existence of an inhibitory factor, capable of preventing seizures, which can be breached by external or internal factors. Lerman (1992) suggested that a precipitating factor was needed to convert the inherited trait into the overt disease.

The marked age dependency of symptoms and almost regular disappearance of seizures and EEG abnormalities at puberty has led Doose and Baier (1989) to postulate an hereditary impairment of brain maturation.

The fact that patients with typical rolandic spikes may develop occipital spikes typical of benign occipital epilepsy (Fig. 13c.1), while patients with typical occipital spikes may develop typical rolandic spikes and generalized spike-waves typical of idiopathic generalized epilepsy (Fig. 13c.4), strongly suggests that there are close links between these disorders (Panayiotopoulos, 1993a).

INVESTIGATION

Neuroimaging procedures are usually considered unnecessary in this benign syndrome, but may be indicated in cases with atypical features such as persistent seizures and/or long duration of active epilepsy. Ambrosetto (1992) reported unilateral rolandic

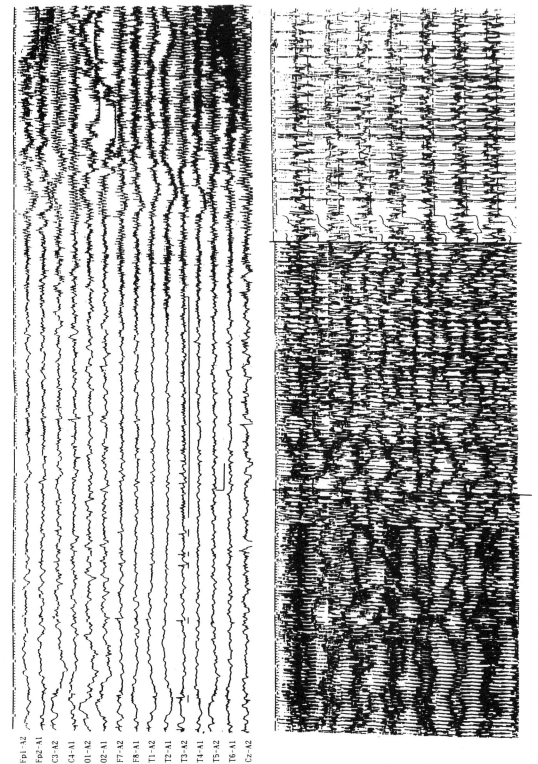

Fig. 13c.2 Ictal EEG of a 9-year-old girl with benign childhood epilepsy with centrotemporal spikes. During stage 2 sleep, low-voltage semirhythmic alpha activity appeared from the left midtemporal region which propagated to other areas with increasing amplitude and decreasing frequency. Seven seconds later, the right corner of her mouth was drawn downward to the right. Ten seconds later, she opened her eyes. Fifteen seconds later, her head rotated to the right, followed by generalized tonic-clonic convulsions.

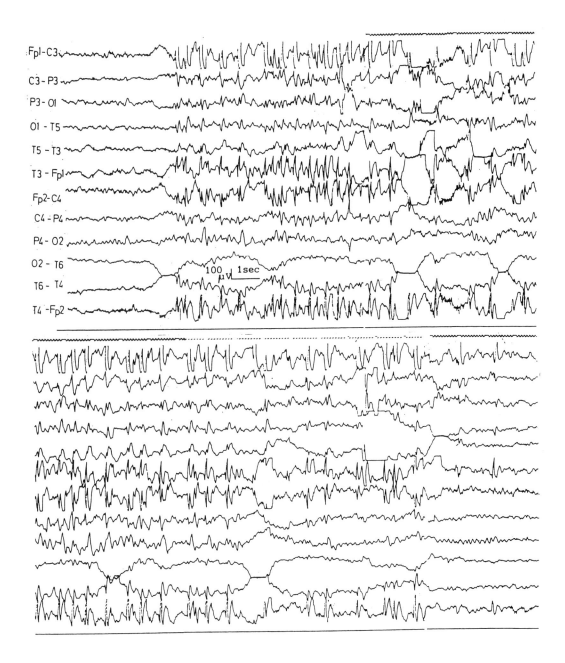

Fig. 13c.3 Ictal EEG of a diurnal simple partial seizure in a 9-year-old girl with benign childhood epilepsy with centrotemporal spikes. A burst of repetitive spikes was observed in the right and left midtemporal and central regions in association with an attack consisting of speech arrest and salivation. The dipole shows negativity in the midtemporal region and positivity in the frontal region.

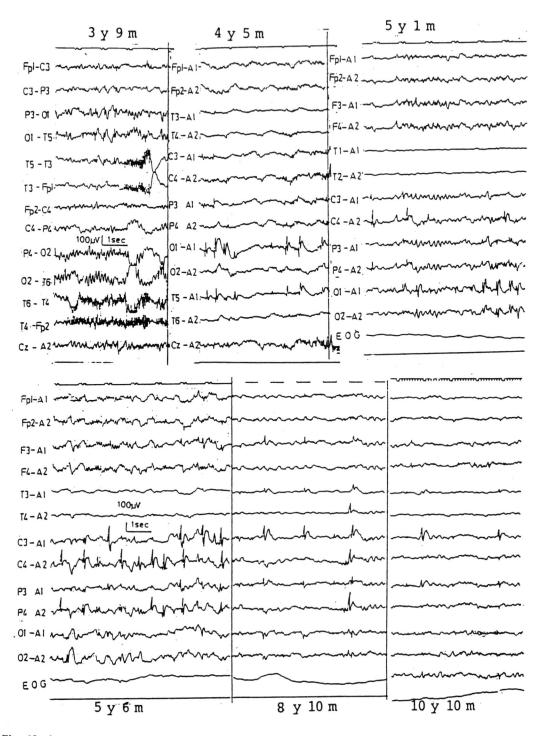

Fig. 13c.4

macrogyria in a patient with BCECT-like epilepsy. Typical rolandic sharp waves may be seen in children with tumors and other organic lesions (Kraschnitz *et al.*, 1988). We have recently had a case of typical BCECT fortuitously associated with a temporal astrocytoma.

Visual and somatosensory evoked potentials have been reported to be of high amplitude with no changes in morphology and latency (Farnarier *et al.*, 1988; Plasmati *et al.*, 1992). Overnight sleep recordings in children with BCECT do not show significant modifications in sleep organization (Clemens and Olah, 1987; Baldy-Moulinier, 1992). Laub *et al.* (1992) found localized hypoperfusion in about 40% of the patients using single photon emission computed tomography (SPECT) with technetium-99m hexamethyl propyleneamine oxime (HMPAO). The significance of their findings is unknown because of the absence of correlation between the localization of the EEG focus and the site of the hypoperfused area.

TREATMENT

In view of the benign nature of the condition, intensive therapy is unnecessary. Treatment should not be instituted after the first seizure. Ambrosetto, Giovanardi Rossi and Tassinari (1987) advise withholding treatment even after the second seizure if it occurs more than 6 months after the first. The same authors reported no differences in seizure frequency, recurrence or duration of active epilepsy between untreated and treated patients with BCECT (Ambrosetto and Tassinari, 1990).

Side-effects of anticonvulsants may be more harmful than seizures. If treatment is initiated, carbamazepine is considered the drug of first choice, although a possible worsening of seizures has rarely been reported with this medication. Phenobarbitone, phenytoin, and valproate have been reported equally effective, but may not be advised because of behavioral, cosmetic, or haematologic side-effects, respectively. Once-daily administration at bedtime may be sufficient in the case of nocturnal seizures. We have also found once-daily administration of a low dose of clonazepam highly effective in some cases. Although most patients respond to a low dose of a single drug, a few are highly drug-resistant. In such cases, monotherapy at a moderate dose with some persisting seizures may be better than high-dose polypharmacy with neurotoxic side-effects (Loiseau, 1993). The duration of treatment may be shorter in some cases than in epilepsy in general, in keeping with the spontaneous disappearance of rolandic spikes between 12 and 15 years of age. Although some authors adovocate continuance of anticonvulsant therapy until the age of 14–16 years (Loiseau, 1993), anticonvulsants may be successfuly discontinued in patients with normal EEGs who have been seizure-free for more than 2 years. Some 80% of patients followed by De Romanis, Feliciani and Ruggieri (1986) became seizure-free, and remained so for at least 6–12 months when drug therapy was discontinued after 2 years of treatment. It is more important to give the parents a full explanation of the benign

---

Fig. 13c.4 This neurologically and developmentally normal 14-year-old boy had had several febrile seizures up to 7 years 6 months, when he developed afebrile nocturnal generalized convulsions. The EEG was normal at 3 years of age. At 3 years 9 months small spikes and slow waves were seen in the left occipital region, becoming more definite and of high voltage at 4 years 5 months. The EEG at 5 years 1 month showed sporadic spikes in the right central area, in addition. At 5 years 6 months abundant spikes were seen in the left or right central and parietal areas, but fewer came from the occipital regions. Occipital spikes were hardly seen at 8 years and at 10 years 10 months only central spikes were demonstrable. The EEG normalized at 12 years and he has been seizure free without treatment for 3 years.

nature of the disorder, in order to avoid unnecessary psychologic reactions than to prescribe drugs (Lerman, 1992).

Spike discharges typically seen in benign partial epilepsies of childhood can also be observed in nonepileptic asymptomatic children with symptoms such as headache, abdominal pain, cyclic vomiting, etc. Such children should not be treated with antiepileptic drugs (Lerman and Kivity, 1992).

PROGNOSIS

Seizures eventually disappear and EEGs normalize irrespective of treatment. The duration of active epilepsy is longer in patients with earlier ages of onset (Loiseau *et al.*, 1988). Seizures are more easily controlled in patients with secondarily generalized seizures than those with only partial seizures (Haga *et al.*, 1992). Rarely (in 1–2% of patients), partial or generalized tonic-clonic seizures recur during adolescence or adulthood (Blom and Heijbel, 1982; Ambrosetto, Tinuper and Baruzzi, 1985: Lerman and Kivity, 1986; Loiseau *et al.*, 1988), which may represent another form of idiopathic epilepsy rather than a relapse of the same syndrome (Loiseau, 1993). The absence of typical EEG sharp waves and seizures characteristic of this syndrome in adults also indicates that this syndrome improves before adulthood.

In patients followed up for long periods, temporal changes in the EEG often make allocation into discrete syndromes impossible (Figs 13c.1, 13c.4, 13c.5). The electroclinical patterns overlap and the determining factor for prognosis is not the location but the morphology of the sharp waves (Loiseau, Duche and Cohadon, 1992).

Morikawa, Seino and Yagi (1992) conducted a longitudinal study of children with partial seizures and rolandic discharges and found that rolandic discharges disappeared in an age-related manner in idiopathic patients, but tended to persist in the sympto-matic ones. They concluded that the presence of rolandic discharges was not a hallmark of a benign outcome, but the presence of sylvian seizures indicated a favorable prognosis.

BENIGN CHILDHOOD EPILEPSY WITH OCCIPITAL PAROXYSMS

DEFINITION

In the International Classification (Commission on Classification and Terminology of the International League Against Epilepsy, 1989), benign childhood epilepsy with occipital paroxysms (BCEOP) is defined as a syndrome generally similar to BCECT, but characterized by seizures which start with visual symptoms (amaurosis, phosphenes, illusions, or hallucinations) and are often followed by a hemiclonic seizure or automatisms. In 25% of cases, the seizures are followed immediately by a migrainous headache. The EEG has paroxysms of high-amplitude spike-waves or sharp waves recurring rhythmically in the occipital and posterior temporal areas of one or both hemispheres, but only when the eyes are closed. During seizures, the occipital discharge may spread to the central or temporal regions. At present, no definite statement on prognosis is possible. Thus, the adjective benign is deleted in the Classification. The current definition is based on the description by Gastaut (1982, 1985), and Gastaut and Zifkin (1987). Some authors have questioned the existence of BCEOP as a distinct clinical entity, and the benign nature of the condition as defined above (Newton and Aicardi, 1983; Aicardi and Newton, 1987; Aso *et al.*, 1987, 1988; Cooper and Lee, 1991; Talwar, Rusk and Torres, 1992). Roger and Bureau (1992) have alluded to the difficulty in diagnosing this syndrome with certainty; they have drawn attention to the nonspecific nature of features on the interictal EEG, as described by Gastaut (1985), findings which can also be observed in symptomatic or cryptogenic partial epilepsies which often

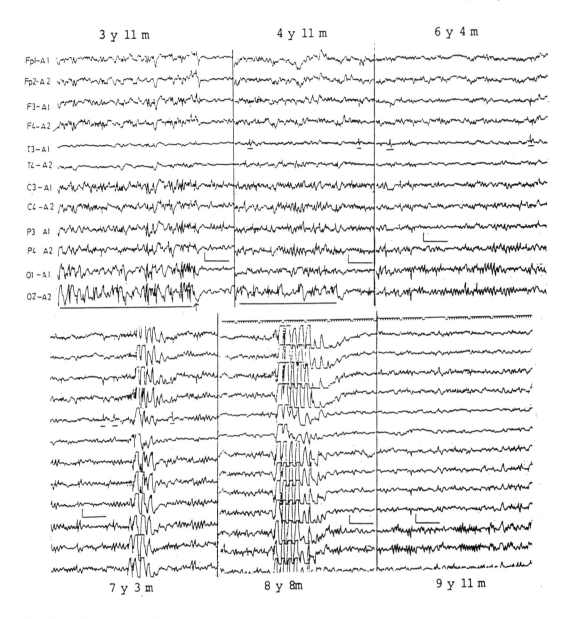

Fig. 13c.5 This neurologically and developmentally normal 12-year-old boy had several febrile seizures starting at 13 months. The EEG showed small spikes in the right occipital region at 3 years 5 months and spike and wave bursts attenuated on eye opening at 3 years and 11 months. Around this time, he developed seizures characterized by deviation of the eyes to the left. At 4 years 4 months, he had an attack consisting of deviation of the eyes to the left, vomiting and stiffening of the body. At 4 years 4 months and 4 years 11 months the EEG displayed focal spikes in the left midtemporal area, in addition to occipital spikes, but occipital spikes disappeared at 6 years 4 months and thereafter. At 7 years 3 months, there were short bursts of generalized spikes and waves in addition to midtemporal spikes; these disappeared at 8 years 8 months. The EEG was normal at 9 years 11 months and thereafter. He has been seizure free without treatment for 3 years.

have unfavorable outcomes. The only selection criterion that they used was the presence of occipital spikes, occurring when the eyes were closed; thus they included patients with organic brain lesions or mental retardation. Moreover, in some of the previous cases, paroxysmal discharges are not increased in slow wave sleep and even disappear during slow wave sleep, which is unusual in BCEOP (Dalla Bernardina *et al.*, 1985, 1992a; Beaumanoir and Thomas, 1992). Only idiopathic patients with normal neurodevelopment status should be considered to have BCEOP.

Much emphasis has been placed on visual symptoms because they were the most frequent ictal manifestation in Gastaut's series (1982). However, the incidence of visual symptoms was low in the series of Panayiotopoulos (1989b), who (Panayiotopoulos, 1989a) delineated a subgroup of BCEOP with an earlier onset than that described by Gastaut (1982, 1985), and characterized by nocturnal partial seizures associated with deviation of the eyes and vomiting, and frequently evolving to hemi- or generalized convulsions. Although the clinicoelectrical features of the early-onset variant may also be observed in symptomatic occipital epilepsy (Aso *et al.*, 1988), the clinical spectrum of BCEOP should be broadened from that described in the current International Classification. The specificity of this syndrome may not be as high as BCECT, since the clinicoelectrical picture of the latter syndrome is rarely seen in symptomatic or cryptogenic partial epilepsy. BCEOP should be defined by stricter criteria.

CLINICAL FEATURES

Although the exact incidence of BCEOP is unknown, Dalla Bernardina, Bandavalli and Colomaria (1985) found 19 (7.3%) patients with BCEOP among 260 with various types of benign partial epilepsies, in contrast to 162 (62.3%) with BCECT.

The age of onset ranges from 15 months to 17 years, with a peak age of onset between 5 and 7 years (Gastaut, 1985; Panayiotopoulos, 1989b). The clinical manifestations differ, depending on the age of onset. The younger children more often present with nocturnal seizures, mainly consisting of motor seizures; whereas the older children, above 8 years of age, have diurnal attacks characterized by visual seizures (Panayiotopoulos, 1989b). Both sexes seem to be equally affected, although either sex is more predominantly affected in different reports (Kivity and Lerman, 1989; Panayiotopoulos, 1989).

Gastaut (1985) elicited a family history of epilepsy in 37% and migraine in 16%, but other authors did not find positive family histories (Panayiotopoulos, 1989b; Fois, Malandrini and Tomaccini, 1988). Kuzniecky and Rosenblatt (1987) postulated an autosomal dominant inheritance for the EEG abnormalities with age-dependent expression and variable penetrance for the seizures. Nagendran, Prior and Rossiter (1989) suggested autosomal dominant inheritance, reporting a familial case in which the mother and two children were affected.

The patients show normal psychomotor development and neurologic examinations. Considering the incidence of BCEOP, fewer children with this syndrome are expected to have incidental mental retardation or neurologic abnormalities than those with BCECT.

Headache and vomiting occur commonly in this syndrome (Gastaut, 1985; Terasaki, Yamatogi and Ohtahara, 1987; Lerman and Kivity, 1991; Talwar, Rask and Torres, 1992). According to Lerman and Kivity (1991), the timing of the headache may be variable: headache was the presenting symptom in 29%, simultaneous with the visual symptoms in 37% and postictal in 33% of their cases. Although postictal migrainous headache is frequent, it is not exclusive to this syndrome. The correlation between epilepsy and migraine is an intricate problem (Panayiotopoulos, 1987; Terzano, Manzani and Parrino, 1987). The conditions seem to be two entirely different disorders, and it is most likely that epileptic discharges trigger migrainous phenomena (Panayiotopoulos, 1987).

SEIZURE MANIFESTATIONS

The clinical manifestations and frequency of seizures depend on the age of onset (Panayiotopoulos, 1993; Vivegano and Ricci, 1993). The early-onset variant is characterized by brief or prolonged, infrequent partial seizures marked by deviation of the eyes and vomiting which begin at the age of 2–8 years. The seizures are usually nocturnal. Consciousness is usually impaired or lost either from the onset or during the course of the seizure, although it may be preserved in some patients. Seizures may last for a few minutes or persist for several hours; they may imitate grave cerebral insults consisting of sudden or gradually evolving impairment and finally loss of consciousness, vomiting, deviation of the eyes and other focal symptomatology, frequently progressing to generalized attacks (Panayiotopoulos and Igoe, 1992; Kivity and Lerman, 1992). Although dramatic and prolonged, seizures occur infrequently and may be solitary. They are usually nocturnal, rarely diurnal, or both. Diurnal seizures are either similar to the nocturnal seizures, simple partial seizures, unclassifiable nonspecific fainting episodes, or infrequent episodes of perceptual abnormalities and automatisms occurring mainly in darkness or when the eyes are closed (Panayiotopoulos, 1993b). Postictal headache, migraine or ictal visual symptoms are extremely rare.

The late-onset type is characterized mainly by diurnal visual symptomatology, often followed by hemiclonic seizures or automatisms and postictal headache. The visual seizures consist of transient partial or complete visual loss in the entire visual field, sometimes preceded by initial hemianopsia, elementary visual hallucinations (i.e. phosphenes or moving flashing spots occupying the half or the entire visual field), complex visual hallucinations, and visual illusions such as micropsia, metamorphosia or palinopsia (Gastaut, 1985). These visual phenomena may be underreported by younger children. Visual symptoms may be followed by: hemiclonic seizures; complex partial seizures with automatisms, indistinguishable from those typical of temporal lobe epilepsy; adversive seizures; and/or secondarily generalized tonic-clonic seizures, followed by postictal diffuse headache, only rarely hemicranial, sometimes associated with nausea and vomiting. This sequence of symptoms may create some difficulties in differentiating migraine and epilepsy (Panayiotopoulos, 1987). The visual epileptic symptoms are predominantly multicolored and circular/spheric in contrast with the predominantly black and white linear pattern of migraine (Panayiotopoulos, 1993b). Seizures may be provoked by light extinction, by entering a dark room, or going from a dark area into a brighter one (Panayiotopoulos, 1981; Lugaresi, Cirignotta and Montagna, 1984; Gastaut, 1985).

EEG FEATURES

The interictal EEG shows characteristic occipital paroxysms on normal background activity (Gastaut, 1985; Panayiotopoulos, 1989b, 1993b). The occipital paroxysms typically consist of high-voltage, repetitive spikes, sharp waves and slow wave complexes over the occipital and posterior temporal regions which are often bilateral, asymmetric and attenuate on eye opening (Fig. 13c.4). Individual complexes consist of a diphasic spike component and a main negative peak on the occipital electrodes, which is followed by a relatively small positive peak and a negative slow wave (Panayiotopoulos, 1989b). The spike component is usually higher in amplitude than the negative slow wave, similar to centrotemporal spikes in benign rolandic epilepsy. The paroxysms are rarely isolated and usually recur pseudorhythmically in bursts of from 1 to 3 Hz or in trains at irregular intervals (Gastaut, 1985). They disappear promptly with opening of the eyes in 94% of cases and reappear 1–20 seconds after eye closure. They are further attenuated by fixation and induced by elimination of central vision (Panayiotopoulos, 1989b). Darkness is not a prerequisite for inducing occipital paroxysms. Thus, the term fixation-off sensitivity is preferable to scotosensitive epilepsy (Panayiotopoulos, 1993b). They are also inhibited by monocular elimination of central vision and monocular fixation. Neither occipital paroxysms nor fixation-off sensitivity is diagnostic of benign occipital epilepsy with occipital paroxysms. Fixation-off sensitivity is not always demonstrable in this syndrome (Panayiotopoulos, 1993b). Polyspikes, small spikes intermixed with slow waves, scattered occipital spikes as seen in photosensitive patients or slow waves which happen to attenuate with eyes open, are not occipital paroxysms in BCEOP (Panayiotopoulos, 1993b). In contrast to Panayiotopoulos (1993b), Vivegano and Ricci (1993) never observed the induction of occipital paroxysms in response to eye closure. Intermittent photic stimulation has an inhibitory effect particularly at high frequencies. Unlike Terasaki, Yamatogi and Ohtahara (1987) and Lerman and Kivity (1991), Gastaut (1985) states that hyperventilation has no activating effect. The effect of sleep is not consistent, in contrast to BCECT where sleep almost always activates spikes. Lerman and Kivity (1991) state that non REM sleep activates or discloses the occipital discharges, but Gastaut (1985) found reinforcement by slow sleep in only 15% of cases. Gastaut and Zifkin (1987) reported that drowsiness and sleep caused the disappearance of occipital paroxysms in 59% of cases, yet, in another series, the discharges occurred more frequently during sleep (Fois, Malandrini and Tomaccini, 1988). In some patients, the occipital paroxysms are associated with generalized bisynchronus spike and waves or focal spikes in other regions such as centro-temporal spikes in the same or subsequent records (Gastaut, 1985; Panayiotopoulos, 1989b). The location of spikes may change during the clinical course and shift from the occipital area to other areas, sometimes showing multifocality (Watanabe, 1989) (Figs 13c.4, 13c.5). Not all children with occipital paroxysms develop clinical seizures (Deonna, Ziegler and Despland, 1984; Herranz-Tanarro, Saenz-Lope and Cristobal-Sassot, 1984).

The ictal EEG of a diurnal seizure recorded by Beaumanoir (1983) disclosed focal rapid spikes, becoming progressively slower. The ictal EEG of nocturnal seizures showed disappearance of interictal occipital paroxysms followed by a tonic discharge of low-voltage spikes of progressively increasing amplitude in an occipital region, followed by spike and waves localized to one or more of the posterior areas.

PATHOPHYSIOLOGY

The varying clinical seizure patterns seen in this syndrome can be explained by the propagation of the occipital ictal discharges to anterior regions (Gastaut 1985). Purely visual seizures are associated with focal occipital discharges limited to the occipital region. Visual auras followed by hemisensory and/or hemiconvulsive seizures are related to the spread of the occipital discharge to the central region. Visual auras followed by psychomotor automatisms are due to the spread of the occipital discharge to the temporal lobe and/or related structures. Seizures without visual phenomena result from the secondary spread of the occipital discharge in which visual symptoms are not reported, or from the discharge of an independent focus away from the primary occipital focus (Gastaut, 1985). Gastaut and Zifkin (1987) suggested a subcortical mechanism for the electrogenesis of occipital paroxysms. They postulated that the postictal migrainous symptoms are due to the persistence, in the territory of the posterior cerebral and basilar arteries, of the initial vasodilatation accompanying the occipital ictal activity, in children with impaired or labile cerebrovascular autoregulation, who are predisposed to migraine.

INVESTIGATION

The occipital paroxysms are not highly specific and may be seen in patients with organic occipital lesions. Gobbi *et al.* (1988) and Giroud *et al.* (1990) reported patients, initially considered to have benign occipital epilepsy, who subsequently showed mental deterioration and worsening of seizures and were found to have occipital calcification. Therefore, neuroimaging studies are necessary, in addition to a careful history and neurologic examination.

TREATMENT

Carbamazepine may be the drug of choice, although almost all of the classic anticonvulsants, chiefly phenobarbitone, valproate and benzodiazepines, are effective (Gastaut, 1985).

PROGNOSIS

The prognosis is usually good, with complete seizure control achieved in 60% of cases. No patients have typical seizures persisting past adolescence, but other types of seizures occur in 5% in adulthood (Gastaut, 1985). The early-onset variant has an excellent prognosis, with remission occurring 1–2 years after onset and before 12 years of age (Panayiotopoulos, 1989b). EEG abnormalities usually outlast the clinical remission for many years, sometimes up to 16 years of age.

BENIGN PARTIAL EPILEPSY WITH AFFECTIVE SYMPTOMATOLOGY

This syndrome was first described by Dalla Bernardina *et al.* (1980, 1992b) and is characterized by ictal affective symptoms, especially fear, as the predominant manifestation and a favorable outcome.

CLINICAL FEATURES

The age of onset in 26 patients reported by Dalla Bernardina *et al.* (1992b) ranged from 2 to 9 years with two peaks at 2–5 years and 6–9 years. The patients were neurologically normal with normal development. CT scans were normal in all cases. A family history of epilepsy was noted in 38% and a past history of febrile convulsions of brief duration in 19%.

SEIZURE MANIFESTATIONS

The predominant feature of the seizure in these 26 patients was sudden fright or terror manifesting itself as screaming, yelling or calling for the mother (46%), clinging to somebody nearby (54%), or trying to hide (12%). The terrorized expression was sometimes associated with either chewing or swallowing movements (23%), distressed laugh (15%), arrest of speech with glottal noises, moans, and salivation (23%) or autonomic symptoms such as pallor, sweating or abdominal pain (27%). Consciousness seemed to be impaired to some extent. The mean duration of the attack was 1–2 minutes, maximally 10 minutes. The seizures took place during sleep and wakefulness and often became frequent soon after the onset, occurring several times a day in 50% of cases. No postictal deficit was observed, although the patient might be sleepy or tired. A few brief nocturnal orofacial clonic seizures were observed at the same period in 15%. No tonic, clonic, tonic-clonic or atonic seizures occurred during the clinical course in any child.

EEG FEATURES

The background activity was normal, with normal organization of sleep, even during periods with frequent seizures. The commonest interictal paroxysmal abnormalities, seen in 73% of cases, were sharp waves or sharp and slow waves, similar to the rolandic spikes of BCECT, occurring in the fronto-temporal or parietotemporal regions of one or both hemispheres and activated by sleep, without changes in morphology. Brief bursts of generalized spike and waves may be observed alone or in association with focal abnormalities. These generalized discharges might appear during drowsiness but never increased in slow wave sleep.

Ictal records usually showed localized discharges in the frontotemporal, centro-temporal or parietal regions, but occasionally more diffuse abnormalities made localization of the initial discharge difficult.

PATHOPHYSIOLOGY

This syndrome is considered to be a benign functional epilepsy because of its similarity to BCECT, i.e. occurrence in normal children, age of onset, high incidence of positive family history, brief seizures, response to treatment, morphology of spikes, sleep enhancement, and brief generalized spike and waves (Dalla Bernardina *et al.*, 1992b), but its pathophysiology is unknown. Fright as a main seizure manifestation is of little value in localizing the seizure origin and may only be a nonspecific response of the child to subjective phenomena. The origin of ictal discharges is also not as specific as in BCECT. Dalla Bernardina *et al.* (1992b) consider that this syndrome does not constitute an independent form of idiopathic partial epilepsy, but probably only a relatively rare variant of BCECT.

TREATMENT

Carbamazepine or phenobarbitone are the most effective drugs. When the seizure frequency is low, medication may not be necessary.

PROGNOSIS

The response to treatment is mostly good. Of 26 patients followed by Dalla Bernardina *et al.*

(1992b), three patients were never treated. Twenty-one of the 26 patients were followed longitudinally (Dalla Bernardina *et al.*, 1992b), 16 of them were eventually seizure-free and off treatment and five patients over 18 years of age had more or less frequent seizures. At the time of frequent seizures, some patients exhibited behavioral and/or intellectual disturbances. Dalla Bernardina *et al.* (1992b) concluded that the presence of symptoms other than affective ones, the absence of typical rolandic spike-like discharges, the presence of a slow wave focus, and poly-morphism of ictal discharges exclude the diagnosis of this syndrome.

NOSOLOGIC PROBLEMS

Inconsistency of the origin of ictal discharges and a poor correlation between the focus and affective symptoms may make it difficult to accept this syndrome as a disease entity. Dalla Bernardina *et al.* (1992b) consider that benign partial epilepsy with affective symp-tomatology (BPEA) does not constitute an independent form of idiopathic partial epi-lepsy but probably only a relatively rare variant of BCECT.

We have also had several patients who showed frequent attacks of sudden fright which responded well to carbamazepine, but the interictal EEG did not show spikes. In spite of treatment for more than 5 years, the anticonvulsant could not be discontinued in some patients, since any attempt at with-drawal resulted in relapse of subjective symptoms. These patients are considered to have frontal lobe epilepsy, judging by their ictal EEGs. In contrast, those who showed similar attacks of terror and interictal rolandic spike-like discharges in the centrotemporal region ultimately became free from seizures and treatment free following the intermittent use of once-daily large doses of diazepam. Thus, this syndrome may be a nonspecific affective response of young children to somatosensory phenomena occurring in rolandic epilepsy or related conditions, and the affective symptoms may themselves not be epileptic manifestations.

REFERENCES

Aarts, J.H.P., Binnie, C.D., Smit, A.M. and Wilkins, A.J. (1984) Selective cognitive impairment during focal and generalized epileptiform EEG activity. *Brain*, **107**, 293–308.

Aicardi, J. and Newton, R. (1987) Clinical findings in children with occipital spike wave complexes suppressed by eye opening, in *Migraine and Epilepsy* (eds F. Andermann and E. Lugaresi), Butterworth, London, pp. 111–24.

Ambrosetto, G. (1992) Unilateral opercular macrogyria and benign childhood epilepsy with centrotemporal (rolandic) spikes: report of a case. *Epilepsia*, **33**, 499–503.

Ambrosetto, G. and Tassinari, C.A. (1990) Antiepileptic drug treatment of benign childhood epilepsy with rolandic spikes: is it neccesary? *Epilepsia*, **31**, 802–5.

Ambrosetto, G., Tinuper, P. and Baruzzi, A. (1985) Relapse of benign partial epilepsy of children in adulthood: report of a case. *Journal of Neurology, Neurosurgery and Psychiatry* **48**, 90.

Ambrosetto, G., Giovanardi Rossi, P. and Tassinari, C.A. (1987) Predictive factors of seizure frequency and duration of antiepileptic treatment in rolandic epilepsy: a retrospective study. *Brain and Development*, **9**, 300–4.

Amit, R. (1987) Benign focal epilepsy of childhood: Individual and intrafamilial multifocality of spikes. *Clinical Electroencephalography*, **18**, 169–72.

Aso, K., Watanabe, K., Negoro, T., *et al.* (1987) Visual seizures in children. *Epilepsy Research*, **1**, 246–53.

Aso, K., Watanabe, K., Negoro, T. *et al.* (1988) Occipital epileptiform discharges in children. *Journal of the Japanese Epileptic Society*, **6**, 103–10.

Baldy-Moulinier, M. (1992) Sleep organization in benign childhood partial epilepsies, in *Benign Localized and Generalized Epilepsies of Early Childhood (Epilepsy Research*, Suppl.6) (eds R. Degen and F.E. Dreifuss), Elsevier, Amsterdam, pp. 121–4.

Beaumanoir, A. (1983) Infantile epilepsy with occipital focus and good prognosis. *European Neurology*, **22**, 43–52.

Beaumanoir, A. and Thomas, P. (1992) Benign epilepsy of childhood with occipital paroxysms, in *Benign Localized and Generalized Epilepsies in Early Childhood* (eds R. Degen, F.E. Dreifuss), Elsevier, Amsterdam, pp. 105–9.

Beaussart, M. (1972) Benign epilepsy of children with rolandic (centrotemporal) paroxysmal foci. A clinical entity. Study of 221 cases. *Epilepsia*, **13**, 795–811.

Beaussart, M. and Faou, R. (1978) Epilepsy with rolandic paroxysmal foci: a study of 324 cases. *Epilepsia*, **19**, 337–42.

Beydoun, A., Garofalo, E.A. and Drury, I. (1992) Generalized spike-waves, multiple loci, and clinical course in children with EEG features of benign epilepsy of childhood with centrotemporal spikes. *Epilepsia*, **33**, 1091–6.

Binnie, C.D., de Silva, M. and Hurst, A. (1992) Rolandic spikes and cognitive function, in *Benign Localized and Generalized Epilepsies of Early Childhood (Epilepsy Reseach*, Suppl.6) (eds R. Degen and F.E. Dreifuss), Elsevier, Amsterdam, pp. 71–3.

Bladin, P.F. (1987) The association of benign rolandic epilepsy with migraine, in *Migraine and Epilepsy* (eds F. Andermann and E. Lugaresi), Butterworths, Boston, London, pp. 145–52.

Blom, S. and Heijbel, J. (1975) Benign epilepsy of children with centrotemporal EEG foci: discharge rate during sleep. *Epilepsia*, **16**, 133–40.

Blom, S. and Heijbel, J. (1982) Benign epilepsy of children with centro-temporal EEG foci: a follow-up study in adulthood of patients initially studied as children. *Epilepsia*, **23**, 629–32.

Blom, S., Heijbel, J. and Bergfors, P.G. (1972) Benign epilepsy of children with centro-temporal EEG foci. Prevalence and follow-up study of 40 patients. *Epilepsia*, **13**, 609–19.

Boulloche, J., Husson, A., Le Luyer, B. and Le Roux, P. (1990) Dysphagie, troubles du langage et pointes ondes centro-temporales. *Archives Francaises de Pediatrie*, **47**, 115 7.

Clemens, B. and Majoros, E. (1987) Sleep studies in benign epilepsy of childhood with rolandic spikes. II. Analysis of discharge frequency and its relation to sleep dynamics. *Epilepsia*, **28**, 24–7.

Clemens, B. and Olah, R. (1987) Sleep studies in benign epilepsy of childhood with rolandic spikes, I. Sleep pathology. *Epilepsia*, **28**, 20–3.

Colamaria, V., Sgrò, V., Caraballo, R. *et al.* (1991) Status epilepticus in benign rolandic epilepsy manifesting as anterior opercular syndrome. *Epilepsia*, **32**, 329–34.

Commission on Classification and Terminology of

the International League Against Epilepsy (1989) Proposal for revised classification of epilepsies and epileptic syndromes. *Epilepsia*, **30**, 389–99.

Cooper, G.W. and Lee, S.I. (1991) Reactive occipital epileptiform activity: is it benign? *Epilepsia*, **32**, 63–8.

D'Alessandro, P., Piccirilli, M., Tiacci, C. *et al.* (1990) Neuropsychological features of benign partial epilepsy in children. *Italian Journal of Neurological Sciences*, **11**, 265–9.

Dalla Bernardina, B. and Beghini, G. (1976) Rolandic spikes in children with and without epilepsy (20 subjects polygraphically studied during sleep). *Epilepsia*, **17**, 161–7.

Dalla Bernardina, B. and Tassinari, C.A. (1975) EEG of a nocturnal seizure in a patient with 'benign epilepsy of childhood with rolandic spikes'. *Epilepsia*, **16**, 497–501.

Dalla-Bernardina, B., Bondavalli, S. and Colomaria, V. (1985) Benign epilepsy of childhood with rolandic spikes (BERS) during sleep, in *Sleep and Epilepsy* (eds M.B. Sterman, M.N. Shouse and P. Passouant), Academic Press, London, pp. 495–506.

Dalla-Bernardina, B., Bureau, M., Dravet, C. *et al.* (1980) Epilepsie bénigne de l'enfant avec crises à sémiologie affective. *Revue d'Electroencephalographie et de Neurophysiologie Clinique*, **10**, 8–18.

Dalla-Bernardina, B., Chiamenti, C., Capovilla, G. and Colomaria V. (1985) Benign partial epilepsies in childhood, in *Epileptic Syndromes in Infancy, Childhood and Adolescence* (eds J. Roger, C. Dravet, M. Bureau *et al.*), John Libbey Eurotext, London, pp. 137–49.

Dalla Bernardina, B., Sgrò, V., Fontana, E. *et al.* (1992a) Idiopathic partial epilepsies in children, in *Epileptic Syndromes in Infancy, Childhood and Adolescence* (eds J. Roger,, M. Bureau, C.Dravet *et al.*), John Libbey, London, pp. 173–88.

Dalla Bernardina, B., Colamaria, V., Chiamenti, C. *et al.* (1992b) Benign partial epilepsy with affective symptoms ('Benign psychomotor epilepsy'), in *Epileptic Syndromes in Infancy, Childhood and Adolescence* (eds J. Roger, M. Bureau, C. Dravet *et al.*), John Libbey, London, pp. 219–23.

De Romanis, F., Feliciani, M. and Ruggieri, S. (1986) Rolandic paroxysmal epilepsy: a long term study in 150 children. *Italian Journal of Neurological Science*, **7**, 77–80.

Degen, R. and Degen, H.-E. (1990) Some genetic aspects of rolandic epilepsy: waking and sleep EEGs in siblings. *Epilepsia*, **31**, 795–801.

Degen, R. and Degen, H.-E. (1992) Contribution to the genetics of rolandic epilepsy: waking and sleep EEGs in siblings, in *Benign Localized and Generalized Epilepsies of Early Childhood* (eds R. Degen and F.E. Dreifuss), Elsevier, Amsterdam, pp. 49–52.

Deonna, Th., Ziegler, A.L. and Despland, P.A. (1984) Paroxysmal visual disturbances of epileptic origin and occipital epilepsy in children. *Neuropediatrics*, **15**, 131–5.

Deonna, T.W., Roulet, E., Fontan, D. and Marcoz, J.-P. (1993) Speech and oromotor deficits of epileptic origin in benign partial epilepsy of childhood with rolandic spikes (BPERS). Relationship to the acquired aphasia-epilepsy syndrome. *Neuropediatrics*, **24**, 83–7.

Doose, A.H. and Baier, W.K. (1989) Benign partial epilepsy and related conditions: multifactorial pathogenesis with hereditary impairment of brain maturation. *European Journal of Pediatrics*, **149**, 152–8.

Drury, I. and Beydoun, A. (1991) Benign partial epilepsy of childhood with monomorphic sharp waves in centrotemporal and other locations. *Epilepsia*, **32**, 662–7.

Eeg-Olofsson, O. (1992) Further genetic aspects in benign localized epilepsies in early childhood, in *Benign Localized and Generalized Epilepsies of Early Childhood* (*Epilepsy Reseach*, Suppl. 6) (eds R. Degen and F.E. Dreifuss), Elsevier, Amsterdam pp. 117–9.

Farnarier, G., Bureau, M., Mancini, J. and Regis, H. (1988) Etude des potentiels evoques multimodalitaires dans les epilepsies partielles de l'enfant. *Neurophysiologie Clinique*, **18**, 243–54.

Fejerman, N. and Di Blasi, A.M. (1987) Status epilepticus of benign partial epilepsies in children: report of two cases. *Epilepsia*, **28**, 351–5.

Fois, A., Malandrini, F. and Tomaccini, D. (1988) Clinical findings in children with occipital paroxysmal discharges. *Epilepsia*, **29**, 620–3.

Frost, Jr J.D., Hrachovy, R.A. and Glaze, D.G. (1992) Spike morphology in childhood focal epilepsy: relationship to syndromic classification. *Epilepsia*, **33**, 531–6.

Gastaut. H. (1982) A new type of epilepsy: benign partial epilepsy of childhood with occipital spike-waves. *Clinical Electroencephalography*, **13**, 13–22.

Gastaut, H. (1985) Benign epilepsy of childhood with occipital paroxysms, in *Epileptic Syndromes in Infancy, Childhood and Adolescence* (eds J. Roger, C. Dravet, M. Bureau, F.E. Dreifuss and P. Wolf), John Libbey Eurotext, London, pp. 159–70.

Gastaut, H. and Zifkin, B.G. (1987) Benign epilepsy of childhood with occipital spike and wave complexes, in *Migraine and Epilepsy* (eds F. Andermann and E. Luagresi), Butterworths, London, pp. 47–81.

Giovanardi Rossi, P., Santucci, M., Gobbi, G. *et al.* (1987) Epidemiological study of migraine in epileptic patients, in *Migraine and Epilepsy* (eds F. Andermann and E. Lugaresi), Butterworths, London, pp. 312–22.

Giroud, M., Borsotti, J.P., Michiel, S.R. *et al.* (1990) Epilepsie et calcifications occipitales bilaterales: 3 cas. *Revue Neurologique*, **146**, 288–92.

Gobbi, G., Sorrenti, G., Santucci, M. *et al.* (1988) Epilepsy with bilateral occipital calcifications: a benign onset with progressive severity. *Neurology*, **38**, 913–20.

Graf, M., Lischka, A. and Gremel, K. (1990) Benign rolandic epilepsy in children. Topographic EEG analysis. *Wiener Klinische Wochenschrift*, **102**, 206–10.

Gregory, D.L. and Wong, P.K. (1984) Topographical analysis of the centrotemporal discharges in benign rolandic epilepsy of childhood. *Epilepsia*, **25**, 705–11.

Guiterrez, A.R., Brick, J.F., Bodensteiner, J. (1990) Dipole reversal: an ictal feature of benign partial epilepsy with centro-temporal spikes. *Epilepsia*, **31**, 544–8.

Haga, Y., Watanabe, K., Negoro, T. *et al.* (1992) Children with centro-temporal EEG foci. *Journal of the Japanese Epileptic Society*, **10**, 113–8.

Heijibel, J., Blom, S. and Bergfors, P.G. (1975) Benign epilepsy of children with centrotemporal EEG foci. A study of incidence rate in outpatient care. *Epilepsia*, **16**, 657–64.

Heijbel, J., Blom, S. and Rasmuson, M. (1975) Benign epilepsy of children with centrotemporal EEG foci. A genetic study. *Epilepsia*, **16**, 285–93.

Herranz-Tanarro F., Saenz-Lope, E. and Cristobal-Sassot, S. (1984) La pointe-onde occipitale avec et sans épilepsie bénigne chez l'enfant. *Revue d'Electroencephalographie et de Neurophysiologie Clinique*, **14**, 1–7.

Holmes, G.L. (1992) Rolandic epilepsy: clinical and electroencephalographic features, in *Benign Localized and Generalized Epilepsies of Early Childhood* (eds R. Degen and F.E. Dreifuss), Elsevier, Amsterdam, pp. 29–43.

Holmes, G.L. (1993) Benign focal epilepsies of childhood. *Epilepsia*, **34** (suppl.3), S49–61.

Hongo, K., Naganuma, Y., Murakami, M. *et al.* (1990) Development of EEG background activity in children with benign partial epilepsy. *Japanese Journal of Psychiatry and Neurology*, **44**, 367–8.

Ishikawa, T., Nakazato, M., Awaya, A. *et al.* (1988) Benign childhood epilepsy with centrotemporal spikes. Evolution of seizure types. *Acta Paediatrica Japonica*, **30**, 73–7.

Kajitani, T., Nakamura, M., Ueoka, K. and Koduchi S. (1980) Three pairs of monozygotic twins with rolandic discharges, in *Advances in Epileptology, The Tenth International Symposium* (eds J.A. Wada and J.K. Penny), Raven Press, New York, pp. 171–5.

Kasteleijn-Nolst Trenité, D.G.A., Bakker, D.J., Binnie, C.D. *et al.* (1988) Psychological effects of subclinical epileptiform EEG discharges. I. Scholastic skills. *Epilepsy Research*, **2**, 111–6.

Kellerman, K. (1978) Recurrent aphasia with subclinical status epilepticus during sleep. *European Journal of Pediatrics*, **128**, 207–12.

Kivity, S. and Lerman, P. (1989) Benign partial epilepsy of childhood with occipital discharges, in *The XVIIth Epilepsy International Symposium (Advances in Epileptology, vol. 17)* (eds J. Manelis, E. Bental, J.N. Loeber and F.E. Dreifuss), Raven Press, New York. pp. 371–3.

Kivity, S. and Lerman, P. (1990) Stormy onset with prolonged loss of consciousness in benign occipital epilepsy of childhood. *Brain and Development*, **12**, 632.

Kivity, S. and Lerman, P. (1992) Stormy onset with prolonged loss of consciousness in benign childhood epilepsy with occipital paroxysms. *Journal of Neurology, Neurosurgery and Psychiatry*, **55**, 45–8.

Kraschnitz, W., Scheer, P., Korner, K. *et al.* (1988) Rolandic spikes als elektroenzephalographische Manifestation eines Oligodendroglioma. *Pädiatrie und Pädologie*, **23**, 313–9.

Kuzniecky, R. and Rosenblatt, B. (1987) Benign occipital epilepsy: a family study. *Epilepsia*, **28**, 346–50.

Laub, M.C., Funke, R., Kirsch, C.-M. and Oberst, U. (1992) BECT: comparison of cerebral flow imaging, neuropsychological testing and long-term EEG monitoring, in *Benign Localized and Generalized Epilepsies of Early Childhood (Epilepsy Research, suppl.6)* (eds R. Degen and F.E. Dreifuss), Elsevier, Amsterdam, pp. 95–8.

Lerman, P. (1992) Benign partial epilepsy with

centro-temporal spikes, in *Epileptic Syndromes in Infancy, Childhood and Adolescence*, 2nd edn (eds J. Roger, M. Bureau, Ch. Dravet *et al.*), John Libbey, London, pp. 189–200.

Lerman, P. and Kivity, S. (1975) Benign focal epilepsy of childhood. A follow up of 100 recovered patients. *Archives of Neurology*, **32**, 261–4.

Lerman, P. and Kivity, S. (1986) The benign focal epilepsies of childhood, in *Recent Advances in Epilepsy*, Vol. 11 (eds T.A. Pedley and B.S. Meldrum), Churchill Livingstone, Edinburgh, pp. 137–56.

Lerman, P. and Kivity, S. (1991) The benign partial nonrolandic epilepsies. *Journal of Clinical Neurophysiology*, **8**, 275–87.

Lerman, P. and Kivity, S. (1992) Focal epileptic EEG discharges in children not suffering from clinical epilepsy, in *Benign Localized and Generalized Epilepsies of Early Childhood* (Epilepsy Research, suppl. 6) (eds R. Degen and F.E. Dreifuss), Elsevier, Amsterdam, pp. 99–103.

Lischka, A. and Graf, M. (1992) Benign rolandic epilepsy of childhood: topographic EEG analysis, in *Benign Localized and Generalized Epilepsies of Early Childhood* (eds R. Degen and F.E. Dreifuss), Elsevier, Amsterdam, pp. 53–8.

Loiseau, P. (1993) Benign focal epilepsies of childhood, in *The Treatment of Epilepsy. Principle and Practice* (ed. E. Wyllie), Lea & Febiger, Philadelphia, pp. 503–12.

Loiseau, P. and Beaussart, M. (1973) The seizures of benign childhood epilepsy with rolandic paroxysmal discharge. *Epilepsia*, **14**, 381–9.

Loiseau, P., Duche, B. and Cohadon, S. (1992) Prognosis of benign localized epilepsy in early childhood, in *Benign Localized and Generalized Epilepsies of Early Childhood* (eds R. Degen and F.E. Dreifuss), Elsevier, Amsterdam, p. 71–7.

Loiseau, P., Duche, B., Cordova, S. *et al.* (1988) Prognosis of benign childhood epilepsy with centro-temporal spikes: a follow-up study of 168 patients. *Epilepsia*, **29**, 229–35.

Lombroso, C.T. (1967) Sylvian seizures and mid temporal spike foci in children. *Archives of Neurology*, **17**, 52–9.

Lüders, H., Lesser, R.P., Dinner, D.S. and Morris, H.H. III (1987) Benign focal epilepsy of childhood, in *Electroclinical Syndromes* (eds H. Luders and R.P. Lesser), Springer-Verlag, Berlin, pp. 303–46.

Lugaresi, J., Cirignotta, F. and Montagna, P. (1984) Occipital lobe epilepsy with scotosensitive seizures: the role of central vision. *Epilepsia*, **25**, 115–20.

Morikawa, T., Seino, M. and Yagi, K. (1992) Is rolandic discharge a hallmark of benign partial epilepsy of childhood?, in *Benign Localized and Generalized Epilepsies of Early Childhood* (*Epilepsy Research*, suppl.6) (eds R. Degen and F.E. Dreifuss), Elsevier, Amsterdam, pp. 59–69.

Nagendran, K., Prior, P.F. and Rossiter, M.A. (1989). Benign occipital epilepsy of childhood: a family study. *Journal of the Royal Society of Medicine*, **82**, 684–85.

Newton, R. and Aicardi, J. (1983) Clinical findings in children with occipital spike wave complexes suppressed by eye opening. *Neurology*, **33**, 1526–9.

Panayiotopoulos, C.P. (1981) Inhibitory effect of central vision on occipital lobe seizure. *Neurology*, **31**, 1331–3.

Panayiotopoulos, C.P. (1987) Difficulties in differentiating migraine and epilepsy based on clinical and electroencephalographic findings, in *Migraine and Epilepsy* (eds F. Andermann and E. Lugaresi), Butterworth, London, pp. 31–46.

Panayiotopoulos, C.P. (1989a) Benign nocturnal childhood epilepsy: a new syndrome with nocturnal seizures, tonic deviation of the eyes, and vomiting. *Journal of Child Neurology*, **4**, 43–8.

Panayiotopoulos, C.P. (1989b) Benign childhood epilepsy with occipital paroxysms. A 15 year prospective study. *Annals of Neurology*, **26**, 51–6.

Panayiotopoulos, C.P. and Igoe, D.M. (1992) Cerebral insult-like partial status epilepticus in the early-onset variant of benign childhood epilepsy with occipital paroxysms. *Seizure*, **1**, 99–102.

Panayiotopoulos, C.P. (1993a) Benign childhood partial epilepsies: benign childhood seizure susceptibility syndrome. *Journal of Neurology, Neurosurgery, and Psychiatry*, **56**, 2–5.

Panayiotopoulos, C.P. (1993b) Benign childhood epilepsy with occipital paroxysms, in *Occipital Seizures and Epilepsies in Children* (eds F. Andermann, A. Beaumanoir, L. Mira *et al.*), John Libbey, London, pp. 151–64.

Petersen, J., Nielsen, C.J. and Gulmann, N.C. (1983) Atypical EEG abnormalities in children with benign partial (rolandic) epilepsy. *Acta Neurologica Scandinavica*, **67** (suppl.), 57–62.

Piccirilli, M., D'Alessandro, P., Tiacci, C. and Ferroni, A. (1988) Language lateralization in children with benign partial epilepsy. *Epilepsia*, **29**, 19–25.

Plasmati, R., Michelucci, R., Forti, A. *et al.* (1992) The neurophysiological features of benign partial epilepsy with rolandic spikes, in *Benign Localized and Generalized Epilepsies of Early Childhood* (*Epilepsy Research* suppl.6) (eds R. Degen and F.E. Dreifuss), Elsevier, Amsterdam, pp. 45–8.

Roger, J. and Bureau, M. (1992) Benign epilepsy of childhood with occipital paroxysms. Up-date, in *Epileptic Syndromes in Infancy, Childhood and Adolescence* (eds J. Roger, M. Bureau, Ch. Dravet *et al.*) John Libbey, London pp. 205–15.

Roger, J., Bureau, M., Genton, P. and Dravet, C. (1990) Idiopathic partial epilepsies, in *Comprehensive Epileptology* (eds M. Dam and L. Gram), Raven Press, New York, pp. 155–70

Roulet, E., Deonna, T. and Despland, P. A. (1989) Prolonged intermittent drooling and oromotor dyspraxia in benign childhood epilepsy with centro-temporal spikes. *Epilepsia*, **30**, 564–8.

Santanelli, P., Bureau, M., Magaudda, A. *et al* (1989) Benign partial epilepsy with centro-temporal (or rolandic) spikes and brain lesion. *Epilepsia*, **30**, 182–8.

Santucci, M., Giovanardi Rossi, P., Ambrosetto, G. *et al.* (1985) Migraine and benign epilepsy with rolandic spikes in childhood: a case-control study. *Developmental Medicine and Child Neurology*, **27**, 60–2.

Septien, L., Pelletier, J.L., Brunotte, F. *et al.* (1991) Migraine in patients with history of centro-temporal epilepsy in childhood: a Hm-PAO SPECT study. *Cephalalgia*, **11**, 281–4.

Talwar, D., Rask, C.A. and Torres, F. (1992) Clinical manifestations in children with occipital spike-wave paroxysms. *Epilepsia*, **33**, 667–4.

Terasaki, T., Yamatogi, Y. and Ohtahara, S. (1987) Electroclinical delineation of occipital lobe epilepsy in childhood, in *Migraine and Epilepsy* (eds F. Andermann and E.Lugaresi), Butterworth, London, pp. 125–37.

Terzano, M.G., Manzoni, G.C. and Parrino, L. (1987) Benign epilepsy with occipital paroxysms and migraine: the question of intercalated attacks, in *Migraine and Epilepsy* (eds F. Andermann and E. Lugaresi), Butterworths, Boston, London, pp. 83–96.

van der Meij, W., Wieneke, G.H. and van Huffelen, A. C. (1993) Dipole source analysis of rolandic spikes in benign rolandic epilepsy and other clinical syndromes. *Brain Topography*, **5**, 203–13.

Vivegano, F. and Ricci, S. (1993) Benign occipital epilepsy of childhood with prolonged seizures and autonomic symptoms, in *Occipital Seizures and Epilepsies in Children* (eds F. Andermann, A. Beaumanoir, L. Mira *et al.*). London: John Libbey, London, pp. 133–40.

Watanabe, K. (1989) The localization related epilepsies: some problems with subclassification. *Japanese Journal of Psychiatry and Neurology*, **43**, 471–5.

Weinberg, H., Wong, P.K.H., Crisp, D. *et al.* (1990) Use of multiple dipole analysis for the classification of benign rolandic epilepsy. *Brain Topography*, **3**, 183–90.

Wong, P.K.H. (1989) Stability of source estimates in rolandic spikes. *Brain Topography*, **2**, 31–6.

Yoshinaga, H., Amano, R., Oka, E., and Ohtahara, S. (1992) Dipole tracing in childhood epilepsy with special reference to rolandic epilepsy. *Brain Topography*, **4**, 193–9.

Thierry Deonna

INTRODUCTION

In many forms of epilepsy, cognitive functions are altered during the seizure itself, the postictal state, and, sometimes, during what is thought to be the normal interictal period. However, for these the cognitive dysfunction is only one amongst other epileptic manifestations and is not recognized or considered the main symptom.

Epilepsies with 'cognitive' symptomatology can be defined as those epilepsies which manifest their effects mainly or exclusively in the cognitive sphere. This means that the cognitive disturbance is the seizure itself, with no other visible epileptic manifestations apart from the altered mental state. In reality, subtle signs may occur, such as brief twitches, changes in posture or color, pupillary dilatation, etc., but these are not the main part of the seizure. It is thus somewhat arbitrary to draw a firm line in the definition of what constitutes a 'cognitive' seizure, and also to separate cognitive from 'affective' epileptic manifestations.

Behavioral disturbances can probably also be the main or only epileptic symptom if the brain systems involved in social behavior and control of emotions are primarily involved in the epileptic process, although this is a much more complex and delicate issue (Gillberg and Schaumann, 1983; Chapter 25). What is certain, however, is that any acquired disruption of cognitive function will have negative consequences on emotional or social behavior, particularly in younger children, so that affective disturbances are often the earliest and, for some time, the only, recognizable manifestation of epilepsy.

In some children with a newly diagnosed 'typical' epilepsy, it is not exceptional to see a rapid unexpected and marked improvement of long-standing behavioral or cognitive problems with the introduction of antiepileptic therapy. These cases suggest an associated direct cognitive effect of epilepsy occurs more often than is usually acknowledged, since one can blame neither the psychologic consequences of the diagnosis of epilepsy nor the side-effects of treatment in these situations.

THE CONCEPT OF COGNITIVE EPILEPSIES

The recognition that specific cognitive and/or behavioral disturbances can be epileptic manifestations requires a drastic conceptual change from the seizures that clinicians usually consider as epileptic.

The nature and organization of higher cortical functions, especially in the developing child, call for another analysis of epileptic symptoms and one must introduce a different time dimension in their evaluation.

Often it is not possible to recognize the typical rapid, paroxysmal change and recovery of function and show clear-cut clinical–EEG

Epilepsy in Children. Edited by Sheila Wallace. Published in 1996 by Chapman & Hall, London. ISBN 0 412 56860 8

correlations, as in usual epileptic manifestations. Frequently, the episodic nature of symptoms, considered characteristic of epilepsy, is not immediately apparent. The clinical disturbances must sometimes be measured in days or weeks, and, in special situations, possibly months or years.

A gradual loss of cognitive functions, arrest or regression in development or a behavioral disorder may thus be the presenting problem with few or no hints of its epileptic origin.

From the electroencephalographic point of view, it must be realized that large parts of the brain which are important for behavior and cognition, such as the temporal and frontal lobes, are far from the brain surface, so that the scalp EEG may be normal, even during clinical seizures. On the other hand, paroxysmal 'epileptic' EEG abnormalities can be found in normal children, or in different pathologic situations, without obvious correlations with the clinical problem.

In this difficult situation, some clinicians remain sceptical about the concept of 'cognitive' epilepsies and legitimately fear the risk of making an unprovable diagnosis with unwarranted practical implications.

This discussion aims to show that there is a need to face the problem and suggests some possible advances in this domain.

COGNITIVE EPILEPSIES IN THE CONTEXT OF MODERN EPILEPTOLOGY

Temporary cognitive disturbances can be due either to focal epileptic discharges in brain areas which mediate a particular cognitive or behavioral function, or to generalized discharges which interfere with more global aspects of mental function (vigilance, execution). The observed deficit corresponds either to the ictal or to the postictal phase. In fact, prolonged cognitive epileptic deficits are probably the consequence of recurrent seizures with prolonged and repeated postictal deficits, with incomplete recovery of function between episodes, rather than true status epilepticus. It is logical to consider that frequent recurrent epileptic discharges in brain areas involved with complex developing mental functions can lead to more lasting consequences on cognition and behavior, without implying a true persistent status epilepticus.

There are two reasons why it is difficult to find these situations in textbooks on epilepsy. Firstly, complex mental symptoms are put on the same conceptual level as simple sensory and motor phenomena, and secondly, any prolonged epileptic manifestation is considered status epilepticus.

The best known of these purely or mainly cognitive manifestations of epilepsy is the **nonconvulsive status epilepticus**. This corresponds to a prolonged alteration of the mental state with continuous or subcontinuous generalized spikes or spike-wave discharges on the EEG. The prototype is the 'absence status' ('petit mal status', 'spike-wave stupor', 'minor epileptic status') (Andermann and Robb, 1972; Manning and Rosenbloom, 1987; see also Chapter 18). In these situations, there is clouding of awareness, but presumably no specific cognitive deficit. Apathy, drowsiness, slowness, inattention, perplexity, strange affect, amnesia, and slow speech are the most obvious abnormal behaviors. It is not clear how much higher-level mental functions are truly preserved and what new memories can be formed during these episodes, because this is virtually never studied in detail. In **complex partial status epilepticus**, only limited purposeful organized activity and responses to outside stimuli are possible and there is usually a total amnesia for the period. The epileptic nature of the disorder is recognized by the presence of automatic motor behavior and vegetative phenomena, although this aspect may be subtle (McBride, Dooling and Openheimer, 1981; Engel, Lufwig and Fetell, 1986).

The cognitive epileptic manifestation which can be considered the 'minimal' cognitive seizure is the **transient cognitive impairment** (so-called 'TCI') observed during electroencephalographic epileptic discharges in children who have otherwise no recognizable clinical sign of seizure activity. It corresponds to a decrease or loss of efficiency of performance during the actual discharge (Aarts *et al.*, 1984; Binnie and Marston, 1992). Such immediate correlation can be achieved only in older cooperative children and is limited to the simple level cognitive processes at work during these brief time intervals (Chapter 24).

Responses to verbal as opposed to non-verbal stimuli are affected differently by left-versus right-sided discharges. From these data, it is possible to extrapolate that other specific cognitive functions can be interfered with by focal 'subclinical' EEG discharges. This notion has important implications (Kasteleijn-Nolst Trénité *et al.*, 1990; Binnie and Marston, 1992).

The cases in which a prolonged specific cognitive or behavioral deficit constitutes the epileptic manifestation are less well recognized. The recently introduced terms of **cognitive status** or **behavioral status** probably refer to some of these situations, although the physiopathology may be different from the classic status epilepticus (Brown and Hussain, 1991).

Various forms of aphasia, apraxia, frontal lobe dysfunction, visuospatial disability, or a selective memory deficit have been reported, although precise detailed observations of these situations in children are rare (Deonna, Fletcher and Voumard, 1982; Matsuoka *et al.*, 1986; Deonna, Cherrie and Hornung, 1987; Boone *et al.*, 1988; Jambaque and Dulac, 1989; Deonna *et al.*, 1993b).

The syndrome of acquired epileptic aphasia (AEA; or Landau–Kleffner syndrome) and dementia with continuous spike-waves during slow wave sleep (DCSWS) deserves a special place in this discussion of cognitive epilepsies (Boel and Casaer, 1989; Hirsch *et al.*, 1990; Deonna, 1991; Roulet-Perez *et al.*, 1993).

These disorders are often progressive and insidious with devastating effects on cognition (language, thinking) and/or behavior, although the children generally have few or sometimes no 'classic' seizures. I.e. the 'visible' seizure disorder is usually 'benign' in conventional terms. No consistent focal brain lesion has been demonstrated and the diagnosis rests on the presence of severe persistent (although fluctuant) focal paroxysmal EEG changes.

This very special situation has led to different and opposite physiopathologic hypotheses, particularly of AEA, which has been studied in more detail. One suggestion is that the abnormal EEG discharges are epiphenomena of a, so far unknown, underlying encephalopathy. Another postulates simply the presence of a secondary focal epilepsy with aphasic symptomatology; a view supported by recent reports of children diagnosed as having AEA, in which various brain lesions (tumor, encephalitis) were found in language areas. A prolonged aphasia can certainly result from a severe focal lesional epilepsy in relevant brain areas (not always seen on brain imaging, e.g. a small focal dysplasia), but the physiopathology of the epilepsy in AEA is probably different.

There are many clinical and EEG similarities between AEA (and DCSWS) and some genetically determined epileptic syndromes, mainly the benign partial epilepsies (Doose, 1989; Doose and Bayer, 1989; Deonna *et al.*, 1993a); in most cases which have been thoroughly studied, no brain lesion has been demonstrable. Clinical data and new evidence drawn from electrophysiologic studies and functional imaging (Hirsch *et al.*, 1990; Maquet *et al.*, 1990) together suggest that the cognitive and behavioral abnormalities are directly related to this particular epileptic dysfunction, which affects specific cortical areas during development and is different, although this is ill-understood, from the usual lesional focal epilepsies (Deonna, 1991; Roulet *et al.*, 1991).

METHODOLOGIC PROBLEMS

Ideally, in order to document and prove beyond doubt the effects of the epileptic activity per se on mental functioning, it is necessary to test the child during and after the episodes suspected to be cognitive ictal or postictal manifestations and show a direct correlation with EEG changes and treatment. Then, the child is his own control. The multiple variables which in group studies usually prevent evaluation of the direct role of epilepsy can thus be excluded (Bourgeois *et al.*, 1983; Besag, 1987; Deonna, 1993). In order to determine which aspects of mental functions are affected during a suspected cognitive seizure (negative symptoms), inter-action with, and not only observation of, the child is necessary. Such systematic studies are difficult to plan (Gloor, 1991). Children certainly do have positive symptoms such as hallucinations, recalled events or acute emotional states (fear, ecstasy). In the adult these can be clearly perceived as abnormal, but the reactions of children may be different: they are usually either unable or unwilling to describe these experiences and such infor-mation as is obtained can only be an under-estimate. Sometimes the behavior of a child who is 'concentrated' on some bizarre sensa-tions, which are being experienced or causing fear, may be interpreted as an absence or a panic reaction.

The practical and methodologic problems of cognitive and behavioral asessment in children who are often 'noncooperative' or 'untestable' and who need repeated EEGs are enormous. In order to document significant changes, it is essential to evaluate the child when he/she is at his/her best and at his/her worst, which is not the period that parents might intuitively think is the most appropri-ate. The emotional reaction of the child to the whole situation may also limit his/her co-operation, but should not prevent attempts at assessment.

These difficulties explain why convincing observations of cognitive epilepsy are only exceptionally found in the literature.

In some special situations, such as the syndrome of acquired epileptic aphasia and dementia with continuous spike-waves during sleep (see above), the epilepsy manifests itself with periods of fluctuating cognitive regres-sion over long periods which are easier to study in a planned manner.

FEATURES SUGGESTIVE OF COGNITIVE SEIZURES

Firstly, it is important to accept that clear-cut paroxysmal clinical changes cannot always be documented, that subtle associated seizures, especially in very young children, are very difficult to diagnose, and that EEG changes are variable and often not conclusive.

The possibility that cognitive seizures are the cause of an acquired learning or behavior disorder may be raised in different contexts. For example, cognitive symptomatology may present in a normally intelligent child with epilepsy, without other previous problems or in a child with symptomatic epilepsy and a fixed cognitive deficit related to the basic underlying pathology. Finally, the cognitive dysfunction may be the first manifestation of the epileptic disease which is not yet recog-nized.

Some features of the history can be sug-gestive of cognitive seizures. Frequent mood changes ('good boy or bad boy'), fluctuating attention, forgetfulness, uneven memory skills ('sometimes forgets everything'), vari-able school results, uneven speed of perform-ance, transient failures in specific domains are sometimes reported by parents and teachers of affected children and are useful hints. Although none of these complaints is specific, their combination and usually, un-explained, sudden occurrence and recurrence can be very suggestive of an unrecognized cognitive seizure interfering with vigilance, attention, or with more specific functions, such as language or memory. Sometimes, the changes resemble those already seen by the parents in the postictal state of previous more clear-cut episodes, and thus can be identified as probable epileptic manifestations. In school children with epilepsy, who must continuously acquire new information, failure to encode, store and consolidate newly formed memories during or after seizures is probably an underscored cause of learning problems. This is particularly likely to occur during occult nocturnal episodes or in children with seizures affecting the limbic areas.

Transient memory impairment as the sole manifestation of a complex partial seizure, known in adults as 'epileptic amnesic attacks' (Galassi *et al.*, 1993), could easily go unrecognized in children, who may not consciously realize the significance of a temporary failure of memory.

It is easy to misinterpret the causes for these fluctuations in behavior or performance. Firstly, one can often find psychologic explanations or blame the antiepileptic therapy, without looking further. Secondly, a long delay may exist between the onset of the cognitive or behavior problem and the diagnosis of epilepsy, during which many psychologic and other reasons can be found to account for the changes. Cognitive seizures must also be considered in children with chronic learning disabilities or behavior disorders secondary to cerebral insults. A recent study in children with congenital hemiplegias suggests that epilepsy can be responsible for or aggravate the chronic cognitive disturbances usually attributed to the basic focal lesion. Such data, and the recently demonstrated possible effects of 'subclinical' focal EEG discharges on cognition, emphasize that close attention should be paid to the possible negative role of epilepsy or paroxysmal EEG discharges on cognitive function in these situations (Varga-Khadem *et al.*, 1992). However, it must be acknowledged that is very difficult to show that fluctuating performances, or regression in a domain which is already weak, can be due to an additional direct effect of epilepsy.

PITFALLS AND PROBLEMS OF TREATMENT OF COGNITIVE EPILEPSIES

The confirmation that a child indeed has cognitive seizures may come from the spectacular results of an antiepileptic drug trial, which may be exceptionally justified in such situations, before the diagnosis is absolutely certain.

Except in the rare cases with an immediate improvement with antiepileptic drugs, the therapy in 'cognitive' epilepsies carries as many difficulties as the diagnosis and deserves special comments. Improvement cannot always be expected to occur more or less immediately. Some time has to be allowed for the effect of treatment to be judged. A clear-cut chronologic correlation between cognitive improvement and change in epileptic activity (as measured by EEG and drug effect) can rarely be demonstrated.

The lack of immediate cognitive or behavior improvement, or even a worsening of symptoms, is often taken as evidence that epilepsy is not the cause of the cognitive symptoms. Such illogical reasoning has often dissuaded clinicians from further drug trials and has probably delayed progress in the recognition of these cognitive epilepsies.

The behavior side-effects noted in the occasional child given any antiepileptic drug may be especially marked when the basic epileptic symptom precisely affects mental functions.

A global cognitive and behavior worsening could also be associated with an increase in the number of seizures, or due to the onset of a new seizure type, as seen in other epilepsies when inappropriate drugs are used. A dissociation between cognitive and behavior responses to treatment is sometimes seen, with the effect being wrongly perceived as globally negative, i.e. the child becomes more difficult to handle, even though he/she is catching up in the cognitive domain.

Prolonged drug trials of uncertain benefit are sometimes necessary; these carry the risk of excessive focusing on the medical management of the child, and reduced attention to the associated educational and psychologic problems. These latter aspects are clearly very important, regardless of the immediate and long-term direct consequences of the epileptic discharges on brain function. Indeed, the child functions with a brain of uncertain and variable efficiency, a situation which has major psychologic consequences.

DEVELOPMENT DISORDERS: THE ROLE OF EPILEPSY

The possibility that epilepsy has a direct causal role in some children who have development disorders, such as developmental dysphasia or autistic disorders and associated clinical seizures (or paroxysmal EEG discharges), is now increasingly considered (Olsson, Steflenberg and Gillberg, 1988; Echenne *et al.*, 1992; Deonna *et al.*, 1993c).

Firstly, experimental data in animals show that focal epileptic discharges early in development can modify the structural development of the brain (Baumbach and Chow, 1981). This suggests that some early-onset epilepsies probably have a negative effect on cognitive development. Secondly, a focal epileptic dysfunction involving a part of the developing cerebral cortex, which mediates a particular cognitive function at a given age, level of experience, and learning, can be expected to produce an aberrant, non-development or loss of that function, regardless of, or in addition to, the effects of any underlying permanent lesion. Considering the variable and uncertain age at onset of the epilepsy, its duration and severity, and the level of commitment of the area (areas) involved by the epileptic process, clear corre-

lations between location (side and site within one hemisphere) of epileptic foci and clinical symptoms would not be expected. The consequences of focal fixed brain lesions sustained prenatally or very early after birth remain very difficult to predict (Bates, Thal and Janowsky, 1992). The situation may be even more complex with focal prolonged but intermittent epileptic dysfunction.

Infantile spasms with hypsarrhythmia (West's syndrome) is the most striking example of the cognitive and behavior consequences of early epilepsy (Chapter 11b). West's syndrome can be seen as a potentially reversible 'epileptic' dementia (Guzzetta *et al.*, 1993). In this situation, cognitive and or behavior changes usually occur before the motor manifestations, and sometimes are the only sign of the disease.

In some children with dysphasia or autism with epilepsy or particular patterns of EEG abnormalities, particularly those who show a stagnation, fluctuation or regression after early normal development, there are several arguments suggesting a direct role of epilepsy (Gesell and Amatruda, 1974; Maccario *et al.*, 1982; Echenne *et al.*, 1992; Deonna *et al.*, 1993c).

At the moment, there are more hypotheses than facts in this domain. However, by extrapolating data obtained in older children with 'cognitive' epilepsies, and knowing the difficulties in diagnosis of subtle seizures in very young children and the limitations of surface EEG recordings, the role of epilepsy may be underestimated (Minshew, 1991).

REFERENCES

Aarts, H.P., Binnie, C.D., Smit, A.M. and Wilkins, A.J. (1984) Selective cognitive impairment during focal and generalized epileptiform EEG activity. *Brain*, **107**, 293–308.

Andermann, F. and Robb, J.P. (1972) Absence status: a reappraisal following review of 38 patients. *Epilepsia*, **13**, 177–87.

Bates, E., Thal, D. and Janowsky, J.J. (1992) Early language development and its neural correlates, in *Handbook of Neuropsychology*, vol. 7, (eds S.J. Segalowitz and I. Rapin), Elsevier, Amsterdam, p. 94.

Baumbach, H.D. and Chow, K.L. (1981) Visuo-cortical epileptiform discharges in rabbits: differential effects on neuronal development in the lateral geniculate nucleus and superior colliculus. *Brain Research*, **209**, 61–76.

Besag, F.M.C. (1987) Cognitive deterioration in children with epilepsy, in *Epilepsy, Behaviour and Cognitive Function*, (eds M. Trimble and E. Reynolds), John Wiley, Chichester, pp. 113–27.

Binnie, C.D. and Marston D. (1992) Cognitive correlates of interictal discharges. *Epilepsia*, **33**(suppl. 6), S11–7.

Boel, M. and Casaer, P. (1989) Continuous spikes and waves during slow wave sleep: a 30 months follow-up study of neuropsychological recovery and EEG findings. *Neuropediatrics*, **20**, 176–80.

Boone, K.B., Miller, B.L., Rosenberg I. *et al.* (1988) Neuropsychological and behavioral abnormalities in an adolescent with frontal lobe seizures. *Neurology*, **38**, 583–6.

Bourgeois, B., Prensky, Y., Palkes, H.S. *et al.* (1983) Intelligence in epilepsy: a perspective in children *Annals of Neurology* **14**, 438–44.

Brown, J.K. and Hussain, I.H.M.I. (1991) Status epilepticus: pathogenesis. *Developmental Medicine and Child Neurology*, **33**, 3–17.

Deonna, T. (1991) Acquired epileptiform aphasia in children. *Journal of Clinical Neurophysiology*, **8**, 288–98.

Deonna, T. (1993) Annotation: cognitive and behavioral correlates of epilepsy in children. *Journal of Child Psychology and Psychiatry*, **34**, 611–20.

Deonna, T., Fletcher, P. and Voumard, C. (1982) Temporary regression during language acquisition: a linguistic analysis of a 2½ year-old child with epileptic aphasia. *Developmental Medicine and Child Neurology*, **24**, 156–63.

Deonna, T., Chevrie, C. and Hornung, E. (1987) Childhood epileptic speech disorder: prolonged isolated deficit of prosodic features. *Developmental Medicine and Child Neurology*, **29**, 100–5.

Deonna, T., Roulet, E., Fontan, D. *et al.* (1993a) Prolonged speech and oromotor deficits of epileptic origin in benign partial epilepsy with rolandic spikes: relationship to acquired epileptic aphasia. *Neuropediatrics*, **24**, 83–87.

Deonna, T., Davidoff, V., Despland, P.A. *et al.* (1993b) Isolated disturbance of written language acquisition as an initial symptom of epileptic aphasia in a 7 year old girl. *Aphasiology*, **7**, 441–50.

Deonna, T, Ziegler, A.L., Moura-Serra, J. and Innocenti, G. (1993c) Autistic regression in relation to limbic pathology and epilepsy: report of 2 cases. *Developmental Medicine and Child Neurology*, **35**, 166–76.

Doose, H. (1989) Symptomatology in children with focal sharp waves of genetic origin. *European Journal of Pediatrics*, **149**, 210–5.

Doose, H. and Baier, W.K. (1989) Benign partial epilepsy and related conditions: multifactorial pathogenesis with hereditary impairment of brain maturation. *European Journal of Pediatrics*, **149**, 152–8.

Echenne, B., Cheminal, R., Rivier, F. *et al.* (1992) Epileptic encephalopathic abnormalities and developmental dysphasias: a study of 32 patients. *Brain and Development*, **14**, 216–25.

Engel J., Lufwig, B.I. and Fetell, M. (1986) Prolonged partial complex status epilepticus: EEG and behavioral observations. *Neurology*, **28**, 863–9.

Galassi, R., Morreale, A., Di Sarro, R. and Lugaresi, E. (1993) Epileptic amnesic syndrome. *Epilepsia*, **33** (suppl. 6), S21–5.

Gesell, A. and Amatruda C. (1974) Developmental diagnosis, in *Autistic, Psychotic and Other Disturbed Behavior*, Harper & Row, London, pp. 321–38.

Gloor, P. (1991) Neurobiological substrates of ictal behavioral discharges. *Advances in Neurology*, **55**, 1–34.

Gillberg, C. and Schaumann, H. (1983) Epilepsy presenting as infantile autism? Two case studies *Neuropediatrics*, **14**, 206–12.

Guzzetta, F., Crisafulli, A. and Isaya Crine, M. (1993) Cognitive assessment of infants with West syndrome. How useful in diagnosis and prognosis? *Developmental Medicine and Child Neurology*, **35**, 379–87.

Hirsch, E., Marescaux, C., Maquet, P. *et al.* (1990) Landau–Kleffner syndrome: a clinical and EEG study of 5 cases. *Epilepsia*, **31**, 768–77.

Jambaque, I. and Dulac, O. (1989) Syndrome frontal réversible et épilepsie chez un enfant de 8 ans. *Archives Françaises de Pediatrie*, **46**, 525–9.

Kasteleijn-Nolst Trénité, D.G.A. Siebelink, B.M., Berends S.G.C. *et al.* (1990) Lateralized effects of subclinical epileptiform discharges on scholastic performance in children. *Epilepsia*, **31**, 740–6.

McBride, M.C., Dooling, E.C. and Oppenheimer, E.H. (1981) Complex partial status epilepticus in young children. *Annals of Neurology*, **9**, 526–30.

Maccario, M., Hefferen, S.J., Keblusek, S.J. and Lipinski, K.A. (1982) Developmental dysphasia and electroencephalographic abnormalities. *Developmental Medicine and Child Neurology*, **24**, 141–55.

Manning, D.J. and Rosenbloom, L. (1987) Non-convulsive status epilepticus. *Archives of Disease in Childhood*, **62**, 37–40.

Maquet, P., Hirsch, E., Dive, D. *et al.* (1990) Cerebral glucose utilization during sleep in Landau–Kleffner syndrome. *Epilepsia*, **31**, 778–83.

Matsuoka, H., Okuma, T., Uen, T. and Saito, H. (1986) Impairment of parietal cortical functions associated with episodic prolonged spike-wave discharges. *Epilepsia*, **27**, 432–6.

Minshew, J.N. (1991) Indices of neural function in autism: clinical and biological implications. *Pediatrics*, **87** (suppl. 1), 775–80.

Olsson, I., Steffenburg, S. and Gillberg, C. (1988) Epilepsy in autism and autistic-like conditions. A population-based study. *Archives of Neurology*, **45**, 666–8.

Roulet, E., Deonna, T., Gaillard, F. *et al.* (1991) Acquired aphasia, dementia and behavior disorder with epilepsy and continous spike-waves during sleep in a child. *Epilepsia*, **32**, 495–503.

Roulet-Perez, E., Davidoff, V., Despland, P.A. and Deonna, T. (1993) Mental deterioration in children with epilepsy and continuous spike-waves during sleep: acquired epileptic frontal syndrome. *Developmental Medicine and Child Neurology*, **35**, 661–74.

Varga-Khadem, F., Isaacs, E., Van Der Werf, S. *et al.* (1992) Development of intelligence and memory in children with hemiplegic cerebral palsy. The deleterious consequences of early seizures. *Brain*, **115**, 315–29.

EPILEPTIC SYNDROMES WITH ONSET IN LATE CHILDHOOD OR EARLY ADOLESCENCE

14

C. P. Panayiotopoulos

Typical absences (TA) as defined by the International League Against Epilepsy (ILAE; Commission on Classification and Terminology of the International League Against Epilepsy, 1981) are not one symptom, but a cluster of clinical features and EEG manifestations which are syndrome related (Panayiotopoulos *et al.*, 1989, 1992; Panayiotopoulos, 1994). Although, by definition, impairment of consciousness is the cardinal clinical sign and 3-Hz spike-wave EEG discharges the required bioelectrical feature, other clinical and EEG manifestations are combined in a nonfortuitous manner characterizing certain epileptic syndromes (Commission on Classification and Terminology of the International League Against Epilepsy, 1989; Panayiotopoulos *et al.*, 1989). The recently proposed hypothesis that all absences constitute a 'biological continuum' (i.e. all absences are the same disease) (Berkovic *et al.*, 1987) may be theoretically attractive and convenient but discourages the diagnostic precision required for correct treatment and prognosis (Panayiotopoulos, 1994).

There are four epileptic syndromes with typical absences recognized by the ILAE (Commission on Classification and Terminology of the International League Against Epilepsy, 1989): childhood absence epilepsy (CAE) (Chapter 13a), juvenile absence epilepsy (JAE), juvenile myoclonic epilepsy (JME) (Chapter 14b) and epilepsy with myoclonic absences (Chapter 13b). The first three (CAE, JAE, JME) are considered to be idiopathic generalized epilepsies, whilst the fourth is categorized amongst the cryptogenic/symptomatic generalized epilepsies. There may be more epileptic syndromes with TA, such as eyelid myoclonia with absences (Jeavons, 1977; Appleton *et al.*, 1993), perioral myoclonia with absences (Panayiotopoulos *et al.*, 1994), stimulus-sensitive absence epilepsies (Chapter 14d) and others awaiting further studies and confirmation.

Many of these syndromes are entirely different in presentation, severity and prognosis. Children with CAE on the whole will remit, those with myoclonic absence epilepsy will suffer or may develop mental and behavior problems, and those with JME will, in their mid-teens, develop lifelong myoclonic jerks and generalized tonic-clonic seizures. Other patients may have subtle clinical manifestations of which they are not aware during the typical 3-Hz spike-wave discharges (phantom absences; Ferner and Panayiotopoulos, 1993; Panayiotopoulos *et al.*, 1995; Giannakodimos *et al.*, 1995). Many of these patients seek medical consultation only after a generalized tonic-clonic seizure develops, probably long after the onset of absences (Panayiotopoulos *et al.*, 1995).

Video-EEG studies in which the level of impairment of consciousness is also assessed are essential to fully evaluate absences and to classify them in syndromes (Panayiotopoulos *et al.*, 1993a).

Epilepsy in Children. Edited by Sheila Wallace. Published in 1996 by Chapman & Hall, London. ISBN 0 412 56860 8

DEFINITION

JAE is broadly defined by the ILAE (Commission on Classification and Terminology of the International League Against Epilepsy, 1989) as follows:

> Onset around puberty. The absences are the same as in childhood absence epilepsy (CAE) but retropulsive movements are less common. Seizure frequency is lower than in CAE. GTCS [generalized tonic-clonic seizures] are common, occur mainly on awakening and may precede the appearance of absences. The patients may also have myoclonic jerks. The prognosis is still unclear but appears worse than CAE. The spike-wave discharge is often faster than 3 Hz. Response to therapy is excellent.

This broad definition of JAE is based mainly on the pioneer work of Doose, Volzke and Scheffner (1965), Janz (1969), and Wolf and Inoue (1984) (for review see Wolf, 1992; Porter, 1993). For Janz (1969) the main criterion for selection is age of onset (after the age of 10 years), while Doose, Volzke and Scheffner (1965) studied the nonpyknoleptic absences (i.e. absences which were not as frequent as in CAE) and found a peak of onset at 10–12 years of age. However, recent investigations with video-EEG recording techniques (Panayiotopoulos *et al.*, 1989, 1992) allow a more precise definition of JAE in which additional clinical and EEG criteria other than simply the age of onset and the frequency of seizures are utilized (Panayiotopoulos, 1994). Also, exclusion criteria appear to be important, allowing the following definition for JAE:

Juvenile absence epilepsy is an idiopathic generalized epileptic syndrome which is mainly characterized by typical absences which are manifested by abrupt and severe impairment of consciousness. In comparison with CAE, the absences of JAE show less severe impairment of cognition (activity may be restored during the ictus), occur less

frequently (1–10 per day) and are of longer duration (16 ± 7 seconds). Random and infrequent myoclonic jerks as well as infrequent generalized tonic-clonic seizures occur in the majority of the patients. However, absences are the predominant clinical feature. Age at onset of absences is between 7–16 years with a peak of 10–12 years. The ictal EEG shows generalized, spike or multiple spike and slow waves at 3 Hz (Figs 14a.1, 14a.2). JAE is a life-long disorder although there is a tendency for the absences to become less severe in terms of impairment of cognition, duration and frequency with age. Elaboration of these characteristics, and details of the exclusion criteria, are given later in this chapter.

Typical case history
An 11-year-old child had frequent (1–10 per day), brief periods of unresponsiveness lasting for 10–20 seconds, described by witnesses as 'the eyes glaze or stare and he is not with it'. There were frequent perioral and limb automatisms which varied in each absence. An EEG confirmed the diagnosis of 'absences' and the diagnosis of 'petit mal' (unsatisfactory term) or 'childhood absence epilepsy' (erroneous diagnosis) was made. Absences responded only when sodium valproate was combined with ethosuximide. Medication was slowly withdrawn after 3 seizure-free years, but a generalized tonic clonic seizure occurred half-an-hour after awakening from a short sleep compounded by the excitement of a planned trip to celebrate the end of school examinations. A video-EEG revealed absences typical of JAE and the patient admitted occasional diurnal mild jerks of the hands, mainly in the evening. Retrospective evaluation of the first EEG revealed that the ictal EEG manifestations consisted of long, 15–22 seconds, generalized discharges of multiple spike and wave at 3.5 Hz and that although the child was usually unresponsive, he could occasionally remember numbers or phrases given to him and kept his eyes closed during the ictus, i.e. ictal

JUVENILE   ABSENCE   EPILEPSY

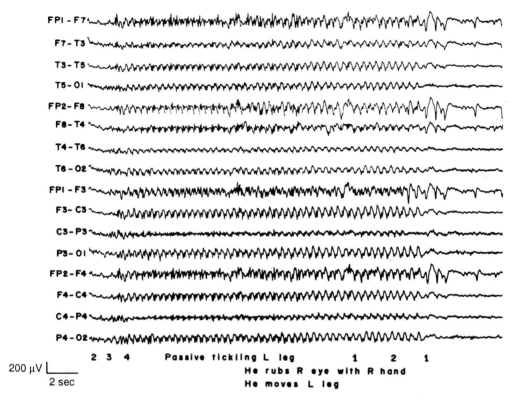

Fig. 14a.1 Video-EEG recording of a typical absence seizure from an 18-year-old patient who had frequent absences daily from age 12 years. His homozygotic twin brother also had JAE. Both brothers had infrequent generalized tonic-clonic seizures together with frequent absences. Breath-counting (annotated with numbers) stopped at the initial phase of the discharge but was resumed, in wrong sequence, 5 seconds before termination. Evoked automatisms from left leg and spontaneous from right hand occurred simultaneously. The EEG discharge is characterized by multiple spike and slow wave complexes without fragmentations. The regularity of the discharge is also apparent. (Reproduced with the permission of the Editor of *Brain* from Panayiotopoulos *et al.*, 1989.)

manifestations favoring juvenile not childhood absence epilepsy.

Reviewed at the age of 37 years, the patient is a solicitor, and has occasional absences, particularly when excited, despite adequate doses of valproate and ethosuximide. He admitted that occasional mild jerks occur randomly during the day. Two generalized tonic-clonic seizures had occurred at ages 18 and 19 years after excessive and unaccustomed alcohol drinking associated *with sleep deprivation on the first and missing his tablets on the second occasion.*

HISTORY

After the establishment of 'pyknolepsy' (an old term implying numerous absences and equated with CAE) as a separate syndrome, epileptologists observed that some older chilren had similar clinical and EEG manifestations to CAE but absences were not

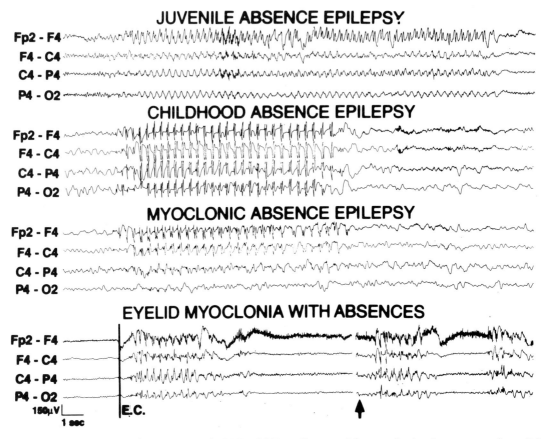

Fig. 14a.2 Video-EEG of patients with JAE, CAE, epilepsy with myoclonic absences, and eyelid myoclonia with absences (E.C. = eye-closure; the discharge following the arrow occurred while the eyes were closed). There are apparent EEG differences between these four epileptic syndromes, but the final diagnosis has to rely also on clinical manifestations during these discharges (see text). Note the long discharges of JAE as opposed to brief ones of eyelid myoclonia with absences, and multiple spikes of eyelid myoclonia with absences and epilepsy with myoclonic absences as opposed to maximum double spikes of CAE.

pyknoleptic in frequency (Janz and Christian, 1957; Doose, Volzke and Scheffner, 1965; Janz, 1969). Only recently has an attempt been made to classify JAE, not only on the basis of frequency of seizures and age of onset, but on a cluster of video-EEG-studied clinical and EEG manifestations (Panayiotopoulos *et al.*, 1989; Panayiotopoulos, 1994).

not identical for all authors. JAE is probably less common than CAE, two to three cases of which will be seen for every one of JAE (Wolf, 1992). At most 10% of adults who suffer from idiopathic generalized epilepsies with absences have JAE (Panayiotopoulos *et al.*, 1995).

PREVALENCE

The exact prevalence of JAE is not known because the criteria and the definitions are

SEX AND AGE

Both sexes are equally affected (Wolf, 1992). Absences start between 7 and 16 years with a peak at 10–12 years. Myoclonic jerks and generalized tonic-clonic seizures usually begin 1–10 years from the onset of absences. However, reports of generalized tonic-clonic seizures preceding absences have been published (Panayiotopoulos *et al.*, 1992; Wolf, 1992).

CLINICAL AND EEG MANIFESTATIONS

Typical absences are the characteristic and the predominant feature of JAE. Although the usual frequency is approximately 1–10 per day, there are cases where absences occur very many times each day (Panayiotopoulos *et al.*, 1989, 1992; Obeid, 1994). The absences show the following features:

1. Ictal clinical manifestations demonstrate profound impairment of consciousness, through it is not as severe as in CAE. Awareness, perception, responsiveness, memory and recollection are deeply but not completely disturbed, with marked variation in severity from seizure to seizure even in the same patient. Some mild awareness and responsiveness may be temporarily and inadequately maintained. Even verbal responses may occur towards the end of the discharge. Automatisms, usually perioral rather than limb, are frequent and are proportional principally to the severity of the impairment of consciousness, but also secondary to the duration of the discharges. Breath-counting during hyperventilation usually stops 3–6 seconds after the onset of the ictal discharge, but may restart, out of order, in the middle, or towards the end, of the EEG paroxysms (Fig. 14a.1). If the eyes are closed during the ictus they may remain closed or they may spontaneously open 3–7 seconds from the onset.
2. The duration of the absences is long (Figs 14a.1, 14a.2), with a mean of 16 ± 7 seconds (range of 3–29 seconds).
3. The ictal EEG discharges consist of a 3–4 Hz generalized spike and/or multiple

spike and slow wave discharge which is regular and continuous (Panayiotopoulos *et al.*, 1989). The frequency at the initial phase of the discharge should be more than 2.5 seconds. There is a gradual and smooth decline in frequency from the initial to the terminal phase. The discharge is regular, with well-formed spikes which retain a constant relation with the slow waves. The interictal EEG is normal or with mild abnormalities only.

The following ictal clinical and EEG exclusion criteria are as important as the inclusion criteria:

Ictal clinical exclusion criteria:

1. Absences with marked eyelid or perioral myoclonus or marked single or rhythmic limb and trunk myoclonic jerks.
2. Absences with exclusively mild or clinically undetectable impairment of consciousness.
3. Visual, photosensitive and other sensory precipitation of absences is against the diagnosis of JAE.

EEG exclusion criteria:

1. Irregular, arrhythmic spike/multiple spike and slow wave discharges with marked variations of the intradischarge frequency.
2. Significant variations between the spike/multiple spike and slow wave relations.
3. Predominantly brief discharges, less than 4 seconds.
4. Markedly abnormal background. Focal abnormalities, particularly as the result of abortive discharges, are accepted.

OTHER TYPES OF SEIZURES

Generalized tonic-clonic seizures occur in 80% of the patients, mainly after awakening, although nocturnal or diurnal generalized tonic-clonic seizures may also be experienced: these are usually infrequent, occurring in noncompliant patients, and often after sleep deprivation, alcohol consumption and/ or fatigue. Myoclonic jerks occur in 15–25% of the patients and are usually mild, infrequent, and of random distribution: they do not occur during the absence ictus. A patient may have all three types of generalized seizures but absences always predominate. Absence status is rare.

GENETICS

There is probably an increased incidence of epileptic disorders in families of patients with JAE (Janz, 1969; Janz, Beck-Managetta and Sander, 1992), and there are reports of identical twins with JAE (Obeid, 1994). The exact mode of inheritance has not yet been established. A multivariant linkage analysis of 25 multiplex families of probands with idiopathic generalized epilepsies (IGE) with absences (JME patients were not included) excluded the EJM1 locus for contributing to the clinical expression of IGEs in these families (Sander *et al.*, 1994).

PROGNOSIS AND TREATMENT

JAE is a lifelong disorder which is not expected to remit, although absences become less severe after the fourth decade. Therefore, although more than 70% become seizure-free with appropriate medication, which is sodium valproate alone or in combination with ethosuximide, the prognosis of JAE is not as good as in CAE. In resistant cases, small doses of lamotrigine 25–50 mg added to sodium valproate resulted in complete cessation of absences in 50% of patients (Ferrie *et al.*, 1995; Panayiotopoulos *et al.*, 1993b). Some authors have advocated the use of amantadine hydrochloride as an add-on drug in generalized epilepsies with absences (Drake *et al.*, 1991). Generalized tonic-clonic seizures and myoclonic jerks occasionally persist, even if absences are well controlled. Vigabatrin, phenytein and carbamazepine

are not indicated because they exaggerate absences. Patients should be warned regarding precipitating factors of GTCS.

DIFFERENTIAL DIAGNOSIS

JAE is easy to differentiate from syndromes with atypical absences which are mainly symptomatic or cryptogenic. However, the differentiation of JAE from other idiopathic generalized epilepsies with absences may pose considerable difficulties without appropriate video-EEG evaluation. It is not possible to diagnose one of these epileptic syndromes on the basis of an EEG with 3-Hz generalized spike and slow wave discharges, although there may be some clear indications in favor of, or against, one or other syndrome (Fig. 14a.2). A diagnosis based on the EEG alone or age at onset or frequency of absences may be convenient but does not justify the basic requirement of a syndromic classification.

In children, it is often difficult to distinguish between CAE and JAE, because features overlap and manifestations are similar. In JAE absences show less severe impairment of cognition, they are less frequent and of longer duration than in CAE. The eyes may remain closed during the ictus and the patient may restore counting or respond to commands in the final seconds before the end of the discharge (Panayiotopoulos *et al.*, 1989). Automatisms are equally prominent in both CAE and JAE. Limb myoclonic jerks (not during the absences) and/or generalized tonic-clonic seizures in the presence of severe absences, indicate JAE.

JAE is distinctly different from eyelid myoclonia with absences. The latter is characterized by brief (3–6 seconds) absences with rapid eyelid myoclonia (fast blinking-like jerks of the eyelids), together with tonic spasm and semi-opening of the eyelids and upwards deviation of the eyes, photosensitivity and an earlier age of onset than in CAE and JAE (Jeavons, 1977; Appleton *et al.*, 1993).

Similarly, JAE is easily differentiated from perioral myoclonia with absences which is characterized by rhythmic perioral myoclonia during the absences, which are rarely associated with severe impairment of cognition and are of shorter duration than in JAE. Absence status and generalized tonic-clonic seizures are common in perioral myoclonic absences (Panayiotopoulos *et al.*, 1994).

The rhythmic myoclonic movements of myoclonic absence epilepsy are characteristic.

In adolescents, the differential diagnosis may be difficult between JAE and JME. However, absences are the major problem in JAE, whereas myoclonic jerks, occurring mainly on awakening, are the main seizure type in JME.

In adults absences are often misdiagnosed as complex partial seizures (Panayiotopoulos *et al.*, 1992).

CONCLUSION

JAE is a syndrome characterized mainly by absences, imitating those of CAE, and infrequent myoclonic jerks and/or generalized tonic-clonic seizures, imitating JME. The phenotypic manifestations of JAE are intermediate between CAE and JME. Whether this is also the case in their genotypes remains to be seen (Janz, Beck-Managetta and Sander, 1992). Irrespective of this, the clinical distinction of patients with JAE from CAE and JME is essential because of the more serious prognosis.

REFERENCES

Appleton, R.E., Panayiotopoulos, C.P., Acomb, B.A. and Beirne, M. (1993) Eyelid myoclonia with typical absences: an epilepsy syndrome. *Journal of Neurology, Neurosurgery and Psychiatry*, **56**, 1312–6.

Berkovic, S.F., Andermann, F., Andermann, E. and Gloor, P. (1987) Concepts of absence epilepsies: discrete syndromes or biological continuum? *Neurology*, **37**, 993–1000.

Commission on Classification and Terminology of the International League Against Epilepsy (1981). Proposed revisions of clinical and electroencephalographic classification of epileptic seizures. *Epilepsia*, **22**, 480–501.

Commission on Classification and Terminology of the International League Against Epilepsy (1989). Proposal for classification of epilepsies and epileptic syndromes. *Epilepsia*, **30**, 389–99.

Doose, H., Volzke, E. and Scheffner, D. (1965) Verlaufsformen Kindlicher Epilepsien mit Spike-Wave-Absencen. *Arch Psychiatr Nervenkrh*, **207**, 394–415.

Drake, M.E. Jr, Pakalnis, A., Denio, L.S. and Philips, B. (1991) Amantadine hydrochloride for refractory generalised epilepsy in adults. *Acta Neurologica Belgica*, **91**, 159–64.

Ferner, R. and Panayiotopoulos, C.P. (1993) 'Phantom' typical absences, absence status and experiential phenomena. *Seizure*, **2**, 253–56.

Ferrie, C.D., Robinson, R.O., Knott, C. and Panayiotopoulos, C.P. (1995) Lamotrigine as an add-on drug in typical absence seizures. *Acta Neurologica Scandinavica*, **91**, 200–2.

Giannakodimos, S., Ferrie, C.D. and Panayiotopoulos, C.P. (1995) Quantitative abnormalities of breath counting during brief 3 Hz spike-wave 'subclinical' discharges. *Clinical Electroencephalography*, **26**, 1–4.

Janz, D. (1969) *Die Epilepsien. Spezielle Pathologie und Therapie*, Georg Thieme, Stuttgart.

Janz, D. and Christian, W. (1957) Impulsiv-Petit mal. *Journal of Neurology*, **176**, 346–86.

Janz, D., Beck-Managetta, G. and Sander, T. (1992) Do idiopathic generalised epilepsies share a common susceptibility gene? *Neurology*, **42**, (suppl. 5), 48–55.

Jeavons, P.M. (1977) Nosological problems of myoclonic epilepsies of childhood and adolescence. *Developmental Medicine and Child Neurology*, **19**, 3–8.

Obeid, T. (1994) Juvenile absence epilepsy. *Journal of Neurology*, **24**, 487–91.

Panayiotopoulos, C.P. (1994) The clinical spectrum of typical absence seizures and absence epilepsies, *Idiopathic Generalised Epilepsies* (eds A. Malafosse *et al.*), John Libbey, London, pp. 75–85.

Panayiotopoulos, C.P., Obeid, T. and Waheed, G. (1989) Differentiation of typical absences in epileptic syndromes. A video EEG study of 224 seizures in 20 patients. *Brain*, **112**, 1039–56.

Panayiotopoulos, C.P., Chroni, E., Daskalopoulos, C. *et al.* (1992) Typical absence seizures in adults: clinical, EEG, video-EEG findings and diagnostic/syndromic considerations. *Journal of Neurology, Neurosurgery and Pyschiatry*, **55**, 1002–8.

Panayiotopoulos, C.P., Baker, A., Grunewald, R. *et al.* (1993a) Breath counting during 3 Hz generalised spike and wave discharges. *Journal of Electrophysiological Technology*, **19**, 15–23.

Panayiotopoulos, C.P., Ferrie, C.D., Robinson, R.O. and Knott, C. (1993b) Interaction of lamotrigine with sodium valproate. *Lancet*, **340**, 1223.

Panayiotopoulos, C.P., Ferrie, C.D., Giannakodimos, S. and Robinson, R.O. (1994) Perioral myoclonia with absences: a new syndrome?, in *Epileptic Seizures and Syndromes* (ed. P. Wolf), John Libbey, London, pp. 143–53..

Panayiotopoulos, C.P., Giannakodimos, S. and Chroni, E. (1995) Typical absences in adults, in *Typical Absences and Related Epileptic Syndromes* (eds J.C. Duncan and C.P. Panayiotopoulos), Churchill Livingstone, London, pp. 289–97.

Porter, R.J. (1993) The absence epilepsies. A review. *Epilepsia*, **34**, (suppl. 3), S42–8.

Sander, T., Hildmann, T., Beck-Managetta, G. *et al.* (1994) Exclusion of linkage between the EJM1 locus and idiopathic generalised epilepsies in absence families, in *Idiopathic Generalised Epilepsies*, International Workshop, Le Bischenberg, Alsace, France (abstracts).

Wolf, P. (1992) Juvenile absence epilepsy, in *Epileptic Syndromes in Infancy, Childhood and Adolescence* (eds J. Roger, M. Bureau, P. Dravet *et al.*), John Libbey, London, pp. 307–12.

Wolf, P. and Inoue, Y. (1984) Therapeutic response of absence seizures in patients of an epilepsy clinic for adolescents and adults. *Journal of Neurology*, **231**, 225–9.

JUVENILE MYOCLONIC EPILEPSY

C.P. Panayiotopoulos

DEFINITION

Juvenile myoclonic epilepsy (JME) is an idiopathic generalized epileptic disorder which is hereditary. Prevalence is 5–11% amongst adult and adolescent patients with other epilepsies, and both sexes are equally affected. JME is characterized by myoclonic jerks on awakening, generalized tonic-clonic seizures, and typical absences, which occur in more than one-third of patients. The seizures have an age-related onset with absences appearing first either in childhood or adolescence followed by myoclonic jerks and generalized tonic-clonic seizures in the middle teens. All seizures are probably life-long, although absences may become less severe with age, jerks and generalized tonic-clonic seizures probably improving after the fourth decade of life. Typical absences of JME manifest with combined clinical and EEG manifestations which are distinctly different from absences of other epileptic syndromes; they are simple with mild impairment of consciousness and 3–6-Hz spike wave discharges which have an unstable intra-discharge frequency with fragmentations and multiple spikes. Seizure-precipitating factors such as sleep deprivation and fatigue, alcohol, photosensitivity, mental and psychologic arousal are prominent.

The EEG in untreated patients is usually abnormal, with generalized discharges of an irregular mixture of 3–6-Hz spike/polyspike and slow wave, with intradischarge fragmentations, unstable intradischarge frequency and no constant relations of the spikes/multiple spikes with the corresponding slow wave of the complexes. One-third of the patients show photoconvulsive responses and one-third may also have focal EEG abnormalities.

Inclusion criteria for JME:

1. Unequivocal clinical evidence of generalized seizures with myoclonic jerks on awakening. Absences, if they occur, are mild. Myoclonic jerks and generalized tonic-clonic seizures, not the absences, are the predominant seizure types.
2. No evidence of neurologic or intellectual deficit, although JME may occur in patients with such deficits caused by other, unrelated, factors.
3. Abnormal EEG in untreated patients with generalized spike and/or multiple spike-slow wave discharges. Focal or background abnormalities should be accepted if other clinical and EEG criteria are strictly justified. Normal EEGs in treated patients are common.
4. Normal brain imaging where performed.

Exclusion criteria for JME:

1. Clinical and/or EEG evidence of myoclonic jerks secondary to brain hypoxia, metabolic diseases, or other structural brain abnormalities.
2. Myoclonic jerks of other epileptic syn-

Epilepsy in Children. Edited by Sheila Wallace. Published in 1996 by Chapman & Hall, London. ISBN 0 412 56860 8

dromes clinically and/or genetically defined (i.e. Baltic-Mediteranean myoclonus, see Chapter 15a), or other epileptic syndromes such as eyelid myoclonia with absences, juvenile absence epilepsy (Chapter 14a), pure forms of photosensitive epilepsy (Chapter 14d), self-induced epilepsy.

3. Generalized seizures, tonic-clonic and/or absences without firm documentation of myoclonic jerks.

4. EEG abnormalities but no clinical evidence of any type of seizures. (Healthy members of JME families with unequivocal generalized spike/polyspike and slow wave discharges should probably be included for the purposes of genetic studies.)

Recent reviews on JME can be found in Dinner *et al.*, 1987; Janz, 1989; Wolf, 1992; Dreifuss, 1989; Penry, Dean and Riela, 1989; Grunewald and Panayiotopoulos, 1993; Janz, Wolf and Delgado-Escueta, 1994; Panayiotopoulos, Obeid and Tahan, 1994.

HISTORY

The first substantial report of a probable case of JME is by Herpin in 1867: myoclonic episodes occurring in a physician's son are described (for an English translation see Grunewald and Panayiotopoulos, 1993).

The best delineation prior to the classical description of this syndrome by Janz and Christian (1957), is by an English physician from a district general hospital who in 1949 accurately diagnosed a 16-year-old patient as suffering from 'Constitutional (i.e. Idiopathic) Myoclonic Epilepsy'.

The following is extracted from notes made in 1949:

Diagnosis: Constitutional Myoclonic Epilepsy. Illness started five years ago (age 16). He began by waking up and shaking violently until falling, but no loss of consciousness. These fits come on also in the morning on getting up, and recently have

recurred several times a week, only on working days except on one occasion; he has not infrequently bruised his head on falling; he often falls whilst walking or drops tin jug of shaving water, but is able to shave. He takes 1 and a ¼ hours from getting out from bed to leaving the house after breakfast.

The one occasion when the falling fits occurred on a Sunday was when he was cycling early to church and fell from his cycle, he felt embarrassed and went to church.

He never has falling fits by day, but he has transient losses of consciousness strongly resembling petit mal.

Phenobarbitone and various other sedations tried by local doctor were not effective.

Seen yesterday evening, half an hour later found in fit near bus stop. Readmitted. Had a major fit during the first night.

The EEG shows frequent high-voltage epileptic discharges throughout, of the type associated with Myoclonic epilepsy. These discharges are inhibited when the eyes are opened. There is no focus of abnormality, and the discharges are seen in both hemispheres without asymmetry.

A detailed description and subsequent diagnostic and therapeutic pitfalls for this didactic case have been reported elsewhere (Grunewald and Panayiotopoulos, 1994).

Janz (1969, 1973, 1985, 1989, 1991; Janz and Christian, 1957) has contributed most to the description and recognition of JME over the last 40 years, justifying the eponym 'Janz syndrome'.

Janz's comments in 1973 are of interest:

What puzzles me is that our description [of JME] has found no echo and little is heard about it, although this form of epilepsy is at least as frequent as the West syndrome or the Lennox syndrome about which many symposium are held and monographs written. I also do not understand why there is no mention of the syndrome in the international classification

PREVALENCE

The reported prevalence of JME in hospital-based clinics has increased since the syndrome was first described, from 2.7% (Janz and Christian, 1957), 4.3% (Janz, 1969) 5.7% (Tsuboi and Christian, 1973), 8.7% (Grune-wald, Chroni and Panayiotopoulos, 1992), to 10.2% (Panayiotopoulos, Obeid and Tahan, 1994). In community-based studies (Sander *et al.*, 1990), the lower reported prevalence probably reflects misdiagnosis which may improve with heightened medical awareness (Editorial, 1992).

AGE AT ONSET

The triad of absences, jerks, and generalized tonic-clonic seizures shows a characteristic age-related onset in JME (Fig. 14b.1). Absences, when a feature, begin between the ages of 5 and 16 years. Myoclonic jerks follow between 1 and 9 years later (mean, 4 years), usually around the age of 14–15 years. They rarely begin after the second decade of life,

and generalized tonic-clonic seizures usually appear a few months later, occasionally earlier, than the myoclonic jerks (Janz, 1985 1989; Delgado-Escueta and Enrile-Bacsal, 1984; Penry, Dean and Riela, 1989; Clement and Wallace, 1990; Panayiotopoulos, Obeid and Tahan, 1994). Whether a late-onset JME exists (Gram *et al.*, 1988) is doubtful.

CLINICAL SYMPTOMS

MYOCLONIC JERKS

The myoclonic jerks of JME generally appear when the patient reaches mid-teens, usually preceding the appearance of generalized tonic-clonic seizures by a few months (Janz, 1985, 1989; Dreifuss, 1989; Clement and Wallace, 1990; Editorial, 1992; Wolf, 1992; Grunewald and Panayiotopoulos, 1993; Panayiotopoulos, Obeid and Tahan, 1994). Some patients (less than 10%) with mild forms of JME never develop generalized tonic-clonic seizures, probably as the result of early diagnosis and treatment.

Myoclonic jerks characteristically occur after awakening, particularly after sleep deprivation and excessive alcohol consumption. Patients who do not demonstrate this

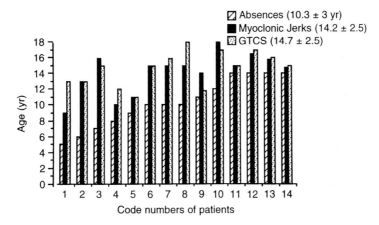

Fig. 14b.1 Age at onset of typical absences, myoclonic jerks and GTCS in 14 patients with absences, generalized tonic-clonic seizures (GTCS) and myoclonic jerks. Typical absences start long before the onset of jerks and generalized tonic-clonic seizures.

circadian pattern probably do not belong to JME but to other syndromes such as juvenile absence epilepsy (Chapter 14a).

The myoclonic jerks of JME are shock-like, irregular and arrhythmic, clonic movements of proximal and distal muscles mainly of the upper extremities, bilaterally. They are of variable amplitude and force. They are sufficiently violent to cause falls in more than half of the patients. In most patients jerks occur in the fingers, making the patient clumsy or prone to drop things unexpectedly. One-fifth of the patients describe their jerks as unilateral, probably because jerks of the dominant hand are more apparent. Video-EEG studies on these patients show that the jerks are bilateral (Fig 14b.2) (Delgado-Escueta and Enrile-Bacsal, 1984)

Consciousness is not impaired during the jerks but patients with pronounced myoclonic jerks and myoclonic status may complain of lack of awareness. This may be due either to the distress caused by the continuous jerks or most likely to absences interspersed with jerks. High-amplitude spikes/ multiple spike and slow wave discharges may occasionally terminate with a massive myoclonic jerk associated with a multiple spike discharge (Fig 14b.3). However, it should be emphasized that myoclonic jerks are independent of typical absences and do not occur during the absence ictus (Figs 14b.4–14b.8), except in the above rare circumstances.

A series of myoclonic jerks often heralds generalized tonic-clonic seizures.

TYPICAL ABSENCES

The clinical and EEG manifestations of typical absences in JME have been detailed by Panayiotopoulos, Obeid and Waheed, 1989a, 1989b; Panayiotopoulos *et al.*, 1992, 1993; Panayiotopoulos, Obeid and Tahan, 1994. They are markedly different from those of other epileptic diseases, i.e. childhood absence epilepsy (CAE) (Chapter 13a), juven-

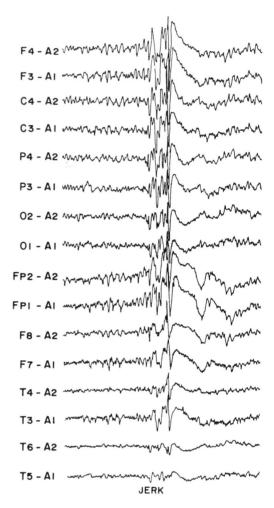

Fig. 14b.2 EEG manifestations during a bilateral myoclonic jerk. (Reproduced with permission from Panayiotopoulos *et al.*, 1994.)

ile absence epilepsy (JAE) (Chapter 14a), myoclonic absence epilepsy (Chapter 13b), eyelid myoclonia with absences, perioral myoclonia with absences (Panayiotopoulos, 1994).

The absences in JME are simple typical absences (Janz, 1969; Commission on Classification and Terminology of the International League Against Epilepsy, 1989; Panayiotopoulos, Obeid and Tahan, 1989a, 1989b), i.e. brief impairment of consciousness with 3–4-Hz spike and slow wave discharges. The

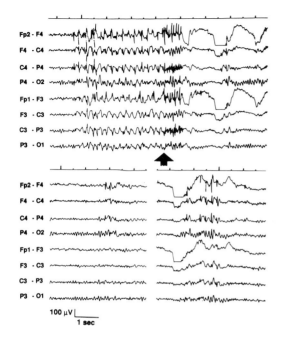

Fig. 14b.3 Video-EEG of a 37-year-old woman with JME. Generalized spike/multiple spike and slow wave discharges terminate in a myoclonic jerk (arrow). Note that the discharges show focal onset from the right.

characteristic JME patient does not jerk, does not have automatisms or other motor clinical manifestations such as eyelid or perioral myoclonia, during the absence ictus. Furthermore, and unlike CAE or JAE, impairment of consciousness is mild (subjectively perceived by the adult patients as 'momentary lack of concentration', 'like in a distance', 'tiny, little blackouts'), and the EEG discharge is characteristically different from that of CAE and JAE (Panayiotopoulos, Obeid and Waheed, 1989b; 1992). The EEG discharge of JME is frequently short and fragmented, the spike and slow wave complexes show intra-discharge frequency variations with multiple spike components (Ws) (Figs 14b.4–14b.8) and other characteristics which are different from those of CAE and JAE (Panayiotopoulos, Obeid and Tahan, 1989a, 1989b, 1994). Longer discharges with the same fragmenta-

tions and Ws as well as no apparent clinical manifestations are less common than the short discharges (Fig. 14b.7).

In our studies typical absences were found in 33.3% of patients, with a mean age at onset of 10.5 years (range 5–16 years). One-third of them appeared before the age of 10 years (Panayiotopoulos, Obeid and Tahan, 1994). Typical absences predated myoclonic jerks and generalized tonic-clonic seizures in all but two patients, who had simultaneous onset of absences and myoclonic jerks at age 16 years.

The clinical severity of absences appeared to be age related (Panayiotopoulos, Obeid and Jahan, 1989a, 1989b).

Early-onset absences (before the age of 10 years)

These are often superficially similar to those of childhood absence epilepsy. They may be pyknoleptic in frequency, with severe impairment of consciousness and occasionally with automatisms. Absences decrease in frequency and become less severe with age. There are no video-EEG studies and detailed observations on these early-onset absences in childhood before the onset of jerks and GTCS. Two of our patients had, in an early stage of their disease, EEG-recorded absences which could probably be differentiated from CAE (Panayiotopoulos, Obeid and Tahan, 1989a, 1989b). This is of significance in the early diagnosis of JME before onset of myoclonic jerks and GTCS, but has to be addressed in future prospective studies.

Late-onset absences

These are usually mild. It is exceptional for the patients to show overt interruption of mental and physical activity and there are no automatisms. Patients usually complain of brief impairment of concentration only, without disturbance of cognition or daily activity (Fig. 14b.6). The frequency of absences is

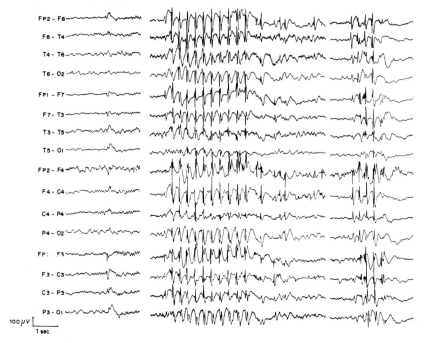

Fig. 14b.4 EEG of a 22-year-old patient. There were no apparent clinical manifestations. Note fragmentation of the discharges, multiple spike complexes (Ws), asymmetries, and frequent focal abnormalities independently right and left. (Reproduced with permission from Panayiotopoulos *et al.*, 1993b.)

difficult to assess and is usually reported by the patients as rare or 1–10 per day.

Asymptomatic absences

One-tenth of patients, predominantly males, do not admit to absences despite generalized spike–slow wave discharges lasting more than 3 seconds.

GENERALIZED TONIC-CLONIC SEIZURES

These are usually preceded by clusters of myoclonic jerks (clonic-tonic-clonic generalized seizures). In other patients, particularly those whose seizures occur in the morning after sleep deprivation and fatigue, myoclonic jerks interspersed with absences, or absences alone may herald a generalized tonic-clonic seizure. In patients on clonazepam alone, generalized tonic-clonic seizures

may be violent and not preceded by myoclonic jerks (Obeid and Panayiotopoulos, 1989). Generalized tonic-clonic seizures are more frequent on awakening, but may also occur at any other time of the day or night (Panayiotopoulos, Obeid and Tahan, 1994).

SEIZURE-PRECIPITATING FACTORS

The most powerful precipitants of jerks and generalized tonic-clonic seizures are sleep deprivation and fatigue, particularly after excessive alcohol intake (Janz, 1989; Asconapé and Penry, 1984; Delgado-Escueta and Enrile-Bacsal, 1984; Penry, Dean and Biela, 1989; Panayiotopoulos, Obeid and Tahan, 1994). Photosensitivity occurs in more than 30% of the patients (Fig. 14b.8). Mental stress, strong emotions, concentration, menstruation and, occasionally, proprioceptive stimuli are also precipitants of seizures.

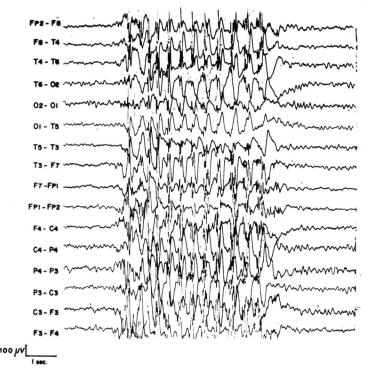

Fig. 14b.5 EEG of a 14-year-old patient with JME. There were no apparent clinical manifestations during the discharge. Note fragmentation of the discharges, multiple spike complexes (Ws), intradischarge irregularities in rhythm and spike/multiple spike–slow wave relations, i.e. features which are unlikely to occur in childhood and juvenile absence epilepsy. (Reproduced with permission from Panayiotopoulos *et al.* 1989a.)

Hyperventilation is another effective precipitant.

EEG FINDINGS

The EEG is nearly always abnormal (Figs 14b.2–14b.8) in untreated patients or in patients with inappropriate antiepileptic medication (Asconape and Penry, 1984; Delgado-Escueta and Enrile-Bacsal, 1984; Janz, 1985, 1989; Cavenini *et al.*, 1993; Aliberti, Grunewald and Panayiotopoulos, 1993; Panayiotopoulos, Obeid and Tahan, 1994; Gentou *et al.*, 1994). A normal EEG in a patient suspected of having JME should prompt an EEG on awakening. Our practice is to ask the patient to wake up at 5 a.m. and to start the EEG at 13:00 hours. This partial,

instead of all-night, sleep deprivation is preferred because of the fear of inducing generalized tonic-clonic seizures. The ideal is an all-night sleep recording extended to one hour after awakening.

In our studies, paroxysmal abnormalities were recorded in 52 out of 66 of patients; 34 (51.5%) had spike/multiple spike–slow wave discharges and 18 had brief generalized bursts of sharp theta activity with occasionally interspersed small spikes (Panayiotopoulos, Obeid and Tahan, 1994).

Morphology and characteristics of the discharges

The discharges consist of spike/double/treble or multiple spikes usually preceding or

Juvenile Myoclonic Epilepsy

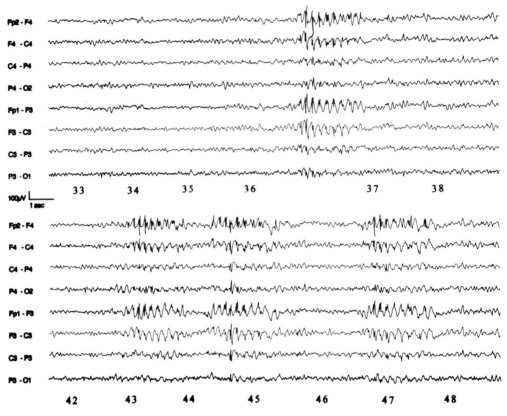

Fig. 14b.6 Video-EEG of an adult patient with JME. She counts her breaths during hyperventilation (annotated numbers). The only detectable clinical abnormality consisted of a delay in pronouncing the number 37 during one of the discharges. Note multiple spikes (Ws) and fragmentations of the discharges.

superimposed on the slow waves. Multiple spikes consist of up to eight spikes with a characteristic 'worm-like' or compressed capital W appearance ('Ws'). The number and amplitude of spikes shows considerable inter- and intra-discharge variation (Figs 14b.4–14b.8). The intra-discharge frequency of the spike/multiple spike–slow wave complexes varies from 2 to 10 Hz, mainly 3 to 5 Hz. The frequency is often higher in the first second from onset (opening phase), with no smooth decrease in frequency from the initial to the terminal phase of the discharge. Fragmentations of the discharge are common

and characteristic (Figs 14b.5–14b.7). These are transient interruptions of individual discharges, either by brief discontinuation of the spike/multiple spike complexes or abrupt changes in the dominant frequency of the discharges (Panayiotopoulos, Obeid and Waheed, 1989a, 1989b). 'Ws' and fragmentation of discharges are observed in all patients, but vary quantitatively between patients and between discharges (Figs 14b.4–14b.8). Fragmentations are more frequent in older, whilst 'Ws' are more abundant in younger patients (Figs 14b.4–14b.8).

Duration of the discharges ranges from 1

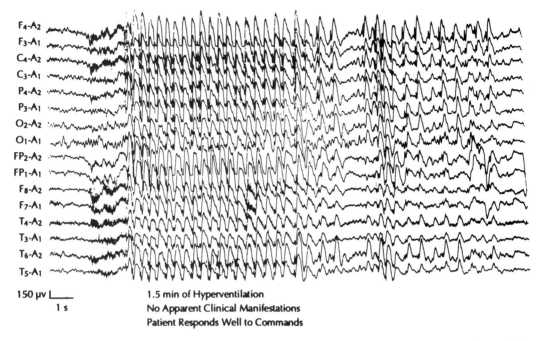

Fig. 14b.7 EEG of an adult patient with JME. A long generalized discharge of multiple spike and slow waves was not associated with apparent clinical manifestations. Note discharge fragmentations and Ws. (Reproduced with permission from Grunewald and Panayiotopoulos, 1993.)

to 20 seconds (mean ± SD = 6.8 ± 4.8 seconds) with frequent Ws and discharge fragmentations. Brief discharges are far more common than long ones (Figs 14b.4–14b.8).

Focal abnormalities are recorded in approximately one-third of patients (Figs 14b.3, 14b.4, 14b.8), of whom half have focal single spikes and spike–slow wave complexes, and half have focal slow waves consisting of sharp, medium- to high-amplitude theta or delta waves, usually independently right or left, but often with a unilateral preponderance. Focal paroxysmal abnormalities are recorded in 9% of patients. These are short transients of localized slow, sharp waves and/or spikes. Focal spikes are either independent or associated with the generalized paroxysms (preceding, following, or interspersed). The same patient may have spikes in multiple locations in the same or a previous EEG. These focal abnormalities are often misinterpreted as evidence of par-

tial seizures with secondary generalization (Aliberti, Grunewald and Panayiotopoulos, 1994).

Photoconvulsive responses (PCR) are evoked in 27% of patients (Fig. 14b.8). In 18 patients with PCR, three had all types of seizures, 13 myoclonic jerks and generalized tonic-clonic seizures, one myoclonic jerks and absences and one absences alone (Panayiotopoulos, Obeid and Tahan, 1994).

Background abnormalities consisting of a moderate excess of theta activity and/or some slowing of the alpha rhythm are recorded in 42.4% of patients.

Hyperventilation accentuates the abnormalities in all patients.

GENETICS

There is unanimous agreement that a family history of JME or other seizure disorders is common in patients with JME (Janz, 1969;

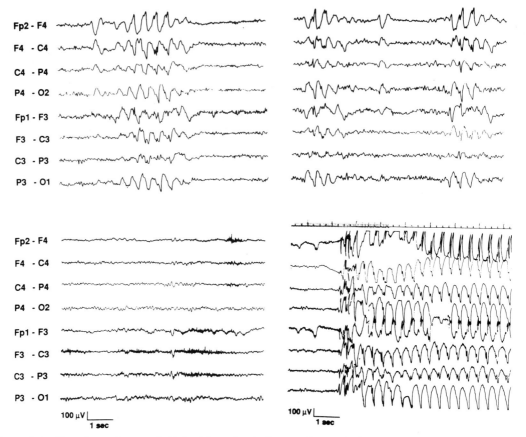

Fig. 14b.8 Female patient with JME. Note focal abnormalities of slow waves in the right anterior temporal electrode (upper traces) and sharp waves in the left anterior temporal electrode (lower left). A generalized discharge of multiple spikes and spike–slow wave at 3 Hz is elicited by intermittent photic stimulation (lower right). (Reproduced with permission from Aliberti, Grunewald and Panayiotopoulos, 1994.)

Tsuboi, 1977; Delgado-Escueta *et al.*, 1989; Janz, 1989; Cavenini *et al.*, 1993) and that in populations with high rates of consanguinity, it may be found in more than 60% (Panayiotopoulos and Obeid, 1989; Panayiotopoulos, Obeid and Tahan, 1994). Various modes of inheritance have been suggested, including polygenic with a lower manifestation threshold for females (Tsuboi, 1977), autosomal dominant with variable penetrance (Delgado-Escueta *et al.*, 1990), a two-locus model with a dominant gene on chromosome 6p and an as-yet unknown recessive gene (Greenberg *et al.*, 1990) or, most possibly, that different genotypes with different modes of inheritance underlie the phenotype (Delgado-Escueta *et al.*, 1990). A majority of families with autosomal recessive mode of inheritance and a minority of families with autosomal dominant mode of inheritance could be admixed with sporadic cases (nonhereditary or dominant new mutations) in the families studied by Delgado-Escueta *et al.* (1993). Using strict phenotypic criteria for JME, a family study in Saudi Arabia found evidence of autosomal recessive inheritance (Panayiotopoulos and Obeid, 1989).

Linkage of JME to the HLA-BF locus

(named as EJM1 locus) on the short arm of chromosome 6 was demonstrated in 34 families with JME (Greenberg *et al.*, 1988) and was replicated in separate groups of families (Weissbecker *et al.*, 1991; Durner *et al.*, 1991, 1993). However, no evidence of linkage was found in other families (Whitehouse *et al.*, 1992; Delgado-Escueta *et al.*, 1993). Genetic heterogeneity of JME is a possible explanation for such discordant observations (Delgado-Escueta *et al.*, 1993), but this has not been supported by other workers (Durner *et al.*, 1993). A possible association of JME and HLA DRW6 was reported in Caucasian (Durner *et al.*, 1992) and Arab (Obeid *et al.*, 1994) patients with JME. Further discussion of genetic aspects of JME can be found in Chapter 8.

DIAGNOSIS

THE RATE OF MISDIAGNOSIS OF JME REMAINS HIGH

We have studied the factors of error in the diagnosis of JME in 70 patients with JME in Riyadh (Panayiotopoulos, Tahan and Obeid, 1991) and 15 patients in London (Grunewald, Chroni and Panayiotopoulos, 1992), and concluded that JME was unrecognized or misdiagnosed for many years in more than 90% of the patients. Factors responsible for this situation included lack of familiarity with JME, failure to elicit a history of myoclonic jerks, misinterpretation of absences as complex partial seizures and jerks reported to be unilateral as motor partial seizures, and high prevalence of focal EEG abnormalities. Myoclonic jerks were sometimes denied by the patients or interpreted as 'nervousness' or 'shakes' in the morning, perhaps related to antiepileptic drugs or alcohol indulgence the night before.

However, the most important factor seems that physicians are not attracted to the syndromic classification of epilepsies. Most of our patients were labeled with vague diagnoses such as 'epilepsy', 'grand mal', or 'epileptic seizures'. The importance of a precise syndromic diagnosis is nowhere more apparent than in patients with JME. It enables optimization of seizure control, an accurate prognosis, probably genetic counseling, and prevents avoidable morbidity. Popular medical practice not to start treatment after the first seizure, to withdraw antiepileptic drugs after a 2–3-year seizure-free period, and to substitute valproate with carbamazepine in women anticipating pregnancy, are all inappropriate in JME (Editorial, 1992).

DIAGNOSING MYOCLONIC JERKS IN JME

Elicitation of the characteristic history of myoclonic jerks is something of an art (Editorial 1992; Panayiotopoulos, 1994). It is often necessary to physically demonstrate mild myoclonic jerks of the fingers and hands, and to enquire about morning clumsiness and tremors. Questions like 'do you spill your morning tea?', 'do you drop things in the morning?', with simultaneous demonstration of how myoclonic jerks produce this effect, may be answered positively by patients who denied myoclonic jerks on direct questioning. Further elaboration is required to confirm that clumsiness was due to genuine myoclonic jerks. If the patient reports normal hypnagogic jactitations, it is reassuring that the concept of myoclonic jerks has been understood. Diagnostic yield may be improved by emphasizing the close relation of jerks to fatigue, alcohol, and sleep deprivation. Some patients do not report their jerks, erroneously assuming that this is a self-inflicted normal phenomenon related to abuse or excess of alcohol and lack of sleep.

DIAGNOSING ABSENCES IN JME

Absences are difficult to reveal and diagnose in JME. In our studies, absence seizures had frequently been unrecognized for years or misdiagnosed as complex partial seizures

(Panayiotopoulos, Tahan and Obeid, 1991, Grunewald, Chroni and Panayiotopoulos, 1992; Panayiotopoulos *et al.*, 1992). Clinically, the absences are perceived by the patients as transient sensations of 'momentary lack of concentration', 'flashes of blackouts', 'going to a distance', 'lack of awareness', which may be misinterpreted as normal sensations; or drug induced in patients who are often overmedicated; or as complex partial seizures. De-realization and fear may be experienced infrequently (Panayiotopoulos *et al.*, 1992).

Clinicians have been trained to identify absences in their classical form, that is of a child with transient episodes of severe impairment/loss of consciousness, and are not familiar with absences in an adult whose level of awareness is not conspicuously impaired during the absence ictus. Similarly, episodes of impairment of consciousness in adults are most likely to be interpreted as complex partial seizures rather than absences.

Furthermore, absences may escape clinical detection even during conventional EEG. Current practice is to test, in an all-or-none manner, the ability of a patient to recall a phrase or number administered during a generalized spike-wave discharge, but this is often inadequate. In patients with spike-wave discharges clinical manifestations (such as slowing down of breath-counting, repetition and mistakes, stuttering) may became apparent only after careful reviews of video-EEG. It is proposed that patients with spike-wave paroxysms should be asked to count their breaths during hyperventilation (Panayiotopoulos *et al.*, 1993); this may show slowing (Fig. 14b.7), discontinuity, errors, repetition and other signs of impairment of consciousness and speech, which otherwise would escape recognition (Giannakodimos, Ferrie and Panayiotopoulos, 1994). This method is sensitive (involves concentration, memory, recollection of learned experience, expressive speech, and other cognitive func-

tions), practical (easy to perform by the patient and easy to evaluate by the observer) and is clinically relevant (reflects impairment of daily-life performance).

PROGNOSIS

Juvenile myoclonic epilepsy is a lifelong disorder but seizures are generally well controlled with appropriate medication in up to 90% of the patients (Janz 1969, 1989, 1991; Covanis, Gupta and Jeavons 1982; Delgado-Escueta and Enrile-Bacsal 1984; Penry, Dean and Riela 1989; Medical Research Council, 1991; Panayiotopoulos, Obeid and Tahan, 1994). However, it is rare for patients with JME to present with seizures after the age of 40 years, implying a decline in seizure susceptibility after the fourth decade (Panayiotopoulos, Obeid and Tahan, 1994).

TREATMENT

Patients should be warned of the common precipitants of seizures. They should be advised to avoid alcohol and to compensate for sleep deprivation caused by staying up late at night by sleeping later the next morning.

Sodium valproate is the most effective anticonvulsant (Covanis, Gupta and Jeavons, 1982; Delgado-Escueta and Enrile-Bacsal, 1984; Christe, 1989; Penry, Dean and Riela, 1989; Panayiotopoulos, Obeid and Tahan, 1994). Patients with persisting violent jerks despite control of generalized tonic-clonic seizures may benefit from the addition of small doses of clonazepam (0.5–2 mg at night) rather than further increases in the dose of valproate (Panayiotopoulos, Obeid and Tahan, 1994). Clonazepam alone may precipitate generalized tonic-clonic seizures; or, by suppressing jerks, deprive patients of the warning of an impending seizure, provided by the jerks (Obeid and Panayiotopoulos, 1989). Monotherapy with clobazam has not been evaluated.

Second-line drugs include primidone, phenobarbitone, and possibly phenytoin (Janz, 1969; Wolf, 1992). Acetazolamide has been used for treating generalized tonic-clonic seizures in cases resistant to conventional treatment, though its use may induce nephrolithiasis (Resor and Resor, 1990).

Carbamazepine is not effective in jerks and absences but its effect in generalized tonic-clonic seizures of idiopathic generalized epilepsies has not been clarified; two of our patients with JME needed carbamazepine as an add-on treatment to sodium valproate for the control of their seizures (Knott and Panayiotopoulos, 1994).

Of the new anticonvulsant drugs, lamotrigine may be effective (Ferrie, Robinson and Panayiotopoulos, 1994).

Lifelong anticonvulsant treatment is usually considered necessary in patients with JME. Withdrawal of medication in well-controlled patients may precipitate isolated seizures and status epilepticus. There is no need to replace old (phenobarbitone, primidone, or phenytoin) with newer drugs in patients who are well controlled and without adverse drug effects. In JME characterized by infrequent seizures, it may be safe to reduce the amount of medication, especially after the fourth decade of life.

In women anticipating pregnancy, the risks of discontinuing treatment with valproate usually outweigh the benefits. Pregnancy does not seem to be associated with an increase in seizure frequency, and maintenance of valproate at the lowest dose as well as prenatal examinations for possible teratogenicity are appropriate.

REFERENCES

Aliberti, B., Grunewald, R. and Panayiotopoulos, C.R. (1994) Focal electroencephalographic abnormalities in juvenile myoclonic epilepsy. *Epilepsia* (in press).

Asconapé, J. and Penry, K. (1984) Some clinical and EEG aspects of benign juvenile myoclonic epilepsy. *Epilepsia*, **25**, 108–14.

Canevini, M., Mai, R., Di Marco, C. *et al.* (1992) Juvenile myoclonic epilepsy of Janz: clinical observations in 60 patients. *Seizure*, **1**, 291–8.

Christe, W. (1989) Valproate in juvenile myoclonic epilepsy, in *Fourth International Symposium on Sodium Valproate and Epilepsy* (ed. D. Chadwick), *International Congress and Symposium Series* (ed. Lord Walton of Detchant), Royal Society of Medicine Services Limited, London, pp. 91–4.

Clement, M.J. and Wallace, S.J. (1990) Juvenile myoclonic epilepsy. *Archives of Disease in Childhood*, **63**, 1049–53.

Commission on Classification and Terminology of the International League Against Epilepsy (1989) Proposal for classification of epilepsies and epileptic syndromes. *Epilepsia*, **30**, 389–99.

Covanis, A., Gupta, A.K. and Jeavons, P.M. (1982) Sodium valproate: monotherapy and polytherapy. *Epilepsia*, **23**, 693–720.

Delgado-Escueta, A.V. and Enrile-Bacsal, F. (1984) Juvenile myoclonic epilepsy of Janz. *Neurology*, **34**, 285–94.

Delgado-Escueta, A.V., Greenberg, D.A., Treiman, L. *et al.* (1989) Mapping the gene for juvenile myoclonic epilepsy. *Epilepsia*, **30** (suppl. 4), S8–18.

Delgado-Escueta, A.V., Greenberg, D., Weissbecker, K. *et al.* (1990) Gene mapping in the idiopathic generalised epilepsies: juvenile myoclonic epilepsy, epilepsy with grand mal seizures, and early childhood myoclonic epilepsy. *Epilepsia*, **31** (suppl.3) S19–29.

Delgado-Escueta, A.V., Liu, A., Serratosa, J.M. *et al.* (1993) Juvenile myoclonic epilepsy: is there heterogeneity?, in *International Workshop on Idiopathic Generalised Epilepsies*, Alsace, France, April 22–25, 1993 (abstr).

Dinner, D.S., Luders, H., Morris, H.H. III and Leser, R.P. (1987) Juvenile myoclonic epilepsy, in *Epilepsy. Electroclinical Syndromes* (eds H. Luders and R.P. Lesser), Springer-Verlag, New York, pp. 131–69.

Dreifuss, F.E. (1989) Juvenile myoclonic epilepsy: characteristics of a primary generalised epilepsy. *Epilepsia*, **30** (suppl. 4) S1–7.

Durner, M., Janz, D., Zingsem, J. and Greenberg, D.A. (1992) Possible association of juvenile myoclonic epilepsy with HLA-DRW6. *Epilepsia*, **33**, 814–6.

Durner, M., Sander, T., Greenberg, D.A. *et al.* (1991) Localisation of idiopathic generalized epilepsy on chromosome 6p in families of juvenile myoclonic epilepsy patients. *Neurology* **41**, 1651–5

Durner, M., Greenberg, D.A., Resor, S. *et al.* (1993). Linkage data from the New York Study Group, in *International Workshop on Idiopathic Generalised Epilepsies*, Alsace, France. April 22–25, 1993 (abstr.).

Editorial (1992) Diagnosing juvenile myoclonic epilepsy. *Lancet*, **340**, 759–60.

Ferrie, C.D., Robinson, R.O., Knott, C. and Panayiotopoulos, C.P. (1994) Lamotrigine as an add-on drug in typical absence seizures. *Acta Neurologica Scandinavica*, **91**, 200–2.

Gentou, P., Salas-Puig, X., Tunon, A. *et al.* (1994) Juvenile myoclonic epilepsy and related syndromes: clinical and neurophysiological aspects, in *Idiopathic Generalised Epilepsies: Clinical, Experimental and Genetic Aspects* (eds A. Malafosse *et al.*), John Libbey, London, pp. 253–65.

Giannakodimos, S., Ferrie, C.D. and Panayiotopoulos, C.P. (1995) Quantitative abnormalities of breath counting during brief 3 Hz spike-wave 'subclinical' discharges. *Clinical Electroencephalography*, **26**, 1–4.

Gram, L., Alving, J., Sagil, J.C. and Dam, M. (1988) Juvenile myoclonic epilepsy in unexpected age groups. *Epilepsy Research*, **2**, 137–40.

Greenberg, D.A., Delgado-Escueta, A.V., Widelitz, H. *et al.* (1988) Juvenile myoclonic epilepsy may be linked to the BF and HLA loci human chromosome. *Americal Journal of Medical Genetics*, **31**, 185–92.

Greenberg, D.A., Durner, M., Delgado-Escueta, A.V. and Janz, D. (1990) Is juvenile myoclonic epilepsy an autosomal recessive disease? *Annals of Neurology*, **28**, 110–11.

Grunewald, R. and Panayiotopoulos, C.P. (1993) Juvenile myoclonic epilepsy. A review. *Archives of Neurology*, **50**, 594–8.

Grunewald, R. and Panayiotopoulos, C.P. (1994) Diagnosing juvenile myoclonic epilepsy in an elderly patient. *Seizure*, **3**, 239–41.

Grunewald, R., Chroni, E. and Panayiotopoulos, C.P. (1992) Delayed diagnosis of juvenile myoclonic epilepsy. *Journal of Neurology, Neurosurgery and Psychiatry*, **55**, 497–9.

Herpin, T.H.. (1867) *Des acces incomplets d'epilepsie*, Ballière, Paris.

Janz, D. (1969) *Die Epilepsien. Spezielle Pathologie and Therapie*, Thieme, Stuttgart.

Janz, D. (1973) The natural history of primary generalised epilepsies with sporadic myoclonias of the 'impulsive petit mal' type, in *Evolution and Prognosis of Epilepsies* (eds E. Lugaresi, P. Pazzaglia and C.A. Tassinari), pp 55–61.

Janz, D. (1985) Epilepsy with impulsive petit mal (juvenile myoclonic epilepsy). *Acta Neurologica Scandinavica*, **72**, 449–559.

Janz, D. (1989) Juvenile myoclonic epilepsy. Epilepsy with impulsive petit mal. *Cleveland Clinic Journal of Medicine*, **56** (suppl., part I), S23–33.

Janz, D. (1991) Remission and relapse in juvenile myoclonic epilepsy. *Boll Lega It Epil*, **76**, 19–28.

Janz, D. and Christian, W. (1957) Impulsive petit-mal. *Dtsch Z Nervenheilk*, **176**, 346–86. See English translation in *Idiopathic Generalised Epilepsies: Clinical, Experimental and Genetic Aspects* (eds A. Malafosse *et al.*), John Libbey, London, pp. 229–51.

Knott, C. and Panayiotopoulos, C.P. (1994) Carbamazepine in the treatment of generalised tonic clonic seizures in juvenile myoclonic epilepsy. *Journal of Neurology, Neurosurgery and Psychiatry*, **57**, 503–6.

Medical Research Council Antiepileptic Drug Withdrawal in Patients in Remission (1991) Randomised study of antiepileptic drug withdrawal in patients in remission. *Lancet*, **337**, 1175–80.

Obeid, T. and Panayiotopoulos, C.P. (1989) Clonazepam in juvenile myoclonic epilepsy. *Epilepsia*, **30**, 603–6.

Obeid, T., El Rab, M.O.G., Daif, A.K. *et al.* (1994) Is HLA-DRW13 (W6) associated with juvenile myoclonic epilepsy in Arab patients? *Epilepsia*, **35**, 319–21.

Panayiotopoulos, C.P. (1994) Juvenile myoclonic epilepsy: an underdiagnosed syndrome, in *Epileptic Seizures and Syndromes* (ed. P. Wolf), John Libbey, London, pp. 221–30.

Panayiotopoulos, C.P. (1994) The clinical spectrum of absence seizures and absence epilepsies, in *Idiopathic Generalised Epilepsies: Clinical, Experimental and Genetic Aspects* (eds A. Malafosse, P. Genton, E. Hirsch *et al.*), John Libbey, London, pp. 75–85.

Panayiotopoulos, C.P. and Obeid, T. (1989) Juvenile myoclonic epilepsy: an autosomal recessive disease. *Annals of Neurology*, **25**, 440–3.

Panayiotopoulos, C.P., Obeid, T. and Waheed, G. (1989a) Absences in juvenile myoclonic epilepsy: a clinical and video-electroencephalographic study. *Annals of Neurology*, **25**, 391–7.

Panayiotopoulos, C.P., Obeid, T. and Waheed, G. (1989b) Differentiation of typical absence seizures in epileptic syndromes. A video EEG study of 224 seizures in 20 patients. *Brain*, **112**, 1039–56.

Panayiotopoulos, C.P., Tahan, R. and Obeid, T. (1991) Juvenile myoclonic epilepsy: factors of error involved in the diagnosis and treatment. *Epilepsia*, **32**, 672–76.

Panayiotopoulos, C.P., Obeid, T. and Tahan, A.R. (1994) Juvenile myoclonic epilepsy: a 5-years prospective study. *Epilepsia*, **35**, 285–96.

Panayiotopoulos, C.P., Chroni, E., Dascalopoulos, C. *et al.* (1992) Typical absences in adults: a clinical, EEG, video-EEG study and syndromic/diagnostic considerations. *Journal of Neurology, Neurosurgery and Psychiatry*, **55**, 1002–8.

Panayiotopoulos, C.P., Baker, A., Grunewald, R. *et al.* (1993) Breath counting during 3 Hz generalised spike and wave discharges. *Journal of Electrophysiological Technology* **19**, 15–23.

Penry, J.K., Dean, J.C. and Riela, A.R. (1989) Juvenile myoclonic epilepsy: long-term response to therapy. *Epilepsia*, **30**(Suppl.4), S19–23.

Resor, S.R. Jr and Resor, L.D. (1990) Chronic acetazolamide monotherapy in the treatment of juvenile myoclonic epilepsy. *Neurology*, **40**, 1677–81.

Sander, J.W.A.S., Hart, Y.M., Johnson, A.L. and Shorvon, S.D. (1990) National General Practice Study of Epilepsy: newly diagnosed epileptic seizures in a general population. *Lancet*, **336**, 1267–71.

Tsuboi, T. (1977) *Primary Generalised Epilepsy with Sporadic Myoclonias of Myoclonic Petit Mal Type*, Thieme, Stuttgart.

Tsuboi, T. and Christian, W. (1973) On the genetics of the primary generalised epilepsy with sporadic myoclonus of impulsive petit mal type. *Human Genetik*, **b19**, 155–82.

Weissbecker, K.A., Durner, M., Janz, D. *et al.* (1991) Confirmation of linkage between juvenile myoclonic epilepsy locus and the HLA region on Chromosome 6. *Americal Journal of Medical Genetics*, **38**, 32–6.

Whitehouse, W.P., Rees, M., Sundqvist, A. and Gardiner, R.M. (1992) Linkage analysis for JME: exclusion data for chromosome 6p including HLA. *Seizure*, **1** (suppl. A), P3/20.

Wolf, P. (1992) Juvenile myoclonic epilepsy, in *Epileptic Syndromes in Infancy, Childhood and Adolescence* (eds J. Roger, M. Bureau, C. Dravet *et al.*), John Libbey, London, pp. 313–27.

C.P. *Panayiotopoulos*

INTRODUCTION

Epileptic seizures consistently occurring on awakening are common. They may occur in any form of partial or generalized, idiopathic or symptomatic seizures. By definition the syndrome of idiopathic generalized tonic-clonic seizures on awakening should be restricted to a pure form with only generalized tonic-clonic seizures which are consistently associated with the awakening phase from sleep, i.e. they occur within 1 or at a maximum 2 hours after awakening. Symptomatic and secondarily generalized tonic-clonic seizures are, by definition, excluded. Furthermore, patients who have absences or myoclonic jerks occurring with or without generalized tonic-clonic seizures on awakening should not be included, as these patients belong to other epileptic syndromes such as juvenile myoclonic epilepsy (Chapter 14b), eyelid myoclonia with absences, or juvenile absence epilepsy (Chapter 14a). Only by adhering to this strict definition of a pure form can 'epilepsy with generalized tonic clonic seizures on awakening' (EGTCSA) be clearly distinguished from other syndromes of idiopathic generalized epilepsies. However, this is a personal view and some epileptologists would propose a broader definition.

Perhaps the biggest conceptual problem in accepting this condition as a separate syndrome is that it is defined almost exclusively on a single positive feature (seizures related to awakening from sleep), which it shares with many other idiopathic generalized epilepsies.

DEFINITION

EGTCSA is classified by the International League Against Epilepsy (Commission on Terminology and Classification of the International League Against Epilepsy, 1989) amongst the idiopathic generalized epilepsies and defined as follows:

> Epilepsy with generalised tonic clonic seizures on awakening is a syndrome with onset occurring mostly in the second decade of life. The GTCS occur exclusively or predominantly (>90% of the time) shortly after awakening regardless of the time of day or in a second seizure peak in the evening period of relaxation. *If other seizures occur they are mostly absence or myoclonic, as in juvenile myoclonic epilepsy.* Seizures may be precipitated by sleep deprivation and other external factors. Genetic predisposition is relatively frequent. The EEG shows one of the patterns of idiopathic generalised epilepsy. *There is a significant correlation with photosensitivity.*

I have purposely italicized part of the above definition in the light of my introductory comments. This seems too broad a

Epilepsy in Children. Edited by Sheila Wallace. Published in 1996 by Chapman & Hall, London. ISBN 0 412 56860 8

definition, which allows excessive overlap with other idiopathic generalized epilepsies and needs revision so that only patients with the pure form of EGTCSA should be included. In addition, video-EEG studies during sleep and awakening are needed for a better understanding of EGTCSA.

CASE HISTORIES

A typical case

A 20-year-old technician presented to the accident and emergency department following a mild head injury caused by a generalized tonic-clonic seizure. This occurred at 9 a.m. as he was getting ready for work. He had been at a wedding the previous night, had become drunk and had only 2 hours sleep. Six previous generalized tonic-clonic seizures had occurred since the age of 16 years; all but one within half an hour of awakening, when he was sleep deprived and drunk. The exception was late in the afternoon while he was relaxing, watching television after a successful job interview.

His EEG, including a video-EEG during sleep and awakening, showed some brief bursts of theta activity. He complies poorly with his medication, currently phenytoin and sodium valproate, is a heavy drinker and frequently stays out late. His maternal half-sister has an interesting form of occipital lobe epilepsy with occipital photosensitivity and infrequent visual partial seizures with secondary generalization occurring mainly during sleep. His father had epileptic seizures but no more details are known.

A probable case

A Cambridge University graduate celebrated his 23rd birthday with an all-night party and many alcoholic drinks. He woke up after 2 hours sleep and within half an hour had a generalized tonic-clonic seizure. A reliable witness described no absences or jerks preceding the seizure. In the previous 4 years he had had two generalized tonic-clonic seizures on awakening under similar conditions of sleep deprivation and alcohol intake. There is no clinical evidence of myoclonic jerks or absences. He considered these episodes to be self-inflicted, and did not wish regular medication but accepted our advice to take valproate 500 mg if he felt at risk. His video-EEG after partial sleep deprivation showed, on awakening, brief, up to 3 seconds, high-amplitude discharges of 3–4-Hz small spikes and slow waves. There were no clinical manifestations during these discharges and breath-counting failed to detect any overt cognitive impairment (Fig. 14c.1).

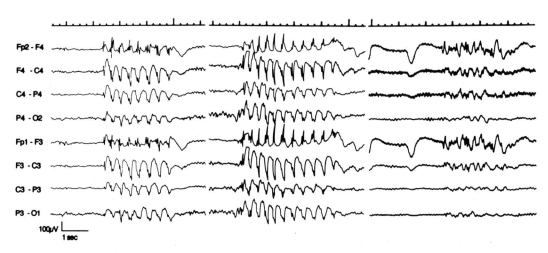

Fig. 14c.1   Video-EEGs of two probable cases of EGTCSA (see text). Generalized 3–4-Hz spike/multiple spike and slow wave discharges without overt clinical manifestations.

This case should be probably considered as EGTCSA despite EEG evidence of 'subclinical absences' (Giannakodimos, Ferrie and Panayiotopoulos, 1995).

PREVALENCE

The reported prevalence of EGTCSA varies from 0% to as high as 17% of patients with epileptic seizures. EGTCSA was not found in a community study (Manford *et al.*, 1992) where underdiagnosis may have occurred. Loiseau, Duchet and Loiseau (1991) found a prevalence of 2.1% in 570 patients of a private practice but none amongst 263 patients seen in the hospital. Schmitz and Wolf (1989) reported a prevalence of 4.6% in 699 hospital patients. Janz (1969) found 'pure' EGTCSA (i.e. generalized tonic-clonic seizures only) in 10% and 'mixed' EGTCSA (i.e. generalized tonic-clonic seizures with absences and/or myoclonic jerks or other seizures) in 17% of 4816 patients. Also the reported prevalence of EGTCSA amongst patients with only generalized tonic-clonic seizures varies markedly (Billiard, 1982; Goosses, 1984; for review see Niedermeyer, 1984; Wolf, 1992).

Personally, from the last 500 patients with epilepsy investigated in St Thomas' Hospital, I have seen only three patients whom I could confidentally classify as having EGTCSA. Many of these patients have had video-EEG (including partial sleep deprivation and EEG on awakening) and MRI. Two of these three patients are described above and the third had clinical and EEG manifestations similar to the Cambridge graduate (Fig. 14c.1). However, the strict definition criteria discussed in the introduction were used and may explain this low prevalence. Cases, who early in their course satisfied the criteria for EGTCSA, but who later developed random diurnal or nocturnal generalized tonic-clonic seizures, have probably been excluded.

For a definite diagnosis of pure EGTCSA, Janz (1994) requires that at least six seizures

have occurred predominantly during awakening or during relaxation.

SEX

It appears that men (55%) are slightly more affected than women (45%). This may be attributed to differences in alcohol exposure and sleep habits. The male to female ratio amongst 88 cases with pure EGTCSA was 1.8 (Janz, 1994).

GENETICS

There is a high incidence of epileptic disorders in families of patients with either the pure (3.8%) or mixed forms of EGTCSA (10.9–12.5%) (Janz 1994; see also Wolf, 1992, and Chapter 8).

AGE

Age at onset varies from 6 to 47 years. There is unanimous agreement that nearly 80% of the cases manifest their first generalized tonic-clonic seizures in the second decade of life, with a peak at 16–17 years.

CLINICAL MANIFESTATIONS, PRECIPITATING FACTORS, AND DIFFERENTIAL DIAGNOSIS

Patients suffer, by definition, from idiopathic generalized tonic-clonic seizures which occur within 1–2 hours after awakening either from nocturnal or diurnal sleep. The seizure may occur while the patient is still in bed or having his breakfast or upon arriving at work. However, seizures may also occur in situations other than awakening. Sometimes they occur during relaxation or leisure and some patients have predominantly 'generalized tonic-clonic seizures at leisure' (Wolf, 1992; Janz, 1994).

Sleep deprivation, fatigue and excessive alcohol consumption are the main seizure precipitants. Shift work, changes in sleep habits, particularly during holidays and celebrations, predispose to generalized tonic-clonic seizures on awakening. With time the interval between seizures becomes shorter and the attacks may become more random (diurnal and nocturnal), either as a result of the evolution of the disease or drug-induced modifications. Thirteen per cent of patients are reported to show photosensitivity on EEG.

The differential diagnosis is mainly from patients with other idiopathic generalized epilepsies which share with EGTCSA the same propensity to seizures after awakening and the same precipitating factors. Juvenile myoclonic epilepsy, juvenile absence epilepsy and eyelid myoclonia with absences are examples of idiopathic generalized epileptic syndromes which may cause diagnostic difficulties (Chapters 14a, 14b). Symptomatic and partial epileptic seizures with secondary generalization may also occur, predominantly on awakening.

ELECTROENCEPHALOGRAPHY

Generalized abnormalities of spike or multiple spike and slow waves are reported in approximately 50% of patients with pure EGTCSA (Fig. 14c.1) and 70% of those with additional absences or myoclonic jerks preceding generalized tonic-clonic seizures. A normal routine EEG should generate a video-EEG performed on sleep and awakening. Myoclonic jerks or, more frequently, absences without seizures will often be revealed and exclude the diagnosis of 'pure' EGTCSA. Focal EEG abnormalities, in the absence of generalized discharges, are rare. Photoconvulsive responses to intermittent photic stimulation (IPS) are reported in 17% of females and 9% of males with EGTCSA (Goosses 1984; Wolf and Goosses, 1986), but whether these patients belong to EGTCSA or to other photosensitive epilepsies is open to debate.

PERSONALITY CHARACTERISTICS AND SLEEP PATTERNS

Generalized tonic-clonic seizures on awakening are heavily influenced by external factors, particularly alcohol and sleep deprivation, which may be avoidable or self-inflicted. Janz (1969, 1994) described patients with EGTCSA as unreliable, unstable and prone to neglect. However, there are patients who remain seizure free after adjusting their lifestyles and their jobs.

The sleep patterns of patients with EGTCSA are particularly unstable and modifiable by external factors (i.e. antiepileptic drugs), and the patients may suffer from chronic sleep deficit (Wolf, 1992; Janz, 1994).

PROGNOSIS

EGTCSA is probably a life-long disease with a high (83%) incidence of relapse on withdrawal of treatment, as in all other types of idiopathic generalized epilepsies with onset in the mid-teens. Characteristically, the intervals between seizures become shorter with time, the precipitating factors less obvious, and, generalized tonic-clonic seizures may become more random and occur also during sleep. This may be a factor contributing to the underdiagnosis of EGTCSA (Janz, 1994).

TREATMENT

Patients should be warned of the common seizure precipitants, sleep deprivation with early awaking and alcohol consumption, and when possible should avoid occupational night shifts. Drug treatment has not been properly evaluated but retrospective open studies suggest that phenobarbitone is more effective than phenytoin or carbamazepine (Janz, 1969; Wolf, 1992). Based on its effectiveness in other forms of idiopathic generalized epilepsies, sodium valproate may be effective. It is interesting that bromide therapy has recently been rediscovered to be useful in resistant cases of EGTCSA (Wolf, 1992). A prophylactic high dose of sodium valproate in patients with strictly defined EGTCSA and infrequent seizures (see 'A probable case' above) may be effective if administered when risk factors are iminent.

CONCLUSION

All types of seizures, partial or generalized, idiopathic, cryptogenic or symptomatic, may be consistently related to the awakening process. However, not all these patients should be classified in the syndrome of idiopathic epilepsy with generalized tonic-clonic seizures on awakening, a diagnosis which should, by definition, be reserved for only those patients with primary, not secondary, idiopathic, not cryptogenic or symptomatic, generalized tonic-clonic seizures without absences or myoclonic jerks. These exclusion criteria may be difficult to apply without video-EEG polygraphic studies during sleep and awakening. There is no conclusive evidence to support that this strictly defined syndrome (pure EGTCSA) is different to other syndromes of idiopathic generalized epilepsies sharing the same precipitating factors and the propensity to seizures on awakening.

REFERENCES

Billiard, M. (1982) Epilepsies and the sleep wake cycle, in *Sleep and Epilepsy* (eds M.B. Sterman, M.N. Shouse and P. Passouant), Academic, New York, pp. 269–86.

Commission on Classification and Terminology of the International League Against Epilepsy (1989) Proposal for classification of epilepsies and epileptic syndromes. *Epilepsia*, **30**, 389–99.

Giannakodimos, S., Ferrie, C.D. and Panayiotopoulos, C.P. (1994) Quantitative abnormalities of breath counting during brief 3 Hz spike-wave 'subclinical' discharges. *Clinical Electroencephalography*, **26**, 1–4.

Goosses, R. (1984) (cited by Wolf, 1992). Die Beziehung der Photosensibilitat zu den verschiedenen epileptiscien Syndromen. West Berlin, Thesis.

Janz, D. (1969) *Die Epilepsien. Spezielle Pathologie und Therapie*. Thieme, Stuttgart.

Janz, D. (1994) Pitfalls in the diagnosis of grand mal on awakening, in *Idiopathic Generalised Epilepsies. Clinical, Experimental and Genetic Aspects* (eds A. Malafosse, P. Genton, E. Hirsch et al.), John Libbey, London (in press).

Loiseau, P., Duchet, B. and Loiseau, J. (1991) Classification of epilepsies and epileptic syndromes in two different samples of patients. *Epilepsia*, **32**, 303–9.

Manford, M., Hart, Y.M., Sander, J.W.A.S. and Shorvon, S.D. (1992) The national general practice study of epilepsy. The syndromic classification of the International League Against Epilepsy applied to epilepsy in a general population. *Archives of Neurology*, **49**, 801–8.

Niedermeyer, E. (1984) Awakening epilepsy (Aufwach-Epilepsie) revisited 30 years later, in *Epilespy, Sleep and Sleep Deprivation* (eds R. Degen and E. Niedermeyer), Elsevier, Amsterdam, pp. 85–96.

Schmitz, B. and Wolf, P. (1989) Epilepsies and epileptic syndromes in a neurological seizure clinic, in *Genetics of the Epilepsies* (eds G. Beck-Mannagetta, V.E. Anderson, H. Doose and D. Janz, Springer, Berlin, pp. 19–22.

Wolf, P. (1992) Epilepsy with grand mal on awakening, in *Epileptic Syndromes in Infancy, Childhood and Adolescence* (eds J. Roger, M. Bureau, P. Dravet et al.), John Libbey, London: pp. 329–41.

Wolf, P. and Goosses, R. (1986) Relation of photosensitivity to epileptic syndromes. *Journal of Neurology, Neurosurgery and Psychiatry*, **49**, 1386–9.

EPILEPSIES CHARACTERIZED BY SEIZURES WITH SPECIFIC MODES OF PRECIPITATION (REFLEX EPILEPSIES)

C.P. Panayiotopoulos

INTRODUCTION

Epileptic seizures can arise in a 'spontaneous' unpredictable fashion without detectable precipitant factors, or they can be provoked by certain recognizable stimuli. The factors which contribute to the generation of a seizure are so numerous, and their interaction so complex, that it is often impossible to define them and thus the seizures appear to arise of their own accord.

Stimuli which contribute towards the initiation of a seizure are provided by the internal and/or external environment of the subject. Hormones, electrolytes, state of consciousness and body temperature are examples of internal factors which alter the epileptogenic threshold. External stimuli may be sensory, electrical and biochemical. A complex interaction between external and internal stimuli may explain why the effectiveness of a well-defined seizure-precipitating stimulus may vary and why a patient may experience both 'spontaneous' and 'stimulus-induced' seizures.

Epileptic seizures which are consistently elicited by a specific stimulus are called stimulus-sensitive (SSE) or reflex or triggered or sensory-evoked epileptic seizures. They have a 4–7% prevalence amongst patients with epilepsies. The Commission of the International League Against Epilepsy (ILAE) has named these SSE as 'Epilepsies characterized by seizures with specific modes of precipitation (reflex epilepsies)' (Commission on Classification and Terminology of the International League Against Epilepsy, 1989).

The stimulus evoking an epileptic seizure is specific for a given patient and may be simple (i.e. flashes of light, elimination of visual fixation, tactile stimuli) or complex (coloured pictures, eating). Stimuli may be extrinsic, as in the above examples, proprioceptive (i.e. movements), or involve higher brain function, emotions and cognition (i.e. thinking, music, arithmetic).

The seizures may be generalized such as typical or atypical absences, myoclonic jerks and generalized tonic/tonic clonic, or they may be partial such as visual, motor or sensory. Generalized tonic-clonic seizures may be either primary or secondary to a partial, simple or complex seizure, or may follow a cluster of absences or myoclonic jerks. Myoclonic jerks are by far the most common type of stimulus-elicited seizures. They may be manifested in the limbs and trunk or localized in a specific muscle group, such as in the jaw muscles (reading epilepsy) or the eyelids (eyelid myoclonia with absences).

EEG is fundamental in establishing the provocative stimulus in SSE because it allows

Epilepsy in Children. Edited by Sheila Wallace. Published in 1996 by Chapman & Hall, London. ISBN 0 412 56860 8

subclinical EEG, or minor clinical ictal, events to be reproduced repeatedly and on demand with application of the appropriate stimulus (Chapter 19). However, there are cases in which the stimulus–seizure relation is difficult to prove. An example is video games-induced seizures. Intermittent photic stimulation elicits photoconvulsive responses in 70% of these patients, demonstrating that the epileptic seizures of these subjects were due to photosensitivity. The provocative factors in the other 30% remain unknown and speculative; sleep deprivation, mental concentration, fatigue, excitement, high-threshold photosensitivity, fixation-off sensitivity, proprioceptive stimuli (praxis) or more complex visual or auditory stimuli, alone or in combination, are all possibilities. There are also epileptic syndromes in which EEG 'epileptogenic activity' is consistently elicited by a specific stimulus but its provocative relevance to the clinical situation is difficult to prove. For example, in the early onset of benign childhood seizures with occipital paroxysms, elimination of fixation and central vision elicits continuous EEG abnormalities of occipital spike and slow wave activity, however, clinically the children appear to have 'unprovoked' seizures consisting of tonic deviation of the eyes, vomiting, impairment of consciousness, and convulsions. The situation in children suffering from benign partial seizures with extreme somatosensory evoked spikes is similar. It is even more difficult to prove that complex, emotional and cognitive stimuli can elicit seizures.

Table 14d.1 lists simple and complex stimuli which have been reported in association with SSE: some of these are well known and common (photosensitive epilepsies), others are extremely rare in humans but may be common in animals (audiogenic epilepsy). Some other forms are only recently described (fixation-off sensitive epilepsies). Visual induced seizures are by far the commonest and are dealt with in this chapter.

Table 14d.1 Stimulus-sensitive epilepsies and the responsible stimuli (for details see Beaumanoir *et al.*, 1989; Gastaut, 1989)

I. Somatosensory stimuli
1. Exteroceptive somatosensory stimuli:
   a. Benign childhood epilepsy with somatosensory evoked spikes
   b. Sensory (tactile) evoked idiopathic myoclonic seizures in infancy
   c. Tapping epilepsy
   d. Tooth-brushing epilepsy

2. Proprioceptive somatosensory stimuli:
   a. Seizures induced by movements
   b. Seizures induced by eye closure and/or eye movements
   c. Paroxysmal kinesigenic choreoathetosis

3. Complex proprioceptive stimuli:
   a. Eating epilepsy.

II. Visual stimuli
1. Simple visual stimuli:
   a. Photosensitive epilepsies
   b. Pattern-sensitive epilepsies
   c. Fixation-off sensitive epilepsies
   d. Scotogenic epilepsy
   e. Self-induced photosensitive epilepsy
   f. Self-induced pattern-sensitive epilepsy

2. Complex visual stimuli and language process
   a. Reading epilepsy
   b. Graphogenic epilepsy

III. Auditory, vestibular and olfactory stimuli
   a. Seizures induced by pure sounds or words
   b. Musicogenic epilepsy (and singing epilepsy)
   c. Olfactorhinencephalic epilepsy
   d. Eating epilepsy triggered by tastes
   e. Seizures triggered by vestibular and auditory stimuli

IV. High-level processes induced seizures (cognitive, emotional, decision-making tasks and other complex stimuli)
   a. Thinking (noogenic) epilepsy
   b. Reflex decision-making epilepsy
   c. Epilepsia arithmetica (mathematica)
   d. Emotional epilepsies
   e. Startle epilepsy

PHOTOSENSITIVE EPILEPSIES

It should be emphasized that 'photosensitive epilepsy' (PE) is a broad term comprising all forms of epilepsies in which seizures are triggered by photic stimulation, and does not correspond to a particular epileptic syndrome. Thus, patients with syndromes of idiopathic generalized epilepsies such as juvenile myoclonic epilepsy (Chapter 14b), or patients with symptomatic epilepsies such as Lafora's disease (Chapter 15a), may have seizures elicited by photic stimulation. Even amongst the pure forms of PE there may be subdivisions, as for example those manifested with generalized or occipital epileptic seizures. Eyelid myoclonia with absences is probably the only well-defined syndrome of a form of PE (Jeavons, 1977; Appleton *et al.*, 1993). Although photosensitivity is usually classified amongst the generalized epilepsies (Commission on Classification and Terminology of the International League Against Epilepsy, 1989), there is evidence that photosensitivity in humans is mainly generated in the occipital lobes and is therefore regional (occipital lobar) epilepsy (Panayiotopoulos, 1972; Wilkins, Andermann and Ives, 1975; Binnie, 1994). In many cases both clinical (visual hallucinations, obscuration of vision and blindness, deviation of the head and eyes) and EEG features show a clear occipital onset (Aso *et al.*, 1988; Michelucci and Tassinari, 1993; Ferrie *et al.*, 1994). It is also possible that in other forms of photosensitivity (eyelid myoclonia with absences may be an example) the onset is in the frontal regions, as is the case in the photosensitive baboon *Papio papio* (see review by Menini and Silva-Barrat, 1989).

Photosensitivity, the propensity to seizures induced by light, is a genetically determined trait (Doose and Gerken, 1973; Waltz, Christen and Doose, 1992) that may be asymptomatic throughout life or manifest with epileptic seizures. Photosensitivity is best demonstrated in EEG with appropriate inter-mittent photic stimulation (IPS) techniques (Jeavons and Harding, 1975; Jeavons, 1982; Wilkins *et al.*, 1980).

An historic review of photosensitive epilepsy and relevant literature before 1970 can be found elsewhere (Panayiotopoulos, 1972; Jeavons and Harding, 1975).

LABORATORY (EEG) AND CLINICAL PHOTOSENSITIVITY

The abnormal responses in their mildest form consist of posterior abnormalities which do not spread into the anterior regions. These are occipital spikes (Fig. 14d.1) which are often time-locked to the flash with a latency of approximately 100 ms (Fig. 14d.2), coinciding with the positive P100 of the visual evoked response (Panayiotopoulos, Jeavons and Harding, 1970a, 1970b), or slow waves intermixed with small, larval spikes. Half of the subjects demonstrating posterior abnormalities also have clinical epileptic seizures (Jeavons and Harding, 1975; Binnie and Jeavons, 1992).

However, it is the photoconvulsive discharges (Figs 14d.3–14d.6) which are highly significantly (90–95%) associated with clinically evident epileptic disorders (Jeavons and Harding, 1975; Reilly and Peters, 1973; Wilkins, Binnie and Darby, 1980; Jayakar and Chiappa, 1990). Video-EEG and close questioning of the patients reveal that clinical manifestations such as mild localized or generalized jerks and/or impairment of cognition or subjective sensations, occur in more than 60% of the photoconvulsive responses (Kasteleijn-Nolst Trenité, 1989). Subjects who, for employment reasons, have an EEG showing photoconvulsive responses but not clinical evidence of epileptic seizures (Grecory, Oates and Merry, 1993) should be reexamined with video-EEG recording and appropriate testing for cognition or other minor ictal symptoms such as eyelid or perioral myoclonia. This may reveal clinical

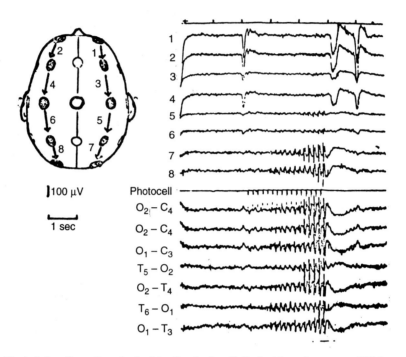

Fig. 14d.1 Occipital spikes, time-locked to the flash, elicited at low frequency IPS in a photosensitive patient. Generalized photoconvulsive responses were elicited at higher frequency IPS. (Reproduced with permission from Panayiotopoulos, 1972.)

manifestations during otherwise silent photoconvulsive responses (Giannakodimos, Ferrie and Panayiotopoulus, 1995).

The photoconvulsive responses consist of generalized spikes or multiple spike and slow wave discharges which are of higher amplitude in the anterior regions (Figs 14d.3–14d.6) but their onset, particularly if patterned IPS is employed, often consists of occipital spikes (Figs 14d.1, 14d.2).

IPS, in order to be maximally provocative, has to employ all potent physical characteristics of the stimulus (intensity, frequency, contrast). Patterned light, a linear grid, not a chequerboard, in front of the stroboscobe may be sufficient (Fig. 14d.4) to increase photosensitivity. Central vision is mandatory (the patient should look at the center of the stroboscope), and IPS on eye closure (Fig. 14d.3) should be tested (Jeavons *et al.*, 1972; Panayiotopoulos, 1972, 1974; Jeavons and Harding, 1975; Wilkins, Binnie and Darby, 1980; Takahashi, 1989). Photosensitivity can also be enhanced by sleep deprivation (Scollo-Lavizarri and Lavizarri, 1974).

Prevalence

Photosensitive epilepsy affects one in 4000 of the population, of whom two-thirds are female. (Video-game-induced seizures occur more often in males.) The onset has a peak age at 12–13 years (Jeavons and Harding, 1975).

The prevalence of EEG photosensitivity is 5% amongst patients with clinically evident

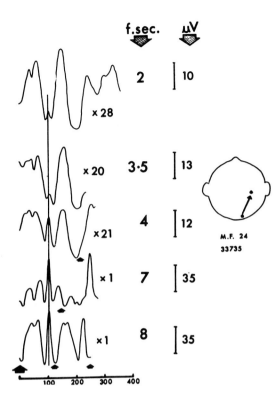

Fig. 14d.2 Responses to photic stimulation in a photosensitive patient. The three upper traces show the visual evoked responses (VER) to 2, 3.5 and 4 flashes/second. The occipital spike elicited at 7 and 8 flashes/second is shown in the two lower traces, coinciding with the negative component of P100. The vertical line crosses the occipital spike as it emerges from the negative component of P100. Arrows show flash frequencies and amplitudes. (Reproduced with permission from Panayiotopoulos, Jeavons and Harding, 1970a.)

epileptic seizures. Amongst patients with photoconvulsive responses and seizures, 42% have only photically induced, and no spontaneous, seizures (pure photosensitive epilepsy), 40% have spontaneous and photosensitive seizures, and the remaining 18% have spontaneous seizures only (Binnie and Jeavons, 1992).

In a recent demographic study the overall annual incidence of cases with a newly presenting seizure and unequivocal photosensitivity in Great Britain was found to be 1.1 per 100 000 (5.7 per 100 000 in the age group from 7–19 years). This means that photosensitivity is found in 2% of patients of all ages presenting with seizures and 10% of patients presenting with seizures in the age range 7–19 years (Fish *et al.*, 1994).

Photosensitivity was found in 48 (0.35%) of 13 625 healthy male candidates, aged 17–25 years, for Royal Air Force crew training (Grecory *et al.*, 1993).

Precipitants of seizures

Television, video-games, visual display units of computers, discotheques, and natural flickering light (shining through trees or reflecting from the sea) are in that order common precipitants of seizures (Jeavons and Harding, 1975; Newmark and Penry, 1979; Wilkins, Binnie and Darby, 1980). Video-game-induced seizures are increasingly common but should not always be equated with photosensitivity, since in only 70% can photosensitivity be confirmed (Ferrie *et al.*, 1994).

Pure photosensitive epilepsy is used only for patients whose seizures are always photically induced and who do not have spontaneous, unprovoked seizures (Jeavons and Harding, 1975). Pure PE has a prevalence of 42% amongst the photosensitive epilepsies. Generalized tonic-clonic seizures are reported far more commonly (87%) than absences (6%), partial seizures (2.5%), and myoclonic jerks (1.5%) (Jeavons and Harding, 1975; Newmark and Penry, 1979; Binnie and Jeavons, 1992). However, experience with video-EEG recordings shows that many patients categorized as having only generalized tonic-clonic seizures, frequently have mild spontaneous or photically induced myoclonic jerks or absences either independ-

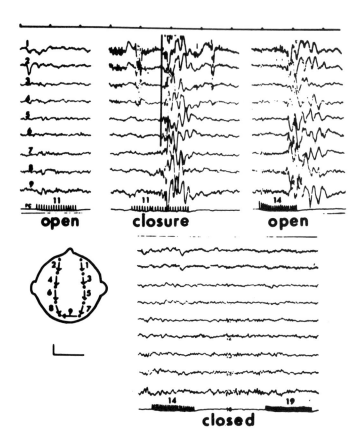

Fig. 14d.3 Photoconclusive responses in a photosensitive patient; elicited mainly after eye closure or when the eyes are opened. No abnormalities at any flash rate when eyes closed. Calibration: 100 μV, 1 second. (Reproduced with permission from Panayiotopoulos, 1974.)

ently or preceding a generalized tonic-clonic seizure, but these are often not reported.

The resting EEG is normal in half of the patients, abnormal photoconvulsive responses occurring only during IPS. Approximately 20% of them show generalized discharges on eye closure (see below the difference between eye closure and eyes-closed states).

The seizures are usually infrequent and the prognosis is often excellent. Avoidance of precipitating factors may be the only treatment necessary (Jeavons and Harding, 1975; Wilkins and Lindsay, 1985).

PHOTOSENSITIVITY AND EPILEPTIC SYNDROMES

A quarter of patients with spontaneous seizures and EEG photosensitivity belong to a variety of syndromes of idiopathic generalized epilepsy, such as juvenile myoclonic epilepsy (Wolf and Goosses, 1986; Wolf, 1992a). Absences with onset in childhood are associated with a higher prevalence (18%) of photosensitivity than absences appearing in the second decade of life (7.5%). Absences combined with photosensitivity have a worse prognosis than those of childhood absence epilepsy (Panayiotopoulos, 1994). A high pre-

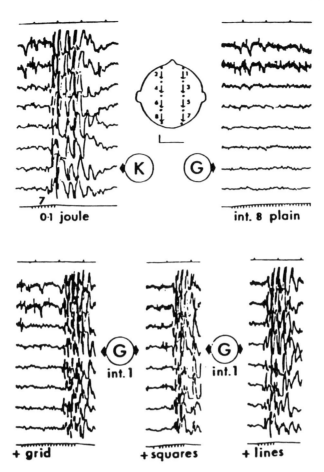

Fig. 14d.4 Effect of IPS combined with patterns. Photoconvulsive responses at 7 flashes/second in one patient under different IPS conditions. Photoconvulsive discharges occurred only when flash combined with linear patterns. No abnormal responses elicited when IPS was given through plain glass despite an eight-fold increase of flash intensity (top right). K = Kaiser stroboscope with protective metal grid (pattern). G = Grass stimulator: unpatterned flash, intensity 8 (top right); pattern flash, intensity 1 (bottom). (Reproduced with permission from Panayiotopoulos, 1972, and Jeavons *et al.*, 1972.)

valence of photosensitivity is also found in certain forms of symptomatic generalized epilepsies, like severe myoclonic epilepsy in infancy (70%), Baltic-Mediterranean myoclonus (90%), and progressive myoclonic epilepsies (Roger *et al.*, 1992).

EYELID MYOCLONIA WITH ABSENCES

This is a syndrome not yet recognized by the ILAE, although vividly described by Jeavons (Jeavons, 1977; see also Dalla Bernardina

et al., 1989; Appleton *et al.*, 1993; Giannakodimos and Panayiotopoulos, 1995). The first case of eyelid myoclonia with absences was probably reported by Radovici, Misirliou and Gluckman (1932): a young man had seizures consisting of rhythmic upward movements of the head with eyelid tremors when he looked at the sun on bright days; two of his seizures were recorded in motion pictures.

In our experience (Appleton *et al.*, 1993; Giannakodimos and Panayiotopoulos, 1995), eyelid myoclonia with absences is a common

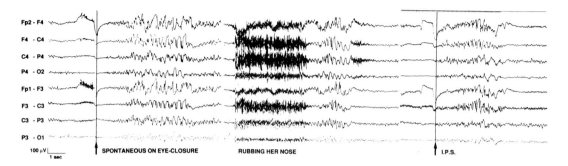

Fig. 14d.5 EEG of a 26-year-old female with JME. Generalized spike and occasionally multiple spike and slow wave discharges occur after eye closure (left) and are also elicited by somatosensory stimulation, e.g. rubbing the nose (middle) or IPS (right). (Reproduced with permission from Panayiotopoulos *et al.*, 1992.)

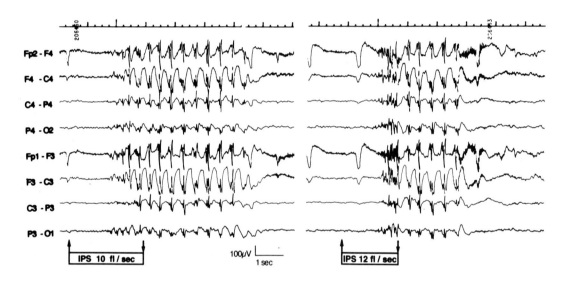

Fig. 14d.6 Video-EEG recorded typical absence seizures evoked in a photosensitive male aged 19 years. Patient is unresponsive and stares.

epileptic syndrome which is frequently misdiagnosed in children as CAE despite marked differences and characteristic features. The following definition is proposed (Panayiotopoulos, 1994): Eyelid myoclonia with absences, is manifested by frequent (pyknolepsy) typical absences with onset in early childhood (2–5 years). The absences are brief (3–6 seconds) and occur after eye closure. There is marked, rhythmic eyelid myoclonia which consists of fast jerks of the eyelids and retropulsion of the eyeballs with an associated tonic component of the involved muscles. The eyelid myoclonia contrasts with the blink-like movements seen in CAE. All patients are highly photosensitive (Jeavons, 1977; Appleton *et al.*, 1993) and self-induction may be seen in a few patients (probably the cases of Radovici, Misirliou and Gluckman, 1932; Binnie *et al.*, 1980; Darby et al., 1980a;

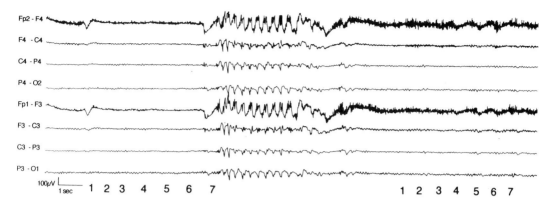

Fig. 14d.7 Eyelid myoclonia with absences. Generalized multiple spike and slow wave discharges occur after eye closure. These are associated with rapid and rhythmic eyelid jerks with retropulsion of the eyeballs and head. Counting (annotated) is interrupted during the discharge.

Kasteleijn-Nolst Trenité *et al.*, 1989; Binnie and Jeavons, 1992).

Generalized tonic-clonic seizures, induced by lights or spontaneously, are probably inevitable and are likely to occur after sleep deprivation, fatigue, and alcohol indulgence. Myoclonic jerks of the limbs may occur in one-fifth of patients (Giannakodimos and Panayiotopoulos, 1995).

Eyelid myoclonia with absences is resistant to monotherapy, does not remit and is probably life-long. However, absences may become less frequent with age, eye-closure EEG abnormalities may persist without photosensitivity, which declines, and eyelid phenomena may occur without EEG accompaniments (Giannakodimos and Panayiotopoulos, 1995).

The EEG ictal manifestations consist mainly of generalized polyspikes/slow wave 3–6 Hz (faster than in CAE), which are more likely to occur after eye closure in an illuminated room (Fig. 14d.7). Total darkness abolishes the eye-closure-related abnormalities. IPS induces photoconvulsive discharges in all patients but may decline with age.

The drugs of choice are sodium valproate combined with ethosuximide.

Comment: Some patients may exhibit marked eyelid myoclonia as in this syndrome but with more marked tonic components of the eyelids and the eyes, which are often deviated to one side. The ictal EEG manifestations consist mainly of generalized polyspikes which are induced either by eye closure (the patients are also photosensitive) or are related to the eyes-closed state (the patients have fixation-off sensitivity, Panayiotopoulos, 1994). The nosologic categorization of these patients is uncertain. Also, eyelid myoclonia with absences may be seen in patients with learning and behavioral problems which, though not belonging in the idiopathic generalized epilepsies, are again difficult to categorize. Some authors have found a high prevalence of self-induction in eyelid myoclonia with absences (Binnie *et al.*, 1980; Darby *et al.*, 1980a; Kasteleijn-Nolst Trenité *et al.*, 1989), which is not our experience (Appleton *et al.*, 1993; Panayiotopoulos, 1994; Giannakodimos and Panayiotopoulos, 1995).

SELF-INDUCED SEIZURES

Self-induction has been well established as a mode of precipitation, but prevalence is disputed from a small number to as high as 30% of photosensitive patients (Andermann *et al.*, 1962; Green, 1966; Panayiotopoulos, 1972; Jeavons and Harding, 1975; Foster 1977; Darby *et al.*, 1980a; Kasteleijn-Nolst Trenité *et al.*, 1989; Tassinari *et al.*, 1989; Binnie and Jeavons, 1992). Self-induction is employed not only by the mentally handicapped, as was initially reported, but also by patients of normal or above-average intelligence. Techniques of self-induction vary from hand-waving the abducted fingers in front of a bright light source, to eyelid blinking, making the television screen roll or viewing geometric patterns (Fig. 14d.8).

Whether eyelid blinking or compulsive attraction to television or bright sun is mainly an attempt at self-induction (Jeavons and Harding, 1975; Kasteleijn-Nolst Trenité *et al.*, 1987; Binnie and Jeavons, 1992) or part of the seizure (Wilkins and Lindsay, 1985; Appleton *et al.*, 1993; Panayiotopoulos, 1994) is presently disputed, although both may be true.

Absences and myoclonic jerks are the commoner types of seizures in self-induction. A generalized tonic-clonic seizure may be induced after a series of absences or jerks (see also Chapter 25).

VIDEO GAME-INDUCED SEIZURES

There is an increasing incidence of seizures induced by playing video games (VGS), and recent media reports have highlighted the risk of VGS (Ferrie *et al.*, 1994). Small hand-held liquid crystal displays and noninterlaced 70-Hz arcade games, as well as games using an interlaced video monitor (TV), are included.

Existing data analysed by Ferrie *et al.* (1994) indicate that photosensitivity is a major precipitating factor (70%), but VGS may also occur in nonphotosensitive patients with idiopathic generalized epilepsies where sleep deprivation, fatigue, cognitive activities, decision making and praxis may alone, or in combination, elicit an epileptic seizure. Occi-

pital lobe epilepsy with, but mainly without photosensitivity, is the second most frequent (29%) type of epilepsy with VGS (Fig. 14d.9). This is more often the case in arcade games. The mechanisms in these patients are not yet known (Ferrie *et al.*, 1994).

VGS may be absences, jerks and generalized tonic-clonic seizures, or visual partial seizures with symptoms such as 'eye fatigue, headache and visual illusions' alone, or preceding a seizure. It should be emphasized that epileptic, mainly occipital lobe, seizures (not only those of VGS) may manifest with symptoms imitating migraine, e.g. headache, vomiting and visual illusions which, as opposed to migraine, are predominantly circular and multicolored (Panayiotopoulos, 1987a, 1994).

In a recent demographic study of VGS by Fish *et al.* (1994), the annual incidence of first or presenting seizures considered to have been triggered by electronic screen game playing was conservatively estimated to be 1.0–1.5 per 100 000 in the age group 7–19 years. The annual incidence of new cases presenting with seizures of any cause in the same 7–19-year age group is 55 per 100 000.

Stimulus-sensitive typical absences

Typical absences may be induced by flickering lights (photosensitive), patterns (pattern sensitivity), elimination of central vision and fixation (fixation-off sensitivity), somatosensory and probably other stimuli (Duncan and Panayiotopoulos, 1995). Absences are common in self-induced seizures. These stimulus-sensitive typical absences are seen either independently or within the broad framework of certain epileptic syndromes (Figs 14d.5, 14d.6).

Pattern-sensitive epilepsy

This is a term used for epileptic seizures and/or EEG abnormalities induced by patterns (Chatrian *et al.*, 1970a, 1970b; Wilkins, Andermann and Ives, 1975; Stefansson *et al.*,

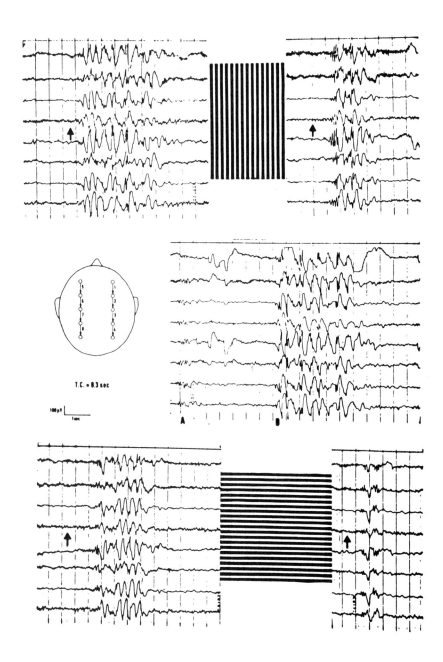

Fig. 14d.8 Self-induced pattern-sensitive epilepsy. High-amplitude discharges of multiple/spike and slow wave induced within 1 second of onset (arrow) of vertical (top) and horizontal pattern stimulation (bottom). Similar responses were induced when the patient looked (B) or glanced at a radiator with linear vertical patterns (middle). The patient was also photosensitive. (Reproduced with permission from Panayiotopoulos, 1979.)

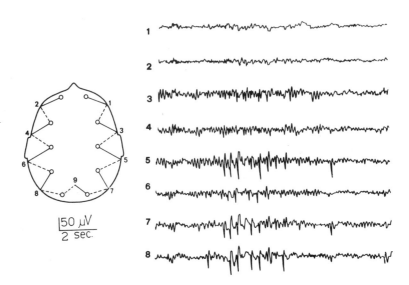

Fig. 14d.9   Occipital spikes in a 9-year-old boy with visual partial seizures and secondary generalization induced by video games. He was not sensitive to lights. (Reproduced with permission from Ferrie *et al.*, 1994.)

1977; Wilkins, Darby and Binnie, 1979; Darby *et al.*, 1980b; Wilkins, Binnie and Darby, 1980; Wilkins *et al.*, 1989; Binnie and Jeavons, 1992). Pattern-sensitive epilepsy is closely related to photosensitivity; nearly all pattern-sensitive patients are also photosensitive, 30% of photosensitive patients are sensitive to stationary continuously illuminated and 70% to appropriately vibrating patterns of stripes. Adding a quadrille pattern of small squares (2 mm × 2 mm) of fine black lines (⅓ mm) in front of a stroboscope increases the photoconvulsive range (Fig. 14d.4) (Panayiotopoulos, 1972; Jeavons *et al.*, 1972). An optimally epileptogenic pattern consists of black and white stripes of equal width and spacing (Fig. 14d.6). Wilkins *et al.* (Wilkins, Andermann and Ives, 1975; Wilkins, Binnie and Darby, 1980; Wilkins *et al.*, 1989) have shown that pattern sensitivity depends on the spatial frequency, orientation, brightness, contrast, and size of the pattern.

Pattern sensitivity without photosensitivity has been reported (Foster, 1977). Patients sensitive to nongeometric patterns are rare and probably nonphotosensitive. Self-induced pattern sensitivity has been described (Fig. 14d.8) (Panayiotopoulos, 1979; Matricardi *et al.*, 1989).

TREATMENT

In patients with pure photosensitive epilepsy, avoidance and protection from the provocative stimulus may be effective. In TV and photosensitive patients with videogame epilepsy, the patient should:

1. Maintain the maximum comfortable viewing distance from the TV screen, which is four to five times the diagonal measurement of the screen, i.e. 2.5 m for a 0.5 m screen.

2. Use the telecontrol and not be close to the screen when changing channels, or switching on and off.
3. Avoid prolonged watching, particularly if sleep deprived and tired.
4. Watch in a well-lit room with a table lamp close to the screen to reduce the relative intensity of the light from the screen.

Polaroid sunglasses may protect from flickering sun-light. Monocular occlusion of one eye should be advised either on watching TV or if the subject is suddenly exposed to flickering lights, i.e. in discotheques. Conditioning treatment has been tried, mainly by Foster (1977).

The drug of choice is sodium valproate which controls all types of seizures induced by light in more than 80% of patients. Clonazepam may be effective, particularly against jerks. Ethosuximide is effective against absences only. Ethosuximide or clonazepam or lamotrigine (in doses smaller than used as monotherapy) added to the therapeutic doses of sodium valproate may be needed, particularly in resistant cases, such as eyelid myoclonia with absences. Lamotrigine in one-dose trials has been effective in suppressing the photoconvulsive responses, but its clinical efficacy has yet to be shown as all patients were also receiving sodium valproate (Binnie *et al.*, 1986).

FIXATION-OFF SENSITIVE EPILEPSIES

Fixation-off sensitivity (FOS) denotes the form/forms of epilepsy and/or EEG abnormalities which are elicited by elimination of central vision and fixation (Panayiotopoulos, 1980, 1987b, 1989, 1994; Cirignotta, Lugaresi and Montagna, 1984).

In routine EEG, performed in an illuminated room and conditions allowing preservation of fixation and central vision, FOS may be suspected if the EEG abnormalities appear and persist as long as the eyes remain closed and disappear when the eyes are opened, i.e.

they show a similar reactivity to that of the alpha-rhythm (Figs. 14d.10, 14d.11).

FOS is related to 'eyes-closed', not 'eye-closure' EEG abnormalities (Figs. 14d.10, 14d.11). It is crucial to differentiate between **eyes-closed** (seen mainly in FOS) and **eye-closure** (seen mainly in photosensitive epilepsies) related abnormalities (Panayiotopoulos, 1972, 1974, 1994).

Eyes-closed related EEG abnormalities of FOS epilepsies are due to the elimination of central vision and fixation by the closed eyelids because (Fig. 14d.11):

1. The EEG paroxysms can also be elicited when eyes are opened in complete darkness or with unpatterned vision, either through plus 10 spherical lenses or through underwater goggles covered with semitransparent paper, i.e. when fixation and central vision are eliminated.
2. The EEG paroxysms disappear on binocular or monocular fixation.

Proprioceptive impulses from ocular and eyelid muscles are not implicated because the EEG paroxysms are not altered when eye closing and eye opening is performed in conditions where fixation and central vision are eliminated. They are inhibited by central vision and fixation.

Darkness is not a prerequisite for eliciting the EEG paroxysms, thus the term scotosensitive epilepsy is not appropriate. Genuine cases of scotosensitivity (Beaumanoir *et al.*, 1989; Pazzaglia, Jabattini and Lugaresi, 1970) may exist, but their documentation would require exclusion of FOS.

EEG ASPECTS OF FIXATION-OFF SENSITIVITY (FIGS 14d.10, 14d.11)

The EEG abnormalities consist of:

1. Occipital paroxysms, i.e. high amplitude, long runs of repetitive occipital spikes/sharp and slow wave complexes, morphologically similar to the centrotemporal

spikes, which are often bilateral and are related to the eyes-closed state, or

2. Generalized discharges of spike/multiple and slow waves which are eyes-closed related, or

3. Generalized slow theta and delta activity intermixed with spikes or multiple spikes which continuously occur as long as the eyes remain closed but disappear as the eyes open.

CLINICAL SYNDROMES OF FIXATION-OFF SENSITIVITY

1. **Benign childhood epilepsy with occipital paroxysms (BCEOP).** FOS is probably more frequently associated with the benign childhood epilepsy with occipital paroxysms than any other epileptic condition (Panayiotopoulos, 1980, 1981, 1989, 1993a, 1993b; Gastaut, 1982; Chapter 13c). BCEOP has been extensively reviewed

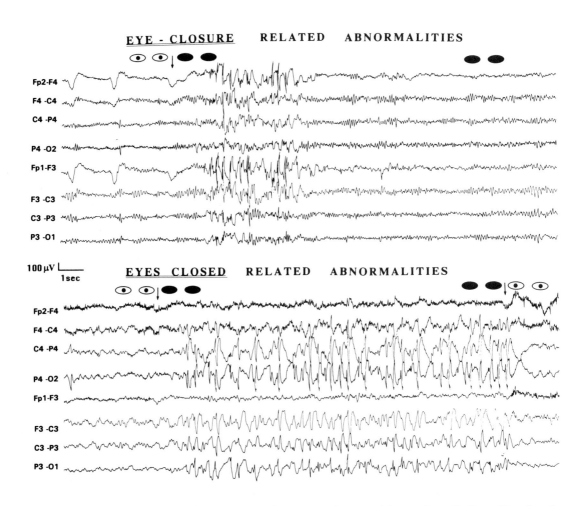

Fig. 14d.10 Top: Eye-closure-related abnormalities in a photosensitive patient. Bottom: Eye-closed-related abnormalities in a boy with benign childhood seizures and occipital paroxysms.

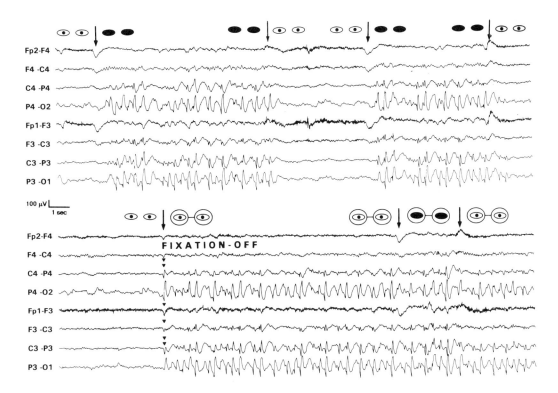

Fig. 14d.11 Video-EEG recording. Fixation-off sensitivity in an 11-year-old boy with benign childhood epilepsy and occipital paroxysms (case 7 in Panayiotopoulos, 1993b.) High-amplitude sharp and slow wave occipital paroxysms are induced by binocular fixation-off. The results are identical whether fixation-off is achieved with closed eyelids or complete darkness or +10 spherical lenses in the presence of light or underwater goggles covered with semitransparent tape. Monocular fixation-off is not effective in eliciting occipital paroxysms, irrespective of the means by which central vision and fixation were eliminated; similarly, occipital paroxysms are inhibited with binocular or monocular fixation. Occipital paroxysms are not inhibited by eyes opened in conditions of elimination of central vision and fixation, thus excluding the contribution of proprioceptive impulses from the eyelids or oculomotor muscles in the activation of the EEG abnormalities (see also Fig. 14d.4). Imaginary fixation (asking the patient to 'look' at his/her thumb) in conditions of elimination of central vision does not alter (does not inhibit) the occipital paroxysms. Arrows indicate when the eyes opened (symbols of open eyes) or closed (symbols of closed eyes). Eyes with glasses indicate that the patient has been deprived central vision and fixation.

recently (Panayiotopoulos, 1993a, 1993b; Roger and Bureau, 1993). Mention should be made of the less well-known form of BCEOP, described by Panayiotopoulos (1980, 1993b), which occurs at a peak age of 5 years and consists of infrequent mainly nocturnal seizures of tonic deviation of the eyes, vomiting with or with-

out impairment of consciousness. This may last for hours before ending in hemi- or generalized convulsions. The prognosis is excellent.

2. **Generalised epilepsies with tonic and clonic manifestations of the eyes and eyelids** (Panayiotopoulos, 1987, 1989, 1994)

PHOTOSENSITIVE VERSUS FIXATION-OFF SENSITIVITY EPILEPSY

Photosensitive epilepsy appears to have opposite mechanisms of excitation and inhibition to that of FOS:

1. The resting EEG of photosensitive patients frequently shows eye closure (not eyes-closed) EEG abnormalities which are inhibited by total darkness and probably by elimination of central vision and fixation (Jeavons, 1966; Panayiotopoulos, 1972, 1974).
2. Photosensitivity is mainly mediated through central vision and fixation (Jeavons, Harding and Panayiotopoulos, 1971b; Jeavons *et al.*, 1972; see also more recent views in Wilkins, Binnie and Darby, 1980; Takahashi, 1989; Binnie, 1994). Photoconvulsive responses are induced only if the patient 'looks' at the center of the stroboscope: 'Sometimes a shift of gaze from the center of the lamp to the edge (12° or 15°) will inhibit responses, including photic driving' (Jeavons, Harding and Panayiotopoulos, 1971a, 1971b).
3. Occipital spikes induced by photic stimulation are elicited when IPS is combined with patterns (Panayiotopoulos, Jeavons and Harding, 1970a, 1970b; Panayiotopoulos, 1972). The occipital spike appears to emerge from the negative component of a triphasic P100 VER (Fig. 14d.2), which suggests that an increase in sensitivity of the occipital cortex is implicated in the pathophysiology of photosensitive epilepsy. This view of a regional or lobar occipital sensitivity has recently been well established (Wilkins, Binnie and Darby, 1980).

READING EPILEPSY

Reading epilepsy (RE) is a distinctive form of idiopathic epilepsy which has been classified amongst the age and localization-related (partial) epilepsies (Foster, 1977; Commission on Classification and Terminology of the International League Against Epilepsy, 1989; Wolf, 1992b). The clinical manifestations are elicited by reading silently or aloud, and consist of brief myoclonic jerks mainly restricted to the masticatory, oral and perioral muscles. They are described as clicking sensations and occur a few minutes to an hour after reading, particularly if difficult or unfamiliar texts are read aloud. Jaw myoclonus is by far the commonest manifestation of RE. One-quarter of the patients also have jaw jerks provoked by talking (particularly if this is fast or argumentative), writing, reading music or chewing. Consciousness is not impaired but if the patient continues reading jaw jerks become more violent, spread to trunk and limb muscles, or generate other seizure manifestations before a generalized tonic-clonic seizure develops. This is usually the only generalized tonic-clonic seizure in the life of the patient, because the condition is effectively treated and the patient learns to stop reading or talking when oral/perioral jerks occur. The sister of one of my patients with RE, who has never sought medical advice for her condition and never had a generalized tonic-clonic seizure controlled her condition by modifying her way of reading and talking. A small number of patients may also have infrequent generalized tonic-clonic seizures, either spontaneous or triggered by other means of precipitation (talking, reading numbers or music, chewing or writing). RE may also rarely present with other types of ictal manifestations (mainly visual hallucinations) in addition to the jaw myoclonic seizures. Hand myoclonic jerks are common in seizures precipitated by writing.

Epileptic ictal difficulty in understanding text (alexia) has also been reported, but whether this is triggered by reading or fortuitous (alexia cannot be experienced unless it is tested by reading) is difficult to prove (Fig. 14d.12). Certainly these cases cannot be categorized as primary RE.

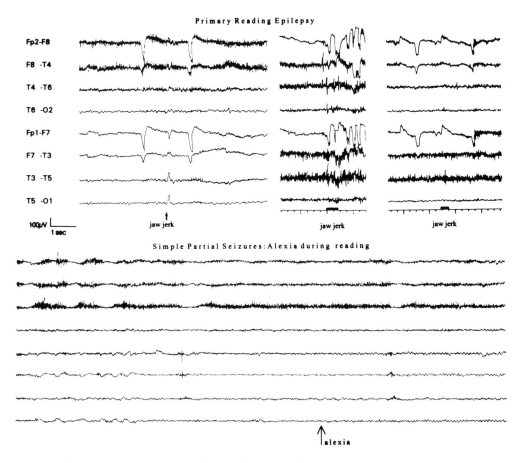

Fig. 14d.12 Three cases of reading epilepsy. Top left: EEG of a female with jaw jerks (arrow) while reading. She had one single generalized tonic-clonic seizure which was induced by reading. She is successfully treated with clonazepam 0.5 mg nocte. Her sister also suffered from jaw jerks, mainly when involved in argumentative and fast talk. Top middle and right: Video-EEG of another female with jaw jerks (bars) while reading. The EEG shows no detectable abnormality when jerks are mild (middle) and possible changes are obscured by muscle activity (right). Bottom: Video-EEG of a 24-year-old man with simple partial seizures manifested with alexia (inability to understand written words) and four nocturnal generalized tonic-clonic seizures. EEG during reading showed sharp and slow wave complexes which were focused in the left temporal regions (midway between middle and posterior temporal electrode). Immediately after this, the patient indicated his inability to understand text (arrow) and the EEG showed low-amplitude fast rhythms localized in the left middle temporal regions. This lasted 70 seconds before clinical recovery. MRI and PET scan were normal. The patient was effectively treated with carbamazepine.

Age at onset of primary RE is usually between 12 and 19 years with a peak in the late teens, i.e. long after reading skills have been acquired. There is a male preponderance of 1.8/1. RE is probably genetically determined and has been reported in identical twins and amongst first-degree relatives.

The interictal EEG is usually normal. Ictal EEG manifestations may be inconspicuous and difficult to detect (Fig. 14d.12) because of muscle activity from the jaw muscles and head (Epstein and Moore, 1982); but, more frequently, they consist of a brief burst of sharp waves which is bilateral, with left side preponderance in the temporoparietal regions (Gastaut and Tassinari, 1966; Foster, 1977; Wolf, 1992b).

The main mechanism of reading which elicits seizures is the transformation and transcoding from written linguistic symbols into phonematic, silent or spoken, speech. This may be enhanced by other superimposed factors such as proprioceptive impulses from oral, perioral and eye muscles involved in reading and difficulty in transcoding script into speech (for review see Wolf, 1992b).

The prognosis of RE appears to be good because seizures are usually minor and they are related to a precipitant stimulus which can be avoidable or modified. Treatment with small doses of sodium valproate or clonazepam (0.5 mg nocte), which is my preference, is highly effective.

REFERENCES

Andermann, K., Oaks, G., Berman, S. *et al.* (1962) Self-induced epilepsy. *Archives of Neurology*, **6**, 49–79.

Appleton, R., Panayiotopoulos, C.P., Acomb, A.B. and Beirne, M. (1993) Eyelid myoclonia with absences: an epilepsy syndrome. *Journal of Neurology, Neurosurgery and Psychiatry*, **56**, 1312–6.

Aso K., Watanabe, K., Negoro, T. *et al.* (1988) Photosensitive partial seizures: the origin of abnormal discharges. *Journal of Epilepsy*, **1**, 87–93.

Beaumanoir, A., Gastaut, H. and Nuquet, R. (1994) *Reflex seizures and reflex epilepsies*. Editions Medicine and Hygiene, Geneva.

Beaumanoir, A., Capizzi, G., Nahori, A. and Yousfi, Y. (1989) Scotogenic seizures, in *Reflex Seizures and Reflex Epilepsies* (eds A. Beaumanoir, H. Gastaut and R. Naquet), Editions Medecine and Hygiene, Geneve, pp. 219–23.

Binnie, C.D. (1994) Simian and human photosensitivity, in *Epileptic Seizures and Syndromes* (ed. P. Wolf), John Libbey Eurotext, London, pp. 49–54.

Binnie, C.D. and Jeavons P.M. (1992) Photosensitive epilepsies, in *Epileptic Syndromes of Infancy, Childhood and Adolescence*, 2nd edn (eds J. Roger, M. Bureau, C. Dravet *et al.*), John Libbey Eurotext, London, pp. 299–305.

Binnie, C.D., Darby, C.E., de Corte, R.A. and Wilkins, A.J. (1980) Self induction of epileptic seizures by eye closure: incidence and recognition. *Journal of Neurology, Neurosurgery and Psychiatry*, **43**, 386–9.

Binnie, C.D., van Emde Boas, W., Kasteleijn-Nolst Trenité, D.G.A. *et al.* (1986) Acute effects of lamotrigine (BW430C) in persons with epilepsy. *Epilepsia*, **27**, 248–54.

Chartrian, G.E., Lettich, E., Miller, L.H. and Green, J.R. (1970a) Pattern-sensitive epilepsy, Part 1. An electroencephalographic study of its mechanisms. *Epilepsia*, **11**, 125–50.

Chatrian, G.E., Lettich, E., Miller, L.H. *et al.* (1970b). Pattern-sensitive epilepsy, Part 2. Clinical changes, tests of responsiveness and motor output, alterations of evoked potentials and therapeutic measures. *Epilepsia*, **11**, 151–62.

Cirignotta, F., Lugaresi, E. and Montagna, P. (1984) Occipital EEG activity induced by darkness: the critical role of central vision, in *Migraine and Epilepsy* (eds F. Andermann and J. Lugaresi), Raven Press, New York, pp. 139–43.

Commission on Classification and Terminology of the International League Against Epilepsy (1989) Proposal for classification of epilepsies and epileptic syndromes. *Epilepsia*, **30**, 389–99.

Dalla Bernardina, B., Sgro, V., Fontana, E. *et al.* (1989) Eyelid myoclonias with absences, in *Reflex Seizures and Reflex Epilepsies* (eds A. Beaumanoir, H. Gastaut and R. Naquet), Editions Medecine and Hygiene, Geneve, pp. 193–200.

Darby, C.E., de Korte, R.A., Binnie, C.D. and Wilkins, A.J. (1980a) The self-induction of epileptic seizures by eye-closure. *Epilepsia*, **21**, 31–41.

Darby, C.E., Wilkins, A.J., Binnie, C.D. and de Korte, R.A. (1980b) A method for the routine testing for pattern sensitivity. *Journal of Electrophysiological Technology*, **6**, 202–11.

Doose, H. and Gerken, H. (1973) On the genetics of EEG-anomalies in childhood. IV. Photoconvulsive reaction. *Neuropaediatrie*, **4**, 162–71.

Duncan, J.S. and Panayiotopoulos, C.P. (1995) Typical absences with specific modes of precipitation/reflex absences, in *Typical absences and related epileptic syndromes* (eds J.S. Duncan and C.P. Panayiotopoulos), Churchill Livingstone, London, pp. 206–12.

Epstein, C.M. and Moore, R.J. (1982) Pseudo-spike-and-wave in reading epilepsy. *Electroencephalography and Clinical Neurophysiology*, **53**, 85P(abstr.).

Ferrie, C.D., De Marco, P., Grunewald R.A. *et al.* (1994) Video game-induced seizures. *Journal of Neurology, Neurosurgery and Psychiatry*, **57**, 925–31.

Fish, D.R., Quirk, J.A., Smith, S.J.M. *et al.* (1994) National survey of photosensitivity and seizures induced by electronic screen games (video games, console games, computer-games) in *Home and Leisure Accident Research Consumer Safety Unit*, Department of Trade and Industry, London, H.M. Stationery Office, July.

Foster, F.M. (1977) *Reflex Epilepsy: Behavioural Therapy and Conditional Reflexes*. C.C. Thomas, Springfield, Illinois.

Gastaut, H. (1982) A new type of epilepsy: benign partial epilepsy of children with occipital spike focus. *Clinical Electroencephalography*, **13**, 13–22.

Gastaut, H. (1989) Synopsis and conclusions of the International Coloquium on Reflex Seizures and Epilepsies, Geneva 1988, in *Reflex Seizures and Reflex Epilepsies* (eds A. Beaumanoir, H. Gastaut and R. Naquet), Editions Medecine and Hygiene, Geneve. pp. 181–91, 497–507.

Gastaut, H. and Tassinari, C.A. (1966) Triggering mechanisms vs epilepsy. The electroclinical point of view. *Epilepsia*, **7**, 85–138.

Giannakodimos, S., Ferrie, C.D. and Panayiotopoulos, C.P. (1995) Qualitative and quantitative EEG abnormalities of breath counting during brief generalised 3 Hz spike and slow wave 'subclinical' discharges. *Clinical Electroencephalography*, **26**, 1–4.

Grecory, R.P., Oates, T. and Merry, R.T.G. (1993) EEG epileptiform abnormalities in candidates for aircrew training. *Electroencephalography and Clinical Neurophysiology*, **86**, 75–7.

Green, J.B. (1966) Self-induced seizures: clinical and electroencephalographic studies. *Archives of Neurology*, **15**, 579–86.

Jayakar, P. and Chiappa, K.H. (1990) Clinical correlations of photoparoxysmal responses. *Electroencephalography and Clinical Neurophysiology*, **75**, 251–4.

Jeavons, P.M. (1966) Summary of papers on abnormalities during photic stimulation. *Proceedings of the Electrophysiological Technological Association*, **13**, 153–7.

Jeavons, P.M. (1977) Nosological problems of myoclonic epilepsies of childhood and adolescence. *Developmental Medicine and Child Neurology*, **19**, 3–8.

Jeavons, P.M. (1982) Photosensitive epilepsy, in *A Textbook of Epilepsy* (eds J. Laidlaw and A. Richens), Churchill Livingstone, London, pp. 195–211.

Jeavons, P.M. and Harding, G.F.A. (1975) *Photosensitive Epilepsy*, Heinemann, London.

Jeavons, P.M., Harding, G.F.A. and Panayiotopoulos, C.P. (1971a) Photosensitive epilepsy and driving. *Lancet*, **i**, 1125.

Jeavons, P.M., Harding, G.F.A. and Panayiotopoulos, C.P. (1971b) The effect of lateral gaze and lateral illumunation on photoconvulsive responses to intermittent photic stimulation. *Electroencephalography and Clinical Neurophysiology*, **32**, 445.

Jeavons, P.M., Harding, G.F.A., Panayiotopoulos, C.P. and Drasdo, N. (1972) The effect of geometric patterns combined with intermittent photic stimulation in photosensitive epilepsy. *Electroencephalography and Clinical Neurophysiology*, **33**, 221–4.

Kasteleijn-Nolst Trenité, D.G.A. (1989) Photosensitivity in epilepsy: electrophysiological and clinical correlates. *Acta Neurologica Scandinavica* (suppl. 125), 3–149.

Kasteleijn-Nolst Trenité, D.G.A., Binnie, C.D. and Meinardi, H. (1987) Photosensitive patients: symptoms and signs during intermittent photic stimulation and their relation to seizures in daily life. *Journal of Neurology, Neurosurgery and Psychiatry*, **50**, 1546–9.

Kasteleijn-Nolst Trenité, D.G.A., Binnie, C.D., Overweg, J. *et al.* (1989) Treatment of self-induction in epileptic patients. Who wants it?, in *Reflex Seizures and Reflex Epilepsies* (eds A. Beaumanoir, H. Gastaut and R. Naquet), Editions Medecine and Hygiene, Geneve, pp. 439–51.

Matricardi, M., Brinciotti, M., Trasatti, G. and Pellicia, A. (1989) Self-induced seizures by spatially structured visual stimuli, in *Reflex Seizures and Reflex Epilepsies* (eds A. Beaumanoir, H. Gastaut and R. Naquet), Editions Medecine and Hygiene, Geneve, pp. 393–5.

Menini, C. and Silva-Barrat, C. (1989) Role of visual afferents in the photosensitive epilepsy of baboons *Papio papio*, in *Reflex Seizures and Reflex Epilepsies* (eds A. Beaumanoir, H. Gastaut and R. Naquet), Editions Medecine and Hygiene, Geneve, pp. 39–48, 395–5.

Michelucci, R. and Tassinari, C.A. (1993) Television-induced occipital seizures, in *Occipital Seizures and Epilepsies in Children* (eds F. Andermann, A. Beaumanoir, L. Mira *et al.*), John Libbey, London, pp. 141–4.

Newmark, M.E. and Penry, J.K. (1979) *Photosensitive Epilepsy: A Review*, Raven Press, New York.

Panayiotopoulos, C.P. (1972) A study of photosensitive epilepsy with particular reference to occipital spikes induced by intermittent photic stimulation. University of Aston in Birmingham, PhD Thesis.

Panayiotopoulos, C.P. (1974) Effectiveness of photic stimulation on various eyes states in photosensitive epilepsy. *Journal of Neurological Science*, **23**, 165–73.

Panayiotopoulos, C.P. (1979) Self-induced pattern-sensitive epilepsy. *Archives of Neurology*, **36**, 48–50.

Panayiotopoulos, C.P. (1980) Basilar migraine? Seizures and severe epileptiform EEG abnormalities. *Neurology*, **30**, 1122–5.

Panayiotopoulos, C.P. (1981) Inhibitory effect of central vision on occipital lobe seizures. *Neurology*, **31**, 1331–3.

Panayiotopoulos, C.P. (1987a) Difficulties in differentiating migraine and epilepsy based on clinical and electroencephalographic findings, in *Migraine and Epilepsy* (eds F. Andermann and J. Lugaresi), Raven Press, New York, pp. 31–46.

Panayiotopoulos, C.P. (1987b) Fixation-off sensitive epilepsy in eye-lid myoclonia with absence seizures. *Annals of Neurology*, **22**, 87–9.

Panayiotopoulos, C.P. (1989) Fixation-off-sensitive epilepsies, in *Reflex Seizures and Reflex Epilepsies* (eds A. Beaumanoir, H. Gastaut and R. Naquet), Editions Medecine and Hygiene Geneve, pp. 203–17.

Panayiotopoulos, C.P. (1993a) Benign childhood partial epilepsies: benign childhood seizure susceptibility syndromes. *Journal of Neurology, Neurosurgery and Psychiatry*, **56**, 2–5.

Panayiotopoulos, C.P. (1993b) Benign childhood epilepsy with occipital paroxysms, in *Occipital Seizures and Epilepsies in Children* (eds F. Andermann, A. Beaumanoir, L. Mira *et al.*), John Libbey, London, pp. 151–64.

Panayiotopoulos, C.P. (1994) Fixation-off sensitive epilepsies, in *Epileptic Seizures and Epilepsies* (ed. P. Wolf), John Libbey, London, pp. 55–66.

Panayiotopoulos, C.P. (1994) The clinical spectrum of absence seizures and absence epilepsies, in: *Idiopathic Generalised Epilepsies: Clinical, Experimental and Genetic Aspects* (eds A. Malafosse, P. Genton, E. Hirsch *et al.*), John Libbey Eurotext, London, pp. 75–85.

Panayiotopoulos, C.P., Jeavons, P.M. and Harding, G.F.A. (1970a) Relation of occipital spikes evoked by intermittent photic stimulation to visual evoked responses in photosensitive epilepsy. *Nature*, **228**, 566–7.

Panayiotopoulos, C.P., Jeavons, P.M. and Harding, G.F.A. (1970b) Occipital spikes and their relation to visual evoked responses in epilepsy with particular reference to photosensitive epilepsy. *Electroencephalography and Clinical Neurophysiology*, **32**, 179–90.

Pazzaglia, P., Sabattini, L. and Lugaresi, E. (1970) Crisi occipitali precipitate dal buio. *Rivista di Neurologia*, **40**, 184–92.

Radovici, A., Misirliou, V. and Gluckman, M. (1932) Epilepsie reflexe provoqué par excitations des rayons solaires. *Revue Neurologique (Paris)*, **1**, 1305–8.

Reilly, E.L. and Peters, J.F. (1973) Relationship of some varieties of EEG photosensitivity to clinical convulsive disorders. *Neurology*, **13**, 1050–7.

Roger, J. and Bureau, M. (1993) Benign epilepsy of childhood with occipital paroxysms: up-date, in *Epileptic Syndromes in Infancy, Childhood and Adolescence* (eds J. Roger, M. Bureau, P. Dravet *et al.*) John Libbey, London, pp. 205–17.

Roger, J., Genton, P., Bureau, M. and Dravet, C. (1992) Progressive myoclonus epilepsies in childhood and adolescence, in *Epileptic Syndromes of Infancy, Childhood and Adolescence*, 2nd edn (eds J. Roger, M. Bureau, C. Dravet, *et al.*), John Libbey Eurotext, London, pp. 381–400.

Scollo-Lavizarri, G. and Lavizarri, G.R. (1974) Sleep, sleep deprivation, photosensitivity and epilepsy. *European Neurology*, **11**, 1–21.

Stefansson, S.B., Darby, C.E., Wilkins, A.J. *et al.* (1977) Television epilepsy and pattern sensitivity. *British Medical Journal*, **2**, 88–90

Takahashi, T. (1989) Techniques of intermittent photic stimulation and paroxysmal responses. *American Journal of EEG Technology*, **29**, 205–8.

Tassinari, C.A., Michelucci, R., Rubboli, G. *et al.* (1989) Self-induced seizures, in *Reflex Seizures and Reflex Epilepsies* (eds A. Beaumanoir, H. Gastaut and R. Naquet), Editions Medecine and Hygiene, Genève, pp. 363–8.

Waltz, S., Christen, H.J. and Doose, H. (1992) The different patterns of photoparoxysmal response – a genetic study. *Electroencephalography and Clinical Neurophysiology*, **83**, 138–45.

Wilkins, A.J. and Lindsay, J. (1985) Common forms of reflex epilepsy: physiological mechanisms and techniques for treatment, in *Recent Advances in Epilepsy, 2* (eds T.A. Pedley and

B.Meldrum), Churchill Livingstone, Edinburgh, pp. 239–71.

Wilkins, A.J., Andermann, F. and Ives, J. (1975) Stripes, complex cells and seizures. An attempt to determine the locus and nature of the trigger mechanism in pattern-sensitive epilepsy. *Brain*, **98,** 365–80.

Wilkins, A.J., Binnie, C.D. and Darby, C.E. (1980) Visually induced seizures. *Progress in Neurobiology*, **15,** 85–117.

Wilkins, A.J., Darby, D. and Binnie, C. (1979) Neurophysiological aspects of pattern-sensitive epilepsy. *Brain*, **102,** 1–25.

Wilkins, A.J., Binnie, C., Darby, D. and Kasteleijn-Nolst Trenité, D.G.A. (1989) Epileptic and non-epileptic sensitivity to light, in *Reflex Seizures and Reflex Epilepsies* (eds A. Beaumanoir, H. Gastaut and R. Naquet), Editions Medecine and Hygiene, Geneve, pp. 153–62.

Wolf, P. (1992a) Juvenile absence epilepsy, in *Epileptic Syndromes of Infancy, Childhood and Adolescence*, 2nd edn (eds J. Roger, M. Bureau, C. Dravet *et al.*), John Libbey Eurotext, London, pp. 307–12.

Wolf, P. (1992b) Reading epilepsy, in *Epileptic Syndromes of Infancy, Childhood and Adolescence*, 2nd edn (eds J. Roger, M. Bureau, C. Dravet *et al.*), John Libbey Eurotext, London, pp. 281–98.

Wolf, P. and Goosses, R. (1986) Relation of photosensitivity to epileptic syndromes. *Journal of Neurology, Neurosurgery and Psychiatry*, **49,** 1386–91.

BENIGN PARTIAL SEIZURES OF ADOLESCENCE

C. P. Panayiotopoulos

DEFINITION

Benign partial seizures of adolescence is an idiopathic, short-lived and transient condition of the second decade of life with a peak at 13–14 years of age. It is manifested by a single or a cluster of two to five partial, mainly motor and sensory, seizures which in half of the cases progress to a secondary generalized tonic-clonic seizure. There are no epileptic events preceding or following this limited seizure period which lasts no more than 36 hours. The seizures are mainly diurnal and predominantly affect male teenagers. Physical and mental states, as well as EEG and brain imaging, are normal.

CASE HISTORIES

A typical case
A 14-year-old boy, 2 weeks after an influenzal-like illness, had a partial motor seizure consisting of tonic deviation of the head to the right, followed by forced circling movements before ending in a generalized tonic-clonic seizure. He was confused postictally for 15 minutes. The neurologist suspected an underlying brain lesion but MRI of the brain was normal; an EEG showed a mild, nonspecific, abnormality consisting of bitemporal theta activity. Treatment with carbamazepine was initiated but the boy was compliant for 2 weeks only, after which he stopped medication.

He remains well with no seizures and a normal EEG 6 years later.

A less typical case
An 18-year-old student rushed to catch the train back home after a hard day's work. He was hungry and thirsty. He looked at a small video display unit of travel information and, after he looked away, the image of the screen persisted in the right upper corner of his vision and nearly simultaneously, started flashing at a rate of 3–5 Hz for 2 seconds. This was followed by the visual perception of the walls of the station and the passengers closing in on him ending in a generalized tonic-clonic seizure. Routine EEG, sleep deprivation EEG and MRI were all normal. No medication was prescribed. Two years later he remained well with no further visual or other seizures.

HISTORY

This condition was described by Loiseau and Orgogozo (1978) as an 'unrecognised syndrome of benign focal epileptic seizures in teenagers'. The most recent review is based on 108 patients (Loiseau and Loiset, 1992).

PREVALENCE, SEX, GENETICS, PRECIPITATING FACTORS, AND CIRCADIAN DISTRIBUTION

According to Loiseau and Loiset (1992), one-quarter of partial seizures with onset between

Epilepsy in Children. Edited by Sheila Wallace. Published in 1996 by Chapman & Hall, London. ISBN 0 412 56860 8

12 and 18 years of age have a benign course, i.e. they are single or occur in a cluster of up to five seizures during 36 hours, never to occur again. There is a 71.2% male preponderance. A family or personal history of seizures is extremely rare. There are no apparent precipitating factors and the seizures are nearly always diurnal (87%). I have retrospectively studied a sample of 120 patients with onset of simple partial seizures in the second decade of life and found nine cases who satisfy the criteria of benign partial seizures of adolescence (see the two cases described above).

AGE

These isolated epileptic events occur between the ages of 10 and 20 years with a peak at 13–15 years (one-third of the cases).

CLINICAL MANIFESTATIONS

The seizures by definition are partial but the temporal lobes are rarely involved. The teenager is fully aware and can give a reliable account of the onset of the clinical manifestations (simple partial seizures) in the majority of episodes (88%). However, consciousness rarely remains intact throughout the whole episode; the seizures usually evolve to impaired cognition, and/or to secondary generalized tonic-clonic convulsions which occur in half of the cases. The commonest ictal clinical manifestations are motor, usually without jacksonian marching, and somatosensory. Visual, vertiginous and autonomic symptoms are reported in one-fifth of the cases. Experiential phenomena like those in temporal lobe seizures practically never occur.

The physical and mental states of the patients are normal.

Laboratory tests and brain imaging are normal. The EEG may show some minor, nonspecific, abnormalities without spikes or focal slowing.

PROGNOSIS

Prognosis is excellent; in 80% of the patients there is a single, isolated seizure event and in the remaining a cluster of two to five seizures all occurring within 36 hours.

CONCLUSION

This is an interesting syndrome of one or a cluster of two to five partial seizures occurring in adolescents. They should not be treated with drugs. However, these patients are difficult to diagnose, as there are no specific features at onset to separate this condition from others with similar clinical manifestations, but of different etiology; particularly, symptomatic or cryptogenic partial epilepsies. My practice is to investigate all adolescents with onset of partial seizures with MRI and EEG which, if normal, would make the diagnosis of benign partial seizures of adolescence more likely. A definitive diagnosis cannot be made before 1–5 years of freedom from seizures.

REFERENCES

Loiseau, P. and Loiset, P. (1992) Benign partial seizures of adolescence, in *Epileptic Syndromes in Infancy, Childhood and Adolescence* (eds J. Roger, M. Bureau, P. Dravet *et al.*) John Libbey, London, pp. 343–45.

Loiseau, P. and Orgogozo, J.M. (1978) An unrecognised syndrome of benign focal epileptic seizures in teenagers. *Lancet*, **ii**, 1070–1.

PROGRESSIVE EPILEPSIES 15

INTRODUCTION

Within the framework of epilepsy the term 'progressive' means an epilepsy which changes with time, becoming more and more severe and becoming associated with other symptoms, mostly neurologic and mental, that also worsen with time. In that sense, many epileptic syndromes have a progressive course, either due to epilepsy itself (early myoclonic encephalopathy (Chapter 11a), West's syndrome (Chapter 11b), severe myoclonic epilepsy (Chapter 11e), Lennox–Gastaut Syndrome (Chapter 12a), for example) or due to the underlying disease (epilepsies related to phacomatoses, Rett's syndrome, progressive myoclonus epilepsies, Kojewnikow's syndrome). There are some diseases, usually secondary to metabolic disorders, with visceral manifestations, lack of psychomotor development and neurologic signs, in which epileptic seizures are only an accessory symptom (Aicardi, 1992). They are actually progressive but we do not consider them as progressive types of epilepsies. Thus, in this chapter only the syndromes in which epilepsy is the main or most significant symptom will be considered. These are essentially represented by the progressive myoclonus epilepsies and Kojewnikow's syndrome.

PROGRESSIVE MYOCLONUS EPILEPSIES 15a

Charlotte Dravet, Pierre Genton, Michelle Bureau and Joseph Roger

The full-blown progressive myoclonus epilepsy (PME) syndrome is characterized by the following association:

1. A myoclonic syndrome, involving a combination of fragmentary or segmental, arrhythmic, asynchronous, symmetric myoclonus and massive myoclonias.
2. An epilepsy, usually with generalized tonic-clonic or clonic seizures; but other types of seizures are also liable to occur.
3. A neurologic syndrome, which nearly always includes cerebellar manifestations.
4. A mental deterioration, culminating in dementia, this last feature being a less constant component of the syndrome (Roger *et al.*, 1992).

The intensity of the various clinical features varies depending on the etiology. Part of the semiology can be quite discrete: in degenerative PMEs such as Unverricht–Lündborg disease (ULD), for instance, the intellectual deficit, if present at all, develops very little, whereas Lafora's disease (LD) evolves rapidly into dementia. In other cases, a wide range of neurologic and sensory symptoms will also be encountered: early blindness due to retinal impairment in juvenile ceroid lipofuscinosis, and deafness or optic atrophy in some mitochondrial encephalomyopathies. The general progression of the disease also varies considerably from one etiology to another:

LD, for instance, progresses rapidly towards death within 5–10 years, whereas ULD can develop slowly over several decades in patients who are not too severely handicapped. The relative intensity of the various symptoms and the speed at which the disease progresses can also vary from one case to another in some forms of PME. The overall prognosis has definitely improved in recent decades, due to better care for these patients.

PMEs in childhood and adolescence are rare conditions which account only for about 1% of patients in the population of the Centre Saint-Paul. The prevalence of the different forms varies from one country, and from one region, to another. Some seem to be focused on a single ethnic group or place (dentato-rubral-pallido-luysian atrophy and galactosidosis in Japan), whereas others have been reported worldwide (Gaucher's disease, mitochondrial encephalomyopathy with ragged red fibers (MERRF)). Other forms have a predilection for some parts of the world: LD in Southern Europe and Southern India, neuronal ceroid lipofuscinosis (NCL) in Scandinavia, ULD in Finland and in the Mediterranean area.

As all the different PMEs cannot yet be classified either according to their etiology or to their genetics, it is possible to present them on the basis of their biologic and morphologic features when these are known (Table 15a.1).

Epilepsy in Children. Edited by Sheila Wallace. Published in 1996 by Chapman & Hall, London. ISBN 0 412 56860 8

Table 15a.1 Various types of PMEs

1. **PMEs related to a known biologic mechanism**
   Sialidosis
   Gaucher's disease
   MERRF
   GM$_2$ gangliosidosis (type III)
   Biopterin deficiency
2. **PMEs with a pathologic marker**
   Neuronal ceroid-lipofuscinosis
   Lafora's disease
3. **PMEs with a genetic marker**
   Unverricht–Lündborg disease
   Huntington's disease
   DRPLA
4. **PMEs without marker**
   Alper's disease

MERFF = mitochondrial encephalomyopathy with ragged red fibers; DRPLA = denato-rubral-pallido-luysian atrophy.

Obviously, in spite of our increasing knowledge, there are still patients who cannot be classified among these different forms even after their death. In this chapter, in order to remain practical, PMEs are listed by age: infancy, early childhood, childhood, and adolescence. The biochemical/metabolic aspects of PMEs are discussed more extensively in Chapter 3c and genetic aspects are covered further in Chapter 8.

PROGRESSIVE MYCLONUS EPILEPSIES IN INFANCY

There are very few syndromes fulfilling the criteria for PME at this age.

EARLY INFANTILE TYPE OF NCL (SANTAVUORI–HALTIA–HAGBERG DISEASE)

This type of NCL was identified by Santavuori, Haltia and Rapola (1974). It occurs between 3 months and 18 months, with hypotonia, arrest of psychomotor development evolving into mental deterioration and autistic features, acquired microcephaly, progressive loss of visual function, and optic atrophy. Massive myoclonias and changes in the EEG suggest the diagnosis. Progressive flattening of the EEG activities described as 'vanishing EEG' occur (Santavuori, 1973; Pampiglione and Harden, 1974). Skin, peripheral nerve or rectal biopsy confirms the diagnosis by showing characteristic inclusions (granular osmiotic deposits). Outcome is always bad with death around 10 years of age. The early infantile type of NCL maps genetically to the short arm of chromosome 1 (Järvela *et al.*, 1991).

TAY–SACHS AND SANDHOFF DISEASES (GM2 GANGLIOSIDOSIS, A AND O VARIANTS)

The first symptom is not epilepsy, since infants present with sudden startles provoked by noises without concomitant EEG modification. Epileptic seizures occur later as spontaneous and induced myoclonic jerks and partial seizures, accompanied by a slowing of the EEG activities and the appearance of multifocal abnormalities (Aicardi, 1992).

BIOPTERIN DEFICIENCY

Hypotonia precedes the onset of erratic myoclonias, which are associated with oculogyric attacks consisting of brief, sudden upward deviation of the eyes (Rey *et al.*, 1977).

POLIODYSTROPHIES (ALPER'S DISEASE)

In the heterogeneous group of the poliodystrophies (Alpers' disease) various types of seizures, myoclonic jerks and neurologic deterioration are the prominent symptoms. One form with associated hepatic dysfunction is progressive neuronal degeneration of childhood with liver disease (Harding *et al.*, 1986). Epilepsy may be the first symptom, characterized by partial seizures, repeated in status and evolving into epilepsia partialis continua, associated with a slowing in psychomotor development and progressive brain atrophy. The hepatic involvement appears at a variably later date, and is sometimes falsely attributed to valproate. EEG is suggestive if performed during a status, showing repetitive small spikes and polyspikes, often unilateral (Boyd *et al.*, 1986).

PROGRESSIVE MYOCLONUS EPILEPSIES IN EARLY CHILDHOOD

Two disorders merit attention in this age group: the childhood form of Huntington's chorea (HC) and the late infantile form of NCL.

JUVENILE MYOCLONIC FORM OF HC

The childhood onset form of HC is rare (Jervis, 1963; Bruyn, 1968); onset is after age 3, with loss of acquired psychomotor skills, cerebellar impairment, rigidity with loss of affect and dystonic posturing; choreic movements are not found. Epilepsy appears in general 2 years after the onset, as tonic-clonic seizures, atypical absences and massive myoclonias; erratic, asymmetric, spontaneous or action myoclonus is present in some cases and coincides mostly with worsening of epilepsy which may culminate in myoclonic or tonic-clonic status (Garrel *et al.*, 1978). The EEG may show clinical photosensitivity even before the onset of seizures; it is later characterized by spontaneous bursts of spike-waves (SWs) and polyspike-waves (PSWs). The prognosis is very poor, death occurring an average of 4 to 6 years after the onset.

The transmission is paternal in these myoclonic forms. HC has recently been mapped to the distal extremity of chromosome 4, 4p16.3 (Macdonald *et al.*, 1993). Preclinical and prenatal diagnosis is now possible but raises very difficult ethical problems.

LATE INFANTILE NCL (JANSKY–BIELSCHOWSKY DISEASE)

The late infantile form of NCL is an autosomal recessive disease that is found in various ethnic groups (Zeman *et al.*, 1970; Aicardi, Plouin and Goutières, 1978; Warburg, 1982). Onset is between ages $1\frac{1}{4}$ and $2\frac{3}{4}$ years; ataxia, speech and gait disturbances with loss of acquired mental skills are the first symptoms. These are soon followed by tonic-clonic seizures and myoclonus; visual impairment is first noted between ages 2 and 5. Progression is fast and children are usually blind, tetraplegic and bedridden by age 5 years. Death occurs at 3–10 years of age.

Optic atrophy can be observed from the age of 3, and the electroretinogram (ERG) is low in amplitude and later extinguished (Harden, Pampiglione and Picton-Robinson, 1973). The EEG shows slowing of background activity, irregular slow waves and polyspikes; single flash photic stimulation provokes very large polyphasic spikes over the posterior regions (Fig. 15a.1 and see Fig 19a.7) Visual evoked potentials (EPs) are accordingly enlarged and this particular response persists throughout the course of the disease (Pampiglione and Harden, 1977); somatosensory EPs may also be enlarged, but less constantly and later on. The electroclinical diagnosis may be confirmed by skin, peripheral nerve or rectal biopsy: the ultrastructural study shows curvilinear profiles and granular inclusions.

A form of NCL intermediate between the late infantile and the juvenile forms has been described as early juvenile NCL by Lake and Cavanagh (1978).

PROGRESSIVE MYOCLONUS EPILEPSIES IN CHILDHOOD AND ADOLESCENCE

JUVENILE NCL (SPIELMEYER–VOGT–SJÖGREN DISEASE)

This form remains the most widespread and relatively common presentation of Batten's disease (Zeman *et al.*, 1970; Sjögren, 1931). It was described as early as in 1826 in Norway (Stengel, 1826) and occurs more frequently in Scandinavia than elsewhere.

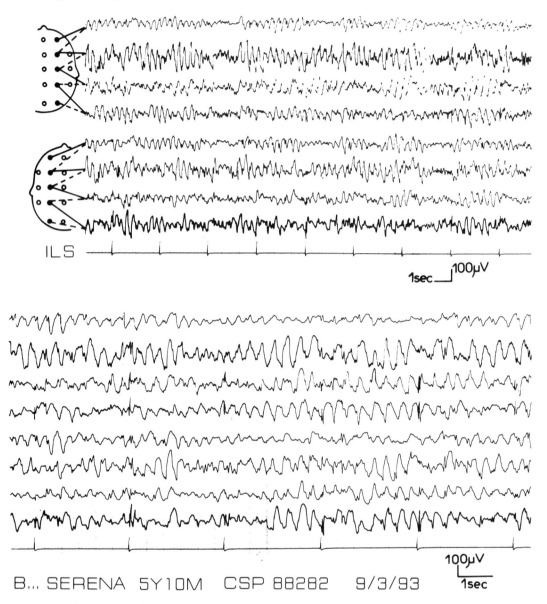

Fig. 15a.1 Characteristic photosensitivity in a girl of 5 years 10 months suffering from a late infantile NCL (Jansky–Bielschowsky). Abnormal potentials are evoked by each flash of stimulation at low frequency, in the posterior areas, sometimes more diffuse spikes are better visible with a high paper speed (bottom).

Onset is between ages 4 and 15 (Sjögren 1931; Sorensen and Parnas, 1979). Sixty per cent of patients present initially with progressive visual loss due to pigmentary degeneration of the retina. Intellectual impairment is less frequent at the onset and progresses slowly; neurologic signs begin generally 2–3 years after the onset. Absences, or more frequently tonic-clonic seizures, occur 1–4 years after the onset; clonic status may be common at the terminal stage. Segmental and later massive myoclonus appear at the same time as the epileptic seizures; myoclonias involving the face may be prominent. According to Berkovic and Andermann (1986), the disease may present at an earlier age in a different sequence, with initially seizures and myoclonus, visual loss appearing later.

The EEG shows early slowing and disruption of the background activity and sharp waves and SWs. The changes are enhanced by sleep. Photic stimulation does not produce EEG or clinical changes. Both ERG and visual evoked responses show a gradual fading; somatosensory EPs are enlarged.

Schooling is usually possible until around age 10; patients later adopt a typical presentation with a stooping gait and dysarthria; motor dyspraxia may be severe and confine the subjects to a wheelchair; psychotic episodes may complicate the evolution of the disease. Death occurs generally around age 20.

The diagnosis is confirmed by the evidence of abnormal storage with the presence of vacuolized circulating lymphocytes (Bagh and Hortling, 1948) and fingerprint membranous profiles on ultrastructural studies of skin biopsy material, or of lymphocytes, sometimes associated with curvilinear and rectilinear bodies.

According to Carpenter *et al.* (1977), four types of inclusions can be found in the biopsy material of patients with NCL: curvilinear bodies (predominating in the late infantile form); fingerprint membranous profiles (in the juvenile form); rectilinear profiles (juvenile form); and granular osmiotic deposits (early infantile form). However, no type is really specific for a clinical form. In contrast it has been found by the group of Gardiner (Eiberg, Gardiner and Mohr, 1989) that the locus for the Spielmeyer–Vogt disease, is on chromosome 16, near the region 16q22, different from that of the Santavuori disease.

Antenatal diagnosis is possible either on cells obtained at amniocentesis (Mac Leod, Nag and Berry, 1988) or on chorionic biopsy material (Conradi *et al.*, 1989).

Based on the biochemical hypothesis of Zeman (1974), an etiologic treatment using antioxidant drugs is now used by some authors in juvenile NCL (Santavuori *et al.*, 1988). It seems to delay the progression of the disease, but does not have the same effect in the other NCL types.

JUVENILE GAUCHER'S DISEASE (TYPE III)

Neither the juvenile form (type I) nor the infantile neuropathic form (type II) of Gaucher's disease (GD) present as PME. A heterogeneous group of patients, with proven histology and biochemistry of GD, have been gathered as a type III (Winkelman *et al.*, 1983). Presenting symptoms are generally myoclonus and saccadic horizontal eye movements; splenomegaly may be present; generalized or partial epileptic seizures, cerebellar impairment and some degree of dementia are usually present. In some families, a prominent, severe action myoclonus, touch myoclonus, and photosensitivity may be found.

The EEG shows a normal or slow background activity and bursts of predominantly posterior, sometimes multifocal, 6–10-Hz PSWs (Nishimura *et al.*, 1980); these are enhanced by sleep. Photic stimulation produces a myoclonic response. Visual EPs are reported to be normal, somatosensory EPs may be enlarged in some patients (Halliday and Halliday, 1980).

Age of onset varies between childhood and early adulthood. Survival ranges between a decade and mid-adulthood. The diagnosis is based on the evidence of storage of β-glucocerebroside in bone marrow (Gaucher cells), in cultured fibroblasts, circulating lymphocytes, and other organs; neuronal storage may be shown on rectal mucosal biopsy or appendicectomy material.

SIALIDOSES

Type I sialidosis is characterized by an autosomal recessively transmitted deficiency in neuraminidase (α-2-6 sialidase) and accounts for the 'cherry-red spot myoclonus' syndrome (Rapin *et al.*, 1978; Thomas *et al.*, 1979; Federico *et al.*, 1980). Age of onset is variable, the mean age being around 15 years. Many variants of sialidosis with the cherry-red spot have been described.

Onset is usually an association or succession of mild visual impairment, epileptic seizures, and systemic neurologic signs ('burning feet' cerebellar impairment) (Steinman *et al.*, 1980). Myoclonus becomes increasingly characteristic: spontaneous, intermittent, irregular myoclonias of the face, around the mouth, that are not stimulus-sensitive and persist during sleep.

The cherry-red spot is found on fundoscopy, but can disappear during the course of the disease. The EEG shows normal or fast and low voltage background activity, which tends to slow down when dementia occurs. There is no photosensitivity. Massive myoclonias are associated with generalized PSWs; facial myoclonias are not associated with EEG changes. Visual EPs are usually decreased, but somatosensory EPs are greatly enhanced. Prenatal diagnosis is possible.

Type II sialidosis, or galactosialidosis, is characterized by an additional partial deficiency in β-galactosidase (Sakuraba *et al.*, 1983). This form has been described mostly in Japanese subjects; it is associated with chondrodystrophy, angiokeratoma, and mild to moderate dementia.

The overall prognosis of sialidoses is poor, as myoclonus becomes rapidly severe and incapacitating, although seizures may respond to antiepileptic drugs.

LAFORA'S DISEASE

(LD) represents a well-defined clinical and neurophysiologic entity with an autosomal recessive inheritance and a known histopathologic marker, the presence of Lafora bodies in brain tissue (Lafora, 1911; Van Heycop Ten Ham and De Jager, 1963; Roger *et al.*, 1967). Deposits of polyglucosans can also be demonstrated in skin, mucosa, liver or muscle biopsy material. The enzyme defect involved in the LD has not yet been elucidated, nor has the gene been located. However, linkage to the location of the ULD gene has been excluded (Lehesjoki *et al.*, 1992).

Case reports have stressed a certain variability in both age of onset (between age 6 and 19) and duration of the disease, sometimes among siblings (Tassinari *et al.*, 1978), although the general progression of the disease remains typical. The clinical picture includes, in typical succession, epileptic seizures, both generalized and focal, visual (Roger *et al.*, 1983); a severe and progressive myoclonic syndrome with erratic resting and action myoclonus; dementia is rapidly progressive, with early and severe impairment of higher cortical functions and marked depression. The clinical course is marked by spontaneous episodes of rapid worsening, followed by periods of apparent stabilization. It is interesting to note that visual partial seizures and photosensitivity are rare in Indian patients (Acharya *et al.*, 1993).

Early EEGs show normal background activity, isolated bursts of SWs, and PSWs with marked clinical photosensitivity; paroxysms are not enhanced during sleep. Erratic myoclonus is not associated with EEG changes. At this very early stage, the characteristics distinguishing these patients from cases with idiopathic generalized epilepsy are the presence of erratic myoclonus (often found on polygraphy before they become clinical) and the lack of activation during sleep. After a few months, sometimes years, the EEG shows typical changes: slowing of the background activity, fast generalized polyspikes and PSWs, focal occipital or multifocal spikes, disappearance of physiologic sleep patterns and persisting erratic myoclonus; photosensitivity may persist throughout the evolution. Brainstem EPs may be delayed; enlarged somatosensory EPs have also been found.

The clinical and EEG features can lead to early diagnosis in isolated cases. Biopsy of axillary skin seems to be the most practical procedure for early diagnosis (Carpenter and Karpati, 1981; Tinuper *et al.*, 1983); the deposits are particularly visible in eccrine sweat duct cells, but also on muscle or liver biopsies. Death occurs within 2–10 years.

MYOCLONUS EPILEPSY WITH RAGGED-RED FIBERS

A group of diseases due to maternally inherited deficiencies in mitochondrial metabolism has been described over the past 15 years (Tsairis, Engel and Kark, 1973; Fukuhara *et al.*, 1980). The frontiers between syndromes remain unclear; the precise relationship between the metabolic defect and its clinical expression has yet to be established. According to Di Mauro *et al.* (1985) 'the usefulness of clinical criteria for identification and classification of mitochondrial myopathies is limited, because there is non-consistent phenotype and because symptoms and signs may be similar in patients with different biochemical defects'.

Among these conditions, the syndrome known as MERRF has emerged as a promising etiology of hitherto unexplained PMEs: several cases diagnosed as Ramsay–Hunt syndrome have been reclassified as mitochondrial encephalopathies (Berkovic and Andermann, 1986). However, most patients with MERRF present with prominent clinical abnormalities besides myoclonus, epilepsy, and dementia. After some years of follow-up, some patients may also show symptoms of the mitochondrial encephalomyopathy with lactic acidosis and stroke-like episodes syndrome (MELAS) (Byrne *et al.*, 1988).

Age of onset varies widely between at least 5 and 42 years, and probably beyond. Myoclonus and ataxia are the most constant features; tonic-clonic seizures and dementia are less constant. A majority of patients present with prominent associated features such as short stature, deafness, optic atrophy (Roger *et al.*, 1982), peripheral neuropathy, pes cavus, and endocrine dysfunction. Muscular symptoms are often very slight, sometimes absent. It is difficult to establish a prognosis in such cases, as the clinical presentation is very variable; overall, the condition seems to follow a relatively benign but nevertheless progressive course.

Skeletal muscle biopsy shows a typical appearance of ragged-red fibers (Di Mauro *et al.*, 1985); swollen/abnormal mitochondria may be present in some tissues (skin) and absent on CNS biopsy material. It has been shown that a single muscular biopsy may be normal in MERRF, although the enzyme defect can be demonstrated on the very same tissue. Conversely, totally or partially asymptomatic family members (e.g. with isolated hearing loss) may show ragged-red fibers on muscle biopsy (Rosing *et al.*, 1985). The biochemical deficit can be located by performing biochemical analysis of the mitochondrial respiratory chain (Bindoff *et al.*, 1991).

The neuropathology of MERRF (Nakano *et al.*, 1982; Sasaki *et al.*, 1983) shows selective neuronal loss of the dentate and inferior olivary nuclei, tract degeneration of superior cerebellar peduncles and posterior columns, as well as gliosis in the brainstem and cerebellum. These findings may cover former descriptions of 'system degeneration' or 'abiotrophy'. Histochemical studies may give more precise clues as to the exact metabolic defect involved and open the way to specific replacement therapy. Patients can be given replacement coenzyme Q, the synthesis of which is blocked in the respiratory chain cycle. The results of initial tests have been promising, but Wallace *et al.* (1991) have pointed out that over-high doses could worsen the symptomatology.

In a study of mitochondrial DNA, Schoffner *et al.* (1990) found a heteroplasmic A/G mutation in position 8,344 in patients affected by MERRF and in some of their relatives. These findings, however, do not necessarily mean that all cases of MERRF are due to the same genetic disorder.

SO-CALLED 'DEGENERATIVE' FORMS OF PME: A MOVING FIELD

This category includes those conditions which can be diagnosed solely on the basis of the clinical and neurophysiologic findings, since no specific biochemical or anatomic markers are so far available. These conditions nevertheless constitute proper diseases, since their genetic, clinical and evolving characteristics have been clearly established. Some typical, familial cases of dentato-rubral-pallido-luysian atrophy have been reported in Japan. On the other hand, numerous patients have presented with a typical form of PME which fits the description of 'Unverricht's myoclonia' very closely. This disease is thought to be rare, but two large groups of patients have been described, the one in Marseille as having myoclonic cerebellar dyssynergy (Ramsay–Hunt syndrome) (Roger, Soulayrol and Hassoun, 1968), dyssynergia cerebellaris myoclonica with epilepsy (Roger *et al.*, 1987), and Mediterranean myoclonus (Genton *et al.*, 1990), and the other in Finland, under the name of either progressive myoclonus epilepsy with no Lafora bodies (Koskiniemi, Toivakka and Donner, 1974) or Baltic myoclonus (Koskiniemi, 1986). Advances in molecular biology have allowed the Finnish group to identify the location of the gene responsible for this condition on the distal part of chromosome 21 band q22.3 (Lehesjoki *et al.*, 1991). A significant linkage for the same markers has been found in the Mediterranean families by our group (Malafosse *et al.*, 1992). Thus it is possible to reassemble these two syndromes under the same heading of Unverricht–Lündborg disease. (Marseille Consensus Group, 1990.) Here, this entity is described on the basis of our most recent series of patients (Genton *et al.*, 1990).

The disease is inherited by recessive autosomal transmission. Age of onset is consistently 6–18 years. The disease begins either insidiously with action myoclonus, noticeable in the morning upon wakening, or more suddenly with nocturnal clonic or clonic-tonic-clonic seizures. The myoclonus gradually becomes incapacitating and few spontaneous jerks occur. Myoclonias make some movements difficult to perform, requiring motor preparation, and being executed only after a period of latency. Eating and drinking become difficult. Some myoclonus attacks are triggered by performing difficult movements and may develop into full-scale clonic or clonic-tonic-clonic seizures, often involving a partial loss of consciousness. Absences have been much less frequently reported.

Ataxia is generally present, to a degree which is variable but difficult to assess because of the jerks. Other neurologic signs are present only in a few patients: pes cavus – a slight but stable symptom – and abolition of the tendon reflexes. In Marseille optic atrophy, sensory disorders, pyramidal or extrapyramidal impairments and amyotrophy have not been observed. The patients' cognitive abilities are not severely affected. Reactional psychologic disorders are, however, both pronounced and frequent.

Myoclonus and ataxia slowly but steadily worsen. The epilepsy, which can be controlled by medication, seems to lessen with time. The patients' condition tends to fluctuate sharply between 'good periods', during which they are only slightly handicapped, and 'bad periods', when the myoclonus becomes more pronounced, not permitting walking, sometimes ending in a seizure or series of seizures. The periods of remission can last from 1 day to several weeks, and they tend to shorten progressively during the evolving phase of the disease.

Depending on the speed at which the disease has progressed, it tends to stabilize once the patient is over 40, and the debilitating effects of the myoclonus in particular also subsequently subside. We have observed no cases where dementia occurs in the course of the disease.

The results of biologic tests are consistently normal. Muscle biopsy is also normal, and MERRF can be ruled out (Tassinari *et al.*, 1989). Mitochondrial DNA does not show the mutation recently found in families with hereditary MERRF (Tassinari *et al.*, 1991).

In the early stages of the disease, the EEG shows normal background activity, with a few slow discharges becoming more frequent as the disease progresses. Short, subclinical generalized SWs are recorded, sometimes associated with massive myoclonias, whereas the action myoclonus is not accompanied by any changes in the EEG. Clinical and EEG sensitivity to photostimulation is observed in almost 90% of all cases. Normal physiologic sleep patterns are present: the paroxysmal anomalies are not noticeably aggravated during slow wave sleep, whereas during REM sleep, fast spike and polyspike discharges occur around the vertex (Tassinari *et al.*, 1974) The amplitude of the somatosensory EPs is found to be abnormally high (Mauguière, Bard and Courjon, 1981; Tassinari *et al.*, 1989). The abnormalities tend to diminish with time. In the longest-established cases, a moderate slowing of the background activity and a slight attenuation of the physiologic sleep patterns during the phases of stage 2 sleep are mainly observed.

Antiepileptic drugs have been successfully used to control the seizures, but the myoclonus responds only transiently to drug therapy. It is advisable to prescribe polytherapy including valproate as the basic medication, a benzodiazepine, and possibly phenobarbitone if generalized seizures are frequent. Alcohol can reduce the intensity of the myoclonias for a few hours, but its effects are short-lived and there is a risk of rapid habituation (Genton and Guerrini, 1990). As with postanoxic myoclonus high doses of piracetam administered orally can be a most effective means of treating ULD (Rémy and Genton, 1991).

In the patients reported by Koskiniemi (1986), some differences could be noted. The course of the disease seemed to be more severe, ending in death within an average of 15 years. Secondary pyramidal symptoms and marked changes in the EEG background activity often occurred. However the Finnish authors now recognize that both the life expectancy and the functional capacities of their patients have improved considerably, thanks to recent changes in the treatment. It now emerges, in particular, that high doses of phenytoin had deleterious effects on a large number of patients (Elridge *et al.*, 1983).

Dentato-rubral-pallido-luysian atrophy (DRPLA)

This disease, with a predominantly autosomal dominant transmission, described in Japan (Naito and Oyanagi, 1982), involves degeneration of both the dentato-rubral and the pallido-luysian systems (Iizuka, Hirayama and Machara, 1984). Diverse clinical pictures have been described and the onset has been reported to occur between 6 and 69 years of age. Nearly half of the cases where the onset occurs between childhood and adulthood present with PME symptoms, sometimes associated with other neurologic disorders, such as choreoathetosis, rapidly developing dementia, and ataxia. The EEG shows slow bursts and generalized SWs, and no consistent pattern of photosensitivity has been observed.

Very recently Japanese authors have identified unstable expansion of a CAG in a gene on chromosome 12 in all the 22 DRPLA patients examined (Koide *et al.*, 1994)

CONCLUSION

PMEs are rare and severe diseases for which our understanding has progressed considerably over the last few years. An accurate diagnosis is now possible in nearly all cases using nonaggressive procedures, first on the

Table 15a.2 Biologic tools for diagnosing the main forms of PMEs

Etiology	Procedure	Biologic/anatomopathologic marker
Lafora's disease	Skin biopsy (armpit)	Lafora bodies (polyglucosans)
Ceroid lipofuscinosis	Biopsy (skin, rectal mucosa, etc. . . .)	Curvilinear granular inclusions + 'fingerprint profiles' + rectilinear profiles and osmiophilic granular profiles
Gaucher's disease (type III)	Lymphocytes, fibroblasts, bone marrow, liver etc . . .	β-Glucosidase deficit β-Cerebroside storage
Sialidosis	Urine, lymphocytes, fibroblasts	Greatly increased urinary oligosaccharide neuraminidase deficit
Galactosialidosis	Lymphocytes, fibroblasts	Associated β-galactosidase deficit
Mitochondrial encephalomyopathy with myoclonus epilepsy (MERRF)	Muscle biopsy	'Ragged-red fibers' Respiratory metabolic chain deficit

basis of clinical and cases histories, later supported by neurophysiologic tests. The diagnosis must be confirmed by searching for biologic markers, mainly by muscle and skin biopsy (Table 15a.2). Treatment involves the judicious use of antiepileptic drugs together with psychosocial care, whereas reversal of the etiologic abnormality is possible in very few patients. Genetic counselling is already possible, as well as prenatal diagnosis, in some diseases.

REFERENCES

Acharya, J.N., Satishchandra, P., Asha, T. and Shankar, S.K. (1993) Lafora's disease in South India: a clinical, electrophysiologic, and pathologic study. *Epilepsia*, **34**, 476–87.

Aicardi, J. (1992) Epilepsy and inborn errors of metabolism, in *Epileptic Syndromes in Infancy, Childhood and Adolescence*, 2nd edn (eds J. Roger M. Bureau, Ch. Dravet *et al.*), John Libbey Eurotext, London, Paris, pp. 97–102.

Aicardi, J., Plouin, P. and Goutières, F. (1978) Les céroide-lipofuscinoses. *Revue d'Electrocephalographie Neurophysiologie Clinique*, **8**, 149–60.

Bagh, K. and Hortling, H. (1948) Blodfynd vid juvenil amaurotisk idioti. *Nordisk Medicin*, **38**, 1072–6.

Berkovic, S.F. and Andermann, F. (1986) The progressive myoclonus epilepsies, in *Recent Advances in Epilepsy*, vol. 3 (eds T.A. Pedley and B.S. Meldrum), Churchill Livingstone, London, pp. 157–87.

Bindoff, L.A., Desnuelle, C., Birch-Machin, M.A. *et al.* (1991) Multiple defects of the mitochondrial respiratory chain in mitochondrial encephalomyopathy (MERRF): a clinical biochemical and molecular study. *Journal of the Neurological Sciences*, **102**, 17–24.

Boyd, S.G., Harden, A., Egger, J. and Pampiglione, G. (1986) Progressive neuronal degeneration of childhood with liver disease ('Alpers' disease'): characteristic neurophysiological features. *Neuropediatrics*, **17**, 75–80.

Bruyn, G.W. (1968) Huntington's chorea: historical, clinical and laboratory synopsis, in *Handbook of Clinical Neurology*, vol.6 (eds P.S. Vinken and G.W. Bruyn), Elsevier North-Holland, Amsterdam, pp. 298–378.

Byrne, E., Trounce, I., Dennett, X *et al.* (1988) Progression from MERFF to MELAS phenotype in a patient with combined complex I and IV deficiencies. *Journal of the Neurological Sciences*, **88**, 327–37.

Carpenter, S. and Karpati, G. (1981) Sweat gland duct cells in Lafora disease: diagnosis by skin biopsy. *Neurology* **31**, 1564–8.

Carpenter, S., Karpati, G., Andermann, F., *et al.* (1977) The ultrastructural characteristics of the abnormal cytosomes in Batten–Kuf's disease. *Brain*, **100**, 137–56.

Conradi, N.G., Uvebrant, P., Hökegård, K.H. *et al.* (1989) First trimester diagnosis of juvenile neuronal ceroid lipofuscinosis by demonstration of fingerprint inclusion in chorionic villi. *Prenatal Diagnosis*, **9**, 283–7.

Di Mauro, S., Bonilla, E., Zeviani, M. *et al.* (1985) Mitochondrial myopathies. *Annals of Neurology*, **17**, 521–38.

Eiberg, H., Gardiner, R.M. and Mohr, J. (1989) Batten disease (Spielmeyer–Sjögren disease) and haptoglobins (HP): indication of linkage and assignment to CH. 16. *Clinical Genetics*, **36**, 217–8.

Elridge, R., Ilvanainen, M., Stern, R. *et al.* (1983) 'Baltic' myoclonus epilepsy: hereditary disorder of childhood made worse by phenytoin. *Lancet* **ii**, 838–42.

Federico, A., Cecio, A., Apponi Battini, G. *et al.* (1980) Macular cherry-red spot and myoclonus syndrome. Juvenile form of sialidosis. *Journal of the Neurological Sciences*, **48**, 57–169.

Fukuhara, N., Tokiguchi, S., Shirakawa, K. and Tsubaki, T. (1980) Myoclonus epilepsy associated with ragged-red fibers (mitochondrial abnormalities): disease entity or a syndrome? *Journal of the Neurological Sciences*, **47**, 117–33.

Garrel, S., Joannard, A., Feuerstein, J. and Serre, F. (1978) Formes myocloniques de la chorée de Huntington. *Revue d'Electroencephalographie et de Neurophysiologie Clinique*, **8**, 123–8.

Genton, P. and Guerrini, R. (1990) Antimyoclonic effects of alcohol in progressive myoclonus epilepsy. *Neurology*, **40**, 1412–6.

Genton, P., Michelucci, R., Tassinari, C.A. and Roger, J. (1990) The Ramsay–Hunt syndrome revisited: Mediterranean myoclonus versus mitochondrial encephalomyopathy with ragged red fibers and Baltic myoclonus. *Acta Neurologica Scandinavica*, **81**, 8–15.

Halliday, A.M. and Halliday, E. (1980) Cerebral somatosensory and visual evoked potentials in different clinical forms of myoclonus, in *Clinical Uses of Cerebral, Brainstem and Spinal Somatosensory Potentials*, vol.17 (ed. J.E. Desmedt), Karger, Basel, pp. 292–310.

Harden, A., Pampiglione, G. and Picton-Robinson, N. (1973) Electroretinogram and visual evoked response in a form of 'neuronal lipidosis' with diagnostic EEG features. *Journal of Neurology, Neurosurgery and Psychiatry*, **36**, 61–7.

Harding, B.N., Egger, J., Portmann, B. and Erdohazi, M. (1986) Progressive neuronal degeneration of childhood with liver disease. *Brain*, **109**, 181–206.

Iizuka, R., Hirayama, K. and Machara, K. (1984) Dentato-rubro-pallido-luysian atrophy: a clinico-pathological study. *Journal of Neurology, Neurosurgery and Psychiatry*, **47**, 1288–98.

Järvela, I., Schleutker, J., Haataja, L. *et al.* (1991) Infantile form of neuronal ceroid lipofuscinosis (CLN 1) maps to the short arm of chromosome 1. *Genomics*, **9**, 170–3.

Jervis, G.A. (1963) Huntington's chorea in childhood. *Archives of Neurology*, **9**, 244–57.

Koide, R., Ikuchi, T., Onodesa, O. *et al.* (1994) Unstable expansion of CAG repeat in hereditary dentatorubral-pallidoluysian atrophy (DRPLA). *Nature Genetics*, **6**, 9–12.

Koskiniemi, M.L. (1986) Baltic myoclonus, in *Myoclonus. Advances in Neurology*, vol.43 (eds S. Fahn, C.D. Marsden and M. Van Woert), Raven Press, New York, pp. 57–64.

Koskiniemi, M. L., Toivakka, E. and Donner, M. (1974) Progressive myoclonus epilepsy. Electroencephalographic findings. *Acta Neurologica Scandinavica*, **50**, 333–59.

Lafora, G.R. (1911) Über das Vorkommen amyloider Körperchen im Inneren der Ganglienzellen. *Virchows Archiv. A, Pathological Anatomy and Histopathology*, 205–95.

Lake, B.D. and Cavanagh, N.P.C. (1978) Early juvenile Batten's disease – a recognizable subgroup distinct from other forms of Batten's disease. *Journal of the Neurological Sciences*, **36**, 265–71.

Lehesjoki, A.E., Koskiniemi, M., Sistonen, P. *et al.* (1991) Localization of a gene for progressive myoclonus epilepsy to chromosome 21q22. *Proceedings of the National Academy of Sciences USA*, **88**, 3606–99.

Lehesjoki, A.E., Koskiniemi, M., Pandolfo, M. *et al.* (1992) Linkage studies in progressive myoclonus epilepsy: Unverricht–Lündborg and Lafora's diseases. *Neurology*, **42**, 1545–50.

Macdonald, M.E., Ambrose, C.M., Duyao, M.P. *et al.* (1993) Novel gene containing a trinucleotide repeat that is expanded and unstable on Huntington's disease chromosomes. *Cell*, **72**, 971–83.

Mac Leod, P.M., Nag, S. and Berry, G. (1988) Ultrastructural studies as a method of prenatal diagnosis of neuronal ceroid lipofuscinosis. *American Journal of Medical Genetics Supplement*, **5**, 93–7.

Malafosse, A., Lehesjoki, A.E., Genton, P. *et al.* (1992) Identical genetic locus for Baltic and Mediterranean myoclonus. *Lancet*, **39**, 1080–1.

Marseille Consensus Group (1990) Classification of

progressive myoclonus epilepsies and related disorders. *Annals of Neurology*, **28**, 113–16.

Mauguière, F., Bard, J. and Courjon, J. (1981) Les potentiels évoqués somesthésiques précoces dans la dyssynergie cérébelleuse myoclonique progressive. *Revue d'Electroencephalographie et de Neurophysiologie Clinique*, **11**, 174–82.

Naito, H. and Oyanagi, S. (1982) Familial myoclonus epilepsy and choreoathetosis: hereditary dentatorubral-pallidoluysian atrophy. *Neurology*, **32**, 798–807.

Nakano, T., Sakai, H., Amano, N. *et al.* (1982) An autopsy case of degenerative type of myoclonus epilepsy associated with Friedreich's ataxia and mitochondrial myopathy. *Brain Nerve*, **34**, 321–32.

Nishimura, R., Omos-Lau, N., Ajmone-Marsan, C. and Barranger, J.A. (1980) Electroencephalographic findings in Gaucher's disease. *Neurology*, **30**, 152–9.

Pampiglione, G. and Harden, A. (1974) An infantile form of neuronal 'storage' disease with characteristic evolution of neurophysiological features. *Brain*, **97**, 355–60.

Pampiglione, G. and Harden, A. (1977) Neurophysiological identification of a late infantile form of 'neuronal lipidosis'. *Journal of Neurology Neurosurgery and Psychiatry*, **36**, 323–30.

Rapin, I., Goldfisher, S., Datzman, R., *et al.* (1978) The cherry-red spot myoclonus syndrome. *Annals of Neurology*, **3**, 234–342.

Remy, C. and Genton, P. (1991). Effect of high doses of oral piracetam on myoclonus in progressive myoclonus epilepsy (Mediterranean myoclonus). *Epilepsia*, **32**, (suppl. 3) 6 (abstr.).

Rey, F., Harpey, J.P., Leeming, R.J. *et al.* (1977) Les hyperphénylalaninémies avec activité normale de la phénylalanine-hydroxylase. *Archives Françaises de Pédiatrie*, **34**, 109–20.

Roger, J., Soulayrol, R. and Hassoun, J. (1968) La dyssynergie cérébelleuse myoclonique (syndrome de Ramsay Hunt). *Revue Neurologique*, **119**, 85–106.

Roger, J., Gastaut, H., Boudouresques, J. *et al.* (1967) Epilepsie myoclonique progressive avec corps de Lafora. Etude clinique et polygraphique. Contrôle anatomique ultrastructural. *Revue Neurologique*, **116**, 197–212.

Roger, J., Pellissier, J.F., Dravet, C. *et al.* (1982) Dégénérescence spino-cérébelleuse. Atrophie optique. Epilepsie-myoclonies. Myopathie mitochondriale. *Revue Neurologique*, **138**, 187–200.

Roger, J., Pellissier, J.F., Bureau, M. *et al.* (1983) Le diagnostic précoce de la maladie de Lafora. Importance des manifestations paroxystiques visuelles et intérêt de la biopsie cutanée. *Revue Neurologique*, **139**, 115–24.

Roger, J., Genton, P., Bureau, M. *et al.* (1987) Dyssynergia cerebellaris myoclonica (Ramsay–Hunt syndrome) associated with epilepsy: a study of 32 cases. *Neuropediatrics*, **18**, 117.

Roger, J., Genton, P., Bureau, M. and Dravet, Ch. (1992) Progressive myoclonus epilepsy in childhood and adolescence, In *Epileptic Syndromes in Infancy, Childhood and Adolescence*, 2nd edn (eds J. Roger, M. Bureau, Ch. Dravet *et al.*), John Libbey Eurotext, London, Paris, pp. 381–400.

Rosing, H.S., Hopkins, L.C., Wallace, D.C. *et al.* (1985) Maternally inherited mitochondrial myopathy and myoclonic epilepsy. *Annals of Neurology*, **17**, 228–37.

Sakuraba, H., Suzuki, Y., Akagi, M. *et al.* (1983) β-Galactosidase-neuraminidase deficiency (galactosialidosis): clinical, pathological and enzymatic studies in postmortem case. *Annals of Neurology*, **13**, 497–503.

Santavuori, P. (1973) EEG in the infantile type of so-called neuronal ceroid lipofuscinosis. *Neuropædiatrie*, **4**, 375–87.

Santavuori, P., Haltia, M. and Rapola, J. (1974) Infantile type of so-called neuronal ceroid lipofuscinosis. *Developmental Medicine and Child Neurology*, **16**, 644–53.

Santavuori, P., Heiskala, H., Westermarck, T. *et al.* (1988) Experience over 17 years with antioxidant treatment in Spielmeyer–Sjögren disease. *American Journal of Medical Genetics Supplement*, **5**, 265–74.

Sasaki, H., Kuzuhara, S., Kanazawa, I. *et al.* (1983) Myoclonus, cerebellar disorder, neuropathy, mitochondrial myopathy and ACTH deficiency. *Neurology*, **33**, 1288–93.

Schoffner, J.M., Lon, M.T., Lezza, A.M.S. *et al.* (1990) Myoclonic epilepsy and ragged red fiber disease (MERRF) is associated with a mitochondrial DNA tRNA Lys mutation. *Cell*, **61**, 931–7.

Sjögren, T. (1931) Die amaurotische Idiotie. Klinische und Erblichkeit medizinische Untersuchungen. *Lund: Hereditas*, **14**, 197–426.

Sorensen, J.B. and Parnas, P. (1979) A clinical study of 44 patients with juvenile amaurotic idiocy. *Acta Psychiatrica Scandinavica*, **59**, 449–61.

Steinman, L., Tharp, B.R., Dorfman, L.J. *et al.* (1980) Peripheral neuropathy in the cherry-red spot-myoclonus syndrome (sialidosis type 1). *Annals of Neurology*, **7**, 450–6.

Stengel, O.C. (1826) Account of a singular illness among four siblings in the vicinity of Røraas. *Eyr (Christiana)*, **1**, 347–52. (English translation reprinted in extenso (1982), in *Ceroid-lipofuscinosis (Batten's disease)* (eds D. Armstrong, N. Koopand and J.A. Rider), Elsevier Biomedical Press, Amsterdam, pp. 17–19.

Tassinari, C.A., Bureau-Paillas, M., Dalla Bernardina, B. *et al.* (1974) Etude électroencéphalographique de la dyssynergie cérébelleuse myoclonique avec épilepsie (syndrome de Ramsay Hunt). *Revue d'Electroencephalographie et de Neurophysiologie Clinique*, **4**, 407–28.

Tassinari, C.A., Bureau-Paillas, M., Dalla Bernardina, B. *et al.* (1978) La maladie de Lafora. *Revue d'Electroencephalographie et de Neurophysiologie Clinique*, **8**, 107–22.

Tassinari, C.A., Michelucci, R. Genton, P. *et al.* (1989) Dyssynergia cerebellaris myoclonica (Ramsay–Hunt syndrome): an autonomous condition unrelated to mitochondrial encephalomyopathies. *Journal of Neurology, Neurosurgery and Psychiatry*, **52**, 262–5.

Tassinari, C.A., Michelucci, R., Forti, A. *et al.* (1991) Ramsay–Hunt syndrome and Merrf: two unrelated conditions as demonstrated by mitochondrial DNA study. *Neurology* **41**, (suppl.1) 281.

Thomas, P.K., Abrams, J.D., Swallow, D. and Stewart, G. (1979) Sialidosis type I: cherry-red spot-myoclonus syndrome with sialidase deficiency and altered electrophoretic mobilities of some enzymes known to be glycoproteins. 1 Clinical findings. *Journal of Neurology, Neurosurgery and Psychiatry*, **42**, 873–80.

Tinuper, P., Aguglia, U., Pellissier, J.F. and

Gastaut, H. (1983) Visual ictal phenomena in a case of Lafora disease proven by skin biopsy. *Epilepsia*, **24**, 214–18.

Tsairis, P., Engel, W.K. and Kark, P. (1973) Familial myoclonic epilepsy syndrome associated with skeletal muscle mitochondrial abnormalities. *Neurology*, **23**, 408.

Van Heycop Ten Ham, M.W. and De Jager, H. (1963) Progressive myoclonus epilepsy with Lafora bodies. Clinical-pathological features. *Epilepsia*, **4**, 95–119.

Wallace, D.C., Shoffner, J.M., Lott, M.T. and Hopkins, L.C. (1991), Myoclonic epilepsy and ragged-red fibers disease (MERRF): a mitochondrial tRNALys mutation responsive to coenzyme Q10(CoQ) therapy. *Neurology*, **41** (suppl.1), 280.

Warburg, M. (1982) The natural history of Jansky–Bielschowsky's and Batten's diseases, in *Ceroid-lipofuscinosis (Batten's disease)* (eds D. Armstrong, N. Koopand and J.A. Rider), Elsevier Biomedical Press, Amsterdam, pp. 35–44.

Winkelman, M.D., Banker, B.Q., Wictor, M. and Moser, H.W. (1983) Non-infantile neuronopathic Gaucher's disease: a clinicopathologic study. *Neurology*, **33**, 994–1008.

Zeman, W., Donahue, S., Dyken, P. and Green, J. (1970) The neuronal ceroid-lipofuscinoses (Batten–Vogt syndrome), in *Handbook of Clinical Neurology* vol. 10 (eds P.S. Vinken and G.W. Bruyn), Elsevier North-Holland, Amsterdam, pp. 588–679.

Zeman, W. (1974) Studies in the neuronal ceroid lipofuscinoses. *Journal of Neuropathology and Experimental Neurology*, **33**, 1.

Charlotte Dravet, Pierre Genton, Michelle Bureau
and Joseph Roger

Kojewnikow's syndrome (KS), which has been extensively studied in a recent book published by F. Andermann (1991), and reviewed by Bancaud (1992) is dealt with more succinctly.

In the International Classification of Epilepsies (Commission on Classification and Terminology of the International League Against Epilepsy, 1989) KS is listed as 'chronic progressive epilepsia partialis continua (EPC) of childhood (Kojewnikow's syndrome)'. The Commission adds:

> Two types of EPC are recognized. The first one is a special epileptic syndrome also known as Rasmussen's syndrome and is related to a chronic focal encephalitis which begins in childhood and has a progressive course. The second type is included in the epilepsies of the motor cortex.

In fact, this comment is confusing because the two types have been well separated by Bancaud *et al.* (1982) into type 1 for the syndrome without progressive course observed at every age, and type 2 for the progressive syndrome which is specific to children. Only the latter will be dealt with here, based on data provided by Andermann (1991), Bancaud (1992), and Dulac *et al.* (1983).

It is a rare condition. Only 10 cases have been seen in 10 years at the Centre Saint-Paul, which specializes in severe epilepsies.

At the Montreal Neurological Institute it represents 1–2% of patients. However the number of cases depends on the definition adopted by the authors. The original definition of EPC, given by Kojewnikow (1895), was 'an association of localized "epileptic jerks" with more or less continuous jacksonian seizures'. In the study by Bancaud (1992) the inclusion criteria were, association of two types of clinical features: (1) localized muscle jerks, semicontinuous or permanent, and most often limited to a small group of muscles; (2) unilateral somatomotor seizures, associated or not with other types of seizures, with an onset before the age of 10. In the study by Dulac *et al.* (1983) the same criteria have been used. On the contrary, in the series studied by the Montreal school only 56% of all cases developed an EPC during the course of the disease. In addition to partial seizures, the main elements of the diagnosis were: onset in childhood; presence of a slowly progressive neurologic deterioration, usually including hemiparesis and mental retardation; dysphasia in involvement of the dominant hemisphere; and radiologic evidence of slowly progressive brain atrophy, predominantly unilateral. The occurrence of EPC was highly suggestive of this diagnosis. All the patients were submitted to surgical treatment and the brain specimens showed a microscopic picture suggestive of a viral encephalitis. The progressive clinical course

Epilepsy in Children. Edited by Sheila Wallace. Published in 1996 by Chapman & Hall, London. ISBN 0 412 56860 8

and the secondary cerebral atrophy also support this hypothesis. Unfortunately no viral agent has yet been identified. It should be noted that an analogous clinical picture can be observed in children with mitochondrial encephalopathy of the MELAS type.

The age of onset is between 14 months and 14 years. The initial seizures are generalized tonic-clonic, simple partial motor or complex partial, as part of a status epilepticus in 20% of patients (Andermann, 1991). When present, EPC appears within the first 2 years after the onset (up to 5 years for Bancaud, 1992). It can be present at the very beginning. After a variable delay seizures become frequent, from several per week to several per day or per hour. They are principally partial motor in type. EPC consists of myoclonic jerks of variable intensity, involving several muscular groups in the same half of the body, in an asynchronous way (upper and lower limbs, face). They are increased by voluntary movements, muscular activity, emotion, and persist during sleep. Simple partial motor seizures do not have a classic jacksonian march. They are associated with complex partial seizures, which sometimes are characterized only by an impairment of consciousness.

Neurologic deterioration appears insidiously, from 1 to 3 years after the onset, with a progressive hemiparesis, predominant in the upper limb. Walking remains possible in most of the patients. Mental retardation and behavioral disturbances develop in parallel. Prior to onset, mental function was normal in 90% of the patients of the Montreal series, but was abnormal at the last examination in 85% in this series, in 88% in the series of Bancaud (1992), and in all the patients of Dulac *et al.* (1983).

The EEGs are not characteristic at the onset. Later they become asymmetric with slow background activity and focal slow waves and spikes in the affected hemisphere, followed by diffuse deterioration. Ictal discharges can be localized in the two hemi-spheres independently. Their onset is difficult to recognize because of muscle activity. There is no relationship between jerks and spikes on the EEG.

Neuroradiologic examinations are abnormal in all patients during the course of the disease, showing signs of cerebral atrophy, usually unilateral. In the three series in the literature, this atrophy was not present in the patients investigated at the onset. MRI was not yet available at the time of these studies. In two patients from Montreal MRI showed an abnormal high intensity signal (in T2-weighted and proton density), in keeping with associated gliosis. The same results have been obtained in two of three recent patients (Peretti *et al.*, 1989).

CSF analysis is normal or shows transient signs of inflammation (high level of proteins, lymphocytes and oligoclonal bands).

Antiepileptic drugs do not control seizures in EPC. Etiologic treatments have been suggested (antiviral agents, immunotherapy). Recently Dulac *et al.* (1991) have reported striking improvement in some patients with corticosteroids used initially in high doses given intravenously.

Surgical therapy did not produce a good outcome in the series of Bancaud (1992). The Montreal experience seems to demonstrate that limited cortical resections are not sufficient to give prolonged control of seizures, while a 'functional' hemispherectomy can lead to complete control in most patients and to a marked reduction in the others. However, this cannot be considered as long as the functional deficit remains mild enough to allow the patient to use his affected limb in daily life (Chapter 23d).

In some patients progression of the disease seems to stop after several years, with persistence of seizures but strong attenuation of EPC and stabilization of neurologic and mental deficits. In others progression continues and some patients have died (one in the Dulac series, three in the Bancaud series, nine in the Montreal series).

REFERENCES

Andermann, F. (1991) *Chronic Encephalitis and Epilepsy: Rasmussen's Syndrome*. Butterworth-Heinemann, London.

Bancaud, J. (1992) Kojewnikow's syndrome (epilepsia partialis continua) in children, in *Epileptic Syndromes in Infancy, Childhood and Adolescence*, 2nd edn (eds J. Roger, M. Bureau, Ch. Dravet *et al.*), John Libbey Eurotext, London, Paris, pp. 363–79.

Bancaud, J., Bonis, A., Trottier, S. *et al.* (1982) L'épilepsie partielle continue: syndrome et maladie. *Revue Neurologique*, **138**, 802–14.

Commission on Classification and Terminology of the International League Against Epilepsy (1989) A revised proposal for the classification of epilepsy and epileptic syndromes. *Epilepsia*, **30**, 268–78.

Dulac, O., Dravet, C., Plouin, P. *et al.* (1983) Aspects nosologiques des épilepsies partielles continues chez l'enfant. *Archives Française de Pediatrie*, **40**, 689–95.

Dulac, O., Robain, O., Chiron, C. *et al.* (1991) High dose steroid treatment of epilepsia partialis continua due to chronic focal encephalitis, in *Chronic Encephalitis and Epilepsy: Rasmussen's Syndrome* (ed. F. Andermann), Butterworths Medical, London.

Kojewnikow, L. (1895) Eine besondere Form von corticaler epilepsie. *Neurologisches Centralblatt*, **14**, 47–8.

Peretti, C., Raybaud, Ch., Dravet, Ch. *et al.* (1989) Magnetic resonance imaging in partial epilepsy of childhood. Seventy-nine cases. *Journal of Neuroradiology*, **16**, 308–16.

Paolo Curatolo

INTRODUCTION

Symptomatic epilepsies and syndromes are considered to be the consequence of a known or strongly suspected disorder of the CNS (Commission on Classification and Terminology of the International League Against Epilepsy, 1989). They include both localization-related epilepsies, in which seizure semiology or findings at investigation disclose a localized origin of the seizures, and generalized epilepsies, in which the first clinical changes indicate initial involvement of both hemispheres and the ictal EEG patterns are apparently bilateral. They are a heterogeneous group of epilepsies with different pathophysiologic mechanisms, causes, and clinical manifestations, including syndromes of great individual variability. Their diagnosis lies not only in the correct identification of seizure types and clinical and EEG features, but also in the anatomic localization of the structural causes and in their etiology, when known (Chapter 7). Nonetheless, epilepsies symptomatic of structural lesions share some common characteristics, including uncertain prognosis, frequent association with neurologic and/or mental abnormalities, and often a certain degree of resistance to drug treatment. Factors associated with a more favorable outcome include absence of neurologic and mental abnormalities, a limited number of seizures, the presence of a single type of seizure, absence of tonic, atonic, and second-arily generalized seizures and of episodes of status epilepticus, a relatively late onset of seizures (i.e. after the age of 3 years) and absence of secondary bilateral synchrony on EEG. The prognosis for children with epilepsies symptomatic of structural lesions is generally poor and depends mainly on the type, extension, and topography of brain abnormalities. Therefore, prognostic studies should be performed on etiologically homogeneous cohorts of individuals. Epidemiologic studies examining the strength of the association between a probable cause of epilepsy and the time of onset of the condition could provide clues to the major and minor etiologic agents and their potential interaction. Systematic study of the etiologies of epilepsy is the key to prevention. Furthermore, since epilepsy, mental retardation, and/or cerebral palsy are often associated in the same child, as a result of the same underlying brain abnormalities, prognostic studies should also be carried out stratifying different homogeneous groups that present only epilepsy or concurrent epilepsy and mental retardation and/or cerebral palsy.

The etiology of some epilepsies can be strongly suspected from clinical and EEG features, but in the majority of children the identification of a structural cause requires the use of neuroimaging techniques, particularly since epilepsies sharing the same cause may have different clinical expressions. An

Epilepsy in Children. Edited by Sheila Wallace. Published in 1996 by Chapman & Hall, London. ISBN 0 412 56860 8

etiologic approach and a careful search for the underlying cause are mandatory in order to compare the natural history and the efficacy of treatment in homogeneous groups of children. Unfortunately, morphologic changes seen in symptomatic epilepsies may have no bearing on the genesis of seizures. Despite the progress in developmental neuropathology, we still do not know of any structural abnormality in neurons which could unquestionably act as a direct cause of seizures. Therefore, the possible morphologic basis of epileptic seizures often remains unknown. Symptomatic epilepsies may be intractable because of a serious associated brain disease. Brain tumors are one possible cause, but any structural lesion of the brain in an epileptogenic area is likely to lead to difficulties in seizure control. Such patients are potential candidates for surgical treatment as discussed in Chapters 20 and 23d.

GENERAL CONSIDERATIONS

CLINICAL FEATURES

The first sign or symptom of a seizure is often the most important indicator of the site of origin of a seizure discharge, whereas the subsequent sequence of ictal events can reflect its further propagation throughout the brain. The total sequence can help in localizing the site of origin. However, one of the major problems is that the initial discharge may start in a clinically silent region; therefore, the first clinically recognizable events occur only after subsequent spread to a site that is more or less distant from the zone of the initial discharge. Another problem is that subtle focal onset of secondary generalized seizures may not be recognized and this seizure may be incorrectly defined as generalized. Many types of generalized seizures, including myoclonic, tonic, and atonic seizures, may complicate different diseases, such as malformations or inborn errors of metabolism. Any type of partial seizure may be

present in epilepsies symptomatic of structural lesions. The following tentative description of syndromes related to anatomic localization summarizes data which include findings from electrocorticographic recordings (see also Chapter 7)

Frontal lobe epilepsies are characterized by simple partial, complex partial or secondarily generalized seizures, or by various combinations of these types of seizures. Seizures often occur several times a day and are characterized by short duration and rapid secondary generalization. They frequently occur during sleep, with prominent motor manifestations that are often tonic or postural. Complex gestural automatisms are common at onset. There is minimal or no postictal confusion. Drop attacks responsible for multiple falls are common when the discharge is bilateral. Status epilepticus is a frequent complication. Supplementary motor seizures are characterized by focal tonic manifestations, with vocalization, speech arrest, and fencing postures. Anterior frontopolar seizure patterns include loss of contact and adversive movements of the head and eyes with possible subsequent evolution, including axial clonic jerks and falls and autonomic signs. Opercular seizures include mastication, salivation, swallowing, speech arrest, epigastric aura, and autonomic phenomena. In frontal lobe seizures interictal EEG recordings may show frontal spikes, sharp waves or slow waves, either unilateral or frequently bilateral. Frontal lobe epilepsies are mainly characterized by a severe course that is frequently resistant to antiepileptic drugs and commonly associated with mental retardation.

Temporal lobe epilepsies are characterized by simple partial seizures, complex partial seizures, and secondary generalized seizures or combinations of these. A family history of seizures is common. Simple partial seizures are typically characterized by both autonomic and psychic symptoms and certain sensory phenomena, such as an epigastric sensation or olfactory and auditory illusions. Complex partial seizures are characterized by motor arrest followed by oroalimentary automatisms. In lateral temporal seizures a language disorder may occur when the focus is located in the dominant hemisphere. Postictal confusion and memory deficits also usually occur. Interictal EEG patterns include unilateral or bilateral temporal spikes, sharp waves and slow waves, often asynchronous. These events are not always confined to the temporal regions.

Parietal lobe epilepsies are usually characterized by simple partial and secondarily generalized seizures. Seizures are predominantly sensory. Positive phenomena include a feeling of electricity that is initially confined, subsequently spreading in a jacksonian manner, facial and tongue sensations, and a desire to move a body part. Metamorphopsia with distortions and parietal lobe visual phenomena, such as hallucinations, may also occur. Negative phenomena include numbness and a loss of awareness of a part of the body. Disorientation in space and vertigo may be indicative of inferior parietal lobe seizures. Seizures in the dominant parietal lobe result in a variety of receptive or conductive language disturbances.

Occipital lobe epilepsies are usually characterized by simple partial and secondarily generalized seizures. Complex partial seizures may occur and may spread beyond the occipital lobe. The clinical manifestations usually include visual phenomena which are either positive, such as flashes and phosphenes, or, more rarely, negative, such as amaurosis, hemianopsia, and scotoma. Disperceptive illusions, including a change in size, distance, or shape may occur. Illusional and hallucinatory visual seizures involve epileptic discharges in the temporo-parieto-occipital junction. The initial signs may also include tonic or clonic deviation of the eyes and head. The discharge may spread to the temporal lobe, producing seizure mani-

festations of lateral temporal or amygdala-hippocampal seizures.

EEG FINDINGS

Video-EEG recording has greatly improved the ability to precisely classify seizures by accurately illustrating the chronologic relationship between seizures and ictal EEG abnormalities. The ictal EEG recording is of great importance. Certain features are generally considered to be indicative of symptomatic partial epilepsies: specifically, rhythmic slow waves or rapid, low-amplitude bilateral activity recorded in frontal epilepsies. However, the anatomic origin of certain epilepsies is sometimes difficult to assign to specific lobes. For example, perirolandic seizures may include both precentral and postcentral symptomatology.

Interictal scalp EEG may be misleading. The absence of interictal abnormalities does not eliminate the possibility of a lesional epilepsy. Furthermore, some focal abnormalities may temporarily disappear during antiepileptic treatment, even in the case of brain tumours. Certain nonparoxysmal abnormalities are of great value because they are generally related to etiology rather than to the epileptic phenomenon. They include abnormal basic rhythm, focal polymorphic or even monomorphic slow waves, localized depression of rhythms in one hemisphere, and asymmetry of rhythms during hyperventilation and sleep. Paroxysmal focal abnormalities may assume the morphology of unifocal spike-waves, multifocal spike-waves, and even bilateral synchronous or asynchronous spike and waves. Multifocal spike-waves recorded on the awake EEG are often asynchronous and blend into slow background activity. They may evolve from a hypsarrhythmic pattern and generally occur in the context of bilateral lesions in severe lesional epilepsies associated with encephalopathy.

Difficulties in accurate topographic localization of epileptogenic foci by visual inspection of the tracings may arise due to the presence of apparently bilateral synchronous EEG abnormalities, associated with multifocal spike-waves, suggesting the possible existence of a secondary bilateral synchrony (SBS). SBS is defined by the occurrence of bilateral synchronous spike-wave or polyspike-wave complexes on EEG recordings, in which spike-wave bursts are immediately preceded by a sequence of focal spikes or sharp waves lasting at least 2 seconds (Blume and Pillay, 1985). SBS is thought to originate from a limited area of abnormal cortex in one hemisphere and to spread rapidly to both sides. This phenomenon is particularly frequent for discharges originating in the frontal regions. The bilateral nature of these abnormalities is probably linked to a number of factors: ease of propagation and bilateralization from a unilateral frontal focus, the existence of multiple foci, and the existence of an epileptic predisposition (Blume and Pillay, 1985; Gastaut *et al.*, 1987). The finding of bilateral synchronous paroxysmal EEG activity should not automatically exclude the possibility of surgical treatment of an epilepsy, at least in the presence of a detectable unilateral lesion. It is well known that in cases of unilateral brain damage, bilateral paroxysmal abnormalites may be present, and they may be larger over the healthy hemisphere where even ictal onset may appear to be located (Sammaritano *et al.*, 1987).

NEW TECHNIQUES IN LOCALIZATION OF STRUCTURAL LESIONS

These techniques are discussed in greater detail in Chapter 20.

MAGNETIC RESONANCE IMAGING

Magnetic resonance imaging (MRI) has undoubtedly facilitated the detection of structural lesions such as subtle cortical alterations and neuronal migration disorders, providing new information and allowing for better identification of the etiology of symptomatic epilepsies. Among children under 15 years of age with normal CT scans who have partial epilepsies, abnormal MRI is found in 38% (Peretti *et al.*, 1989). In a recent retrospective study in 44 children with intractable partial epilepsies who underwent surgical treatment, MRI revealed abnormalities that were consistent with the clinical and EEG data in 84% of patients (Kuzniecky *et al.*, 1993). The pathologic findings were abnormalities of neuronal migration (Chapter 4a), particularly of the sensori-motor cortex, in 25% of patients, and hippocampal sclerosis in 50% of patients with temporal lobe resection. Thus MRI is sensitive in the detection of pathologic abnormalities in most children who receive surgery. However, the exact relationship between electroclinical semiology and abnormal images often remains unclear, even in the presence of a well-documented brain lesion. Even localized morphologic findings detected by CT and MRI are not necessarily in topographic concordance with an epileptogenic lesion. Therefore, in these cases it is necessary to apply other techniques, such as MR spectroscopy, SPECT and PET (see below). When imaging fails to show a well-defined lesion in the child with intractable epilepsy, interictal and ictal scalp EEG localization are not sufficient to indicate whether or not surgery would be appropriate and the focus of abnormality should be further confirmed by chronic intracranial EEG monitoring with depth or subdural electrodes.

SINGLE PHOTON EMISSION COMPUTED TOMOGRAPHY AND POSITRON EMISSION TOMOGRAPHY

Functional imaging, using single photon emission computed tomography (SPECT) with xenon-13 and, more recently, with HMPAO technetium, and positron emission tomography (PET) with F-desoxyglucose and oxygen-15, have made valuable contributions to the better localization of lesions. SPECT hypofixation and PET hypometabolism are found during the interictal stage, and hyperfixation and hypermetabolism during the ictal and postictal phases respectively (Chugani, Shewmon and Phelps, 1990). The correlation of SPECT and PET data with clinical data, especially for complex partial seizures originating in the temporal lobe, and with ictal and interictal EEG data and MRI are satisfactory (Theodore *et al.*, 1989, 1990; Vles *et al.*, 1990; Ryvlin *et al.*, 1992). PET may also provide details on the degree of hypometabolism in epilepsies that are apparently generalized, as shown in West's and Lennox–Gastaut syndromes. Of 36 children with infantile spasms, PET revealed focal abnormalities in 26, whereas the combined use of CT and MRI revealed focal abnormalities in only 10 of these infants (Chugani *et al.*, 1990b). Such findings have practical implications since focal resections in infants with intractable spasms have resulted in cessation of seizures and developmental improvement. In the Lennox-Gastaut syndrome, PET studies have shown four subtypes based on the patterns of cerebral glucose utilization: unilateral focal, unilateral diffuse and bilateral diffuse hypometabolism, and normal patterns (Chugani *et al.*, 1987). Children with focal hypometabolism on PET corresponding to focal epileptiform discharges on EEG should be further evaluated for focal cortical resection.

In children with intractable seizures and normal radiologic studies, PET can be of great value in localizing the seizure focus and is highly sensitive and superior to CT and MRI in localizing focal areas of cortical dysplasia and other structural abnormalities corresponding to surface EEG localization of epileptogenic zones (Adelson *et al.*, 1992).

TOPOGRAPHIC MAPPING OF THE EEG

EEG mapping is designed to precisely identify and characterize epileptogenic areas of the brain. Such zones may be single or multiple, point-like or diffuse, and may be near to or distant from the recording electrodes. The resulting measured electric fields are used to obtain information which, when analysed in the light of all the complementary clinical information, provides a valuable adjunct to conventional EEG, and is thus considered to be a supplementary tool in presurgical evaluation (Ebersole and Wade, 1991). The combined use of spike voltage topography, dipole localization methods, and small interchannel time difference estimation applied to interictal discharges may provide important clues for understanding the spatiotemporal dynamics of epileptogenic discharges, even in cases with apparently synchronous spike wave bursts. Dipole localization methods may help to differentiate epilepsies of mesial and lateral temporal origin. EEG techniques are discussed further in Chapter 19.

MAGNETOENCEPHALOGRAPHY

Recently magnetoencephalography (MEG) recordings have led to important achievements in source localization, complementing structural information provided by MRI in children with localization-related symptomatic epilepsies. The time resolution of MEG is in the millisecond scale, making it possible to follow spatiotemporal changes reflecting signal processing in the brain. Progress in MEG technology has also made it possible to achieve a good spatial resolution, up to 1–2 mm under favorable conditions. In focal epilepsies, MEG provides reliable and noninvasive three-dimensional localization of the source. MEG is sensitive in detecting tangential dipoles missed by EEG, but may miss foci located over gyri. Furthermore, since it is difficult to capture ictal events on MEG, localization is usually restricted to interictal spike data. Therefore, EEG and MEG are complementary in the study of epilepsy associated with structural lesions: their combined use may allow for identification of both radial and tangential dipoles and distinction between cortical and deep sources.

LOCALIZATION-RELATED SYMPTOMATIC EPILEPSIES WITH SPECIFIC ETIOLOGY

Epileptic seizures may complicate many disease states. Diseases in which seizures are a presenting or predominant feature are included under this heading.

CEREBRAL PALSY

Cerebral palsy (CP) is a chronic disability of CNS origin, characterized by abnormal control of movement or posture, appearing early in life. CP is not a single disease, but a group of disorders resulting from nonprogressive abnormalities in the developing brain, occurring prenatally or acquired peri- or postnatally. The risk of epilepsy is increased among children with CP particularly in those who are mentally retarded. CP and epilepsy may have an intricate multifactorial relationship involving adverse pre- or perinatal events. Neuropathologic states that occur in pre- or perinatal hypoxic-ischemic brain injury and that may account for both CP and epilepsy include focal and multifocal ischemic brain injuries, selective neuronal necrosis, and parasagittal cerebral injury, as discussed in Chapter 5.

Epilepsy is estimated to occur in 10–40% of children with CP. However, the prevalence is generally lower when epilepsy is defined as recurrent afebrile seizures than when single seizures are included in the definition (Nelson and Ellenberg, 1986). Seizures are common in spastic CP, especially in congenital hemiplegia, in which half of the patients have seizures. Athetoid, ataxic, and diplegic CP are only rarely associated with seizures. Children with quadriplegic CP almost always have multifocal or secondarily generalized seizures, those with hemipareses are more likely to show partial jacksonian or generalized tonic-clonic seizures. Compared with children who are seizure-free, those who have epilepsy are more likely to be mentally retarded, especially it left-sided hemiparesis or tetraplegia coexist. The onset of seizures is most frequently in the first 2 years of life, but is sometimes much later, and is characterized by generalized seizures of focal or multifocal origin. However, almost any form of seizure may occur. Tonic-clonic, myoclonic, and atonic seizures are relatively common among severely retarded children and may be intractable. Among the epilepsies observed in children with CP, startle epilepsy is a well-defined clinical entity related to early lesions of the motor cortex (Chauvel *et al.*, 1987). Complex partial seizures may be symptomatic of parieto-occipital lesions secondary to circulatory disorders occurring during the perinatal period.

A family history of seizures is commoner among hemiplegic children who develop epilepsy compared with those who do not. Thus genetic susceptibility may be a contributory factor. A familial predisposition to epilepsy is not uncommon among children with CP and symptomatic epilepsy, supporting the view that the manifestation of epileptic attacks results from the interaction of endogenous genetic factors and exogenous brain damage mechanisms (Curatolo *et al.*, 1991a). Some children with similar paroxysmal EEG manifestations to those who have clinical seizures never have clinical problems; a situation which is difficult to explain. In a case-control study of risk factors for partial epilepsies with onset in the first 3 years in children with CP and mental retardation, we found a surprisingly high family history of epilepsy in first-degree relatives, suggesting that genetic transmission plays an important role in these children. Other risk factors associated with partial epilepsy in children with CP and mental retardation were placental pathologies, low gestational age, low birth weight for gestational age, cardiopulmonary resuscitation, and neonatal convulsions. However, only epidemiologic studies carried out on homogeneous populations, not only for the type of seizures but also for age at onset, can improve identification of risk factors for partial epilepsy associated with CP and provide clues for their prevention.

Prognosis for seizures varies according to the type, extension, and topography of the brain abnormalities underlying both CP and epilepsy. Therefore, a detailed investigation of lesions is essential in all children.

Seizures commonly occur following hypoxic-ischemic cerebral injury, especially in the full-term infant. The prognosis for seizure control is influenced by the underlying cause. Spasms associated with periventricular leukomalacia have a better prognosis than those associated with hypoxic-ischemic brain injury in the term infant. Perfusion failure and hypoxia during the second half of gestation are associated both with epilepsy and CP. Unfortunately, a diagnosis of prenatal brain ischemia is sometimes difficult after the event, even by MRI. Some children show neuroradiologic findings of both cerebral malformations and hypoxic-ischemic insult.

Prenatal perfusion failures occurring after the end of neuronal migration and before the establishment of the gyration may cause microgyria associated with the early onset of severe epilepsy and with poor prognosis (Curatolo *et al.*, 1989). However, the nature and pathogenesis of ischemic disturbances affecting prenatal development of the CNS remain largely unknown. Factors relevant to labor and delivery appear to contribute little to childhood seizure disorders. Due to the human cost of caring for these individuals and treating these conditions, further studies on the etiology and on the co-occurrence of these conditions are needed. Identification of antecedents may be helpful in the development of preventive measures. Given the strong and consistent association between CP and epilepsy, prevention of CP should reduce the incidence of epilepsy among children.

HEAD INJURY

Head trauma caused by accidents is becoming increasingly common during infancy, childhood, and adolescence. However, epilepsy develops in only a small percentage of head-injured patients. Head trauma is a potentially preventable risk factor for epilepsy. Identification of patients with head trauma at risk for epilepsy is of practical importance.

Approximately 5% of children hospitalized for head injuries have a seizure within the first week. A family history of seizures is commoner amongst individuals who develop epilepsy rather than those who do not, suggesting that genetic susceptibility contributes to seizure occurrence. Seizures may occur predominantly in the first 24 hours following the trauma. These early seizures are likely to be focal, and 75% are partial motor in type. They may be followed by localizing signs and associated with temporary alterations in consciousness. Status epilepticus following head trauma is common (22%) in children less than 5 years old (Jennett, 1973). Nevertheless, approximately one-third of affected patients have only one attack. Thus, the earliest seizures often remain isolated, and, consequently, should not be regarded as epilepsy. Early post-traumatic epilepsy does not indicate the presence of a neurosurgical complication, but is often a precursor of late post-traumatic epilepsy. All seizures that occur more than 1 week after head trauma are termed late post-traumatic epilepsy; this can develop at any time following trauma, but the relative risk decreases after the first 2 years. Late seizures are more often complex partial or apparently generalized, mainly with frontal or fronto-temporal lesions.

An increased risk for early post-traumatic epilepsy exists when the following occur: penetrating cranial trauma, early post-traumatic seizures, acute intracranial hemorrhage, focal neurological signs, unconsciousness for more than 24 hours, depressed fracture with dural laceration, and fractures at the base of the skull (Jacobi, 1992).

The EEG is only marginally useful in the prediction of late epilepsy. Persistence of focal abnormalities related to the site of the trauma is usually associated with late epilepsy, although localized paroxysmal abnormalities can persist for up to 10 years or more without the patient ever developing seizures.

Prophylactic treatment is based on the concept that antiepileptic drugs given early enough after trauma can prevent the development of an epileptic focus. However, there is no proven basis for this concept. Decisions in relation to treatment must take into account the likely benefit and risk of this strategy in terms of adverse behavioral effects.

The pathogenesis of post-traumatic epilepsy remains unknown, despite the standard explanations suggesting that meningocerebral scars and focal ischemic lesions may be factors. Early post-traumatic seizures have been linked with focal injury to the brain and with local ischemia and metabolic changes. Late epilepsy has been attributed to scarring and has been associated with tissue distortion, vascular involvement, and mechanical irritation of the brain. Iron deposition following hemorrhage is also considered a possible risk factor. Pathological considerations are examined in detail in Chapter 5.

HYDROCEPHALUS

Seizures are relatively common in children with congenital hydrocephalus. The reported incidence is 48% in children with congenital hydrocephalus and up to 16% in children with myelomeningocele and hydrocephalus (Noetzel and Blake, 1991, 1992). When children with hydrocephalus are considered as a group, including those with posthemorrhagic and other pathologies, the incidence of seizures is approximately 50%. Within this group, there are variable risks, related to the pathologic condition producing hydro-

cephalus: e.g. injury to the cortex as a result of shunt insertion; damage from shunt complications, such as infection or obstruction resulting in higher intracranial pressure; other intracerebral abnormalities, e.g. neuronal migration disorders; posthemorrhagic or periventricular ischemic lesions etc. Seizures are not related to site of shunt insertion, number of shunt revisions, number of shunt infections, or age at shunt insertion (Stellman, Bannister and Hillier, 1986).

Some patients have seizures following an episode of shunt dysfunction. The location of EEG foci has been found to correspond to the location of the ventricular catheter. However, the cause of hydrocephalus may also be responsible for the epilepsy, and a topographic correlation between EEG foci and the position of the catheter has not been confirmed by all authors.

Mental retardation, often in combination with cerebral malformation other than hydrocephalus, is associated with seizure occurrence and seizure persistence. Approximately one-third of children with epilepsy in association with isolated hydrocephalus continue to have frequent seizures despite treatment. In contrast, in the vast majority of children with hydrocephalus and myelomeningocele there is an excellent prognosis for seizure control, and discontinuation of drug treatment after relatively brief seizure-free periods does not increase the risk of recurrent convulsions. However, in children with congenital hydrocephalus who are of normal intelligence, and, who, as a result of anticonvulsants, have been seizure-free for 3 years, it is safe to discontinue therapy.

INTRACRANIAL TUMORS

Brain tumors are uncommon causes of epilepsy in children. However, hemispheric tumors may present with epileptic seizures which may remain the only clinical symptom for prolonged periods, ranging from a few months to many years. Generally, such

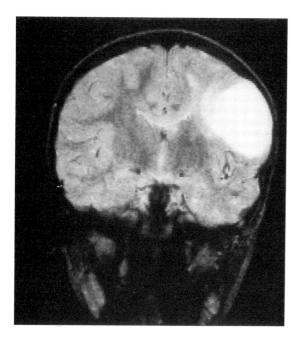

Fig. 16.1 MRI of a 2-year-old girl who had three partial motor seizures. Large area of hyperdensity of the left rolandic area was shown to be a low-grade astrocytoma. After surgical removal, the seizures disappeared.

seizures are not immediately associated with other neurologic signs and symptoms, especially in patients with normal intellect (Blume, Girvin and Kaufmann, 1982), which may be very important from a practical point of view. Tumors located close to the brain surface have a greater propensity to cause seizures than deep subcortical tumors. Seizures are more commonly associated with slower growing tumors, than rapidly growing lesions. Since most tumors that give rise to seizures are benign (e.g. low-grade astrocytomas and oligodendrogliomas), early diagnosis is important because many children can completely recover following surgical treatment (Fig. 16.1). Therefore, identification of those few children whose attacks are likely to be caused by brain tumors is very important. In the past the mean interval between the first seizure and the diagnosis of

a tumor has been 5.6 years (Aicardi *et al.*, 1970) and intervals as long as 20 years have been reported (Spencer *et al.*, 1984). The main factors considered to be responsible for this delay are: initial EEG normal or soon normalized after the onset of the treatment, misinterpretation of CT, and remission of seizures with or without antiepileptic drug treatment (Sjors, Blennow and Lantz, 1993).

Epilepsies caused by hemispheric tumors are mainly characterized by simple or complex partial seizures; but, apparently generalized seizures and bilaterally synchronous interictal EEG abnormalities may also be present. Some seizures are described as generalized because the localizing symptoms are missed or they originate from a clinically silent zone of the brain. Suspicion should be heightened when seizures are partial and refractory, particularly if intelligence and physical examination are normal or if there is a progressive deterioration in behavior. Localized EEG foci of polymorphic slow waves or sharp waves on a slow disorganized EEG background are suggestive of a tumor (Fig. 16.2).

In a recent series of 20 children with seizures who had histologically confirmed cerebral tumors mainly involving the temporal and the frontal lobes, 40% were aged 15 months or younger at onset of the first partial seizure (Williams, Abbott and Manson, 1992). Initial misdiagnosis occurred in 25% of these infants. Examination was normal in 75%. EEG at onset revealed focal abnormalities in 62% and generalized abnormalities in 25%. CT scan findings were not diagnostic in 40%; conversely, MRI confirmed the presence of tumors in all children. Although MRI findings are not specific, such imaging has made the diagnosis of brain tumors easier and faster, allowing for an accurate evaluation of all regions.

Outcome with regard to seizures is generally considered favorable. Postoperative freedom from seizures is probable when complete or near-complete resection of epi-

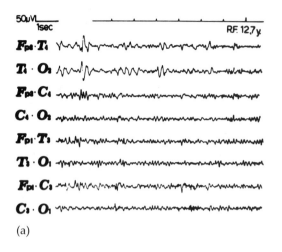

(a)

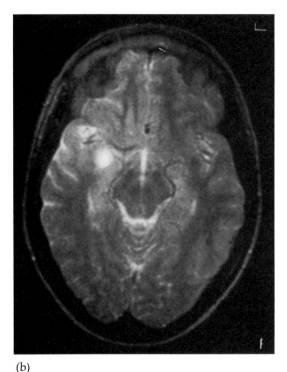

(b)

Fig. 16.2 (a) Interictal EEG showing sporadic sharp waves over the right anterior temporal region in a 12-year-old boy with seizures characterized by olfactory-gustatory aura, oral automatisms, and loss of contact. (b) Hyperdense signal of the right temporal region detected by MRI is an oligodendroglioma.

leptogenic cortex is achieved. A clear trend towards improvement of neuropsychologic and cognitive functions is also noted (Adelson *et al.*, 1992). Tumors are further considered in Chapters 5 (pathology) and 23d (surgery).

Gelastic epilepsy

Seizures begin before 3 years of age, and often before 1 year of age. At the onset or during evolution the ictus is characterized by laughter, eventually followed by a more complex event characterized by head and eye deviation and automatisms. The seizures are brief, but very frequent. Neurologic examination is generally normal.

Gelastic epilepsy should always arouse a strong suspicion of a tumor of the floor of the third ventricle, especially a hamartoma (Curatolo *et al.*, 1984). The onset of gelastic epilepsy and precocious puberty in childhood is potentially serious since, rarely, this combination has been reported to be associated with a low-grade astrocytoma. However, the most common association is with a posterior hypothalamic hamartoma, a tumor-like collection of normal tissue lodged in an abnormal location. The attacks of laughter can be confused with behavioral or emotional disorders, but their stereotyped recurrence, the absence of any precipitating factor, other manifestations of epilepsy (generalized, temporal-lobe, and psychomotor seizures), and no other obvious cause for the pathologic laughter make the diagnosis of gelastic epilepsy highly probable. Ictal and interictal awake EEG show localized discharges of spikes, predominantly originating in the temporal or frontotemporal areas, and generalized slow spike and wave discharges (Curatolo *et al.*, 1984). Investigation with MRI or CT may confirm the diagnosis by detecting a posterior hypothalamic tumor. MRI is superior to CT in showing the exact size and anatomic location of the hamartomata (Fig. 16.3). These lesions are not expansive and are not readily accessible to surgery. The evolu-

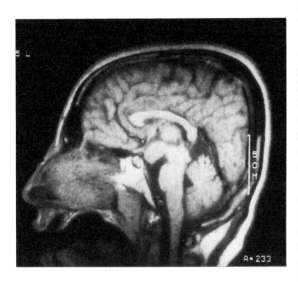

Fig. 16.3 Sagittal MRI showing hypothalamic hamartoma in a boy with precocious puberty and gelastic epilepsy from the age of 2 years.

tion is characterized by the persistence of seizures, mental retardation, and behavioral problems.

Dysembryoplastic neuroepithelial tumors

Dysembryoplastic neuroepithelial tumors are newly described, pathologically benign, tumors originating in the supratentorial cortex and having an invariable association with intractable partial complex seizures. Age at onset of the partial seizures ranges from 2 to 19 years. MRI demonstrates a well-circumscribed focal cortical mass, located in the temporal lobe or more rarely in the occipital lobe. These lesions have an increased signal intensity on T2-weighted images and may simulate benign cysts or low-grade astrocytomata (Koeller and Dillon, 1992).

NEUROCUTANEOUS SYNDROMES

Advances in neuroimaging and developmental neuropathology are providing new and exciting information on the structure of the brain in neurocutaneous syndromes (NCS). Previously unknown relationships with the neurologic complications of NCS, including seizures, are becoming apparent. A large number of NCS are associated with migrational disorders (Chapter 4a) accounting for the coexistence of brain and skin pigmentary pathology. On occasions, seizures are the presenting symptoms or contribute significantly to the severity of the disease.

The prognosis for seizure control and neurologic development is influenced particularly by the underlying cause. For example, in children with tuberous sclerosis spasms have a very poor outcome, but spasms associated with neurofibromatosis have an excellent prognosis.

Tuberous sclerosis

Tuberous sclerosis (TS) is a congenital hamartomatosis with variable expression in multiple organs, and is transmitted by autosomal dominant inheritance. TS shows genetic heterogeneity with linkage to 9q34 and 16p13. Pathologically, TS is a disorder of cellular migration, proliferation, and differentiation. Cortical tubers constitute the hallmark of the disease and are pathognomonic of cerebral TS. There is variability in the range and extent of the neurologic problems, of which seizures are the most common, occurring in 92% of patients.

Epilepsy in TS often begins in the first year of life, and, in most cases, in the very first months of life, when the commonest types of seizure are partial motor and infantile spasms (Chapter 11b). The high incidence of infantile spasms and hypsarrhythmia has long been emphasized, but it is now clear that infants with TS exhibit some specific clinical, and interictal and ictal EEG features, which distinguish them from those with classic infantile spasms and hypsarrhythmia. In the same child partial seizures may precede, coexist with, or evolve into infantile spasms.

A vast number of subtle partial seizures such as unilateral tonic or clonic phenomena, mainly localized to the face or limbs, and other subtle lateralizing features, such as tonic eye deviation, head turning, and unilateral grimacing can be missed by the parents until the third or fourth month of life when infantile spasms occur.

The awake EEG, at the onset, shows multifocal or focal spike discharges and irregular slow focal activity. Although EEG foci can be located in any region of the brain, the commonest locations for focal EEG discharges, at the age when infantile spasms occur, are the posterior temporal and occipital regions. During sleep, an increase in epileptiform activity is usually observed, and the multifocal abnormalities tend to generalize, giving a semblance of hypsarrhythmia.

Video-EEG monitoring and polygraphic recordings of the spasms have shown that the ictal phenomenon is a single seizure. Each spasm consists of a combination of both focal and bilateral manifestations. The ictal EEG starts with a focal discharge of spikes and polyspikes, often originating from the temporal, rolandic, or occipital regions, and is followed by a generalized irregular slow transient and an abrupt flattening of the background activity in all regions.

The vast majority of patients who have infantile spasms at onset later manifest either partial motor or complex partial seizures or apparently generalized seizures. In the EEG of older patients, the pseudotype pattern of hypsarrhythmia tends to disappear, and tracings tend to exhibit bifocal or multifocal spikes or slowing. After 2 years of age, additional foci with a frontal localization become progressively evident.

Cortical tubers detected by MRI represent the epileptogenic foci of TS, and a topographic relationship exists between EEG abnormalities and the largest MRI high-signal lesions (Curatolo and Cusmai, 1988). MRI lesions in the occipital lobes show the best correlation with the EEG foci, while the weakest correlation is in the frontal lobes (Cusmai *et al.*, 1990a; Tamaki *et al.*, 1990). The age of seizure onset and the age of occurrence of EEG foci may depend on the localization of cortical tubers, with an earlier expression for parietal and occipital lesions than for frontal ones. This may result from maturational phenomena. Since perfusion of the occipital lobes decreases with age and frontal areas reach complete maturation only in the second year of life, it is not paradoxical that cortical lesions which are associated with infantile spasms are not epileptogenic as the child gets older; and, that, in the same child, complex partial seizures originating from a more anterior tuber may become evident only a number of years later. Patients with multiple lesions may have a greater tendency to show hypsarrhythmia at an early age with subsequent development of bilateral synchronization. In the tubers, disarray of the neuronal architecture is associated with malformed neurons and astrocytes and neural cells of indeterminate identity, suggesting a defect in neuronal and glial differentiation and migration (Chapter 4a) and providing a likely anatomic substrate for epilepsy (Huttenlocher and Wolman, 1991).

A consistent association between seizures and mental retardation has been observed. Both the number and the localization of cortical tubers play important roles in mental outcome, suggesting that epilepsy and mental retardation reflect the underlying brain dysfunction caused by cortical tubers (Curatolo *et al.*, 1991b). In our series, late-onset partial seizures or transient infantile spasms were the only seizure types observed in the nonretarded individuals. All the patients with favorable evolutions of their epilepsy had normal psychomotor development before the onset of the first seizure and generally showed only one seizure type. Children with normal intelligence showed small sized isolated cortical tubers, mainly localized to the parietal and rolandic regions. By contrast, patients with mental retardation

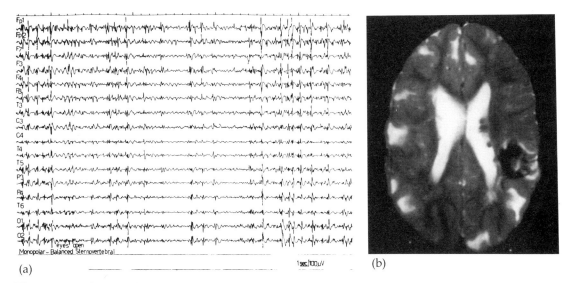

Fig. 16.4 (a) Interictal EEG showing apparently generalized spike and wave discharges in a girl with tuberous sclerosis, intractable epilepsy, and severe mental retardation. (b) MRI reveals multiple tubers in both hemispheres.

suffered from frequent partial seizures, developing into multifocal or secondary generalized epilepsy, and showed multiple bilateral cortical tubers on MRI (Fig. 16.4). Progressive mental deterioration observed in children with intractable seizures may be due to a particular epileptogenicity of parasagittal frontal tubers.

Difficulties in accurate topographic localization of epileptogenic foci by visual inspection of the tracing may arise due to the presence of apparently bisynchronous EEG abnormalities. This phenomenon is particularly frequent for discharges originating in the frontal regions. Children with bilateral involvement with three or more affected lobes on MRI are more likely to show bilateral synchronization on EEG, when, mainly during sleep, a multifocal frontally dominant pattern of bursts of bilateral and more synchronous slow spike waves, tending to assume the appearance of a Lennox–Gastaut pattern, is characteristic.

In children with apparently bilateral synchronous spike-wave bursts on standard EEG, high time resolution topographic spike mapping enables the recognition of a focal frontal onset with propagation to the contralateral homologous region, in topographic concordance with the site of a prominent MRI lesion (Curatolo *et al.*, 1993). These findings support the concept that apparently generalized spike-wave discharges are of focal origin in most children, with a subsequent phenomenon of secondary bilateral synchrony. This has important implications not only in the clinical management, but also in the therapeutic approach, since the presence of multifocal and generalized interictal EEG abnormalities and/or multiple areas of cerebral involvement is not an automatic basis for exclusion for surgical treatment.

Correlations between cortical tubers and epileptogenic areas are far from being definitive in TS. The combined use of topographic mapping of EEG and dipole-localization methods may provide important clues to localization of epileptogenic areas even in cases with apparently synchronous spike-wave bursts. Mapping the results on a three-dimensional MRI reconstruction can provide a more accurate localization of the zone of the cortical focal abnormalities and can help the surgeon to make tailored and conservative resections in children with intractable seizures. However, MRI is not yet able to detect all the cortical tubers that may be identified pathologically. Therefore, the disturbance of cerebral function may be more extensive than indicated by morphologic imaging alone.

Neurofibromatosis

Neurofibromatosis 1 (NF1) (previously known as von Recklinghausen's neurofibromatosis) is an autosomal dominant disorder affecting about one in 3000 individuals. It is characterized by multiple hyperpigmented areas and peripheral neurofibromata. Anomalous migration and localization of neural crest cells occurs (Chapter 4a). The gene for NF1 has been mapped on chromosome 17. Brain findings include cortical architectural abnormalities, with random orientations of neurons and disarray of normal cortical lamination, heterotopic neurons within the cortical molecular layer in the subcortical or deep cerebral white matter, and gross cerebral malformations such as polymicrogyria, pachygyria, and hemimegalencephaly (Cusmai *et al.*, 1990b). In recent years MRI has improved the diagnosis of brain abnormalities in NF1, particularly in relation to dysembryoplastic lesions and heterotopic foci. The incidental discovery of high-signal MRI lesions localized in the basal ganglia, brainstem, and cerebellum has been reported in as many as 60% of children. Since MRI abnormalities have been detected both in children affected by early-onset partial seizures and in asymptomatic individuals, these findings do not seem to have any correlation with neurologic dysfunction.

Seizures are 10 times more frequent in NF1 than in the general population, but are rarely the presenting symptom. They are generally sporadic and respond rapidly to drug treatment.

Infantile spasms (Chapter 11b) with onset between 4 and 6 months and associated with an EEG pattern of hypsarrhythmia have been observed in children with NF1; they are usually associated with a favorable evolution and a normal developmental outcome. Discontinuation of anticonvulsants is possible in the vast majority of patients.

Sturge–Weber syndrome

Sturge–Weber syndrome is characterized by a nevus of the upper face; ipsilateral leptomeningeal angiomatosis; contralateral hemiparesis or hemianopia; contralateral partial or secondary generalized seizures; and, frequently, mental retardation. The association and localization of aberrant vasculature in the facial skin, eyes, and meninges are compatible with a single early localized defect in vascular morphogenesis at a very early stage of development in the tissue from which the vasculature of these three regions eventually develops. The degree of CNS involvement is variable. Seizures most commonly begin between 2 and 7 months of age and are often the presenting symptom, usually preceding the motor deficit and mental retardation. Partial motor and/or secondary generalized seizures occur in almost all patients; infantile spasms are rarely reported. The first seizure is often asymmetric or unilateral, long-lasting and followed by a transient paralysis. EEG is characterized by decreased amplitude and frequency of background electrocerebral activity over the affected hemisphere. Unilateral or diffuse multiple independent spike foci are commonly associated. As time goes on there is a notable increase in seizure frequency and severity, with progressive worsening of the hemiparesis, and dementia; generalized tonic, tonic-clonic or myoclonic seizures may become manifest and may be refractory to drug treatment. Despite the topographic localization of the intracranial angioma in the occipital region, visual seizures and complex partial seizures are rare.

Seizures occur in about 75% of individuals affected by Sturge–Weber syndrome. In a retrospective study of 102 patients, 88 individuals had one cerebral hemisphere affected, and 14 showed bilateral hemispheric involvement (Bebin and Gomez, 1988). Sixty-three of the 88 patients with unilateral hemispheric disease had seizures, with a mean age of seizure onset of 24 months; whereas 13 of 14 individuals with bilateral hemispheric lesions had seizure disorders, with a mean age of seizure onset of 6 months. Mental retardation was present in about half of the patients and was generally more severe in patients with bihemispheric lesions and persistence of seizures. By contrast, 25 patients with unihemispheric leptomeningeal involvement who did not have seizures were all of average intelligence. Therefore, seizures must play some role in determining mental retardation and in causing deterioration of mental function.

CT, MRI, SPECT, and PET can be used to define the extent of the intracerebral angioma and to carefully select candidates for early focal resection. Serial PET scanning can be useful in documenting the progression of the disease. The delineation of hypoperfusion or hypometabolism in the region of the angioma can provide an accurate definition of the epileptogenic zone to be resected in children with early-onset intractable seizures (Chiron *et al.*, 1989; Chugani, Mazziotta and Phelps, 1989).

Other neurocutaneous syndromes

Epidermal nevus syndrome. Epidermal nevus is a sporadic congenital skin lesion characterized by a slightly raised, yellow-brown plaque usually located in the midline of the forehead and nose, associated with congenital abnormalities of the brain and other systems. A subgroup of patients with a recognizable neurologic variant has been described (Pavone *et al.*, 1991). This syndrome consists of facial epidermal nevi, ipsilateral hemi-megalencephaly, gyral malformation, contralateral hemiparesis, mental retardation, seizures, and often facial hemihypertrophy. Seizures may begin between birth and 6 months. Both partial seizures and infantile spasms are commonly reported. EEG abnormalities at the onset are usually ipsilateral to the major brain abnormality.

Hypomelanosis of Ito. Hypomelanosis of Ito is characterized by areas of skin hypopigmentation in the form of streaks or whorls. Neurologic abnormalities such as mental retardation and seizures are present in more than half of the reported cases and can probably be explained by abnormal neuronal migration (Chapter 4a). A large spectrum of brain abnormalities, including pachygyria, multiple gray matter heterotopias, and hemimegalencephaly has been reported in individuals with hypomelanosis of Ito, supporting the concept that the basis of the CNS lesions is probably neuronal migration disorder. Seizures (infantile spasms or partial seizures) usually become manifest during the first year of life and tend to be refractory to anticonvulsants. Abnormal rhythmic EEG activity and radiologic images of neuronal migration defects also seem to be correlated (Esquival, Pitt and Boyd, 1991).

Incontinentia pigmenti. Incontinentia pigmenti is probably transmitted as an X-linked dominant trait, affecting females in 95% of cases. The syndrome is characterized by various hyperpigmented skin lesions that are apparent at birth or during the first weeks of life as vesiculobullous lesions, becoming hyperpigmented gray-brown macular lesions during the first years of life. Most patients have symptoms and signs of neurologic abnormalities, manifested by developmental delay, spastic cerebral palsies and seizures. Seizures are observed in about 20% of individuals. Partial seizures or infantile spasms may begin during the first months of life and may persist with great frequency and severity during the first year. Mental retardation, observed in a minority of individuals, is most frequent in association with early seizures and with structural changes in the brain.

Incontinentia pigmenti achromians. Incontinentia pigmenti achromians is characterized by bilateral, asymmetric, hypopigmented whorls associated with CNS abnormalities, including seizures, mental retardation, and motor system dysfunction. Abnormalities of neuronal migration, such as micropolygyria, are also reported.

REFERENCES

Adelson, P.D., Peacock, W.J., Chugani, H.T. *et al.* (1992) Temporal and extended temporal resections for the treatment of intractable seizures in early childhood. *Pediatric Neurosurgery*, **18**, 169–78.

Aicardi, J., Praud, E., Bancaud, J. *et al.* (1970) Epilepsies cliniquement primitives et tumeurs cerebrales chez l'enfant. *Archives Française Pediatrie*, **27**, 1041–55.

Bebin, E.M. and Gomez, M.R. (1988) Prognosis in Sturge–Weber disease: comparison of unihemispheric and bihemispheric involvement. *Journal of Child Neurology*, **3**, 181–4.

Blume, W.T. and Pillay, N. (1985) Electrographic and clinical correlates of secondary bilateral synchrony. *Epilepsia*, **26**, 636–41.

Blume, W.T., Girvin, J.P. and Kaufmann, J.C.E. (1982) Childhood brain tumors presenting as chronic uncontrolled focal seizure disorder. *Annals of Neurology*, **12**, 538–41.

Chauvel, P., Vignal, J.P., Liegeois-Chauvel, C. *et al.* (1987) Startle epilepsy with infantile brain damage: clinical and neurophysiological rationale for surgical therapy, in *Presurgical Evaluation of Epilepsies* (eds H.G. Wieser and C.E. Elger), Springer-Verlag, Berlin, pp. 306–7.

Chiron, C., Raynaud, C., Tzourio, N. *et al.* (1989) Regional cerebral blood flow by SPECT imaging in Sturge–Weber disease: an aid for diagnosis. *Journal of Neurology, Neurosurgery and Psychiatry*, **52**, 1402–9.

Chugani, H.T., Mazziotta, J.C. and Phelps, M.E. (1989) Sturge–Weber syndrome: a study of cerebral glucose utilization with PET. *Journal of Pediatrics*, **114**, 244–53.

Chugani, H.T., Shewmon, D.A. and Phelps, M.E. (1990) Ictal patterns of cerebral glucose utilization in children with epilepsy. *Epilepsia*, **31**, 626.

Chugani, H.T., Mazziotta, J.C., Engel, J. and Phelps, M.E. (1987) Lennox–Gastaut syndrome: metabolic subtypes determined by 18FDG positron emission tomography. *Annals of Neurology*, **21**, 4–13.

Chugani, H.T., Shields, W.D., Shewmon, A. *et al.* (1990) Infantile spasms: PET identifies focal cortical dysgenesis in cryptogenic cases for surgical treatment. *Annals of Neurology*, **27**, 406–14.

Commission on Classification and Terminology of the International League against Epilepsy (1989) Proposal for revised classification of epilepsies and epileptic syndromes. *Epilepsia*, **30**, 389–99.

Curatolo, P. and Cusmai, R. (1988) MRI in Bourneville disease: relationship with EEG findings. *Neurophysiologie Clinique*, **18**, 149–57.

Curatolo, P., Seri, S. and Cerquiglini, A. (1993) Topographic spike mapping of EEG in tuberous sclerosis. *Neuropediatrics*, **24**, 178.

Curatolo, P., Cusmai, R., Finocchi, G. and Boscherini, B. (1984) Gelastic epilepsy and true precocious puberty due to hypothalamic hamartoma. *Developmental Medicine and Child Neurology*, **26**, 509–14.

Curatolo, P., Cusmai, R., Pruna, D. and Feliciani, M. (1989) Polymicrogyria: a case detected by MRI. *Brain and Development*, **11**, 257–59.

Curatolo, P., Arpino, C., Stazi, M.A. and Medda, E. (1991a) Risk factors for early symptomatic localized epilesies. *Epilepsia*, **32**, 22.

Curatolo, P., Cusmai, R., Cortesi, F. *et al.* (1991b) Neuropsychiatric aspects of tuberous sclerosis. *Annals of the New York Academy of Sciences*, **615**, 8–16.

Cusmai, R., Chiron, C., Curatolo, P. *et al.* (1990a) Topographic comparative study of MRI and EEG in 34 children with tuberous sclerosis. *Epilepsia*, **31**, 747–55.

Cusmai, R., Curatolo, P., Mangano, S. *et al.* (1990b) Hemimegalencephaly and neurofibromatosis. *Neuropediatrics*, **21**, 179–82.

Ebersole, J. and Wade, P.B. (1991) Spike voltage topography identifies two types of frontotemporal epileptic foci. *Neurology*, **41**, 1425–33.

Esquival, E.E., Pitt,. M.C. and Boyd, S.G. (1991). EEG findings in hypomelanosis of Ito. *Neuropediatrics*, **22**, 216–9.

Gastaut, H., Zifkin, B., Magaudda, A. and Mariani, E. (1987) Symptomatic partial epilepsies with secondary bilateral synchrony: differentiation from symptomatic generalized epilepsies of the Lennox–Gastaut type, in *Presurgical Evaluation of*

Epilepsies (eds H. G. Wieser and C.E. Elger), Springer Verlag, Berlin, pp. 308–16.

Huttenlocher, P.R., Wolman, R.L. (1991) Cellular neuropathology of tuberous sclerosis. *Annals of the New York Academy of Sciences*, **615**, 140–8.

Jacobi, G. (1992) Post-traumatic epilepsy. *Monatsschrift Kinderheilkunde*, **140**, 619–23.

Jennett, B. (1973) Trauma as a cause of epilepsy in childhood. *Developmental Medicine and Child Neurology*, **15**, 56–72.

Koeller, K.K. and Dillon, W.P. (1992) Dysembryoplastic neuroepithelial tumors: MRI appearance. *American Journal of Neuroradiology*, **13**, 1319–25.

Kuzniecky, R., Muroo, A., King, D. *et al.* (1993) MRI in childhood intractable partial epilepsies: pathologic correlations. *Neurology*, **43**, 681–7.

Nelson, K.B. and Ellenberg, J.K. (1986) Antecedents of seizure disorders in early childhood. *American Journal of Diseases of Children* **140**, 1053–61.

Noetzel, M. and Blake, J.N. (1991) Prognosis for seizure control and remission in children with myelomeningocele. *Developmental Medicine and Child Neurology*, **33**, 803–10.

Noetzel, M.J. and Blake, J.N. (1992) Seizures in children with congenital hydrocephalus: long term outcome. *Neurology*, **42**, 1277–81.

Pavone, L., Curatolo, P., Rizzo, R. *et al.* (1991) Epidermal nevus syndrome: a neurologic variant with hemimegalencephaly, gyral malformation, mental retardation, seizures and facial hemihypertrophy. *Neurology*, **4**, 266–71.

Peretti, P., Dravet, C., Raybaud, Ch. *et al.* (1989) L'IRM dans les epilepsies partielles ayant debute' avant 15 ans. *Epilepsies*, **1**, 227–33.

Ryvlin, P., Garcia Larrea, L., Philippon, B. *et al.* (1992) High signal intensity of T2-weighted MRI correlates with hypoperfusion in temporal lobe epilepsy. *Epilepsia*, **33**, 28–35.

Sammaritano, M., De Lobiniere, A., Andermann, F. *et al.* (1987) False lateralization by surface EEG of seizure onset in patients with temporal lobe epilepsy and gross focal cerebral lesions. *Annals of Neurology*, **21**, 361–9.

Sjors, K., Blennow, G., and Lantz G. (1993) Seizures as the presenting symptom of brain tumors in children. *Acta Paediatrica*, **82**, 66–70.

Spencer, D.D., Spencer, S.S., Mattson, R.H. and Williamson, P.D. (1984) Intracerebral masses in patients with intractable partial epilepsy. *Neurology*, **34**, 432–6.

Stellman, G.R., Bannister, C.M. and Hillier, V. (1986) The incidence of seizure disorder in children with acquired and congenital hydrocephalus. *Zeitschrift fur Kinderchirurgie*, **41**, 38–41.

Tamaki, K., Okuno, T., Ito, M. *et al.* (1990) MRI in relation to EEG epileptic foci in tuberous sclerosis. *Brain and Development*, **12**, 316–20.

Theodore, W.H., Dorwart, R., Holmes, M. *et al.* (1989) Neuroimaging in refractory partial seizures: comparison of PET, CT and MRI. *Neurology*, **36**, 750–9.

Theodore, W.H., Katz, D., Kufta, C. *et al.* (1990) Pathology of temporal lobe foci: correlation with CT, MRI and PET. *Neurology*, **40**, 797–803.

Vles, J.S., Demandt, E., Ceulemans, B. *et al.* (1990) Single photon emission computed tomography (SPECT) in seizure disorders in childhood. *Brain and Development*, **12**, 385–9.

Williams, B.A., Abbott, K.J. and Manson, J.I. (1992) Cerebral tumors in children presenting with epilepsy. *Journal of Child Neurology*, **7**, 291–4.

EPILEPSY IN THE MENTALLY RETARDED

Matti Sillanpää

INTRODUCTION

Epilepsy and mental retardation (MR) are among the most common major neuro-developmental disabilities. MR is a chronic or life-long disorder, which is generally defined as an inability to care for oneself in a manner which would be comparable to one's peers, based on a low intelligence level (<70) at the age of less than 18. When associated with MR, repeated unprovoked epileptic seizures, or epilepsy, also tend to be difficult to treat or completely intractable. Therefore, a combination of epilepsy and MR constitutes a considerable challenge, and, also an economic load to the health care system. Investments in prevention, early diagnosis, treatment and management of both MR and epilepsy may markedly diminish institutionalization and other costs of care, and help patients to become less dependent on other people.

EPIDEMIOLOGIC ASPECTS

The association of epilepsy with MR may be approached in many ways. Several studies deal with the prevalence of epilepsy in selected, institutionalized subjects with MR or patients seen in hospital (Illingworth, 1959; Iivanainen, 1974; Mariani *et al.*, 1993). Data are available on the prevalence of MR from population studies of epilepsy (Sillanpää, 1983; von Wendt *et al.*, 1985; Ellenberg, Hirtz and Nelson, 1986) or on the prevalence of

epilepsy and MR from population studies of cerebral palsy (CP) (Lagergren, 1981). Overall aspects of the epidemiology of epilepsy are considered in Chapter 3.

Studies related to the occurrence of epilepsy in mentally retarded populations are often cross-sectional, yielding a point prevalence, or period prevalence of an 'active' epilepsy (Drillien, Jameson and Wilkinson, 1966; Forsgren *et al.*, 1990; Gustavson *et al.*, 1977a; Richardson *et al.*, 1980). Figures are markedly different when different criteria are used; in the study of Corbett, Harris and Robinson (1975), in MR children up to age 14 at least one epileptic seizure had occurred in 32%, but the period prevalence of 1 year was only 19%. In studying a life-time prevalence or, better still, a cumulative incidence of epilepsy in people with MR, only unselected prospective cohort studies can give reliable data on the epidemiology of epilepsy in MR. An overall prevalence of epilepsy is approximately 15% in patients with mild MR (IQ 50–69) (Drillien, Jameson and Wilkinson, 1966; Blomquist, Gustavson and Holmgren, 1981; Hagberg *et al.*, 1981) and 30% in those with severe MR (IQ<50) (Drillien, Jameson and Wilkinson, 1966; Corbett, Harris and Robinson, 1975; Gustavson *et al.*, 1977a, 1977b).

The prevalence of epilepsy is higher in institutionalized than unselected populations. Illingworth (1959) found epilepsy in 34.2% of 816 consecutive MR patients seen in

Epilepsy in Children. Edited by Sheila Wallace. Published in 1996 by Chapman & Hall, London. ISBN 0 412 56860 8

Table 17.1　Occurrence of various types of epileptic seizures in mentally retarded (MR) patients with or without cerebral palsy (CP) in percentages

Author(s)/year	No.	Seizures in IQ groups		Seizure		Seizures	
		69–50	<50	GTCS	Total	Without CP	With CP
Hospital-based prevalence studies							
Illingworth, 1959	816	22.8	53.7		34.2	31.3	37.5
Iivanainen, 1974	334			18.3	62.9	27.6	72.4
Mariani et al., 1993	1 024			19.9	31.8		
Population-based prevalence studies							
Forsgren et al., 1990	1 479	11.2	23.3	13.8	20.2	43.1	
Jacobson and Janicki, 1983	10 471					18.1	51.6
Population-based cumulative incidence studies							
Goulden et al., 1993	221	10.1	34.8		15.3	5.2	37.5

GTCS = generalized tonic-clonic seizures; PS = partial seizures.

hospital (Table 17.1). Seizures were more common in patients with any degree of MR and CP compared with those without CP (37.5% vs. 31.3%), and in severe MR with CP (53.7% vs. 46.8%).

Iivanainen (1974) retrospectively studied 338 out of 1000 patients consecutively admitted to an institution for the mentally retarded during the years 1943 to 1966 and who were still alive at the end of 1966. The life-time prevalence of epilepsy was 62.1%. The seizures were classified as focal in 22.4%, generalized in 18.0%, and miscellaneous in 48.6%. In the whole group of 1000, including those still surviving and those who had died, the life-time prevalence was 44.2% (Iivanainen, 1985).

In a recent retrospective study of 1023 institutionalized MR patients with an encephalopathy (Mariani et al., 1993), 326 (31.9%) patients had epilepsy. Generalized seizures were markedly more common than partial types (62.5% vs. 32.5%).

The prevalence of MR in patients with epilepsy in epidemiologic studies seems to be of the same order as epilepsy in MR. Sillanpää (1983) reported severe MR in 33.3% and mild MR in 6.6% in Finland. In another Finnish study (von Wendt et al., 1985), the

corresponding figures were 15.4% and 5.8%. In a large National Collaborative Perinatal Project (NCPP), Ellenberg, Hirtz and Nelson (1986) reported MR in 14.3% of children with epilepsy followed up to the age 7 compared with 5.1% in their siblings, but no difference in case–sibling pairs, if both were neurologically normal on early examinations. The full-scale intelligence quotient was not significantly affected by the occurrence of seizures.

Gustavson et al. (1977b) retrospectively investigated the occurrence of severe MR (IQ<50) in an unselected population aged 5–16 years in Sweden. The prevalence of severe MR was 3.9‰, increasing from 3.1‰ in the age group of 5–8 years to 5.3‰ in the group aged 13–16 years. Altogether 84 out of 161 (52.2%) had epilepsy. The prevalence of mild MR in the same area was found to be 4.2‰ in the same age groups. Epilepsy was less frequent in mild than in severe MR (Blomquist, Gustavson and Holmgren, 1981): only 36 of 171 (21.1%) had had repeated afebrile epileptic seizures.

Forsgren et al. (1990) found 20.2% of 1479 patients to have 'active' epilepsy on the prevalence day. In the age group 0–9 years, the prevalence rate was higher for girls, while in other age groups there was a male majority. Epilepsy was found in 11.2% of patients with mild MR and in 23.3% of those severely mentally retarded.

Richardson *et al.* (1980) analyzed a child population, born in 1951 through 1955 and resident in a British city in 1962, for MR. Using two reference groups, one with borderline intelligence, and another with normal intelligence and matched for age and sex, they found the corresponding figures for the occurrence of one or more epileptic seizures to be 27%, 11%, and 4%. Within the group with MR, the more severe MR was associated with more frequent seizures at a younger age and over a longer time span than those with a mild MR.

In their prospective cohort of 221 children with MR (the Aberdeen study, Scotland), Goulden *et al.* (1991) found two or more unprovoked epileptic seizures, considered to be epilepsy, in 33 (15%) and one febrile or afebrile seizure in an additional 16 (7%) children by the age of 22 years. The cumulative incidence of epilepsy was 9%, 11%, 13%, and 15% at 5, 10, 15, and 22 years, respectively. In patients with severe MR, two or more seizures occurred in 35% and one or more in 44%. Another, comparable study from the UK (Camberwell, South London) showed similar results (Corbett, Harris and Robinson, 1975; Corbett, 1993), at least one seizure having occurred in 32% in patients with severe MR.

Age at onset of epilepsy is as early as or earlier than in the general population (Richardson *et al.*, 1980; Forsgren *et al.*, 1990; Goulden *et al.*, 1991). Seizure frequency is usually high, with 60–70% having annual seizures (Forsgren *et al.*, 1990).

EPILEPTIC SEIZURES, EPILEPSIES, AND EPILEPTIC SYNDROMES IN THE MENTALLY RETARDED

Classification of seizures in people with MR is met by several difficulties, not least because of inadequate or defective verbal communica-

tion resulting in underestimation of, especially, partial seizures. Generalized convulsive seizures are most easily identifiable and reportedly commonest in population-based studies, varying from 58% to 68% (von Wendt *et al.*, 1985; Forsgren *et al.*, 1990; Baldev and Towle, 1993; Marcus, 1993), while patients with partial seizures with or without secondary generalization may be preferentially selected in studies derived from institutions for the mentally retarded, making the distribution of seizure types less clear (Matilainen *et al.*, 1988; Mariani *et al.*, 1993). Partial, rather than primary generalized epilepsies, are associated with more severe handicaps and institutionalization.

Since seizure types are age related, they vary in distribution, particularly in childhood. In addition, most patients with MR have mixed seizure types. As age increases, the proportions of generalized convulsive and partial seizures increase markedly, while seizures typical of early childhood decrease (Forsgren *et al.*, 1990). Convulsive status epilepticus occurred in 56 of 299 (18.7%) patients in Forsgren's study.

The International Classification of Epilepsies and Epileptic Syndromes is given in Chapter 7, but is not easily applicable for MR patients with seizures. Manford *et al.* (1992) could classify only 34% and Mariani *et al.* (1993) 28% into specific types. However, some epilepsies and epileptic syndromes are of importance in association with MR.

Ohtahara's syndrome, or early infantile epileptic encephalopathy (Chapter 11a), presents with very early onset and drug-resistant tonic spasms and suppression burst in the EEG, associated with early death or MR and with frequent evolution to infantile spasms and further to Lennox–Gastaut syndrome. The etiology is heterogeneous but always of lesional or metabolic origin.

Infantile spasms, hypsarrhythmia, and MR make up the typical triad of West's syndrome (chapter 11b), of which the incidence is about 40/100 000 live births (Riikonen and Donner,

1979), 3.3–4.9% of epilepsies in an unselected population-based study (Sillanpää, 1973; von Wendt *et al.*, 1985) and 7.0% in a MR population with onset of epilepsy during the first year of life (Forsgren *et al.*, 1990). Association with MR is almost invariable, occurring in 70–90% of cases. Ninety per cent have an organic etiology. Seizures are persistent in 40% of patients.

Lennox–Gastaut syndrome (Chapter 12a) although often a continuation of West's syndrome, may occur as an independent syndrome with axial tonic and other types of seizures (atypical absences, atonic or myoatonic falls), combined with MR, severe personality disturbances, and drug resistance. Tonic seizures have been reported in 90% (Beaumanoir and Dravet, 1992).

EPILEPSY IN CERTAIN MENTAL RETARDATION SYNDROMES

CHROMOSOMAL ABNORMALITIES (see also Chapter 4b)

Down's syndrome is the most common chromosomal cause of MR but also shows several other neurologic abnormalities of a progressive nature. The vast majority of patients with Down's syndrome develop similar neuropathologic changes to those found in Alzheimer's disease at middle age, and, later clinical signs of dementia. They also tend to have sensorineural hearing loss, nystagmus and cervical spinal cord injuries as a result of atlantoaxial subluxation.

Down's syndrome was not associated with epilepsy by Down himself (1866) nor other earlier authors (Illingworth, 1959; Shuttleworth, 1909; Wilmarth, 1890). Later, the reported prevalence of epilepsy has varied considerably, from 1 to 9% (Engler, 1949; Kirman, 1951; Ellingson, Menolascino and Eisen, 1970), probably depending on small patient series, definition of epilepsy, nature of source population, difficulties in case identification and age of the subjects.

Based on his large series of 1654 patients, Veall (1974) reported an age-related incidence with a bimodal distribution of age at onset, the first peak occurring between 16 and 23 and the second one between 35 and 54 years of age. The age-related higher incidence was ascribed to the occurrence of Alzheimer's disease-like alterations in the brain, which have been reported to occur in Down's syndrome in early or presenile dementia (Lott and Lai, 1982; Sim, Turner and Smith, 1966). Further evidence for the association of seizures with presenile dementia in Down's syndrome was obtained by Collacott (1993). In his 351 patient series, onset of epilepsy at 35 or more was significantly associated with dementia, which was also indicated by significantly reduced Adaptive Behaviour Scale scores. Contrary to the report of Veall (1974), the incidence was remarkably low between 30 and 49 years of age.

The incidence of epilepsy in patients with Alzheimer's disease but without Down's syndrome is 10% (Hauser *et al.*, 1986), but in patients with Down's syndrome and Alzheimer-like dementia 75% or more (Lai and Williams, 1989), suggesting a specific epileptogenic factor in Down's patients (Stafstrom, 1993).

Fragile X syndrome is an X-linked chromosomal disorder with MR, facial dysmorphism, macro-orchidism, and language and learning disorders. Recurrent partial and generalized convulsive seizures and infantile spasms may occur in 25% (Wisniewski *et al.*, 1985; Forsgren *et al.*, 1990).

DYSPLASTIC CONDITIONS (see also Chapter 4a, Chapter 16)

In many neurocutaneous syndromes, MR is the rule and epilepsy is almost invariable. This is true, for example, for tuberous sclerosis and Sturge–Weber syndrome, both of which are characterized by drug-refractory and deteriorating epilepsy syndromes of West's and Lennox–Gastaut. Aicardi's syndrome, megalencephaly and other cerebral malformations also present with West's, Lennox–Gastaut or other epilepsy syndromes. In these conditions, 41–100% suffer from epilepsy (Corbett, Harris and Robinson, 1975).

NEUROMETABOLIC AND DEGENERATIVE ABNORMALITIES (see also Chapters 4c, 15a)

Neuronal ceroid lipofuscinosis is a group of syndromes, which are characterized by the storage of material similar to ceroid and lipofuscin and cause, among other things, MR, blindness due to retinal atrophy, ataxia, and pyramidal and extrapyramidal symptoms. Several clinical types may be differentiated: infantile, late infantile, juvenile, and adult types. Epileptic seizures occur in most pediatric forms. Myoclonic seizures are invariably found in children with infantile types of ceroid lipofuscinosis.

Rett's syndrome characteristically occurs in girls aged 5–10 years with gradual loss of acquired skills up to 3 years, mental deterioration, peculiar hand-writhing and hand-mouthing behavior, gait apraxia, jerky truncal ataxia, and often breathing dysfunction. Epileptic seizures usually start at age 3–5 years, but very early onset is possible. The incidence of epilepsy with partial or generalized seizures, or possibly atypical infantile spasms, is 70–80% (Hagberg, 1993).

Other metabolic abnormalities with frequent epilepsy are phenylketonuria, maple syrup urine disease, metachromatic leucodystrophy, and several organic acidemias. In the Camberwell study, 41% of patients with a metabolic disease and MR had epilepsy (Corbett, Harris and Robinson, 1975).

CONCOMITANT HANDICAPS

Marcus (1993) could not find any firm relationship between the occurrence of epilepsy and, on the other hand, degree of MR, neurologic disability, or electroencephalogram. However, in numerous cohort studies with long-term follow-up, MR has proved to be a significant independent risk factor in the occurrence or persistence of seizures. In many investigations, the risk of epilepsy has been shown to bear a positive relationship to the severity of MR.

Illingworth (1959) retrospectively studied 816 children with MR, 285 of whom also had CP. Epilepsy occurred in 32.5% with CP and in 31.3% of those without CP. If MR was mild (IQ $\geqslant$50), the corresponding figures were 22.8% and 16.3%. In cases of severe MR (IQ <50) the prevalence of epilepsy was 53.7% or 46.8%, depending on whether or not CP was associated. The age at onset of epilepsy was similar, regardless of possible combined CP.

In the Camberwell study (Corbett, Harris and Robinson, 1975), the risk of epilepsy was three-fold (60% vs. 20%) in patients with MR and CP compared to those without CP.

Jacobson and Janicki (1983) collected data on 43 692 persons, 95% of whom had MR. Epilepsy occurred in 23% and CP in 16% of persons less than 22 years of age. The prevalence of epilepsy increased from 9% in mild MR to 43% in profound MR. The corresponding figures for CP were 9% and 29%.

In mildly affected patients a combination of MR and CP slightly raised the prevalence of epilepsy, when compared with patients with MR but not CP, in the retrospective study of Blomquist, Gustavson and Holmgren (1981) (22.2% vs. 18.8%); but in severe MR the co-existence of CP had a less obvious effect (55.2% vs. 46.4%; Gustavson *et al.* 1977b).

In another retrospective study from the same Swedish area including both children and adults with MR (age range not given; Forsgren *et al.*, 1990), 20.2% of 1479 patients with MR had epilepsy. The prevalence of epilepsy was 33.4%, when CP was combined with MR.

In the prospective cohort study of Goulden *et al.* (1991), previously reported in part by Richardson *et al.* (1980), 15% of 221 patients with MR had developed epilepsy. The etiology of MR played a major role. The incidence of epilepsy was unrelated to the severity of MR in the subgroup of MR only; but it was about seven-fold (38% vs. 5%) in children with MR and CP and 15-fold (75% vs. 5%) in children with MR and a postnatal injury, when compared with the cumulative incidence of epilepsy in patients with MR only. It is concluded that a significantly increased incidence of epilepsy in severe compared with mild MR (35% vs. 10%) may be due to the occurrence of CP, and even more so to a postnatal brain lesion. The cumulative incidence of febrile seizures was 9%. One-third (32%) of the patients with febrile seizures later developed epilepsy. The predictive value of febrile seizures to the incidence of epilepsy in this population remained unclear.

In 100 children examined by Voutilainen (1992), who developed expansive hydrocephalus at age less than 1 year, epilepsy was significantly more frequent in children with MR (IQ <70) than in those without MR (74% vs. 28%).

ADAPTIVE BEHAVIORAL PROBLEMS

Espie *et al.* (1989) studied 15 institutionalized adults who suffered from MR and epilepsy and reported poorer life skills compared with matched controls without epilepsy. Behavioral problems are substantially more frequent and severe in epileptic patients with MR than in those of normal intelligence. Aggression, and emotional and self-injurious problems are greater and social competence less than in nonretarded people with epilepsy (Corbett, Harris and Robinson 1975; Hermann, 1982). In the Camberwell study, behavior disorder occurred in 40%, temper tantrums in 38%, hyperkinesis in 30%, and childhood autism in 15% (Corbett, Harris and Robinson, 1975). Behavioral disturbances are more severe if seizures are drug resistant (Espie *et al.*, 1989).

COMMON PROBLEMS OF IDENTIFICATION AND CLASSIFICATION OF SEIZURES

Epileptic seizures are more difficult to diagnose in the mentally retarded than in others because of problems with expression of subjective symptoms and sensations, specifically in relation to auras and aspects of ictal consciousness. Still greater difficulties are present in differentiating epileptic from nonepileptic seizures (see also Chapter 2). An attempt to classify nonepileptic seizures on the basis of the underlying principal mechanism has been made in Table 17.2. Keeping in mind the possibility of their occurrence, most of these conditions can be identified without difficulty. Problems may arise particularly with emotionally triggered pseudoepileptic seizures, such as aggressive and rage attacks, staring-like unresponsiveness and masturbation, as well as nocturnal phenomena. A multifaceted psychopathology may be hidden behind these disorders, including anxiety, dissociative, psychotic and factitious disorders, malingering and rarely rage attacks (Kloster, 1993).

Patients with MR frequently suffer from sleep deprivation and other sleep disturbances, which precipitate the occurrence of seizures (Aird, 1983; Papini *et al.*, 1984). In addition, antiepileptic drug therapy may predispose to sleep disturbances.

It is important to recognize that nonepileptic attacks may often, and in MR patients in particular, be combined with epileptic seizures (Metrick *et al.*, 1991), and accordingly be less easily detectable. Pseudoepileptic seizures may be generalized tonic-clonic, partial or absence seizures, or even pseudo-status epilepticus. Major motor seizures are more common in patients with pseudo-epileptic seizures only, compared with those with a combination of pseudo-seizures with real ones (Kloster, 1993).

The following signs are characteristic but not pathognomonic of pseudo-epileptic seizures: duration of 3 minutes or more and a

Table 17.2 Differential diagnosis of epileptic seizures in mental retardation

1. Cerebral hypoxic states
   1.1 Reflex and mechanical syncope
   1.2 Transient global cerebral ischemia
   1.3 Cardiogenic
   1.4 Migraine
2. Disturbed homeostasis
   2.1 Hypoglycemia
   2.2 Electrolyte imbalance
   2.3 Disturbed thermoregulation
3. Involuntary paroxysmal movements
   3.1 Paroxysmal dystonia or choreoathetosis
   3.2 Drug-related dyskinesias
   3.3 Startle reponses
   3.4 Nystagmus and other oculomotor disorders
   3.5 Tic
   3.6 Stereotypic rocking and hand-waving
4. Sleep disorders
   4.1 Night terrors
   4.2 Pavor nocturnus
   4.3 Head banging
   4.4 REM sleep-related violence
   4.5 Somnambulism
   4.6 Benign nocturnal myoclonus
   4.7 Sleep apnea
5. Diurnal psychogenic episodes
   5.1 Episodic rage attacks
   5.2 Hyperventilation syndrome
   5.3 Masturbation
   5.4 Self-injurious behavior
   5.5 Panic attacks
   5.6 Breath-holding spells
6. Gastrointestinal disorders
   6.1 Vomiting, regurgitation, and rumination
   6.2 Gastroesophageal reflux
   6.3 Urinary and stool incontinence
7. Other
   7.1 Unresponsiveness or 'staring'
   7.2 Tonic episodes due to brainstem compression
   7.3 Self-induced seizures

gradual termination; discontinuance by verbal suggestion; absence of cyanosis; whole-body rigidity with typical tossing pelvic movements; no clear-cut postictal phase. Nevertheless, it is often difficult to differentiate between pseudo-epileptic seizures and temporal or frontal focal-onset seizures.

A video-EEG recording is often necessary for a correct diagnosis. The serum prolactin level may contribute. Peak concentrations of prolactin are mostly found about 15 minutes after seizures, with the highest levels occurring after generalized tonic-clonic seizures and complex partial seizures of temporal lobe origin. Levels are rarely raised in association with complex partial seizures of extratemporal origin, simple partial seizures, or pseudo-epileptic seizures (Kloster, 1993).

Self-induced seizures are usually a sign of photosensitive epilepsy. Flickering is elicited in bright light by waving a hand rhythmically against the eyes. Apparently, self-provoked seizures produce pleasure and the patient is often reluctant to discontinue seizure-provoking behaviour.

ETIOLOGY OF EPILEPSY IN MENTALLY RETARDED PEOPLE

The etiology of severe MR is reportedly prenatal in 55–72%, perinatal in 8–15%, postnatal in 1–12%, and unknown in 13–22% (Gustavson *et al.*, 1977a; Hagberg and Kyllerman, 1983; Linna, 1989). The corresponding figures for mild MR are 23–43%, 7–18%, 4–5%, and 43–55% (Blomquist, Gustavson and Holmgren, 1981; Hagberg and Kyllerman, 1983). The etiology of the epilepsy cannot be separated from that of MR. Epilepsy may be regarded as a result of any pre-, or postnatal brain injury, which is a presumed cause of MR. However, every abnormal event in the pre-, peri- or postnatal history is not necessarily of importance.

TREATMENT AND MANAGEMENT

It is now generally accepted that antiepileptic drugs with clear-cut sedative side-effects, such as phenobarbitone and phenytoin (Corbett, Trimble and Nichol, 1985), should be avoided in the therapy of epilepsy in patients with MR. These drugs may further weaken the patients' mental capacity even at acceptable blood levels. Discontinuation of phenobarbitone does not necessarily worsen and can improve seizure control and behavior patterns (Pointdexter, Berglund and Kolstoe, 1993). Phenytoin-induced cerebellar atrophy has been reported in MR patients (Iivanainen, Viukari and Helle, 1977). Children with multihandicapped MR appear to be especially sensitive to phenytoin (Zielinski, 1989). In MR side-effects may be masked by pre-existing neurologic abnormalities and are therefore less easily detectable.

Monotherapy should always be preferred to polypharmacotherapy. However, difficult-to-treat epilepsies, special epileptic syndromes such as refractory atypical absences and epilepsy with multiple seizure types, may require two or more antiepileptic drugs. If seizures are drug resistant despite trials of several combinations, a reduction of polytherapy may not change the seizure frequency but may diminish side-effects. If the epilepsy is getting worse, the patient must be carefully observed for possible drug toxicity and also for poor compliance, and the rare development of an intracranial tumor or raised intracranial pressure.

Valproate, carbamazepine, oxcarbazepine, and ethosuximide can be regarded as drugs of choice. However, when on valproate therapy, MR children with a metabolic disease including liver involvement, are at high risk of developing a life-threatening condition. The risk for an idiosyncratic reaction is particularly high in mentally handicapped children aged 2–4 years or less (Scheffner *et al.*, 1988; Dreifuss *et al.*, 1989). Up to the end of 1991, 129 fatal valproate-treated cases were reported (Scheffner and König, 1992). Dementia is also possible as a valproate side-effect (Zaret and Cohen, 1986).

Recently, vigabatrin has been shown to be effective as add-on therapy in patients with drug-resistant seizures (Matilainen *et al.*, 1988). More than 50% reduction in seizure frequency was achieved in 43% of seizures of partial onset and in 33% of generalized seizures. Adverse effects were mild, and there was no need to interrupt the add-on therapy. Lamotrigine can be helpful for atypical absences and drop attacks.

Seizures in neuronal ceroid lipofuscinosis may not be reduced by carbamazepine and may get worse on phenytoin therapy. Exceptionally, phenobarbitone can be used in this disease due to its antioxidant properties. Valproate is often effective, but its side-effects must be kept in mind in these children. Furthermore, benzodiazepines are of use, especially for myoclonic seizures.

Epileptic seizures associated with Rett's syndrome may be very therapy resistant; and the patients, even, in an unexplainable way, sensitive to antiepileptic drugs, only to become later, and surprisingly, spontaneously seizure free (Hagberg, 1993)

Although it is most important, antiepileptic drug therapy given by the doctor is not the only way to care for epilepsy in patients with MR. A multidisciplinary approach and team work are needed to train professionals of various categories, and families, to observe seizures, side-effects, and long-term neurologic and behavior changes in order to minimize the adverse effects of drugs.

Surgical intervention may be indicated in resistant epilepsy if there is unilateral spike-and-wave activity, which should be prevented from spreading to the other hemisphere. In these cases, corpus callosotomy or commissurotomy could be the preferential approach, but in some cases, cortical resection, lobectomy or hemispherectomy will be feasible (Chapter 23d).

In the management of patients with MR and epilepsy, several specific aspects must be considered. These may be associated with MR or seizures or both, and include risks of aspiration, drowning for example in bath water, nutritional deficiencies due to swallowing difficulties, and gastrointestinal disorders arising from constipation or other dysfunctions. Fatal and nonfatal, seizure-related and other injuries should be prevented by avoidance of identified risk factors, enhanced staff supervision, minimizing risks in the environment, and developing reasonable activities for patients to decrease boredom and restlessness.

PROGNOSIS

The association of MR with epilepsy has generally been regarded as unfavorable (Aicardi, 1986; Brorson and Wranne, 1987; Sillanpää, 1990), but some authors have not found any difference in outcome related to the severity of MR in patients on or off medication (Theodore, Schulman and Pumer, 1983; Shinnar *et al.*, 1985). Rowan *et al.* (1980) retrospectively compared 44 institutionalized subnormal patients with at least 50 convulsive seizures during the first 9 months of the year 1976, with 29 matched controls who had had no seizures during the same period of time. A seizure outcome after 20–22 years of follow-up was predictable with an 80% probability on the basis of admission EEG characteristics and clinical findings. In the group with a poor outcome, early-onset seizures with high initial frequency, multiple seizure types and severe mental retardation predominated, combined with absence of posterior dominant rhythmic activity, generalized delta activity and frequent generalized paroxysmal discharges on the EEG.

Goulden *et al.* (1991) reported seizure freedom for 5 months on or off medication in 39% of the patients with MR by age 22. The etiology of MR was clearly related to the prognosis of the epilepsy. The remission rate was 56% in the subgroup of MR only, 47% in the MR and CP group, and 11% in patients with MR resulting from a perinatal brain injury.

Contrary to a generally held view, Marcus (1993) could not find any correlation between seizure control and level of MR, abnormal neurologic status or EEG abnormalities.

Litzinger, Duvall and Little (1993) showed that medically fragile patients with severe MR and complex epilepsy could be successfully relocated from an institution into the community by early initiation of drug therapy, reducing polypharmacotherapy, and improving staff education.

REFERENCES

Aicardi, J. (1986) *Epilepsy in Children*. Raven Press, New York.

Aird, R.B. (1983) The importance of seizure-inducing factors in the control of refractory forms of epilepsy. *Epilepsia*, **24**, 567–83.

Baldev, K.S. and Towle, P.O. (1993) Antiepileptic drug status in adult outpatients with mental retardation. *American Journal of Mental Retardation*, **98** (Suppl.), 41–6.

Beaumanoir, A, and Dravet, C. (1992) The Lennox–Gastaut syndrome, in *Epileptic Syndromes in Infancy, Childhood and Adolescence*, 2nd revised edn (eds J. Roger, M. Bureau, C. Dravet *et al.*), John Libbey, London, pp. 115–32.

Blomquist, H.K. (1982) Mental retardation in children. An epidemiological and etiological study of mentally retarded children born 1959–1970 in a northern Swedish county. *Umeå University Medical Dissertations. New Series*, **76**/1982, 1–145.

Blomquist, H.K., Gustavson, K.H., and Holmgren, G. (1981) Mild mental retardation in children in a Northern Swedish county. *Journal of Mental Deficiency Research*, **25**, 92–109.

Brorson, L.O. and Wranne, L. (1987) Long-term prognosis of childhood epilepsy: survival and seizure prognosis. *Epilepsia*, **28**, 324–30.

Collacott, R.A. (1993) Epilepsy, dementia and adaptive behaviour in Down's syndrome. *Journal of Intellectual Disability Research*, **37**, 153–160.

Corbett, J. (1993) Epilepsy and mental handicap, in *A Textbook of Epilepsy* (eds J. Laidlaw, A. Richens and D. Chadwick), Churchill Livingstone, Edinburgh, pp. 631–6.

Corbett, J.A., Harris, R. and Robinson, R. (1975) Epilepsy, in *Mental Retardation and Developmental Disabilities*, vol. VII (ed J. Wortis), Raven Press, New York, pp. 79–111.

Corbett, J.A., Trimble, M.R. and Nichol, T. (1985) Behavioral and cognitive impairment in children with epilepsy: the long-term effects of anticonvulsant therapy. *Journal of the American Academy of Child Psychiatry*, **23**, 17–23.

Down, J.L.H. (1866) Observations on an ethnic classification of idiots. *London Hospital, Clinical Lectures and Reports*, **3**, 259–62.

Dreifuss, F.E., Langer, E.H., Moline, K.A. *et al.*

(1989) Valproic acid fatalities. II. US experience since 1984. *Neurology*, **39**, 201–7.

Drillien, C.M., Jameson, S. and Wilkinson, E.M. (1966) Studies in mental handicap. Part I: Prevalence and distribution by clinical type and severity of defect. *Archives of Disease in Childhood*, **41**, 528–38.

Ellenberg, J.H., Hirtz, D.G. and Nelson, K.B. (1986) Do seizures cause intellectual deterioration? *New England Journal of Medicine*, **314**, 1085–8.

Ellingson, R.J., Menolascino, F.J. and Eisen, J.D. (1970) Clinical–E.E.G. relationships in mongoloids confirmed by karyotype. *American Journal of Mental Deficiency*, **74**, 645–50.

Engler, M. (1949) *Mongolism*, John Wright, Bristol.

Espie, C.A., Pashley, A.S., Bonham, K.G. *et al.* (1989) The mentally handicapped person with epilepsy: a comparative study investigating psychosocial functioning. *Journal of Mental Deficiency Research*, **33**, 123–35.

Forsgren, L., Edvinsson, S.O., Blomquist, H.K. *et al.* (1990) Epilepsy in a population of mentally retarded children and adults. *Epilepsy Research*, **6**, 234–48.

Goulden, K.J., Shinnar, S, Koller, H. *et al.* (1991) Epilepsy in children with mental retardation: a cohort study *Epilepsia*, **32**, 690–7.

Gustavson, K.H., Hagberg, B., Hagberg, G. *et al.* (1977a) Severe mental retardation in a Swedish county I. Epidemiology, gestational age, birthweight and associated CNS handicaps in children born 1959–70. *Acta Paediatrica Scandinavica*, **66**, 373–9.

Gustavson, K.H., Holmgren, G., Jonsell, R. *et al.* (1977b) Severe mental retardation in children in a Northern Swedish county. *Journal of Mental Deficiency Research*, **21**, 161–80.

Hagberg, B. (1993) Clinical criteria, stages and natural history, in *Rett syndrome – Clinical and Biological Aspects, Clinics in Developmental Medicine*, No. 127 (ed. B. Hagberg), MacKeith Press, London, pp. 4–20.

Hagberg, B. and Kyllerman, M. (1983) Epidemiology of mental retardation – a Swedish survey. *Brain and Development*, **5**, 441–9.

Hagberg, B., Hagberg, G., Lewerth, A. *et al.* (1981) Mild mental retardation in Swedish school children. II. Etiologic and pathogenetic aspects. *Acta Paediatrica Scandinavica*, **70**, 445–52.

Hauser, W.A., Morris, M.L., Heston, L.L. *et al.* (1986) Seizures and myoclonus in patients with Alzheimer's disease. *Neurology*, **36**, 1226–30.

Hermann, B.P. (1982) Neuropsychological functioning and psychopathology in children with epilepsy. *Epilepsia*, **23**, 545–54.

Iivanainen, M. (1974) A study of origins of mental retardation, in *Clinics in Developmental Medicine*, No. 51, Spastics International Publications, William Heinemann Medical Books, London.

Iivanainen, M. (1985) *Brain Developmental Disorders Leading to Mental Retardation. Modern Principles of Diagnosis*, C.C. Thomas, Springfield, IL.

Iivanainen, M., Viukari, M. and Helle, E.P. (1977) Cerebellar atrophy in phenytoin-treated mentally retarded epileptics. *Epilepsia*, **18**, 375–85.

Illingworth, R. S. (1959) Convulsions in mentally retarded children with or without cerebral palsy. *Journal of Mental Deficiency Research*, **3**, 88–93.

Jacobson, J.W. and Janicki, M.P. (1983) Observed prevalence in multiple mental disabilities. *Mental Retardation*, **21**, 87–94.

Kirman, B.H. (1951) Epilepsy in mongolism. *Archives of Disease in Childhood*, **26**, 501–3.

Kloster, R. (1993) Pseudo-epileptic v. epileptic seizures: a comparison, in *Pseudo-epileptic Seizures* (eds. L. Gram, S.I. Johannessen, P.O. Osterman and M. Sillanpää), Wrightson Medical Publishing, Petersfield, pp. 3–16.

Lagergren, J. (1981) Children with motor handicaps: epidemiological, medical and sociopaediatric aspects of motor handicapped children in a Swedish county. *Acta Paediatrica Scandinavica*, **70**(suppl. 289), 1–71.

Lai, F. and Williams, R.S. (1989) A prospective study of Alzheimer disease in Down syndrome. *Archives of Neurology*, **46**, 849–53.

Linna, S.L. (1989) Prevalence, aetiology, associated handicaps and self care ability in 5–19-year-old severely mentally retarded. University of Oulu, PhD thesis, pp. 1–166.

Lizinger, M.J., Duvall, B. and Little, P. (1993) Movement of individuals with complex epilepsy from an institution into the community: seizure control and functional outcomes, *American Journal on Mental Retardation*, **98**, 52–7.

Lott, I.T. and Lai, F. (1982) Dementia in Down's syndrome: observations from a neurology clinic. *Applied Research in Mental Retardation*, **3**, 233–9.

Manford, M., Hart, Y.M., Sander, J.W.A.S. *et al.* (1992) The national general practice study of epilepsy: the syndromic classification of the International League Against Epilepsy in a general population. *Archives of Neurology*, **49**, 801–8.

Marcus, J.C. (1993) Control of epilepsy in a mentally retarded population: lack of correlation with IQ, neurological status, and electroencephalogram. *American Journal of Mental Retardation*, **98**(suppl.), 47–51.

Mariani, E., Ferini-Strambi, L., Sala, M. *et al.* (1993) Epilepsy in institutionalized patients with encephalopathy: clinical aspects and nosological considerations. *American Journal of Mental Retardation*, **98**(suppl.), 27–33.

Matilainen, R., Pitkänen, A., Ruutiainen, T. *et al.* (1988) Effect of vigabatrin on epilepsy in mentally retarded patients: a 7-month follow-up study. *Neurology*, **38**, 743–47.

Metrick, M.E., Ritter, F.J. Gates, J.R. *et al.* (1991) Nonepileptic events in childhood. *Epilepsia*, **32**, 322–8.

Papini, M., Pasquinelli, A., Armellini, M. *et al.* (1984) Alertness and incidence of seizures in patients with Gastaut–Lennox syndrome. *Epilepsia*, **25**, 161–7.

Pointdexter, A.R., Berglund, J.A. and Kolstoe, P.D. (1993) Changes in antiepileptic drug prescribing patterns in large institutions: preliminary results of a five-year experience, *American Journal of Mental Retardation*, **98**, 34–40.

Richardson, S.A., Koller, H., Katz, M. *et al.* (1980) Seizures and epilepsy in a mentally retarded population over the first 22 years of life. *Applied Research in Mental Retardation*, **1**, 123–38.

Riikonen, R. and Donner, M. (1979) Incidence and aetiology of infantile spasms from 1960 to 1976. A population study in Finland. *Developmental Medicine and Child Neurology*, **21**, 333–43.

Rowan, A.J., Overveg, J., Sadikoglu, S. *et al.* (1980) Seizure prognosis in long-stay mentally subnormal epileptic patients: interrater EEG and clinical studies. *Epilepsia*, **21**, 219–26.

Scheffner, D. and König, St. (1992) Hepatotoxische Nebenwirkungen von Valproinsäure. Allgemeine klinishe Gesichtspunkte, in *Valproinsäure* (eds. G. Krämer and M.C. Laub), Springer Verlag, Berlin, pp. 266–70.

Scheffner, D., König, St., Rauterberg-Ruland, I. *et al.* (1988) Fatal liver failure in 16 children on valproate therapy. *Epilepsia*, **29**, 530–41.

Shinnar, S.S., Vining, E.P.G., Mellits, E. *et al.* (1985) Discontinuing antiepileptic medication in children with epilepsy after two years without seizures. *New England Journal of Medicine*, **313**, 976–80.

Shuttleworth, G.E. (1909). Mongolian imbecility. *British Medical Journal*, **2**, 661–5.

Sillanpää, M. (1973) Medico-social prognosis of children with epilepsy. Epidemiological study and analysis of 245 cases. *Acta Paediatrica Scandinavica, Supplement*, **237**, 1–104.

Sillanpää, M. (1983) Social functioning and seizure status of young adults with onset of epilepsy in childhood. An epidemiologic 20 year follow-up study. *Acta Neurologica Scandinavica*, **68**(suppl. 96), 1–77.

Sillanpaa, M. (1990) Children with epilepsy as adults: outcome after 30 years of follow-up. *Acta Paediatrica Scandinavica*, **7**, Supplement 368, 1–78.

Sim, M., Turner, E. and Smith, W.T. (1966) Cerebral biopsy in the investigation of presenile dementia. I. Clinical aspects. *British Journal of Psychiatry*, **112**, 119–25.

Stafstrom, C.E. (1993) Epilepsy in Down syndrome: clinical aspects and possible mechanisms. *American Journal of Mental Retardation*, **98**, 12–26.

Theodore, W.H., Schulman, E.A. and Porter, R.J. (1983) Intractable seizures: long-term follow-up after prolonged inpatient treatment in an epilepsy unit. *Epilepsia*, **24**, 336–43.

Veall, R.M. (1974) The prevalence of epilepsy among mongols related to age. *Journal of Mental Deficiency Research*, **18**, 99–106.

Voutilainen, A. (1992) Lapsuusiän hydrokefalian esiintyvyys, etiologia ja ennuste aikuisikään saakka (Incidence, etiology and outcome up to adulthood of infantile hydrocephalus.) Helsinki, PhD Thesis, pp. 1–143. (In Finnish).

von Wendt, L., Rantakallio, P., Saukkonen, A.-L. *et al.* (1985) Epilepsy and associated handicaps in a 1 year birth cohort in Northern Finland. *European Journal of Paediatrics*, **144**, 149–51.

Wilmarth, A.W. (1890) Report on the examination of one hundred brains of feeble-minded children. *Alienist and Neurologist*, **11**, 520–33.

Wisniewski, K.E., Laure-Kamionowska, M., Connell, F. and Wen, G.Y. (1985) Neuronal density and synaptogenesis in the postnatal stage of brain maturation in Down's syndrome, in *The Neurobiology of Down Syndrome* (ed. C.J. Epstein), Raven Press, New York, pp. 29–44.

Zaret, B.S. and Cohen, R.A. (1986) Reversible valproic acid dementia: a case report. *Epilepsia*, **27**, 234–40.

Zielinski, J.J. (1989) Childhood epilepsy and mental retardation, in *Childhood Epilepsies: Neuropsychological, Psychosocial and Intervention Aspects* (eds B.P. Hermann and M. Seidenberg), John Wiley, Chichester, pp. 221–45.

John Livingston

Status epilepticus (SE) is common in pediatric practice. In the USA, it has been estimated to occur between 50 000 and 60 000 times per year in patients of all ages (Hauser, 1990). Twenty per cent of cases of SE occur in the first year of life and 60% in the first 5 years (Aicardi and Chevrie, 1970; Dunn, 1988; Maytal *et al.*, 1989; Philips and Shanahan, 1989). Convulsive SE is a life-threatening medical emergency that demands prompt recognition and treatment.

DEFINITIONS

The most widely quoted definition states that 'SE is a condition in which epileptic seizures are sufficiently prolonged or repeated at such frequent intervals as to produce an enduring epileptic condition' (Gastaut, 1973). As an operational tool this is not precise enough and more recent definitions have been more specific about the duration and nature of seizures that constitute SE.

Most authors now define SE as recurrent epileptic seizures continuing for more than 30 minutes without full recovery of consciousness before the next seizure begins, or continuous clinical and/or electrical seizure activity lasting for more than 30 minutes whether or not consciousness is impaired (Treiman, 1993).

Earlier reports defined SE as seizures persisting for 60 minutes or longer (Aicardi and Chevrie, 1970). However, most recent studies have used a time limit of 30 minutes, recog-

nizing that early aggressive treatment will be effective in most cases and that irreversible damage may occur in seizures persisting longer than 1 hour.

CLASSIFICATION

There are as many types of SE as there are types of seizures (Gastaut, 1983). SE can be classified using the model of the 1981 ILAE classification of epileptic seizures. However a more empirical classification is into convulsive and nonconvulsive SE (Delgado-Escueta, Swartz and Abad-Herrera, 1990) (Table 18.1). In this classification, tonic SE is included as a form of convulsive SE.

Included under the heading of nonconvulsive SE (NCSE) is electrical SE. This refers to continuous EEG seizure activity without any obvious clinical change. This occurs particularly in the syndromes of continuous spike and wave activity during slow sleep and in the Landau–Kleffner syndrome (Chapter 13d).

Hypsarrhythmia has been considered by some authors to be a form of NCSE (Doose, 1983; Livingston and Brown, 1988) and has been included in this classification.

Those patients with convulsive SE who are pharmacologically paralyzed or anesthetized but continue to show SE on the EEG, are not included under electrical SE. Nonparalyzed patients who develop so-called subtle generalized convulsive SE with electromechanic dissociation can show a similar pattern, which is thought to occur in severe encephalopathies,

Epilepsy in Children. Edited by Sheila Wallace. Published in 1996 by Chapman & Hall, London. ISBN 0 412 56860 8

Table 18.1 Classification of status epilepticus (SE)

	Convulsive status epilepticus	*Nonconvulsive status epilepticus*
Generalized	Tonic Tonic-clonic Clonic Myoclonic	Absence { typical / atypical
Partial	Simple partial motor Simple partial motor with secondary generalization Epilepsia partialis continua	Simple partial SE with sensory symptomatology affective symptomatology Complex partial SE
Other		CSWSS Hypsarrhythmia

CSWSS = continuous spike and wave during slow sleep.

or as a result of inadequately treated overt generalized convulsive SE (Treiman, 1993).

ETIOLOGY (Table 18.2)

Most studies of SE have included all types, although the largest group represented is always convulsive SE. SE can be etiologically classified into four approximately equal groups. The two largest reported series, those of Aicardi and Chevrie (1970) and Maytal *et al.* (1989), although separated by two decades, show remarkably similar proportions when examined by etiology.

Table 18.2 Etiology of status epilepticus

Febrile	20–29%
Idiopathic	16–39%
Chronic static CNS disorder (remote symptomatic)	14–23%
Acute symptomatic	23–40%
CNS infection	
CNS trauma	
Hypoxic-ischemic damage	
Cerebrovascular	
Intoxication	
Metabolic/electrolyte disturbance	
Tumor	
Acute AED withdrawal	
Progressive encephalopathy	2–6%

Data from Aicardi and Chevrie (1970); Dunn (1988); Maytal *et al.* (1989); Philips and Shanahan (1989).

The following groups can be defined: (1) febrile; (2) idiopathic; (3) chronic static encephalopathy (remote symptomatic); and (4) acute symptomatic. Progressive encephalopathies, such as neurodegenerative diseases or some tumors, account for a small group (2–6% of all cases), and, should be considered separately from the static encephalopathies because of their different outcomes.

The etiology of SE is age dependent. In the first year of life, acute symptomatic causes account for up to 50% of cases. Between 1 and 3 years, febrile SE is the commonest group (see Chapter 10). In older children chronic CNS disorder (see Chapter 16) and idiopathic SE are the most important groups.

1. **Febrile SE** refers to SE occurring in febrile children with no previous history of non-febrile seizures, and no evidence of CNS infection or other acute CNS process. This group is considered to be the extreme end of the spectrum of complex febrile seizures (Ellenberg and Nelson, 1978; Maytal and Shinnar, 1990).
2. **Idiopathic SE** occurs in the absence of any acute CNS or systematic insult in neurologically normal children, and includes SE in children with a past history of epilepsy for which no cause has been found.
3. **Chronic static encephalopathy (remote symptomatic SE)**. Affected children have

a known prior neurological insult, with, or without, a past history of epilepsy. The prior insult may be infection, malformation, hypoxic ischemic encephalopathy, trauma, or stroke. Most of these children will have cerebral palsy and/or mental retardation, or other neurological abnormalities.

4. **Acute symptomatic SE** occurs during the course of an acute illness affecting the CNS. From 25 to 50% cases of SE are acute symptomatic (Aicardi and Chevrie, 1970; Maytal *et al.* 1989; Dunn, 1988; Dulac *et al.*, 1985). Most of the mortality of SE occurs in this group, which accounts for many cases with seizures lasting longer than 1 hour. There are many different etiologies, including CNS infection, head trauma, cerebrovascular accident, hypoxic ischemic encephalopathy, systemic metabolic derangement, and intoxication. Acute withdrawal of antiepileptic drug (AED) treatment is included in this group by many authors.

Toxin ingestion accounts for a small proportion of cases. Many different agents can be causative. The commonest are theophylline derivatives, tricyclic antidepressants, anticonvulsant drugs themselves, insulin, and amphetamines (Tunik and Young, 1992)

SYSTEMIC AND METABOLIC EFFECTS

The clinical effects of convulsive SE are initially compensatory with increase in sympathetic output resulting in tachycardia, hypertension, increased intracranial pressure, hyperglycemia, and hyperpyrexia. Metabolic acidosis may develop, secondary to a release of lactic acid. As the seizure continues, decompensation begins to occur with the development of hypotension, cardiac arrhythmias, hypoglycemia, pulmonary edema, hypoxia, and hypoventilation (Wasterlain *et al.*, 1993) Rhabdomyolysis and myoglobinuria with renal failure may occur. Leucocytosis and CSF pleocytosis are common (Aminoff and Simon, 1980)

There is a three- to four-fold increase in cerebral blood flow, with a comparable increase in the metabolic rate (Chapman, Meldrum and Siesjo, 1977). ATP levels and energy reserves fall somewhat after prolonged seizures. Eventually neuronal damage will begin to occur in selectively vulnerable areas.

Experimental evidence suggests that after 30–60 minutes of seizure activity, maladaptive changes occur that make neuronal damage much more likely. These include mismatch between blood flow and metabolism, self-sustaining seizure activity, and calcium-mediated excitotoxicity leading to neuronal injury (Wasterlain *et al.*, 1993).

These effects still occur but to a lesser degree, in well-oxygenated, ventilated and paralyzed experimental animals (Meldrum, Vigouroux and Brierley, 1973; Nevander *et al.*, 1984). Cellular mechanisms and subsequent pathology are presented in Chapters 5 and 6.

CLINICAL FEATURES

CONVULSIVE STATUS EPILEPTICUS

Although in the majority of reported series, generalized convulsive SE is commonest, it is probable that partial seizures with secondary generalization are underrecognized, particularly in the acute symptomatic group.

Generalized tonic-clonic SE comprises either a series of generalized tonic-clonic seizures or a more or less continuous clonic seizure (Aicardi, 1986) With repetitive generalized tonic-clonic seizures the attacks usually last 1–3 minutes and the patient is in a coma interictally. The tonic phase may become less conspicuous as the status continues. This type of seizure may then evolve into continuous clonic SE.

Although usually described as generalized, it has often been noted that these seizures will shift from side to side, wax and wane in intensity and involve different segments of the body at different times (Aicardi, 1986;

Roger, Lob and Tassinari, 1974). The EEG in generalized tonic-clonic SE may show repetitive seizure discharges, or in clonic status, rhythmic slow wave or spike-wave complexes.

TONIC STATUS EPILEPTICUS

Tonic SE is relatively uncommon and occurs predominantly, if not exclusively, in children with previous epilepsy, particularly the Lennox–Gastaut syndrome. Tonic SE may be prolonged, lasting up to several days. Individual seizures are typical tonic seizures but as the status progresses the motor seizure may become less and less prominent. Hypoventilation, salivation, and cyanosis are often marked. Tonic SE can be precipitated by intravenous benzodiazepines (Prior *et al.*, 1972; Tassinari *et al.*, 1972).

MYOCLONIC STATUS EPILEPTICUS

Myoclonic SE is characterized by repeated massive myoclonic jerks. It may occur in a child with a previous history of myoclonic or generalized epilepsy, or as part of one of the progressive myoclonic epilepsy syndromes (Chapter 15c).

PARTIAL CONVULSIVE STATUS EPILEPTICUS

Partial SE refers to convulsive SE localized to one part of one side of the body. It has been suggested that it be separated from unilateral SE where the whole of one side of the body may be involved. Unilateral SE often occurs during an attack of generalized SE (Aicardi, 1986). In practice, this may be a difficult distinction to make. Many episodes of partial SE may become secondary generalized.

Acute focal CNS lesions (e.g. hemorrhage, ischemia) may produce a pure partial motor SE. Consciousness is not disturbed in partial motor SE. However consciousness will be impaired when unilateral seizure activity occurs as part of generalized SE.

The commonest form of partial motor SE is

Table 18.3 Differential diagnosis of convulsive status epilepticus

Tonic extensor spasms:
Tentorial herniation
Acute brainstem dysfunction
Rigors
Acute dystonic reaction
Chorea/ballismus
Paroxysmal dyskinesia
Pseudo-status epilepticus:
Emotional/psychiatric disorders

partial clonic status with continuous jerks of an extremity or one side of the face.

Other more subtle forms of partial SE involve: eye deviation, ipsiversive or contraversive; eye jerking or oculo-clonic status; oculogyric status; or unusual movements such as trunk rotation. In such cases EEG verification may be required.

Epilepsia partialis continua is a form of continuous motor status and is considered elsewhere in this volume (Chapter 15b).

DIFFERENTIAL DIAGNOSIS OF CONVULSIVE STATUS EPILEPTICUS (Table 18.3)

There are a large number of nonepileptic paroxysmal disorders that may be mistaken for epileptic seizures (Chapter 2). When these are repeated frequently, are continuous or occur in a comatose child, they may be mistaken for SE.

Repetitive tonic extensor spasms in a child in coma are usually due to acute brainstem dysfunction, secondary to tentorial herniation, ischemia, severe metabolic disturbance, or a combination of these factors. Such movements occurring in a comatose child with other signs of brainstem dysfunction are highly unlikely to be epileptic seizures. It is very important that these signs are not mistaken for SE, since aggressive AED treatment may cause hypoventilation and hypotension, which can further exacerbate an already critical state.

Rigors are usually easily identified. However, when they occur in a comatose febrile child they may be mistaken for seizures.

True tonic SE usually occurs in the context of a severe preexisting epilepsy, when other types of convulsive movements or seizures may be present, but not always readily recognizable.

Acute dystonic reactions to drugs, particularly phenothiazines or butyrophenones, may produce florid motor features, usually without alteration of consciousness, and usually with a clear temporal association with drug ingestion. Such episodes are likely to be self-limiting, or will respond to intravenous procyclidine or benzhexol.

Chorea, ballismus, and paroxysmal dyskinesia may suggest SE. However the movements should be readily distinguishable, and consciousness is preserved. Such movements may develop during acute encephalopathic illnesses or following trauma. In such cases it may be difficult to exclude SE without EEG verification.

Fictitious epilepsy may take the form of prolonged 'pseudo-status epilepticus'. This has been recognized increasingly in adults (Betts and Boden, 1992) and undoubtedly occurs in childhood.

Prolonged nocturnal seizures with prominent motor features suggestive of sexual behavior have been reported in young women following sexual abuse (Betts and Boden, 1992). However, similar movements may occur in frontal lobe seizures.

In this context, EEG recorded during attacks is essential when there is doubt about diagnosis, and is advisable prior to initiating drug therapy.

MANAGEMENT OF CONVULSIVE STATUS EPILEPTICUS

Recent studies show a decline in the morbidity and mortality of SE, due, at least in part, to improvement in emergency management of acutely ill children and more widespread availability of pediatric intensive care facilities, providing full neurointensive care. Nevertheless, SE is a pediatric emergency which still has significant morbidity and mortality (Gross-Tsur and Shinnar, 1993).

A well-designed protocol with which the staff in the emergency department, the ward, and the intensive care unit (ICU) are familiar is more important than the choice of one AED rather than another. The aims of treatment are to control seizures within 30–60 minutes and to treat any reversible cause. Protocols usually recommend proceeding to general anesthesia after 60 minutes of SE. However, this requires the support of pediatric anesthetic staff, and, monitoring in a pediatric ICU that can provide continuous EEG and cardiopulmonary monitoring.

Earlier recourse to general anesthetics should be avoided, since it is important that the morbidity of treatment does not exceed that of the condition itself (Freeman, 1989). The management of convulsive SE can be divided into four stages (Table 18.4) and these are detailed below.

INITIAL STABILIZATION

It is essential to document the time at which treatment commences. The first priority is protection of the airway. Suction of the pharynx and positioning of the head usually achieve this. Insertion of an airway may be helpful but the mouth should not be forced open.

A nasogastric tube should be passed to decompress the stomach. Oxygen at 100% should be administered by facemask to all patients. Oxygen saturation and heart rate should be monitored. If there is evidence of hypoventilation, bag and mask ventilation should be initiated. If this does not provide adequate ventilation, the child should be intubated. In certain situations, including severe head injury, evidence of raised intracranial pressure, and severe acute CNS insults, early intubation should be considered.

Table 18.4 Management of status epilepticus

Immediate stabilization and resuscitation
Check airway
Suction
Nasogastric tube
100% oxygen by mask
Monitor oxygen saturation
Assess ventilation
Assess circulation
Establish IV access
Blood tests – glucose
                urea and electrolytes
                calcium
                magnesium
                AED level
Start IV infusion 5% dextrose/0.45% saline

Confirmation of diagnosis of SE
Observation of ictal behavior
Documentation of duration
If in doubt, further observation and EEG

Initial evaluation (Table 18.5)
History
Examination
Investigation

Treatment (Tables 18.6, 18.7)

It is difficult to assess the depth of coma in a child with SE and the coma scale cannot be used during the status. Circulation should be assessed, by measuring capillary return, blood pressure, and heart rate. If there are signs of hypovolemia or hypotension these should be treated. Early vascular access is important both for optimal administration of AEDs and for continued resuscitation and treatment.

An IV infusion of 0.45% saline and 5% dextrose should be started at normal maintenance rates (unless otherwise indicated).

As there may be difficulty in finding IV access in small convulsing children, other routes of drug administration are often used (intramuscular, rectal). However it is essential to have good vascular access as optimal treatment may require full circulatory support as well as AED treatment. If peripheral cannulation is not possible, a central line should be inserted. Intraosseous infusion has been used with success in children under 6 years of age when vascular access cannot be found (Lathers, Jim and Spivy, 1989; Tunik and Young, 1992).

CONFIRMATION OF DIAGNOSIS

During initial assessment the clinician will be able to observe the ictal behavior and decide whether it is consistent with SE or not. Documentation of the duration of the seizure prior to start of treatment is essential. If the patient is having repetitive seizures then at least two cycles of seizures should be observed, with confirmation that consciousness has not been regained between seizures (Delgado-Escueta, Swartz and Abad-Herrera, 1990).

If the behavior is not typical of SE, further evaluation is required before instituting aggressive treatment. In particular, an emergency EEG should be obtained.

Repetitive tonic extensor spasms should be managed and investigated as for incipient tentorial herniation, until proved otherwise.

INITIAL EVALUATION

This will have taken place during the first two stages. It is important to take a history and carry out a brief clinical examination, documenting the features outlined in Table 18.5.

Investigations that should be sent for all patients, and those to be considered in selected cases, are detailed in Table 18.5.

If the cause of the SE is unknown, blood and urine collected on presentation should be sent for toxicology and a metabolic screen, including amino acids, organic acids, and ammonia. In all unexplained cases of SE an urgent CT scan should be performed, particularly if there are focal neurologic signs.

Meningitis is an important cause of SE, especially in infants. In young children who present in SE with a fever, high-dose broad-spectrum antibiotics (e.g. cefotaxime or ceftriaxone) should be started until the child is

Table 18.5 Initial evaluation of patient in status epilepticus

History
Recent trauma
Recent infection
Ingestion
Drug history
Past history of seizures
Medical history
Development history
Family history

Examination
Heart rate
Blood pressure
Temperature
Respiratory rate
Pupils
Brainstem reflexes
Tone, posture and movement of limbs
Signs of trauma
Rashes/neurocutaneous stigmata

Investigations

*All patients**	*Selected patients*
Blood – Glucose	Toxicology
Urea/electrolytes	Ammonia
Calcium	Amino acids
Magnesium	
AED	
Blood gas	
Urine	Organic acids
	Toxicology
CSF	Micro + culture

*Immediate glucose stick test on arrival.

stabilized and a lumbar puncture can be performed safely. Lumbar puncture should be deferred until SE has been controlled and the level of consciousness improves; or, raised intracranial pressure and brain swelling have been excluded or treated.

TREATMENT OF STATUS EPILEPTICUS

The aim of drug treatment is to bring the seizures under control as quickly as possible. The ideal drug should: enter the brain rapidly; have a long distribution half-life; a short elimination half-life; and should not produce cardiac or respiratory depression or sedation (Delgado-Escueta, Swartz and Abad-Herrera, 1990). Such a drug does not yet exist. Clear guide-lines for how long to allow a drug to take effect before moving onto the next stage of the protocol, and the appropriate dose of the AED to be given at the outset of treatment, are essential.

The first-line drugs used for SE are benzodiazepines, phenytoin, and phenobarbitone, giving three choices for initial management: lorazepam alone, diazepam plus phenytoin, or phenobarbitone alone (Table 18.6). Lorazepam has a number of advantages and is now the first choice of many clinicians. A suggested protocol is shown in Fig. 18.1.

Individual first-line drugs are considered in more detail below.

Benzodiazepines

These are extremely potent AEDs which enter the brain rapidly but have short distribution half-lives. The main adverse effects are respiratory depression and sedation. These occur particularly when benzodiazepines are used in conjunction with phenobarbitone, or in a child with brain swelling and raised intracranial pressure on presentation.

Diazepam

This is probably still the most widely used initial treatment. Its onset of action is within 1–3 minutes. Eighty per cent of cases are controlled within 5 minutes of administration (Treiman, 1990), but there is a very short duration of action and seizures often recur after 15–20 minutes, because of rapid distribution to other tissues. Therefore, diazepam is not recommended as a single agent, but should be given with a longer acting AED, such as phenytoin. The initial dose of diazepam recommended is 0.2–0.3 mg/kg by slow IV injection.

Clonazepam

Clonazepam has a very similar spectrum of activity to diazepam with a comparable short

Table 18.6 First-line drugs for the treatment of status epilepticus

Drug	Route	Dosage and administration	Time to peak effect	Duration of action	Adverse effect
Diazepam	IV	0.2–0.3 mg/kg	1.5 min	15–20 min	Respiratory depression Sedation
Lorazepam	IV	0.05–0.1 mg/kg	1–5 min	12–48 h	Respiratory depression Sedation
Midazolam*	IV/IM	0.1–0.2 mg/kg max dose 5 mg	1–5 min	1–5 h	Respiratory depression Sedation
Phenytoin	IV	20 mg/kg slow infusion no faster than 1 mg/kg/min	10–30 min	12–24 h	Cardiac effect if infused too rapidly
Phenobarbitone	IV	20–25 mg/kg infused no faster than 100 mg/min	10–20 min	24–72 h	Cardiorespiratory depression if infused too rapidly Sedation

*Midazolam not recommended as first-line drug, but if no IV access, can be given IM.

duration of action. It has no particular advantage over diazepam.

Lorazepam

Lorazepam has a rapid onset of action but is less lipophilic and has a smaller volume of distribution than diazepam. Its duration of action is consequently longer, lasting from a minimum of several hours up to 48 hours (Crawford, Mitchell and Snodgrass, 1987; Treiman, 1990). The initial dose is 0.05–0.1 mg/kg with a maximum dose of 4 mg. It can be repeated after 15 minutes. In comparative studies, lorazepam was as effective as other benzodiazepines and as phenytoin (Lacey *et al.*, 1986; Crawford, Mitchell and Snodgrass, 1987; Giang and Mcbride 1988; Treiman, 1990)

Midazolam

This is an extremely potent short-acting benzodiazepine that has been used to treat SE. Several case reports indicate that it is effective treatment, but no comparative or controlled studies have been done (Reves *et al.*, 1985; Mayhue, 1988; Kumar and Bleck, 1992) It is short acting and needs to be given

by frequent boluses or infusion. The main advantage is that midazolam can be given safely and effectively intramuscularly. The loading dose is 0.1–0.3 mg/kg.

Phenytoin

Phenytoin is very effective, and can control SE in 70–80% of patients (Wilder *et al.*, 1977; Cranford *et al.*, 1979). Peak activity in the brain occurs in 10–30 minutes. However, because the infusion may take 20 minutes, the total time until maximal clinical effect may be as long as 50 minutes.

Intravenous phenytoin must be given by slow infusion at a rate no faster than 0.5–1 mg/kg/min with continuous monitoring of ECG and blood pressure. Hypotension, bradycardia and arrhythmias may be precipitated if the infusion is too rapid. Phenytoin is highly alkaline and poorly soluble in water and should be diluted in normal saline (Tunik and Young, 1992). The normal loading dose is 18–20 mg/kg. In patients with epilepsy on long term treatment with phenytoin it is usually safe to give a full loading dose on presentation with SE (Simon, 1985).

Maintenance doses are not usually required until 12 hours after intravenous loading.

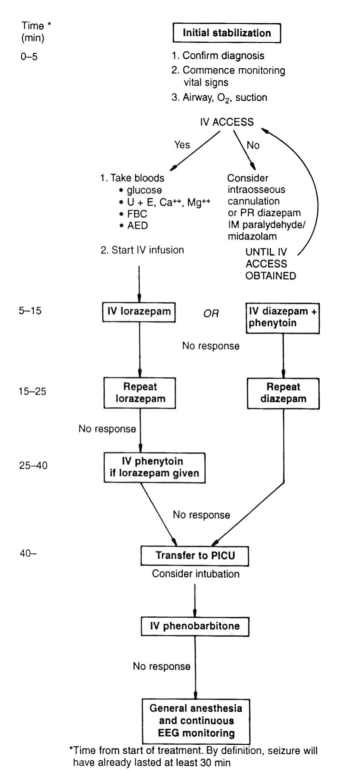

Fig. 18.1 A protocol for the management of status epilepticus. PICU = pediatric intensive care unit.

Prediction of the subsequent maintenance dose required may be difficult. Recent studies have attempted to produce guidelines based on early blood level monitoring (Rivello *et al.*, 1991; Richard *et al.*, 1993). The generally effective serum level is 40 to 80 μmol/l (10 to 20 mg/l)

The main advantage of phenytoin is its lack of sedative side effects, but because of its relatively slow onset of action, it should be given with a benzodiazepine.

Phenobarbitone

Phenobarbitone is a very effective agent for the treatment of SE and has been used for many years. It is relatively nontoxic (Shaner *et al.*, 1988; Dunn, 1990). Peak activity occurs 10–20 minutes after an IV loading dose. It has a very long half-life, up to 120 hours, and thus a long duration of action after a single dose.

The initial loading dose is 20 mg/kg at a rate no faster than 100 mg/min. If seizures persist, a second dose may be given (Shields, 1989).

The main disadvantages of phenobarbitone are depression of conscious level, respiration and blood pressure. These are particularly likely to occur if benzodiazepines have already been given.

FURTHER APPROACHES

A trial of intravenous pyridoxine 100 mg should be given to all infants who have SE that is resistant to AED treatment or recurs.

If problems have been encountered finding intravenous access, an intramuscular injection of midazolam or paraldehyde can be given. Paraldehyde, given by deep intramuscular injection into the thigh in a dose of 1 ml/year of age, is relatively slowly absorbed, and may cause a sterile 'abscess'. Administration of drugs rectally for treatment of SE is, on the whole, not recommended because of erratic absorption, and, sometimes, delayed effects. However admin-

istration of rectal diazepam by parents or nonmedical personnel has been shown to be effective. Diazepam is well absorbed from the rectum, with peak levels and control of seizures within 6–10 minutes. The initial dose is 0.5 mg/kg, and can be repeated after 15 minutes.

Rectal paraldehyde may be given in a dose of 1 ml per year of age (or 0.1 ml/kg) diluted in a 1:1 solution of arachis or peanut oil. Absorption is erratic and slow and a much lower peak concentration of paraldehyde is achieved than for the intramuscular or intravenous routes (Browne, 1983). It is therefore not recommended for treatment for SE.

Rectal valproic acid has been used for SE (Snead and Miles, 1985), but absorption and onset of action are slow.

REFRACTORY STATUS EPILEPTICUS

General anesthesia is recommended for SE that has not come under control after 1 hour, despite adequate doses of first-line drugs. General anesthesia carries significant risks, particularly of cardiac depression, and vigorous circulatory support may be necessary. There are also risks associated with artificial ventilation and pharmacologic paralysis.

Once the child is anesthetized, it is essential that continuous EEG monitoring is commenced, to check on both depth of anesthesia and persistence of seizures. There is no entirely adequate system currently available for continuous monitoring of the EEG in the ICU. Cerebral function monitors (CFM or CFAM) do however allow detection of most seizures and assessment of the depth of anesthesia (Fig. 18.2).

Children should be managed in a unit that is skilled in pediatric and neurointensive care, and able to provide full circulatory support.

There are no controlled trials of the anesthetic agents that have been used for SE. The ideal agent should be able to bring seizures under control rapidly, without major adverse

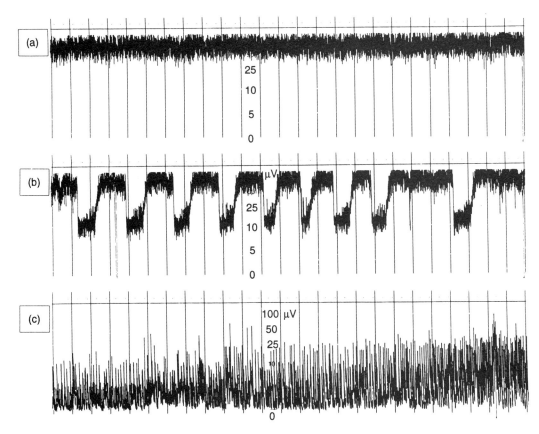

Fig. 18.2   Cerebral function monitor (CFM) recording during barbiturate anesthesia for status epilepticus. (a) Continuous high-amplitude seizure activity. (b) Seizure activity becoming intermittent. (c) Cessation of seizure activity with suppression of background activity to a burst suppression pattern.

effects. The aim of anesthesia is to control the seizures and produce a burst suppression pattern on the EEG (Fig. 18.2). This is maintained for at least 2 hours before being slowly withdrawn (Tunik and Young, 1992). If the seizures relapse, anesthesia is reinduced.

The most widely reported agents are barbiturates (thiopentone, pentobarbitone, and phenobarbitone) and inhalational agents such as isoflurane (Table 18.7).

Recently propofol has been reported as effective (Mackenzie, Kapadia and Grant, 1990; De Riu *et al.*, 1992), but a number of deaths have been associated with propofol infusion in children (Parke *et al.*, 1992), and it is not currently recommended for SE.

No evidence exists that any one of the above agents is superior to another. The most important factors are that the staff managing the child are familiar with the agent employed, and that full hemodynamic and EEG monitoring are available.

OTHER AGENTS THAT MAY BE EFFECTIVE IN STATUS EPILEPTICUS

The following agents may be effective in SE but cannot be regarded as first-line drugs. These should be used in refractory SE and therefore not outside the intensive care setting. None have been subjected to controlled studies.

Table 18.7 Agents used for general anesthesia in control of refractory status epilepticus

Drug	Loading dose	Maintenance	Comment	Reference
Thiopentone	5–30 mg/kg	2–10 mg/kg/h continuous infusion	Hypotension frequent complication. Inotrope support often needed but not on lower dose regimen	Tasker *et al.* (1989) Amit *et al.* (1988) Orlowski, Erenberg and Haus (1984)
Pentobarbital	5 mg/kg	1–5 mg/kg/h continuous infusion	Hypotension Pulmonary edema Ileus	Lockman (1990) Rashkin, Youngs and Penovich (1987) Van Ness (1990)
Phenobarbitone	10–20 mg/kg repeated boluses every 30–60 min until control			Crawford *et al.* (1988)
Isoflurane	0.5–3.0% inhalational anesthetic		Circulatory support necessary in all patients reported by Kofke *et al.*	Kofke *et al.* (1981) Meeke, Solifer and Gels (1989)

Lignocaine is given as an initial IV bolus of 1–2 mg/kg followed by an infusion of 6 mg/kg/h. It has been reported to be effective (Browne, 1983; Pascual *et al.*, 1988). The effects are rapid but short lived; seizures may be induced if the dose is too high, and arrhythmias and cardiac depression may occur.

Chlormethiazole is a sedative hypnotic that may be effective in generalized and partial SE (Harvey, Higenbottom and Loh, 1975; Lingam *et al.*, 1980; Browne 1983). A recommended dose has not been agreed. It cannot be given by rapid bolus because of the risk of apnea, therefore, slow infusion is necessary. The suggested rate of infusion is 5–10 mg/h. Chlormethiazole is available as a 0.8% solution which can therefore be infused at a rate of 1 ml/kg/h. It has many adverse effects, including fever, sedation, hypotension, apnea, thrombophlebitis, hiccups, and severe headaches. Whilst it may have some role in drug-resistant SE, its many adverse effects limit its usefulness (Lingam *et al.*, 1980).

Intravenous valproate has been used in uncontrolled studies of SE following head injury (Price, 1989) It appears safe, but the dosage has not been finalized. Further studies are necessary.

OUTCOME OF CONVULSIVE STATUS EPILEPTICUS

SE can result in death or serious long-term morbidity. However, the outcome is determined primarily by the cause. Thus acute symptomatic SE carries a significant risk of death or long-term sequelae. The outcome is worse in infants, corresponding to the higher proportion of acute symptomatic cases in this age group (Philips and Shanahan, 1989; Gross-Tsur and Shinnar, 1993).

MORTALITY

Aicardi and Chevrie (1970) reported an overall mortality of 11% for all causes of SE. More recent studies have shown mortality rates of between 3.6 and 7% (Dunn, 1988; Maytal *et al.* 1989; Philips and Shanahan, 1989).

Death occurs primarily in those with acute symptomatic SE or progressive encephalopathy.

In the series of Maytal *et al.* (1989), there were no deaths due to either febrile or unprovoked SE. On the other hand, Philips and Shanahan (1989) reported one child who died following febrile SE.

MORBIDITY

Morbidity is probably also declining. Aicardi and Chevrie (1970) reported neurologic sequelae in 20% and mental retardation in 33% of survivors. Recent morbidity rates are 9–28% (Dunn, 1988; Maytal *et al.* 1989; Philips and Shanahan, 1989). Morbidity is very low in the febrile or idiopathic groups. Maytal *et al.* (1989) reported no neurologic abnormalities in 67 children who had idiopathic, remote symptomatic, or febrile SE. The syndrome of hemiconvulsion, hemiplegia and epilepsy described in older series following prolonged SE was not reported in a recent study (Gross-Tsur and Shinnar, 1993).

The development of new-onset epilepsy after SE is determined by the etiology. In children presenting with idiopathic SE as their first seizure there is a 25% chance of seizure recurrence, which does not differ from the risk of epilepsy following an initial short seizure (Hauser *et al.*, 1990; Shinnar *et al.*, 1990).

Epilepsy after febrile SE occurred in 4% of cases of Maytal and Shinnar (1990). Overall epilepsy follows acute symptomatic SE in 15–30% of patients, which is probably comparable to the risk of epilepsy following acute CNS injury in which SE does not occur.

Patients with a preceding chronic neurologic disorder (remote symptomatic) who present with SE as a first seizure have a very high risk of subsequent epilepsy and recurrent SE (Berg and Shinnar, 1991; Gross-Tsur and Shinnar, 1993).

RECURRENT STATUS EPILEPTICUS

The risk of a further episode of SE is between 11 and 25% (Shinnar *et al.*, 1992; Gross-Tsur and Shinnar, 1993), and is primarily related to the presence of neurologic abnormalities predating the original SE. In the remote symptomatic or progressive encephalopathies group, the risk of recurrent SE is 50%.

Long-term AED therapy is not always recommended after SE (Freeman, 1989). The risk of subsequent epilepsy is low in most groups. In the acute symptomatic group, there is no evidence that long-term AED treatment reduces the subsequent likelihood of developing epilepsy. However, the high risk of recurrent SE in the remote symptomatic group means that long-term AED treatment is recommended for these patients (Gross-Tsur and Shinnar, 1993).

NONCONVULSIVE STATUS EPILEPTICUS

COMPLEX PARTIAL STATUS EPILEPTICUS

There are few reports of complex partial status epilepticus (CPSE) in children (Mayeux and Lueders, 1978; McBride, Dooling and Oppenheimer, 1981). However, CPSE is increasingly reported in the adult literature. Delgado-Escueta, Swartz and Abad-Herrera (1990) believe that CPSE should no longer be considered rare.

Characteristically, fluctuating impairment of consciousness, staring, speech arrest, and automatisms occur. There is a lack of interaction with familiar people; staring alternates with wandering movements of the eyes and motor automatisms such as picking at clothes or lip-smacking. Focal clonic or motor components are common. Two forms of CPSE have been identified: frequently occurring complex partial seizures without complete return to normal between attacks; and continuous long-lasting confusion and altered behavior (Delgado-Escueta, Swartz and Abad-Herrera, 1990). CPSE may occur in children who have had no prior seizure (Mayeux and Lueders 1978) or may occur in the context of preexisting epilepsy.

The clinical manifestations are subtle, so

EEG confirmation is necessary. The EEG characteristically shows the features of individual complex partial seizures; or sometimes low-voltage activity followed by a build up of higher amplitude slow wave frequency is recorded. Spike and slow wave activity in the temporal or occipital regions, which may wax and wane and be replaced by continuous slow wave activity, can occur.

A high level of suspicion is needed to diagnose CPSE. It should be considered in any situation where there is an unexplained prolonged change in a child's behavior (Mayeux and Lueders, 1978; McBride, Dooling and Oppenheimer, 1981; Ballenger, King and Gallagher, 1983; Shalev and Amir, 1983).

OTHER FORMS OF NONCONVULSIVE PARTIAL STATUS EPILEPTICUS

Other forms of simple partial SE with nonconvulsive SE have been reported. These are prolonged simple partial seizures with sensory or affective symptomatology, and include such symptoms as isolated fear, simple auditory sensations, cognitive symptoms, and true dysphasia (De Pasquet *et al.*, 1976; McLachlan and Blume, 1980; Dinner *et al.*, 1981; Nakada *et al.*, 1984; Wieser *et al.*, 1985).

ABSENCE STATUS EPILEPTICUS

Absence SE is a form of generalized nonconvulsive SE. It has been defined as a prolonged period of diminished awareness associated with generalized spike and wave discharges (Gastaut, 1970). Other terms used are petit mal status, spike-wave stupor, and prolonged epileptic twilight state (Niedermeyer and Kalifeh, 1962; Porter and Penry, 1983; Zappoli, 1955). In children, absence SE occurring during the course of childhood absence epilepsy or another idiopathic generalized epilepsy is very uncommon. Absence SE is much more frequent in patients with severe mixed epilepsy syndromes, and occurs par-

ticularly in those with Lennox–Gastaut syndrome, myoclonic astatic epilepsy, severe polymorphic epilepsy, or following West's syndrome. Therefore in childhood, absence SE is usually subdivided into typical absence SE and atypical absence SE. Typical absence SE occurs in children with idiopathic generalized epilepsy or childhood absence epilepsy with generalized (synchronous/symmetric) 3-Hz spike and wave on the EEG, and has recently been described in a child following reflex anoxic seizures (Battaglia, Guerrrini and Gastaut, 1989). In adults absence SE has also been described as a de novo occurrence particularly related to acute benzodiazepine withdrawal (Thomas *et al.*, 1992).

Atypical absence SE, on the other hand, occurs in children with severe mixed epilepsies. The clinical features range from obvious to very subtle. The child appears to 'switch off' and lose contact with the external environment, responses are very delayed, speech may be lost, drooling and feeding difficulties are common and the gait may deteriorate with pseudo-ataxia and loss of ambulation. In addition, there may be frequent motor components such as brief headnods, jerks of the face, limbs and trunk, and eyelid myoclonias, which have been termed minor epileptic status (Brett, 1966; Ohtahara *et al.*, 1979). The diagnosis may be difficult, since affected children often have preexisting cognitive problems, making recognition of subtle changes problematic. In children on polytherapy, adverse effects from the AEDs can produce a very similar picture.

EEG diagnosis may also be difficult. The interictal EEG of such children can be very abnormal, with an incomplete relationship between clinical and EEG changes. Often there is continuous generalized slow spike and wave activity, which may be synchronous and rhythmic, but is more likely to be very irregular with asynchronous spike and wave bursts, sometimes approaching a hypsarrhythmic pattern.

Long-term monitoring and serial cognitive

Table 18.8 Differential diagnosis of nonconvulsive status epilepticus

Chronic intoxication
Prolonged postictal state
Progressive ataxia (when associated with
  depressed conscious level)
    Intoxication
    Hydrocephalus
    Tumors
    Metabolic disease
Dementia
    Neurodegenerative disease
    Metabolic disease
    Subacute sclerosing panencephalitis
Psychiatric disease

tests may be necessary to identify truly ictal changes (Stores, 1986).

DIFFERENTIAL DIAGNOSIS OF NONCONVULSIVE STATUS EPILEPTICUS
(Table 18.8)

Nonconvulsive status epilepticus (NCSE) is becoming increasingly recognized as a cause of behavioral or cognitive changes in children; but is often overlooked, while other less satisfactory explanations are entertained.

Many different processes can produce similar behavioral changes. These include intoxications (particularly iatrogenic, with AEDs); any cause of progressive ataxia, particularly when accompanied by drowsiness; diseases leading to dementia such as neurodegenerative disorders or metabolic derangements. Occasionally prolonged postictal confusion may be mistaken for NCSE. Psychiatric disorders may suggest NCSE.

In practice it is common for alternative diagnoses to be considered and NCSE to be overlooked (Stores, 1986). An EEG should be recorded early in the work-up of children with an acute onset of altered behaviour, confusion, or loss of cognitive skills, and any very abnormal record evaluated further with NCSE in mind.

TREATMENT OF NONCONVULSIVE STATUS EPILEPTICUS

NCSE is not a life-threatening emergency, but there is some evidence that it may result in long-term irreversible sequelae. It should be treated aggressively.

COMPLEX PARTIAL STATUS EPILEPTICUS

In most patients CPSE will respond rapidly to intravenous phenytoin or benzodiazepines (Mayeux and Lueders, 1978; Treiman and Delgado-Escueta, 1983).

ABSENCE STATUS EPILEPTICUS

Typical absence status responds rapidly and completely to intravenous benzodiazepines. Valproate may be equally effective (Shields, 1989; Porter and Penry, 1983).

ATYPICAL ABSENCE STATUS

This may prove very resistant to treatment. Response to treatment can be difficult to monitor, since atypical absence status may stop suddenly and spontaneously.

Benzodiazepines are much less effective in this type of SE than in all other types (Livingston and Brown, 1987; Tassinari *et al.*, 1983). In addition, benzodiazepines may precipitate tonic status in children with the Lennox–Gastaut syndrome.

Sodium valproate may be effective. Lamotrigine is very effective against atypical absences, but, in order to avoid allergic side-effects, it is started at a low dose, with gradual escalation, which limits its usefulness for acute management of NCSE. Nevertheless rapid oral loading with lamotrigine has been reported in a 17 year old with tonic SE, without adverse effects (Pisani, Gallitto and Di Perri, 1991).

Occasionally steroids or ACTH may be

effective, but relapse on discontinuation of treatment and severe side-effects may occur.

OUTCOME OF NONCONVULSIVE STATUS EPILEPTICUS

COMPLEX PARTIAL STATUS EPILEPTICUS

There is little data on long-term outcome of CPSE. However, there are several well-documented reports of patients who developed long-term neurologic and behavioral problems after CPSE. In particular, memory deficits have been documented (Engel, Ludwig and Fettell, 1978; Treiman, Delgado-Escueta and Clark, 1981). Experimental evidence suggests that CPSE may cause permanent damage and dysfunction (McIntyre, Nathanson and Edson, 1982). Nevertheless, some patients recover without sequelae (Williamson *et al.*, 1985).

ABSENCE STATUS EPILEPTICUS

Distinction between typical and atypical absence SE is essential when considering the prognosis after absence SE. Typical absence SE has a good long-term outlook in most patients.

Livingston *et al.* (1965) suggested that episodes of absence status were responsible for dementia in six out of 11 patients who had 'petit mal status'. However details of what constituted dementia, and of the preexisting status of these children, were not given, and there was little information on the five children who did not develop dementia.

Children who have atypical absence status later have a high incidence of severe epilepsy and cognitive impairment. Many deteriorate in intellectual ability (Brett, 1966; Doose and Volzke, 1979; Stores, 1986), but it is difficult to demonstrate that this is due entirely to NCSE. Nevertheless, Beaumanoir *et al.* (1988) did not find evidence of cognitive deterioration in their patients with Lennox–Gastaut syndrome who developed NCSE.

Atypical absence SE certainly causes immediate disruption to the child's life, and cumulative episodes lead to lost learning opportunities. Separation of the effects of the NCSE from the effects of frequent short seizures, drug therapy, or the underlying condition can be very difficult.

There is experimental evidence that NCSE is detrimental (Wasterlain, 1976; Meldrum, 1983). However, the models used are paralyzed and ventilated animals, and are not valid for absence SE in humans.

In conclusion, many children who have had atypical absence SE have long-term cognitive difficulties, but currently there is no proof that these are due to the SE itself.

PREVENTION OF STATUS EPILEPTICUS

Prevention of SE is mostly likely to be achieved by targeting the disorders which cause chronic neurologic damage, some of which also cause acute symptomatic SE.

Immunization programs reduce the incidence of meningitis and encephalitis. Road safety programs may be able to reduce the incidence of head trauma and health education, the ingestion of toxins. Improvement in pre- and perinatal care may have some impact on the incidence of cerebral palsy.

Better understanding of the large number of genetic disorders that lead to chronic or progressive CNS disease will allow prevention or treatment of some of these conditions.

Improved patient education and support for families of children with epilepsy are likely to improve compliance and decrease the likelihood of acute withdrawal of AEDs. In future, new AEDs could be developed that do not have major withdrawal effects on acute discontinuation.

ACKNOWLEDGMENTS

I would like to thank Dr Debbie Murdoch-Eaton for her invaluable help in preparing the tables and illustrations and reading the manuscript and Mrs Janine Madden for typing the manuscript.

REFERENCES

Aicardi, J. (1986) Status epilepticus, in *Epilepsy in Children*, Raven Press, New York, pp. 240–59.

Aicardi, J. and Chevrie, J.J. (1970) Convulsive status epilepticus in infants and children: a study of 239 cases. *Epilepsia*, **11**, 187–97.

Aminoff, M.J. and Simon, R.P. (1980) Status epilepticus. Causes, clinical features and consequences in 98 patients. *American Journal of Medicine*, **69**, 657–66.

Amit, R., Goitein, K.J., Mathot, I. and Yatziu, S. (1988) Prolonged electrocerebral silent barbiturate coma in intractable seizure disorders. *Epilepsia*, **29**, 63–6.

Ballenger, C.E., King, D.W. and Gallagher, B.B. (1983) Partial complex status epilepticus. *Neurology*, **33**, 1545–52.

Battaglia, A., Guerrini, R. and Gastaut, H. (1989) Epileptic seizures induced by syncopal attacks. *Journal of Epilepsy*, **2**, 137–45.

Beaumanoir, A., Foletti, G., Magistris, M. *et al.* (1988) Status epilepticus in the Lennox–Gastaut syndrome, in *The Lennox–Gastaut Syndrome* (eds E. Niedermeyer and R. Degen), Alan R. Liss, New York, pp. 283–99.

Berg, A.T. and Shinnar, S. (1991) The risk of recurrence following a first unprovoked seizure: a metanalysis. *Neurology*, **41**, 965–72.

Betts, T. and Boden, S. (1992) Diagnosis, management and prognosis of a group of 128 patients with non epileptic attack disorder. *Seizure*, **1**, 19–32.

Brett, E. (1966) Minor epileptic status. *Journal of the Neurological Sciences*, **3**, 52–75.

Browne, T.R. (1983) Paraldehyde, chlomethiazole and lidocaine for treatment of status epilepticus, in *Advances in Neurology*, vol. 34, *Status Epilepticus* (eds A.V. Delgado-Escueta, C.G. Wasterlain, D.M. Treiman and R.J. Porter), Raven Press, New York, pp. 509–17.

Chapman, A.G., Meldrum, B.S. and Siesjo, B.K. (1977) Cerebral metabolic changes during prolonged epileptic seizures in rats. *Journal of Neurochemistry*, **28**, 1025–35.

Cranford, R.E., Leppik, I.E., Patrick, B. *et al.* (1979) Intravenous phenytoin in acute management of seizures. *Neurology*, **29**, 1474–9.

Crawford, T.O., Mitchell, W.G. and Snodgrass, S.R. (1987) Lorazepam in childhood status epilepticus and serial seizures: effectiveness and tachyphylaxis *Neurology*, **37**, 190–5.

Crawford, T.O., Mitchell, W.G., Fishman, L.S. *et al.* (1988) Very high dose phenobarbital for refractory status epilepticus in children. *Neurology*, **38**, 1035–40.

Delgado-Escueta, A.V., Swartz, B. and Abad-Herrera, P. (1990) Status epilepticus, in *Comprehensive Epileptology* (eds M. Dam and L. Gram), Raven Press, New York, pp. 251–70.

De Pasquet, E., Gaudin, E., Bianchi, A. and De Zmendilaharsu, S. (1976) Prolonged and mono-symptomatic dysphasic status epilepticus. *Neurology*, **25**, 244–7.

De Riu, P.L., Petruzzi, V., Testa, C. *et al.* (1992) Propofol anticonvulsant activity in experimental epileptic status. *British Journal of Anaesthesia*, **69**, 177–81.

Dinner, D.S., Lueders, H., Lederman, R. and Gretter, T.E. (1981) Aphasic status epilepticus; a case report. *Neurology*, **31**, 888–91.

Doose, H. (1983) Non-convulsive status epilepticus in childhood: clinical aspects and classification, in *Advances in Neurology* vol. 34, *Status Epilepticus* (eds A.V. Delgado-Escueta, C.G. Wasterlain, D.M. Treiman and R.J. Porter), Raven Press, New York, pp 83–92.

Doose, H. and Volzke, E. (1979) Petit mal status and early childhood dementia. *Neuropadiatrie*, **10**, 10–14.

Dulac, O., Aubourg, P., Chercoury, A. *et al.* (1985) Infantile status epilepticus, etiological and prognostic aspects. *Revue d'Electroencephalographie et de Neurophysiologie*, **14**, 255–62.

Dunn, D.W. (1988) Status epilepticus in children: etiology, clinical features and outcome. *Journal of Child Neurology*, **3**, 167–73.

Dunn D.W. (1990) Status epilepticus in infancy and childhood. *Neurologic Clinics*, **8**, 647–57.

Ellenberg, J.H. and Nelson, K.B. (1978) Febrile seizures and later intellectual performance. *Archives of Neurology*, **35**, 17–21.

Engel, J.E. Jr, Ludwig, B.I. and Fettell, M. (1978) Prolonged partial complex status epilepticus. EEG and behavioural observation. *Neurology*, **28**, 863–9.

Freeman, J.M. (1989) Status epilepticus: it's not what we've thought or taught. *Pediatrics*, **83**, 444–5.

Gastaut, H. (1970) Clinical and electroencephalographical classification of epileptic seizures. *Epilepsia*, **11**, 102–13.

Gastaut, H. (1973) *Dictionary of Epilepsy. Part 1. Definitions*, World Health Organisation, Geneva.

Gastaut, H. (1983) Classification of status epilepticus, in *Status Epilepticus: Mechanisms of Brain Damage and Treatment* (eds A.V. Delgado-Escueta, C.G. Wasterlain, D.M. Treiman and R.J. Porter), Raven Press, New York, pp. 15–35.

Giang, D.W. and McBride, M.C. (1988) Lorazepam versus diazepam for the treatment of status epilepticus. *Pediatric Neurology*, **4**, 358–61.

Gross-Tsur, V. and Shinnar, S. (1993) Convulsive status epilepticus in children. *Epilepsia*, **34** (suppl. 1), S12–20.

Harvey, P.K., Higenbottom, T.M. and Loh, L. (1975) Chlormethiazole in the treatment of status epilepticus. *British Medical Journal*, **2**, 603–5.

Hauser, W.A. (1990) Status epilepticus: epidemiologic considerations *Neurology*, **40** (suppl. 2), 9–13.

Hauser, W.A., Rich, S.S., Annegers, J.F. and Anderson, V.E. (1990) Seizure recurrence following a first unprovoked seizure: an extended follow up. *Neurology*, **40**, 1163–70.

Kofke, W.A., Young, R.S.K., Davis, P. *et al.* (1989) Isoflurane for refractory status epilepticus: a clinical series. *Anesthesiology*, **71**, 653–9.

Kumar, A. and Bleck, T.P. (1992) Intravenous midazolam for the treatment of refractory status epilepticus. *Critical Care Medicine*, **20**, 483–8.

Lacey, D.J., Singer, W.D., Horwitz, S.J. *et al.* (1986) Lorazepam therapy of status epilepticus in children and adolescents. *Journal of Pediatrics*, **108**, 771–4.

Lathers, C.M., Jim, K.F. and Spivey, W.H. (1989) A comparison of intraosseous and intravenous routes of administration for antiseizure agents. *Epilepsia*, **30**, 472–9.

Lingam, S., Bertwhistle, H., Ellison, H.M. and Wilson, J. (1980) Problems with intravenous chlormethiazole (hemineverin) in status epilepticus. *British Medical Journal*, **280**, 155–6.

Livingston, J.H. and Brown, J.K. (1987) Non convulsive status epilepticus resistant to benzodiazepines. *Archives of Disease in Childhood*, **62**, 41–4.

Livingston, J.H. and Brown, J.K. (1988) Diagnosis and managment of non convulsive status epilepticus. *Pediatric Review Communications*, **2**, 283–315.

Livingston, S., Torres, I., Pauli, L. *et al.* (1965) Petit mal epilepsy: results of a prolonged follow up study of 117 patients. *Journal of the American Medical Association*, **194**, 227–32.

Lockman, L.A. (1990) Treatment of status epilepticus in children. *Neurology*, **40**(suppl. 2), 43–6.

Mackenzie, S.J., Kapadia, F. and Grant, I.S. (1990) Propofol infusion for control of status epilepticus. *Anaesthesia*, **45**, 1043–5.

Mayeux, R. and Lueders, H. (1978) Complex partial status epilepticus, case report and proposal for diagnostic criteria. *Neurology*, **28**, 957–61.

Mayhue, F.E. (1988) IM midazolam for status epilepticus in the emergency department. *Annals of Emergency Medicine*, **17**, 643–5.

Maytal, J. and Shinnar, S. (1990) Febrile status epilepticus. *Pediatrics*, **86**, 611–16.

Maytal, J., Shinnar, S., Moshe, S.L., Alvarez, L.A. (1989) Low morbidity and mortality of status epilepticus in children. *Pediatrics*, **83**, 323–31.

McBride, M.C., Dooling, E.C. and Oppenheimer, E.Y. (1981) Complex partial status epilepticus in young children. *Annals of Neurology*, **9**, 526–30.

McIntyre, D.C., Nathanson, D. and Edson, N. (1982) A new model of partial status epilepticus based on kindling. *Brain Research*, **250**, 53–63.

McLachlan, R.S. and Blume, W.T. (1980) Isolated fear in complex partial status epilepticus. *Annals of Neurology*, **8**, 639–41.

Meeke, R.I., Soifer, B.E. and Gelb, A.W. (1989) Isoflurane for managment of status epilepticus. *DICP*, **23**, 579–81.

Meldrum, B. (1983) Metabolic factors during prolonged seizures and their relation to nerve cell death, in *Advances in Neurology*, vol. 34, *Status Epilepticus* (eds A.V. Delgado-Escueta, C.G. Wasterlain, D.M. Treiman and R.J. Porter), Raven Press, New York, pp. 261–77.

Meldrum, B.S., Vigouroux, R.A. and Brierley, J.B. (1973) Systemic factors and epileptic brain damage. Prolonged seizures in paralysed artifically ventilated baboons. *Archives of Neurology*, **29**, 82–7.

Nakada, T., Lee, H., Kwee, I.L. and Lerner, A.M. (1984) Epileptic Kluver–Bucy syndrome: case report. *Journal of Psychiatry*, **45**, 87–8.

Nevander, G., Ingvar, M., Auer, R. and Siesjö, B.K. (1984) Status epilepticus in well oxygenated rats causes neuronal necrosis. *Annals of Neurology*, **18**, 281–90.

Niedermeyer, E. and Kalifeh, R. (1965) Petit mal status ('spike wave stupor'). An electro clinical appraisal. *Epilepsia*, **6**, 250–62.

Ohtahara, S., Oka, E., Yamatogi, Y. *et al.* (1979) Non convulsive status epilepticus in children. *Folia Psychiatrica Neurologica (Japan)*, **33**, 345–51.

Orlowski, J.P., Erenberg, G. and Hans, L. (1984) Hypothermia and barbiturate coma for refractory status epilepticus. *Critical Care Medicine*, **12**, 367–72.

Parke, J.J., Stevens, J.E., Rice, A.S.C. *et al.* (1992) Metabolic acidosis and fatal myocardial failure after propofol infusion in children: five case reports. *British Medical Journal*, **305**, 613–6.

Pascual, J., Sedano, M.J., Polo, J.M. *et al.* (1988) Intravenous lidocaine for status epilepticus. *Epilepsia*, **29**, 584–9.

Philips, S.A. and Shanahan, R.J. (1989) Etiology and mortality of status epilepticus in children: a recent update. *Archives of Neurology*, **46**, 74–6.

Pisani, F., Gallitto, G. and Di Perri, R. (1991) Could lamotrigine be useful in status epilepticus? A case report. *Journal of Neurology, Neurosurgery and Psychiatry*, **54**, 845–6.

Porter, R.J. and Penry, J.K. (1983) Petit mal status, in *Advances in Neurology*, vol. 34, *Status Epilepticus*, (eds A.V. Delgado-Escueta, C.G. Wasterlain, D.M. Treiman and R.J. Porter), Raven Press, New York pp. 61–8.

Price, D.J. (1989) Intravenous valproate: experience in neurosurgery, in *Fourth International Symposium on Sodium Valproate and Epilepsy* (ed. D. Chadwick), Royal Society of Medicine, International Congress and Symposium Series, London, pp. 197–203.

Prior, P.F., McLaine, G.N., Scott, D.F. and Laurance, B.M. (1972) Tonic status epilepticus precipitated by intravenous diazepam in a child with petit mal status. *Epilepsia*, **13**, 467–72.

Rashkin, M.C., Youngs, C. and Penovich, P. (1987) Pentobarbital treatment of refractory status epilepticus. *Neurology*, **37**, 500–3.

Reves, J.G., Fragen, R.J., Vinik, H.R. *et al.* (1985) Midazolam: pharmacology and uses. *Anesthesiology*, **62**, 310–24.

Richard, M.O., Chiron, C., d'Athis, P. *et al.* (1993) Phenytoin monitoring in status epilepticus in infants and children. *Epilepsia*, **34**, 144–50.

Riviello, J.J. Jr, Roe, E.J. Jr, Sapin, J.J. and Grover, W.D. (1991) Timing of maintainance phenytoin therapy after intravenous loading dose. *Pediatric Neurology*, **7**, 262–5.

Roger, J., Lob, H. and Tassinari, C.A. (1974) Status epilepticus, in *Handbook of Neurology*, vol. 15, *The Epilepsies* (eds P.J. Vinken and G.W. Bruyn), North Holland, Amsterdam, pp. 145–88.

Shalev, R.S. and Amir, N. (1983) Complex partial status epilepticus. *Archives of Neurology*, **40**, 90–2.

Shaner, D.M., McCurdy, S.A., Herring, M.O. *et al.* (1988) Treatment of status epilepticus: a prospective comparison of diazepam and phenytoin versus phenobarbital and optional phenytoin. *Neurology*, **38**, 202–7.

Shields, W.D. (1989) Status epilepticus. *Pediatric Clinics of North America*, **36**, 383–93.

Shinnar, S., Berg, A.T., Moshe, S.L. *et al.* (1990) The risk of seizure recurrence following a first unprovoked seizure in childhood, a prospective study, *Pediatrics*, **85**, 1076–85.

Shinnar, S., Maytal, J., Krasnoff, L. and Moshe, S.L. (1992) Recurrent status epilepticus in children. *Annals of Neurology*, **31**, 598–604.

Simon, R. P. (1985) Managment of status epilepticus, in *Recent Advances in Epilepsy*, 2 (eds T.A. Pedley and B.S. Meldrum), Churchill Livingstone, Edinburgh, pp. 137–60.

Snead, O.C. and Miles, M.V. (1985) Treatment of status epilepticus in children with rectal sodium valproate. *Journal of Pediatrics*, **106**, 323–5.

Stores, G. (1986) Non convulsive status epilepticus in children, in *Recent advances in Epilepsy*, 3 (eds T.A. Pedley and B.S. Meldrum), Churchill Livingstone, Edinburgh, pp 295–310.

Tasker, R.C., Boyd, S.G., Harden, A. and Matthew, D.J. (1989) EEG monitoring of prolonged thiopentone administration for intractible seizures and status epilepticus in infants and young children. *Neuropediatrics*, **20**, 147–53.

Tassinari, C.A., Dravet, C., Roger, J. *et al.* (1972) Tonic status epilepticus precipitated by intravenous benzodiazepine in five patients with Lennox–Gastaut syndrome. *Epilepsia*, **13**, 421–35.

Tassinari, C.A., Daniele, O., Michelucci, R. *et al.* (1983) Benzodiazepines: efficacy in status epilepticus, in *Advances in Neurology*, vol. 34, *Status Epilepticus* (eds A.V. Delgado-Escueta, C.G. Wasterlain, D.M. Treiman and R.J. Porter), Raven Press, New York, pp. 465–76.

Thomas, P., Beaumanoir, A., Genton, P. *et al.* (1992) 'De novo' absence status of late onset: report of 11 cases. *Neurology*, **42**, 104–10.

Treiman, D.M., Delgado-Escueta, A.V. and Clark, M.A. (1981) Impairment of memory following prolonged complex partial status epilepticus. *Neurology*, **31**, 109.

Treiman, D.M. (1990) The role of benzodiazepines in the management of status epilepticus. *Neurology*, **40**, (suppl. 2), 32–42.

Treiman, D.M. (1993) Generalised convulsive status epilepticus in adults. *Epilepsia*, **34,** (suppl. 1), S2–11.

Treiman, D.M. and Delgado-Escueta, A. V. (1983) Complex partial status epilepticus, in *Advances in Neurology*, vol. 34, *Status Epilepticus* (eds A.V. Delgado-Escueta, C.G. Wasterlain, D.M. Treiman, R.J. Porter), Raven Press, New York, pp. 69–82.

Tunik, M.G. and Young, G.M. (1992) Status epilepticus in children: the acute management. *Pediatric Clinics of North America*, **39,** 1007–30.

Van Ness, P.C. (1990) Pentobarbital and EEG burst suppression in treatment of status epilepticus refractory to benzodiazepines and phenytoin. *Epilepsia*, **31,** 61–7.

Wasterlain, C.G. (1976) Inhibition of cerebral protein synthesis by epileptic seizures without motor manifestation. *Neurology (Minn)*, **24,** 175–80.

Wasterlain, C.G., Fujikawa, D.G., Penix, L. and Sankar, R. (1993) Pathophysiological mechanisms of brain damage from status epilepticus. *Epilepsia*, **34**(suppl. 1.). S37–53.

Wieser, H.G., Hailemariam, S., Regard, M. and Landis, T. (1985) Unilateral limbic epileptic status activity: stereo EEG, behavioural and cognitive data. *Epilepsia*, **26,** 19–29.

Wilder, B.J., Ramsay, R.E., Willmore, L.J. *et al.* (1977) Efficacy of intravenous phenytoin in the treatment of status epilepticus: kinetics of central nervous system penetration. *Annals of Neurology*, **1,** 511–8.

Williamson, P.P., Spencer, D.D., Spencer, S.S. *et al.* (1985) Complex partial status epilepticus: a depth electrode study. *Annals of Neurology*, **18,** 647–54.

Zappoli, R. (1955) Prolonged epileptic twilight state with almost continuous 'wave-spikes'. *Electroencephalography and Clinical Neurophysiology*, **3,** 421–23.

NEUROPHYSIOLOGIC INVESTIGATION

19

ELECTROENCEPHALOGRAPHY

Sheila J. Wallace

INTRODUCTION

It is clearly beyond the scope of this chapter to consider, in depth, the electrophysiologic mechanisms or the highly technical procedures underlying the generation and recording of the EEG. Aspects of the cellular mechanisms involved in the pathophysiology of epilepsy are discussed in Chapter 6. A brief overview of the basic principles of the EEG and its clinical applications is followed by a section on the appearances of the normal EEG throughout infancy and childhood. The EEG findings in specific conditions, e.g. epilepsy syndromes and degenerative disorders, will be presented. Special techniques for exploiting information obtained from the EEG are discussed.

BASIC PRINCIPLES OF THE EEG AND ITS CLINICAL APPLICATIONS

Historic aspects of the development of the EEG are considered by Niedermeyer (1993a). Initial recordings of brain electrical activity were made directly from the cortices of rabbits 120 years ago, using a galvanometer and reflected light beams. Forty years later, Russian physiologists demonstrated, in dogs, regular rhythms which slowed on asphyxia: a string galvanometer was used. Another 17 years passed before Hans Berger produced the first report on the human EEG in a paper in 1929, which described alpha rhythm. He used a double coil galvanometer, chlorinated silver needle electrodes, and platinum wires. Berger's pioneering work included observa-

tions of changes of the EEG during alterations in consciousness; sleep; hypoxia; and, various diffuse and localized brain disorders. So far as epilepsy is concerned, the work of Erna and Frederic Gibbs and William Lennox in the early 1930s has been crucial. The paper by Gibbs and Davis (1935), demonstrating the EEG changes in absence epilepsy of childhood (Chapter 13a), was a landmark in the recognition of the EEG as a tool for the investigation of epileptic seizures.

During the past 50 years, the developments of intracranial recordings using depth electrodes (late 1940s), automatic frequency analysis (late 1940s), microelectrode techniques (1950s), sleep research (1950s), EEG computerization (1960s), evoked potential techniques (1970s), and computerized brain mapping (1980s) have confirmed the importance of the place of the EEG and its applications in the investigation of the patient with epilepsy and other functional brain disorders.

The 'routine' EEG is recorded using scalp electrodes. In adults and older children, 20 electrodes are usual, but, in keeping with the smaller head size, fewer electrodes may be employed in childhood. A minimum of four recording channels are necessary to compare right and left, and anterior and posterior activity. The limitations of the EEG must be constantly recognized. The electrodes are relatively enormous in comparison with the many millions of neurons from which they are recording, thus the EEG signals are but a

Epilepsy in Children. Edited by Sheila Wallace. Published in 1996 by Chapman & Hall, London. ISBN 0 412 56860 8

crude representation of the underlying cerebral electrical activity. Slow postsynaptic potentials of 5–50 milliseconds' (ms) duration contribute most to the EEG. Briefer action potentials, which last approximately 1 ms, do not generate fields recordable at sufficient distances from their sites of origin to make further significant contributions. In keeping with the very high numbers of neurons to each electrode, only synchronous activity from many neurons is recorded on EEG. Abnormal synchronous neuronal discharges are the pathophysiologic hallmark of epilepsy.

The EEG mainly records changes in the activity of vertically orientated neurons; whereas activity generated in tangentially orientated neurons can be recorded via the magnetencephalogram (MEG), which measures alterations in cerebral magnetic fields (Chapter 19c). Further details of the physiologic basis of the EEG have been summarized by Binnie (1991). In the vertically orientated neurons changes in the membrane potential may occur either in the cell body, deep in the cortex, or in the more superficially placed dendrites, with the resultant formation of a dipole, i.e. a potential difference between the deep and superficial layers of the cortex. Dependent on the orientation of the dipole in relation to the overlying electrode, there is greater or lesser registration of this potential difference on the EEG. Thus, if the abnormal cortex is in the wall of a sulcus, resulting in orientation of the dipole tangentially to the surface of the brain, there may be no detectable change on the EEG.

The complexities of the relationships between the EEG waves and the activities of the underlying neurons have been emphasized by Binniè (1991), who records them as dependent on:

1. The nature of the change, i.e. whether there is increased negativity within the cell with inhibitory postsynaptic potentials, or decreased negativity with excitatory postsynaptic potentials.
2. The parts of the neurons experiencing changes in membrane potential (i.e. the cell body or the dendrites) – dendritic EPSPs are likely to produce negative, and EPSPs on the soma, positive EEG changes.
3. The rate of spread from one part of the cell to another – the surface EEG changes with a polarity opposite to that inside the cell body when intracellular changes are slow, but, when the latter are rapid, the intracellular and EEG polarities tend to be in phase.

Thus, fast negative spikes on the EEG may reflect cellular excitation and depolarization, whereas surface negative slow waves can indicate hyperpolarization due to inhibition. For the clinician, it is probably more useful to concentrate on the EEG tracings than on the underlying neurophysiology.

EEGs are recorded either using a common reference derivation, when each of 8–20 channels records the potential difference between one scalp electrode and a common reference point which is the same for all channels, or with a bipolar derivation, when recordings from consecutive pairs of electrodes are obtained.

The EEG is assessed in three main domains: background activity, episodic changes and responses to activating procedures. All activity is analyzed for both amplitude and frequency. Four frequency bands have been defined: delta, up to 4 waves/s (Hz); theta, 4–8 Hz; alpha, 8–14 Hz; and beta, greater than 14 Hz. The scalp EEG gives a somewhat attenuated version of changes which can be more dramatically visualized using depth electrodes.

NORMAL EEG IN INFANTS AND CHILDREN

In keeping with structural and neurophysiologic maturation of the CNS the 'normal' EEG varies considerably during infancy and childhood. The changes seen during the development of waking and sleep patterns are well summarized by Niedermeyer (1993b). Significant contributions to knowledge of the EEG in childhood have been made by Dreyfus-Brisac and Monod (1975), Benda, Engel and Zhang (1989), and Hughes, Fino and Hart (1987) for premature infants; by Parmalee *et al.* (1968), Schulte, Hinze and Schrempf (1971), Varner, Peters and Ellingson (1978), and Kuks, Vos and O'Brien (1988) for infants born about term; by Dreyfus-Brisac and Curzi-Dascalova (1975) during the first year of life; by many workers, including Kellaway and Fox (1952) and Eeg-Olofsson (1971a), for children from 1–3 years; by Eeg-Olofsson (1971a), Eeg-Olofsson, Petersén and Sellden (1971), and Petersén and Eeg-Olofsson (1971) for those aged 3–12 years; and by Eeg-Olofsson (1971b) for adolescents. The following is a distillation of their findings, as tabulated by Niedermeyer (1993b).

In the **premature infant of 24–27 weeks' gestation**, the background activity is discontinuous with long flat stretches, interhemispheric synchrony is present in short bursts, waking and sleeping EEGs are undifferentiated, no posterior basic rhythms are recorded, during the awake and sleeping states very slow bursts of high voltage are seen, temporal theta waves are present and increasing, and occipital theta activity is present. There is very little beta activity. No *tracé alternant*, spindles, vertex waves, K complexes, or positive occipital sharp transients are seen. REM sleep is undifferentiated. There is no 14- and 6-Hz positive spike or rhythmical frontal theta activity, but some intermixed sharp activity, occurring in bursts, is a normal finding.

From **28–31 weeks' gestation**, the background activity is discontinuous; interhemispheric activity is mostly asynchronous; waking and sleep EEGs are undifferentiated; posterior basic rhythms are not seen; very slow activity predominates; temporal theta activity is prominent; and occipital theta is decreasing in comparison with less mature

infants. Frequent ripples or brushes of activity at around 16 Hz are seen, as are flat stretches, which are mainly asynchronous. The EEG remains undifferentiated during drowsiness. No *tracé alternant*, spindles, vertex waves, K complexes, or positive occipital transients of sleep are seen. During sleep, the plentiful slow activity is more irregular than in the younger infant and a little fast activity is recorded. During REM sleep, the EEG remains undifferentiated; and no rhythmic frontal theta activity or 14- and 6-Hz positive spikes are noted. Some intermixed sharp activity is normal.

In the premature **infant of 32–36 weeks' gestation**, the background activity is now continuous in the waking and REM sleep states, but remains discontinuous (*tracé alternant*) in non-REM sleep; interhemispheric activity is partially synchronous, particularly in the occipital channels; the waking record can be distinguished from that during sleep, and differentiation of the activities of REM and non-REM sleep develops; delta activity is maximal occipitally; temporal theta decreases and disappears; and occipital theta becomes less prominent. Frequent ripples or brushes at 16 Hz are observed. A low-voltage recording at this age is suggestive of serious cerebral pathology. Drowsiness remains undifferentiated. Spindles, vertex waves, K complexes, and positive occipital sharp transients of sleep do not occur; but irregular slow activity, predominantly in the occipital regions is recorded during sleep. REM sleep is identifiable oculographically. Neither rhythmic frontal theta activity nor 14- and 6-Hz positive spikes are recorded. Prominent sharp waves or spikes are common in EEGs from normal babies of this gestational range.

The EEG of the **full-term newborn (36–41 weeks)** shows a continuous background activity, except for *tracé alternant* during non-REM sleep; minor interhemispheric asynchrony; good differentiation of waking and sleeping; and no posterior basic rhythm; moderate voltage delta activity when awake;

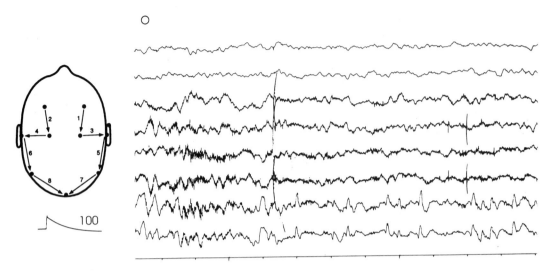

Fig. 19a.1   Normal record, age 5 months. Note the prominent lambda waves over the occipital region. The large spiky components seen over the temporal regions are sucking artefacts, a characteristic EMG pattern at this age. O = eyes open; calibration = 100 microvolts/cm; paper speed (time marker) 3 cm/s.

rare or no temporal theta activity; and no occipital theta. Ripples are decreasing and fast activity is sparse. Very low voltage EEGs are of serious pathologic import. During intermittent photic stimulation (IPS) a driving response may occur below 4 flashes/s, this is difficult to elicit. Drowsiness remains un-differentiated. *Tracé alternant* is present in non-REM sleep; delta and theta activities are continuously present during REM sleep. No sleep spindles, vertex waves, K complexes, or positive occipital sharp transients of sleep are seen. During REM sleep, which now occupies more time than non-REM sleep, there is continuous slow activity. Rhythmic frontal theta and 14- and 6 Hz positive spikes are not seen. Minor sharp transients can still be seen in records from normal babies; but spikes are now abnormal and are more prominent and consistent, when present.

During **infancy (2–12 months, postnatally)**, the background rhythms are continuous, there is interhemispheric synchrony, and good differentiation between sleeping and waking. Posterior basic 4-Hz rhythms be-

come visible at 3–4 months, reaching about 6 Hz at 12 months. Prominent lambda waves over the occipital region are normal (Fig. 19a.1) Considerable slow activity is observed. Temporal and occipital theta activity disappears, and does not reappear during the rest of childhood and adolescence. There is a moderate amount of fast activity. Low-voltage activity is uncommon and usually abnormal. After the age of 6 months, driving to low flash frequencies on IPS improves. Rhythmic theta begins to appear with drowsiness, at about 6 months. *Tracé alternant* disappears during the first month. Sleep spindles, which are sharp and shifting, at 12–16 Hz, appear after the second month; fairly large and blunt vertex waves and K complexes are seen from 5 months; but positive occipital sharp transients of sleep are not yet observed. During sleep, much diffuse 0.75–3 Hz activity, maximal posteriorly, and moderate amounts of fast activity are recorded. The REM portion of sleep is less evident than in the neonate, and consists mainly of slow activity. No rhythmic frontal theta nor 14- and 6-Hz positive spikes are seen. Sharp waves and spikes are abnormal.

Between 12 and 36 months, the background activity is continuous, there is no significant asynchrony and differentiation of sleep and waking is good. The posterior basic rhythm rises from 5 to 6 Hz, or rarely 9 Hz, but considerable slow activity remains during wakefulness. Fast activity is usually moderate; low-voltage activity is uncommon and is mostly abnormal; and there is marked 'hypnagogic' rhythmic 4- to 6-Hz activity during drowsiness. During IPS, a good driving response is often found to low flash rates. *Tracé alternant* is no longer seen, and does not reappear throughout childhood. During the second year, sleep spindles are sharp and shifting; later they become symmetric and maximal at the vertex. Vertex waves and K complexes are large and become more pointed, and poorly defined positive occipital sharp transients of sleep begin to appear. During sleep, there is marked predominance of slow activity posteriorly, often accompanied by a lot of fast activity. During REM sleep, the EEG mostly shows slow activity which is becoming less synchronized. Rhythmic frontal theta is seldom seen in the the third year of life, and 14- and 6-Hz positive spikes are rare. Spikes, mainly occipital, but sometimes rolandic, may be observed in seizure-free children.

During **the preschool years, age 3–5**, the background activity remains continuous and synchronous, with good wake/sleep differentiation (Fig. 19a.2). The posterior basic rhythms rise from 6–8 Hz, to 7–9 Hz, with a marked admixture of slow activity. Fast activity is mostly moderate. Low voltage usually indicates abnormality. Hyperventilation can now be used as an activating mechanism and is often associated with a marked delta response. There is often a good driving response to low flash rates during IPS. During sleep, slow activity continues to predominate, but is less obviously maximal in the posterior regions. In REM sleep, there

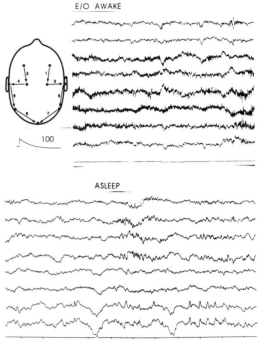

E/O AWAKE

100

ASLEEP

Fig. 19a.2 Normal records, waking and sleeping, age 5 years. Upper: Normal mixture of activities with EMG activity over the temporal regions. Lower: Note the sharp waves over the occipital region. These are POSTS (positive occipital sharp transients of sleep) and are a normal phenomenon. Note also the sleep spindles over the frontocentral regions.

is slow activity, with some desynchronization. Both rhythmic frontal theta activity and 14- and 6-Hz positive spikes may occur, but are uncommon. The EEGs of seizure-free children can show spikes, usually in the occipital, but sometimes in the rolandic, areas.

In **older children, aged 6–12 years**, the background activity is still continuous, with no significant interhemispheric asynchrony, and there is good differentiation between sleep and waking. The posterior basic rhythms reach 10 Hz by 10 years. Varying degrees of posterior slow activity are mixed with the alpha rhythms, and there is a moderate amount of fast activity when

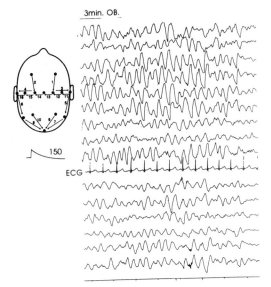

Fig. 19a.3 Normal response to overbreathing in a 9 year old. Note the calibration of 150 microvolts/cm.

awake. Low-voltage activity is occasionally seen as a normal variant. There is often a marked delta response to hyperventilation (Fig. 19a.3). With intermittent photic stimulation (IPS), a good driving response is frequently seen, mainly at medium (8–16/second) flash rates. During drowsiness, there is a gradual alpha drop-out, with increase in slow activity. Vertex waves and K complexes are large with prominent sharp components. Positive occipital sharp transients of sleep remain poorly defined, but evolve throughout this age range. During sleep, there is much diffuse slowing, with some slight decrease in voltage with increasing age. Throughout childhood, in REM sleep, slowing becomes less and desynchronization greater; rhythmic frontal theta becomes rather more common, and 14- and 6-Hz positive spokes are fairly frequent. Spikes in seizure-free children are now mainly rolandic (central to midtemporal). Physiologic occipital spikes may also be seen in records from congenitally blind children.

The background activity in **adolescents** is continuous and synchronous and shows good differentiation between waking and sleep. On average, the posterior basic rhythms are 10 Hz, and posterior slow activity during wakefulness diminishes with age. With the exception of low-voltage fast rhythms, which are commoner at the end of the teenage period than earlier, fast activity is usually moderate in amount. Delta responses to hyperventilation become less impressive. IPS often produces a good driving response, especially at medium flash frequencies. During drowsiness, there is a gradual alpha drop-out, with low-voltage stretches which mainly contain slow activity. Vertex waves and K complexes are smaller than in younger children, and the sharp components are less prominent, whereas positive occipital sharp transients of sleep are often well developed. During sleep, there is much diffuse slowing and the voltage becomes more attenuated than in childhood. There is more desynchronization during REM sleep. Rhythmic frontal theta is commoner than in younger chidren, and tends to decline again towards the end of the second decade; 14- and 6-Hz positive spikes, although remaining rare, are commoner than in childhood. Benign rolandic spikes usually disappear before the age of 13 years.

There is some evidence that, for the individual, the predominant EEG rhythms are genetically determined (Niedermeyer, 1993c).

ACTIVATION OF THE EEG: NORMAL RESPONSES

Although activation methods are used particularly to precipitate abnormalities on the EEG (Takahashi, 1993), it is important to recognize changes which are physiologic.

Hyperventilation causes an increase in bilaterally synchronous slow activity in 70% of children aged 3–5 years, but the response is most abrupt and dramatic between 8 and 12 years of age (Fig. 19a.3). In young children, delta waves appear initially in the posterior regions and spread forwards; they are more prominent if the child is erect, rather than reclining; and they disappear rapidly after cessation of hyperventilation.

IPS induces the physiologic response of photic driving which can be seen in full-term and older infants, but is more readily demonstrated in children of 6 years or more. Photic driving consists of rhythmic activity elicited over the posterior regions in time-locked association (either frequency identical or harmonically related to the stimulus frequency) with IPS. The frequencies involved are about 5–30/second. The amplitude of photic driving is greater in children than adults, and can be enhanced by using either red flicker or a flickering dot pattern. Isolated photomyoclonic responses to IPS are considered to be nonepileptic in nature.

Apart from IPS, other visual stimuli may lead to alterations in the EEG. Children are particularly likely to produce posterior slow wave transients on eye-closure. Dot patterns are likely to evoke lambda waves and/or posterior slow activity, particularly in patients with strong photic driving responses.

EPILEPTIC AND PAROXYSMAL EEG PATTERNS

Epileptic and paroxysmal patterns found on the EEG are reviewed by Niedermeyer (1993d). The distinctions between ictal-clinical, ictal-subclinical and interictal paroxysmal EEG activity are sometimes made only with great difficulty. Sudden changes in frequency, and sudden either loss of voltage or increase in voltage are highly suggestive of ictal events. Although spikes are the EEG events most likely to indicate epilepsy, the sudden changes in frequency may not be seen as spiky in character. Electrodecremental, i.e. sudden loss of voltage, events are those commonest in the infantile spasms of West's syndrome (Ohtahara and Yamatogi, 1990; Chapter 11b). A typical example of sudden increase in voltage is provided by the 3-Hz spike and wave seen in childhood absence epilepsy (Chapter 13a).

The following may be seen at times when no seizure can be identified clinically. A spike is defined as a transient, clearly distinguishable from the background activity with a pointed peak, at conventional paper speed. The duration is from 20 to less than 70 ms; the amplitude is variable; and the main component is usually negative. Less than 50% of children with occipital spikes have seizures, and of those with rolandic spikes clinical seizures occur in only approximately half. Frontal or multifocal spikes are of much more significant import for clinical seizures. Sharp waves are also transients, clearly distinguishable from the background activity, with the main component generally negative, but with a longer duration than spikes, i.e. 70–200 ms. Polyspikes are now officially referred to as multiple spike complexes; they consist of the close association of two or more diphasic spikes occurring more or less rhythmically in bursts, usually with large amplitudes. Multiple spike complexes can be associated with myoclonus, particularly in primary generalized epilepsies, especially where there is associated photosensitivity.

Runs of rapid spikes, i.e. bursts of spikes occurring at a rate of 10–25/s, may be seen, only in sleep, in older children and adolescents, but not younger children. They occur exclusively in the Lennox–Gautaut syndrome (Niedermeyer, 1988; Chapter 12a). Spike-wave complexes are defined simply as patterns of spikes followed by slow waves. In keeping with the fact that the initial description of spike-waves related to the 3-Hz changes seen in childhood absence epilepsy, (Chapter 13a), this frequency is termed 'classic'. However, it is important to recognize that 3-Hz spike-wave (or spike and wave) is also seen in association with epilepsy with myoclonic absences (Chapter 13b) and in the absences which occur as a component of juvenile myoclonic epilepsy (Chapter 14b).

Spike-wave complexes can also be termed slow. Slow spike-wave implies a frequency of 1–2.5 Hz. This pattern is of serious import, and tends to be associated with severe epileptic conditions with multiple seizure types, particularly the Lennox–Gastaut syndrome (Chapter 12a). Fast spike-wave complexes, occurring at 4 or 4–5/s, tend to occur in adolescence; when accompanied by clinical seizures, they are associated with juvenile absence epilepsy (Chapter 14a), eyelid myoclonia with absences (Chapter 14d), or the absences seen as a component of juvenile myoclonic epilepsy (Chapter 14b).

The 6/s spike-wave complex must be differentiated from 14- and 6-Hz positive spike discharges. The former rarely occurs in childhood, only 50–60% of patients have definite seizures (usually generalized tonic-clonic episodes); but syncopal attacks, post-traumatic states and psychiatric problems are common in the remainder, when adults are considered. Rudimentary spike-wave complexes are generalized, or nearly generalized, 3–4-Hz waves, with a poorly developed spike in the positive trough between the slow waves. This pattern is found only in drowsiness; is particulary prominent over the parietal areas; occurs only in infancy and early childhood in association with marked rhythmic theta activity; and, there is often a history of febrile seizures (Chapter 10). Small sharp spikes, also known as benign epileptiform transients of sleep, do not occur in childhood.

Needle-like occipital spikes of the blind have a characteristic appearance and are present in most congenitally blind children. The 14- and 6-Hz positive spike discharges seen in children, adolescents and young adults, mainly over the temporal areas uni- or bilaterally during sleep, appear to have no epileptic connotations, but this pattern has also been observed in advanced states of metabolic encephalopathies, especially in hepatic coma. Rhythmic temporal theta bursts may be seen in older children and adolescents, but are commoner in adults.

Although there is a definitely paroxysmal appearance to these bursts, there seems to be little association with epilepsy.

Ictal recordings can be difficult to obtain, since movement artefact mars the traces, particularly in tonic-clonic seizures. The events during partial seizures have been outlined by Binnie (1991). During ictal recordings of partial seizures, assuming that sufficient, accessible, vertically orientated neurons are firing, there is initially a high frequency discharge at 60-Hz or faster; or, less often, alternating spikes and waves. Alternatively, an isolated spike of 100–200 ms duration; a spike followed by a slower wave; or, more rarely, reduction in amplitude of the background rhythms, or even loss of previous interictal spiky transients, may present at the onset of the ictus. On the whole, as the seizure progresses, the discharges decrease in frequency and amplitude, allowing the identification of discrete spikes at 20–10-Hz; later spike and wave activity appears, followed by irregular spike discharges, loss of spikes, predominance of slow or very low amplitude activity; and, finally, the record is dominated by high-voltage waves of low frequency. Subsequently, there is a gradual return to the interictal pattern. The changes seen during neonatal seizures are discussed in Chapter 9. A further example is given in Fig. 19a.4.

During tonic attacks in the Lennox–Gastaut syndrome, massive fast spike activity occurs; or there may be simple flattening and desynchronization of all activity, or rhythmic activity at 10 Hz, and a diffuse delta wave pattern (Niedermeyer, 1993c). In brief atonic seizures (drop attacks), the EEG shows generalized polyspike-waves or spike-waves. In longer-lasting atonic seizures, rhythmic spikes around 10 Hz with intermixed slow activity are observed, or rhythmic slow spike activity may occur. The EEG during the spasms of West's syndrome shows sudden generalized flattening and desynchroniza-

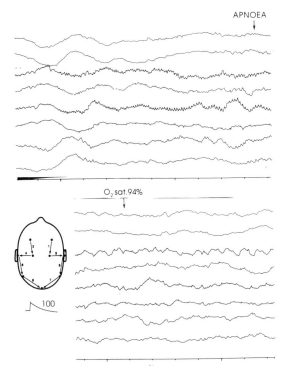

APNOEA

O₂ sat.94%

100

Fig. 19a.4 Seizure recorded in a full-term infant of 5 days. Note the run of rhythmic activity over the right temporal region preceding the apnea and desaturation. Typical findings in neonatal seizures and particularly those which present with apnea.

tion; or rapid spike discharges of high voltage in all leads; or no ictal alteration of the ongoing hypsarrhythmic EEG activity (Chapter 11b).

Rhythms considered to be of genetic significance in nonparoxysmal abnormal EEG patterns are: posterior 4–5 Hz rhythms (which must be carefully distinguished from other types of posterior activity); parieto-occipital delta rhythms (Gerken and Doose, 1972); and 'abnormal theta rhythms' (Doose, Gerken and Volzke, 1972). The possibilities that 3-Hz generalized spike and wave discharges (Chapter 13a), paroxysmal flicker sensitivity (the photoconvulsive response) (Chapter 14d), and rolandic spikes in childhood (Chapter 13c) are genetically determined has been considered by Niedermeyer (1993c).

ACTIVATION OF THE EEG: ABNORMAL RESPONSES

Methods of activation of the EEG are reviewed by Takahashi (1993). They are mainly intended to produce epileptic patterns; physiologic responses are considered above.

Hyperventilation is particularly effective in precipitating generalized, synchronized seizure discharges and in provoking clinical classic absence seizures. Seizures and epileptic syndromes where there is sensitivity to IPS are considered in Chapter 14d, as are seizures precipitated by patterns or reading. Activation of seizure discharges by auditory stimuli is rare; when found, such discharges are mainly over the temporal areas. There are isolated reports of the appearances of paroxysmal discharges over the temporal or frontal areas in response to hearing spoken language or music. In the presence of hyperexcitability of areas of the primary sensorimotor cortex, contralateral afferent stimulation may trigger focal spikes, with or without partial seizures. Olfactory stimulation has been reported to exaggerate spiking in the temporal areas in patients with known pathology in these regions. Isolated cases of seizures precipitated by gustatory or vestibular stimulation are also reviewed by Takahashi (1993).

The use of strong convulsants, such as metrazol, is totally unacceptable in attempts to identify seizure origin, or an underlying propensity to epilepsy, in childhood. However, chlorpromazine may occasionally be of value in enhancing abnormal discharges in doubtful cases. Reenactment of the triggering situation with simultaneous video and EEG recordings should always be considered when seizures are believed to be secondary to a specific stimulus.

PERIODIC DISCHARGES

Periodic discharges are not necessarily associated with epileptic seizures, but are more a feature of severe ongoing CNS disease (Niedermeyer, 1993c). Such discharges are

KK Age 7y.
SSPE

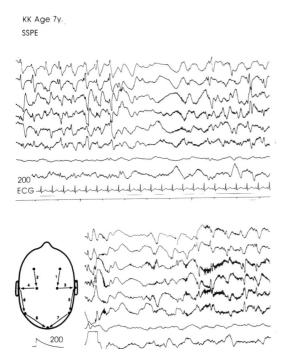

200
ECG

200

ECG

Fig. 19a.5 SSPE. At first sight, the most prominent features of this EEG are the frequent sharp waves associated with slower components, suggesting that the underlying problem is one of epilepsy in this 7 year old with a history of falling and of impaired school performance. However, the brief pauses in this activity were noted to have a relatively stereotyped outline (seen best in the first two channels) and the diagnosis of SSPE was subsequently confirmed.

always of large amplitude, usually in the range of 100–300 μV. If they are sharp waves, the duration is usually more than 150 ms. They may be compounded and polymorphic. They can be focal, scattered, or generally synchronous. A review of periodic discharges has been tabulated by Spehlmann (1981). The periodic discharges seen in the EEGs of children with subacute sclerosing panencephalitis (SSPE) are virtually diagnostic of this condition (Fig. 19a.5). They are found during stage 2 of SSPE, and are of 0.5– 3 seconds' duration. They consist of two or

more waves with a mean amplitude of 500 μV (100–1000 μV). Their periodicity becomes more obvious as the disease progresses. The actual elements of the discharge vary, but, typically, a giant slow wave is mixed with several sharp waves. These, although generalized, have a fronto-central or vertical predominance. Complexes occur at regular intervals, with a frequency of between 4 and 16 per minute. Discharges tend to be particularly evident during waking and are accompanied by more or less synchronous myoclonus.

Periodic complexes may also be seen in advanced herpes simplex encephalitis and in the adult slow virus infection, Jakob– Creutzfeldt disease. A variety of acute neurologic conditions can cause periodic lateralized epileptiform discharges, but this type of abnormality is relatively uncommon in childhood. Acute cerebral anoxia may lead to a pattern of repetitive simple or compounded sharp waves in generalized synchrony on a flat background, which probably, usually, is an aborted suppression burst recording.

CLINICAL APPLICATIONS OF THE EEG

Clearly, from the aforegoing, the greatest clinical applications of the EEG are found in epileptology. EEGs do not always show paroxysmal abnormalities, in particular, spikes or sharp waves, in patients suffering from epilepsy, even in those who have recordings during the ictus; but if multiple ictal recordings are obtained, if the attacks are epileptic in nature, some change is usually evident. Those epileptic seizures which are most difficult to record on EEG usually start in deep structures, for example, in the cortex lining the interhemispheric fissure. Unfortunately, these seizures also often have rather bizarre clinical features, leading to erroneous conclusions that a primary psychiatric condition might be present.

The characterization of epileptic syndromes depends partly on the EEG findings. It is probably unwise to use the normal EEG as a definitive means of excluding epilepsy, though a normal recording can be useful additional information when considering other diagnoses which might mimic epileptic seizures (Chapter 2).

In the presence of brain tumors and other space-occupying lesions which might present with epileptic seizures, the EEG may suggest there is a structural lesion by demonstrating a persisting slow wave focus. The EEG can also give information on the functioning of the brain, as a whole, under these circumstances. The EEG can contribute to the investigation of cerebral inflammatory processes, cerebrovascular disorders, degenerative and metabolic disorders affecting the CNS, craniocerebral trauma, pre- and perinatal brain disorders, nontherapeutic and accidental drug ingestion, cerebral anoxia, and toxic states. It is worth considering the EEG when planning investigation of any systemic condition which includes CNS dysfunction, and particularly when seizures are part of the illness.

EEGS IN DISORDERS LIKELY TO BE COMPLICATED BY SEIZURES

Most acute cerebral inflammatory disorders, i.e. meningitis or encephalitis, cause slowing of the background rhythms, whether they are due to viral, bacterial, rickettsial, fungal or parasitic causes (Westmoreland, 1993). Epileptiform abnormalities occur rarely in acute infectious mononucleosis; and periodic, localized discharges can be found in herpes simplex encephalitis. Spikes and sharp waves may also be observed in the chronic encephalopathies associated with prenatal cytomegalovirus, toxoplasma or rubella infections.

In association with an acute stroke, the EEG can show a localized functional disturbance, with high-voltage slow activity, before the CT scan demonstrates structural change. Changes typical of moya-moya disease are seen in Fig. 19a.6.

The following is a summary of the EEG

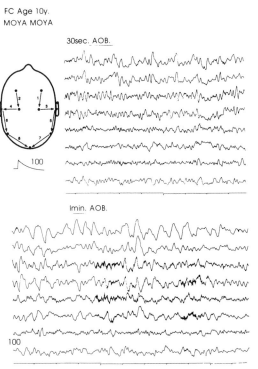

FC Age 10y.
MOYA MOYA

30sec. AOB.

1min. AOB.

Fig. 19a.6 Moya-moya disease. This 10 year old presented with a history of attacks interpreted as complex partial seizures. On overbreathing, the EEG changes were mild but some slow components appeared over the upper frontal regions 30 seconds after overbreathing ceased. This increased in amount and amplitude, especially over the right over the next 30 seconds. This 'rebuild-up' phenomenon is typical of moya-moya disease, which was later confirmed on angiography.

changes noted in degenerative disorders of the CNS many of which are associated with seizures (see Naidu and Niedermeyer, 1993). In Tay–Sachs disease, the EEG is initially normal, but high-voltage delta bursts with sharply contoured potentials and widespread spike and wave activity gradually appear. Seizures usually occur in GM_1 gangliosidosis; this disease is associated with prominent rhythmic 4–5-Hz activity, maximal over the temporal areas. Sialidosis type I is considered in Chapter 15a: the EEG shows rhythmic positive spiking over the vertex, on a poorly defined low-voltage background. In sialidosis type II, the EEG does not alter during myoclonus, though occasional generalized 4–6-Hz paroxysms occur. In types II and III of Gaucher's disease, seizures may occur at presentation, but paroxysmal EEG abnormalities can be observed before the onset of seizures in those with other initial symptoms. Since Farber's disease may be complicated by infantile spasms, severe generalized EEG changes are usual. Hypsarrhythmia-like patterns may also be present in the middle stages of Krabbe's disease, but, in the terminal stages, the EEG is almost flat in all leads. EEG changes are unremarkable in metachromatic leukodystrophy and Fabry's disease. In association with Schindler's disease, there are diffuse and multifocal paroxysmal discharges, accompanied by slowing, particularly over the centro-parieto-occipital regions. High-voltage polymorphic delta activity, especially over the temporo-occipital areas is observed in adrenoleukodystrophy.

Zellweger's syndrome is associated with the early onset of seizures, and the EEG shows either bilateral spiking, mainly over the temporal regions, or continuous spike and wave activity. In the mitochondrial syndromes of MELAS and MERRF, bursts of spikes or spike and wave activity may be found. Severe abnormalities on the EEG, including multifocal spikes, spike-waves, sharp waves, and slowing, are observed when seizures complicate urea cycle disorders. Phenylketonuria may present with infantile spasms and hypsarrhythmia. Multifocal sharp activity can be found in the oculocerebrorenal syndrome. Nonketotic hyperglycinemia is discussed in detail in Chapters 4c and 11a; suppression burst patterns are usual in the neonatal period, with slowing and multifocal spikes and polyspikes occurring later. Despite the presence of seizures and severe progressive neuropathologic changes, the EEG is often normal in Canavan's disease. In cerebrotendinous xanthomatosis, there is background slowing, with associated high-voltage delta bursts,

spikes, sharp waves, and polyspikes. Abnormal EEGs with excessive slowing have been observed in galactosemia. The findings in the various types of neuronal ceroid lipofuscinosis are discussed in Chapters 4c and 15a: EEGs are particularly helpful in these disorders. Typical findings in the late infantile variant are shown in Fig. 19a.7, which demonstrates the precipitation of spikes by slow flash frequencies. Multifocal abnormalities and hypsarrhythmia occur in Menkes' disease. In Alper's disease, the EEG characteristically shows continuous anterior high-voltage 1–3 Hz spike-wave-like activity, regardless of ongoing focal motor seizures; terminally, there is gradual diminution of the paroxysmal activity and overall slowing.

The EEG findings in some chromosomal disorders have been identified (Naidu and Niedermeyer, 1993; Chapter 4b). The recordings in Angelman's syndrome show very large discharges, facilitated by eye closure, with a tendency to normalize after 8 years of age (Fig. 19a.8). In Aicardi's syndrome, in the first 6 months, multifocal paroxysmal discharges are similar to suppression burst with the exception that there is total asymmetry between the hemispheres; later multiple epileptic foci are seen. Epilepsy occurs in 70–80% of girls with Rett's syndrome, where spikes are common and most often noted over the central regions, particularly in sleep; slow spike-wave complexes may also be seen. In the late stages of Rett's syndrome, diffuse slowing, without additional spikes, is usual.

There are specific EEG changes in some brain abnormalities of early childhood. These have been reviewed by Nogueira de Melo and Niedermeyer (1993). In hydranencephaly, when compared with severe hydrocephalus, the EEG tends to be of very low voltage and featureless, whereas there is much more, often very abnormal, activity in hydrocephalus. The EEG in lissencephaly, a severe neuronal migration disorder (Chapter 4a), shows very high voltage rapid frequen-

MS Age 4y
LATE INF. BATTENS

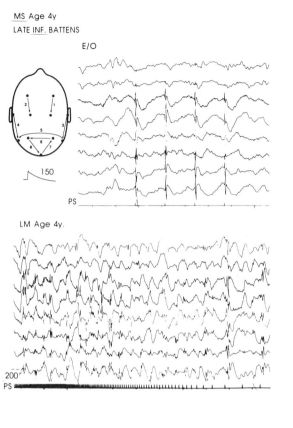

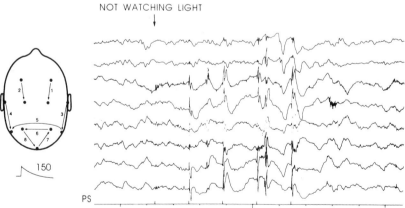

Fig. 19a.7 Four-year-old with late infantile neuronal ceroid lipofuscinosis (Batten's disease). Typical EEG findings in the late infantile form of Batten's disease. Note the distinctive 1 to 1 relationship of the spikes and the photic stimulation ((a) upper trace) is lost when more conventional rates of flash are used ((a) lower trace). Note also the failure to elicit the response when the child looks away (b). Attention to the details of data collection is essential if these EEG signs, suggesting that the problem is not simply one of epilepsy, are not to be missed.

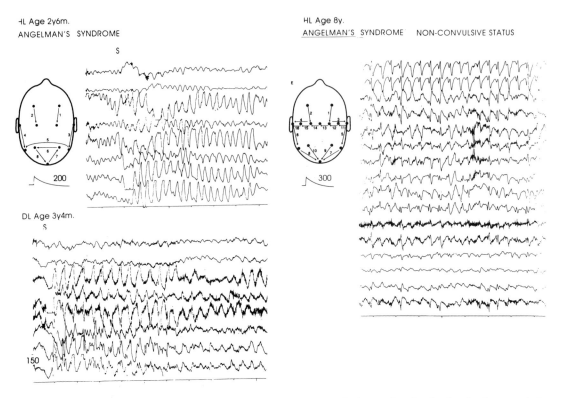

HL Age 2y6m.
ANGELMAN'S SYNDROME

DL Age 3y4m.

HL Age 8y.
ANGELMAN'S SYNDROME   NON-CONVULSIVE STATUS

Fig. 19a.8 (a) Features of Angelman's syndrome. Upper: High-amplitude rhythmic theta activity. Lower: Sharp waves and ill-defined spikes seen over the occipital and posterior temporal regions, facilitated by eye closure. (b) Nonconvulsive status epilepticus. Seen in many children with seizures complicating other disorders, including Lennox–Gastaut syndrome and, as here, in Angelman's syndrome. Note the calibration (300 microvolts/cm).

cies, over 10 Hz and usually faster than this, mixed with delta waves and infrequent spikes (Fig. 19a.9). There may be no abnormality on the EEG in association with agenesis of the corpus callosum. Most children with hemimegalencephaly (Chapter 4a) present either with seizures or development delay; their EEGs show 'alpha-like' activity, triphasic waves and suppression burst patterns.

Seizures often accompany reduced awareness in the acute stages of post-traumatic coma. The background EEG shows increasing amounts of delta and superimposed fast activities as the coma deepens. Once hemispheric death has occurred, the record becomes flat, but it is essential to allow all

drugs to be eliminated before life support is discontinued.

The EEGs found in the various epileptic syndromes are itemized in Chapters 11–15. It is possible to make generalizations in relation to some characteristics, but the records of all the children with the syndromes indicated do not necessarily show these features. Normal background activity for age is usual in benign myoclonic epilepsy in infants, myoclonic astatic epilepsy in childhood (abnormal theta rhythms may be prominent), childhood absence epilepsy, juvenile absence epilepsy, epilepsy with myoclonic absences, benign epilepsy of childhood with occipital paroxysms and other benign partial epilepsies of

AM Age 6y.
NMD

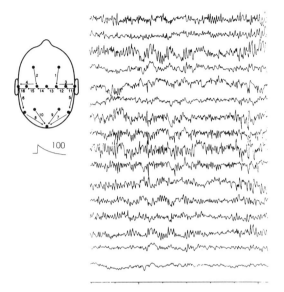

Fig. 19a.9 Neuronal migration disorder. The markedly rhythmic theta/alpha activity seen over a wide area is fairly typical of the changes which may be associated with severe degrees of neuronal migration defects. This activity is most distinctive in the first year of age, but, as here, can persist into later childhood.

childhood and adolescence, juvenile myoclonic epilepsy, and epilepsy with generalized tonic-clonic seizures on awakening. Photosensitivity can be found in benign epilepsies such as benign myoclonic epilepsy in infants, childhood and juvenile absence epilepsy, primary generalized tonic-clonic seizures on awakening; but also in severe myoclonic epilepsy in infants, where the photosensitivity can be evident very early in life; myoclonic astatic epilepsy; and in many of the progressive myoclonic epilepsies (Chapter 15a). A minority of photosensitive children have seizures only when exposed to IPS.

In the contexts of both treating epilepsy and the investigation of the comatose patient, it is important to be aware of the effects that drugs can have on the EEG (Wallquier, 1993;

Bauer, 1993). Most psychotropic agents, including neuroleptics, psychostimulants, anxiolytics, hypnotics, and nootropics, will produce a noticeable increase in fast activity ($\geq$13 Hz); and, sedative hypnotics and neuroleptics will also lead to more delta activity. Benzodiazepines and barbiturates increase beta activity. Hydantoins enhance slow waves without increasing fast activity. Carbamazepine can cause diffuse slowing as well as an increase in paroxysmal abnormalities, though the latter is not necessarily associated with a parallel increase in clinical seizures. Most anti-epileptic drugs normalize and stabilize sleep patterns; but, ethosuximide may encourage light sleep, and thus be associated with more awakenings. Carbamazepine has little effect on sleep patterns.

SPECIAL TECHNIQUES

All the foregoing parts of this chapter refer to EEG tracings obtainable using scalp electrodes. A number of more sophisticated techniques have been developed. In addition, recording in the EEG laboratory, with immediate tracing on to paper, can now be supplemented by ambulatory collection of data which are stored and analyzed at a later date.

Ambulatory monitoring allows acquisition of the EEG over long periods of time and with the patient carrying out normal day-to-day activities including sleep. Initially the numbers of channels were very restricted, but more recently, this problem has been largely overcome. Other channels within the system can be adapted for the recording of ECGs and other physiologic parameters. The montage is, of course, fixed during the recording; thus it is important to target this as accurately as possible. EEG signals are recorded and stored on cassette magnetic tape. Where definite events take place, or the EEG is of interest only in specific circumstances, only these portions of the recordings need to be examined. Playback is usually via a rapid viewing system on to a video screen, but may be on to paper. In systems with large numbers of channels (up to 24 are now available), there can be in-built mechanisms for selectively recording only those epochs or events which are likely to be of interest. Ambulatory EEG monitoring can be used for: documentation of the electrical correlates of clinically suspicious events, particularly when these are not obtained during ordinary recordings; confirmation of the nature of new attacks in patients; lateralization, localization, distribution, and classification of EEG abnormalities; quantification of discharges, both ictal and interictal, during circadian cycles; and evaluation of therapeutic measures. Electrodes other than those on the scalp can be used for recording, as mentioned below. Interpretation must take into account the vulnerability to movement and other artefacts. Combined video and EEG monitoring is a particularly useful association in the investigation of suspected pseudo-seizures.

Additional electrodes can be added to the usual 10–20 montage. Most of these are designed to get better recordings from the temporal lobes. Most involve invasive techniques, and are thus unsuitable for the young unanesthetized child. In the past, sphenoidal electrodes enjoyed the greatest popularity. They are inserted between the zygoma and the sigmoid notch in the mandible until they come into contact with the base of the skull lateral to the foramen ovale. More recently, electrodes have been inserted through the foramen ovale. In the investigation of patients who might benefit from surgery, other depth recordings, using tresses formed from strands of thin wires, can explore EEG changes arising in the frontal or temporal lobes.

Stereoencephalography (Wieser, 1993) aims to measure brain activity in a three-dimensional way. It involves simultaneous recording of surface and depth EEGs, with the subsequent minimization of problems inherent in isolated depth recordings, where exact localization of the origins of abnormal discharges may be difficult. Better precision in the identification of lesions which might be suitable for surgery is possible.

Electrocorticography implies direct recording from the cortex, and is used as an explorative method for mapping interictal epileptic activity during surgery for epilepsy. It can be difficult to interpret.

In the work-up for epilepsy surgery (Chapter 23d), many operators now use **subdural grid and strip electrodes**. After raising a bone flap, these can be inserted over the cortex to be investigated; the flap is replaced and chronic recording using an ambulatory monitor can take place. Both interictal and ictal events may, thus, be analyzed.

Increasing sophistication of the apparatus used for recording of the EEG, and for its analysis, has lead to the need for reappraisal of some of the previous tenets.

Figure 19a.10 shows that, visually, propagation of spikes may appear synchronous in the hemispheres, but computer processing demonstrates that very short time differences are present (Allen, Smith and Scott, 1992). In addition to cassette recordings, long-term EEG can be collected by cable telemetry, transmission by telephone line, radiotelemetry and the use of fiber optics, but these are, on the whole, less versatile.

The contents of this short chapter are based on the assumption that analysis of the EEG will remain, as at present, largely a visual exercise of examination of paper traces or video playbacks. The development of more sophisticated recording and analytic tools has already enhanced topographic mapping of the EEG, so that foci of specific frequencies can be mapped visually (and usually colorfully). In future, it seems likely that epilepsy monitoring will be computerized and the EEG digitized, i.e. paperless.

COMPUTER ANALYSIS·SHOWS SEIZURE PROPAGATION

Fig. 19a.10 (a) The problem of detecting propagation of spikes by visual inspection. (b) The results of computer processing (Allen, Smith and Scott, 1992), displaying the very short time differences found in the apparently synchronous discharges. (Courtesy of Dr Shelagh Smith.)

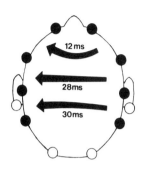

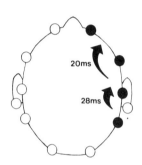

EEG APPEARS SYNCHRONOUS TO VISUAL INSPECTION

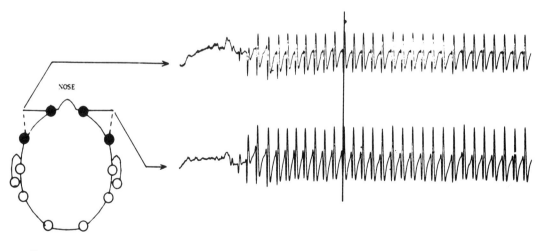

PLAN VIEW OF HEAD

ACKNOWLEDGMENTS

The figures and their legends were provided by Dr Stewart Boyd, Department of Clinical Neurophysiology, Great Ormond Street Hospital for Children, London.

REFERENCES

Allen, P.J., Smith, S.J.M. and Scott, C.A. (1992) Measurement of interhemispheric time differences in generalised spike-and-wave. *Electroencephalography and Clinical Neurophysiology*, **82**, 81–4.

Bauer, G. (1993) EEG, drug effects and central nervous system poisoning, in *Electroencephalography: Basic Principles, Clinical Applications and Related Fields* 3rd edn, (eds E. Niedermeyer, and F. Lopes da Silva), Williams and Wilkins, Baltimore. pp. 631–42.

Benda, C.I., Engel, R.C.H. and Zhang, Y. (1989) Prolonged inactive phases during discontinuous pattern of prematurity in the electroencephalogram of very-low-birthweight infants. *Electroencephalography and Clinical Neurophysiology*, **72**, 189–197.

Binnie, C.D. (1991) Electroencephalography, in *A Textbook of Epilepsy*, 4th edn. (eds J. Laidlaw, A. Richens and D. Chadwick), Churchill Livingstone, Edinburgh, pp. 277–348.

Doose, H., Gerken, H. and Volzke, E. (1972) On the genetics of EEG anomalies in childhood. I Abnormal theta rhythms. *Neuropaediatrie*, **3**, 386–401.

Dreyfus-Brisac, C. and Curzi-Dascalova, L. (1975) The EEG during the first year of life, in *Handbook of Electroencephalography and Clinical Neurophysiology*, vol. 6B (ed. A. Remond), Elsevier, Amsterdam, pp. 24–30.

Dreyfus-Brisac, C. and Monod, N. (1975) Electroencephalogram of full-term newborns and premature infants, *Handbook of Electroencephalography and Clinical Neurolphysiology*, vol. 6B (ed. A. Remond), Elsevier, Amsterdam, pp. 6–23.

Eeg-Olofsson, O. (1971a) The development of the EEG in normal children from 1 to 15 years. The 14 and 6Hz positive spike phenomenon. *Neuropaediatrie*, **2**, 405–27.

Eeg-Olofsson, O. (1971b) The development of the electroencephalogram in normal adolescents from age 16 through 21 years. *Neuropaediatrie*, **2**, 11–45.

Eeg-Olofsson, O., Petersén, I. and Selldén, U. (1971) The development of the electroencephalogram in normal children from the age of 1 through 15 years. Paroxysmal activity. *Neuropaediatrie*, **2**, 375–404.

Gerken, H. and Doose, H. (1972) On the genetics of EEG anomalies in childhood. II Occipital 2–4/s rhythms. *Neuropaediatrie*, **3**, 437–54.

Gibbs, F.A. and Davis, H. (1935) Changes in the human electroencephalogram associated with loss of consciousness. *American Journal of Neurophysiology*, **113**, 49–50.

Hughes, J.R., Fino, J.J. and Hart, L.A. (1987) Premature temporal theta (PTth). *Electroencephalography and Clinical Neurophysiology*, **67**, 7–15.

Kellaway, P. and Fox, B.J. (1952) Electroencephalographic diagnosis of cerebral pathology in infants during sleep. I Rationale, technique and the characteristics of normal sleep in infants. *Journal of Pediatrics*, **41**, 262–87.

Kuks, J.B.M., Vos, J.E. and O'Brien, M.J. (1988) EEG coherence function for normal newborns in relation to their sleep state. *Electroencephalography and Clinical Neurophysiology*, **69**, 295–302.

Naidu, S. and Niedermeyer, E. (1993) Degenerative disorders of the central nervous system, in *Electroencephalography: Basic Principles, Clinical Applications and Related Fields*, 3rd edn (eds E. Niedermeyer and F. Lopes da Silva), Williams and Wilkins, Baltimore, pp. 351–71.

Niedermeyer, E. (1988) The electroencephalogram in the differential diagnosis of the Lennox–Gastaut syndrome, in *The Lennox–Gastaut Syndrome* (eds E. Niedermeyer and R. Degen), Alan R. Liss, New York, pp. 177–220.

Niedermeyer, E. (1993a) Historical aspects, in *Electroencephalography: Basic Principles, Clinical Applications and Related Fields*, 3rd edn (eds E. Niedermeyer and F. Lopes da Silva), Williams and Wilkins, Baltimore, pp. 1–14.

Niedermeyer, E. (1993b) Maturation of the EEG: development of waking and sleep patterns, in *Electroencephalography: Basic Principles, Clinical Applications and Related Fields*, 3rd edn (eds E. Niedermeyer and F. Lopes da Silva), Williams and Wilkins, Baltimore, pp. 167–91.

Niedermeyer, E. (1993c) EEG patterns and genetics, in *Electroencephalography: Basic Principles, Clinical Applications and Related Fields*, 3rd edn (eds E. Niedermeyer and F. Lopes da Silva), Williams and Wilkins, Baltimore, pp. 192–5.

Niedermeyer, E. (1993d) Abnormal EEG patterns: epileptic and paroxysmal, in *Electroencephalo-*

graphy: Basic Principles, Clinical Applications and Related Fields, 3rd edn, (eds E. Niedermeyer and F. Lopes da Silva), Williams and Wilkins, Baltimore, pp. 217–41.

Nogueira de Melo, A. and Niedermeyer, E. (1993) The EEG in infantile brain damage, cerebral palsy and minor cerebral dysfunctions of childhood, in *Electroencephalography: Basic Principles, Clinical Applications and Related Fields*, 3rd edn, (eds E. Niedermeyer and F. Lopes da Silva), Williams and Wilkins, Baltimore, pp. 373–81.

Ohtahara, S. and Yamatogi, Y. (1990) Evolution of seizures and EEG abnormalities in childhood onset epilepsy, in *Handbook of Electroencephalography and Clinical Neurophysiology, Revised Series*, vol. 4 (eds J.A. Wada and R.J. Ellington), Elsevier, Amsterdam, pp. 457–77.

Parmalee, A.H., Akiyama, Y., Wenner, W. *et al.* (1968) The electroencephalogram in active and quiet sleep in infants, in *Clinical Electroencephalography in Children* (eds P. Kellaway and I. Petersén), Grune and Stratton, New York, pp. 77–88.

Petersén, I. and Eeg-Olofsson, O. (1971) The development of the electroencephalogram in normal chilren from the age of 1 through 15 years. *Neuropaediatrie*, **2**, 247–304.

Schulte, F.J., Hinze, G. and Schrempf, G. (1971) Maternal toxemia, fetal malnutrition and bio-electric brain activity in the newborn. *Neuropaediatrie*, **2**, 439–60.

Spehlmann, R. (1981) *EEG Primer*, Elsevier, Amsterdam.

Takahashi, T. (1993) Activation methods, in, *Electroencephalography: Basic Principles, Clinical Applications and Related Fields*, 3rd edn, Williams and Wilkins, Baltimore, pp. 241–62.

Varner, J.L., Peters, J.F. and Ellingson, R.J. (1978) Interhemispheric synchrony in the EEG of full-term newborns. *Electroencephalography and Clinical Neurophysiology*, **45**, 641–7.

Wallquier, A. (1993) EEG and neuropharmacology, in *Electroencephalography: Basic Principles, Clinical Applications and Related Fields*, 3rd edn, (eds E. Niedermeyer and F. Lopes da Silva), Williams and Wilkins, Baltimore, pp. 619–629.

Westmoreland, B.F. (1993) The EEG in cerebral inflammatory processes, in *Electroencephalography: Basic Principles, Clinical Applications and Related Fields*, 3rd edn, (eds E. Niedermeyer and F. Lopes da Silva), Williams and Wilkins, Baltimore, pp. 291–304.

Wieser, H.G. (1993) Stereoencephalography and foramen ovale recording, in *Electroencephalography: Basic Principles, Clinical Applications and Related Fields*, 3rd edn, (eds E. Niedermeyer and F. Lopes da Silva), Williams and Wilkins, Baltimore, pp. 679–93.

MAGNETOENCEPHALOGRAPHY

Sheila J. Wallace

Weak magnetic fields outside the head were first noted in the 1960s, but only with the development of a superconducting quantum interference device (SQUID) has it become possible to use these fields for investigative purposes. Recent developments and clinical applications are reviewed by Hari (1993).

At source, EEG and MEG waveforms are similar. MEG has the advantage that the skull and other extracerebral tissues do not interfere with the conduction of magnetic fields. In addition, it is reference free (i.e. there is no need to refer to a reference point, as is essential for EEG). This allows improved localization of the source of any abnormality. MEG detects currents particularly in the tangential plane, whereas the EEG mainly reflects activity in radially orientated neurons. Thus MEG and EEG provide complementary information. However, MEG has more sophisticated laboratory requirements than EEG.

For MEG, the recording room must be magnetically shielded. The subject lies with the head supported by a vacuum cast. The squid sensors are housed in a helium container which is placed as near the head as possible, without touching it.

The magnetic field is picked up from several locations simultaneously. Probe-position indicators give exact sites for the measurements of these fields, and allow the position of the magnetometer, with respect to external markings on the head, to be determined with 2–3 mm accuracy. Magnetometers with from seven to 37 sensors are available. The results resemble conventional EEG traces, but are often presented as field maps, most dramatically in three-dimensional form.

In epilepsy, studies with MEG are still at an experimental, rather than clinical, level. Foci of abnormal activity, associated with partial seizures, can be sharply localized. Multiple irritative areas can be defined; however, differentiation between ictal and interictal spikes can be problematic. Since the subject must remain completely still during examination, ictal recordings of motor seizures are not possible. MEG can be used in the study of evoked potentials. Sources of evoked potentials can then be utilized as landmarks for localizing foci of abnormal activity in patients with epilepsy, particularly in those for whom surgery is being considered.

In summary, MEG is still at an early stage of exploitation, but has clear potential in epileptology. At the moment its applications in childhood epilepsy are somewhat constrained by the need for complete immobility during recording.

REFERENCE

Hari, R. (1993) Magnetoencephalography as a tool of clinical neurophysiology, in *Electroencephalography: Basic Principles, Clinical Applications and Related Fields*, 3rd edn, (eds E. Niedermeyer and F. Lopes da Silva). Williams and Wilkins, Baltimore, pp. 1035–61.

Epilepsy in Children. Edited by Sheila Wallace. Published in 1996 by Chapman & Hall, London. ISBN 0 412 56860 8

Sheila J. Wallace

The roles of the visual evoked potential, electroretinogram, and brainstem auditory and somatosensory evoked potentials in investigation of the child with epilepsy will be considered briefly. Interpretation of all evoked potential studies must take the child's age into consideration: this is particularly important in infancy. A comprehensive review of such studies in childhood can be found in Krumholz (1993).

It is fundamental to the understanding of the place of evoked potentials in investigation to know that the test merely assesses the competence of neuronal pathways, and does not give information about cognition. For example, pathways used for visual evoked potentials might be intact, but the child may not be able to interpret visual stimuli and therefore, effectively, is blind.

VISUALLY EVOKED POTENTIALS

The visually evoked potential (VEP) is recorded via scalp electrodes during presentation of chequered patterns, or flashes, to the eyes. The physiologic changes which occur during repeated stimulation, and are recorded over the occipital region, are summated to give a recognizable pattern of positive-negative deflections.

In adults, the most frequent waves seen are N70 (a negative wave occurring at about 70 ms) and P100 (a positive wave occurring at around 100 ms). Sometimes a positive wave, P50, appears at about 50 ms. In addition to

relationship to age, VEP latencies tend to be shorter in females than in males. In patients, particularly those with cerebral pathology, latencies are unlikely to be exactly 70 ms for the N wave and 100 ms for the P wave, and the conventional presentation of results is to designate the wave by N or P and give the latency immediately afterwards. The early components of the response seem related to cortical reception of primary visual information and thus provide knowledge of the transit time through the brain, whereas the later components, after about 200 ms, are thought to possibly reflect higher cognitive processing of visual information.

The use of pattern stimulation gives a more stable VEP, but requires continuous visual fixation. Therefore, in infants and young children, a flash stimulus is usually employed. Before 30 weeks of gestation, a primitive response to flash can be obtained; this becomes more stable after about 32 weeks and a P latency reaches about 150–200 ms by full term. Subsequently the latencies of the various components of the VEP shorten progressively throughout childhood, attaining adult levels at about 20 years. The amplitude of the VEP is greatest in premature infants, but the various components are not well defined at this time.

The VEP is particularly likely to be abnormal in disorders which affect myelin. Thus children who have seizures in association with leukodystrophies are likely to have long

Epilepsy in Children. Edited by Sheila Wallace. Published in 1996 by Chapman & Hall, London. ISBN 0 412 56860 8

P latencies. The VEP is an essential test in providing supportive evidence of the presence of ceroid neuronal lipofuscinoses and in differentiating between the infantile, late infantile and juvenile types of this condition. Full details are given in Chapters 4c and 15a.

Seizures are much commoner in childhood-than in adult-onset multiple sclerosis: VEPs are likely to be abnormal in this condition.

In summary, the VEP, if abnormal, can suggest that seizures are secondary to widespread brain pathology.

ELECTRORETINOGRAMS

The electroretinogram (ERG) is evoked by bright flashes and consists of high-amplitude potentials generated by the photoreceptors and by the retinal glial cells. Using sequential stimuli varying from blue to white in the dark-adapted state, and from white to blue-green in the light-adapted state, it is possible to separate the contributions of the rod and cone systems to the ERG, but for the purposes of investigation of children with epilepsy, such sophistication is not usually necessary. The ERG can be recorded via electrodes positioned on the skin, close to the eyes. To flashes, it consists of negative-positive deflections labelled 'a wave', 'b wave', and 'c wave'. The amplitudes and latencies of the a and b waves are quantifiable.

ERG is particularly useful in the diagnoses of the ceroid lipofuscinoses and in the distinction between the various types (Chapters 4c, 15a). In children with seizures complicating disorders of peroxisomal function, the ERG is likely to be abnormal.

In summary, the ERG can be utilized as a pointer to the presence of specific diagnoses in children with degenerative disorders of the CNS, but additional information from the EEG and VEPs is usually needed to complement the ERG findings.

BRAINSTEM AUDITORY EVOKED POTENTIALS

Brainstem auditory evoked potentials (BAEPs) are useful in the examination of the auditory pathways, but also as determinants of structural lesions in the brainstem; e.g. in disorders of myelin, and in some systemic or degenerative neurologic disorders. BAEPs are very stable: they do not vary with state of consciousness or level of sedation. The various components have been related to specific source generators in the brainstem auditory pathway: wave I – auditory nerve action potential; wave II – cochlear nucleus; wave III – superior olivary complex; wave IV – ascending auditory pathways in dorsal and rostral pons; wave V – superior to wave IV, in the mesencephalon, possibly around the inferior colliculus; wave VI – medial lemniscus; wave VII – primary auditory cortex. The origins of waves VI and VII are still somewhat speculative. Thus BAEPs are much less useful than VEPs in assessing generalized brain disturbances, but can be helpful in diagnostic work-ups of children whose seizures are considered secondary to degenerative diseases.

The auditory stimulus, a series of clicks, is delivered through headphones. The BAEP is recorded via electrodes at the vertex and the ear lobe (or mastoid process) ipsilateral to the ear stimulated. Prior to 28–30 weeks' gestation, reproducible responses may not be obtained, but by 40 weeks, all components of the BAEP should be visible. Thereafter, the latencies of the individual BAEP waves and their interpeak intervals decrease with age.

The stability of the BAEP, even under conditions of extreme sedation, such as barbiturate coma, which might be used in seriously refractory status epilepticus, allows this investigation to be employed for monitoring brainstem function when other tests might be inappropriate. Abnormalities of the BAEP can be found early in the course of leukodystrophies, e.g. Pelizaeus Merzbacher disease, metachromatic leukodystrophy and adrenoleukodystrophy, or may be found in mitochondrial cytopathies.

SOMATOSENSORY EVOKED POTENTIALS

These potentials combine information on the peripheral and central nervous systems. Stimuli are presented to the peripheral nerve, usually the median or posterior tibial. Depending on the choice of channels, recording electrodes are placed over the chosen nerve, working proximally, whilst scalp electrodes, placed frontally, centrally or parietally, are used for the more central parts of the recording. Thus, in addition to travelling along the peripheral nerve, these potentials traverse large areas of the brain. Latencies in the potentials are likely to be abnormal when systemic or generalized diseases which affect the central and/or peripheral nervous systems are present. Changes are seen particularly if there is an associated disorder of myelin.

As for other evoked potentials, latencies are much longer in infants and young children than in adults. Values approaching those in adults are attained by about 3 years.

Somatosensory evoked potentials (SSEPs) are sometimes abnormally enlarged in epilepsies with myoclonic seizures and cerebral degeneration, e.g. in late infantile and juvenile ceroid lipofuscinoses and Lafora's disease. (Chapter 15a). Otherwise SSEPs are likely to be abnormal in children with epilepsy, if brainstem death has occurred, or if the underlying condition is a leukodystrophy.

REFERENCE

Krumholz, A. (1993) Evoked potentials in infancy and childhood, in *Electroencephalography: Basic Principles, Clinical Applications and Related Fields,* 3rd edn, (eds E. Niedermeyer and F. Lopes da Silva), Williams and Wilkins, Baltimore, pp. 975–88.

Sheila J. Wallace

Examination in children is almost invariably with surface electrodes. Sensory conduction velocities are measured by peripheral stimulation of the nerve and recording of the sensory action potential at a convenient position proximally. The sensory conduction velocity is calculated by measuring the distance between stimulus and recording points, and the time taken for the stimulus to travel between these points. Compound muscle action potentials and motor nerve conduction velocities are assessed by stimulation of a motor nerve and recording peripherally over the relevant muscle.

Nerve conduction studies are only indicated in the diagnostic work-up of children with epilepsy when a multisystem disorder, such as a mitochondrial cytopathy, is suspected. Thus examination of the peripheral nervous system could be relevant when a progressive myoclonus epilepsy presents (Chapter 15a). Peripheral neuropathies are also components of some degenerative neurologic disorders, such as Krabbe's disease and metachromatic leukodystrophy; but these conditions rarely present with seizures, though the latter are fairly frequent in the later stages of the conditions.

The velocities of conduction within the peripheral nerves increase with age (Payan, 1991). They reach levels comparable with those of adults by about 18–24 months.

REFERENCE

Payan, J. (1991) Clinical electromyography in infancy and childhood, in *Paediatric Neurology*, 2nd edn, (ed. E.M. Brett), Churchill Livingstone, Edinburgh: pp. 797–829.

Epilepsy in Children. Edited by Sheila Wallace. Published in 1996 by Chapman & Hall, London. ISBN 0 412 56860 8

ELECTROMYOGRAPHY

Sheila J. Wallace

Electromyography (EMG) is a method for studying the function of the motor unit. Detection of, and distinction between, disorders of the anterior horn cell, nerve root, plexus, peripheral nerve, neuromuscular junction, and muscle are possible. Such sophistication is not usually necessary in children with epilepsy, where the EMG is most frequently used as part of polygraphic recording designed to demonstrate the presence of muscle jerks during EEGs and to note their coincidence, or otherwise, with EEG changes.

When sophisticated information on the motor unit is required, a bipolar needle electrode, inserted into the muscle chosen for examination, is usually employed. For the purpose of determining whether or not a muscular contraction has or has not occurred, without further analysis of the function of the motor unit, surface pad electrodes suffice. When indicated, analysis of the motor unit potential includes assessment of its form, duration, amplitude, stability and firing rate, and relaxation after effort. Most of these factors are assessed by observational methods. The durations of motor unit potentials vary in different muscles and become greater with age (Payan, 1991).

As indicated above and demonstrated in figures in Chapter 13b, surface EMG can be useful in demonstrating brief muscle contractions. In particular, when there is doubt as to whether myoclonic jerks are components of epileptic seizures or due to other causes, simultaneous EMG and EEG can be very helpful. EMG is also useful in highlighting motor components when children are in nonconvulsive status epilepticus, by giving the clinician an indication of minor motor phenomena. Such information can be helpful in the later management, when targeted observation of motor changes may indicate relapse in circumstances where there is little other alteration in the child.

When epilepsy is symptomatic of a generalized systemic disease, EMG can indicate specific involvement of the motor unit. Recording by needle is then necessary. Situations where EMG could be useful in diagnosis include mitochondrial cytopathies, Leigh's syndrome, and in indicating denervation in degenerative disorders where peripheral neuropathy is part of the clinical picture.

REFERENCE

Payan, J. (1991) Clinical electromyography in infancy and childhood, in *Paediatric Neurology*, 2nd edn, (ed. E.M. Brett), Churchill Livingstone, Edinburgh, pp. 797–829.

Epilepsy in Children. Edited by Sheila Wallace. Published in 1996 by Chapman & Hall, London. ISBN 0 412 56860 8

Sheila J. Wallace

The simultaneous recording of several physiologic and/or behavioral variables can be extremely helpful in the correct categorization of sudden-onset attacks, particularly when primary cardiac or psychogenic conditions are considered to be possible alternative diagnoses. Polygraphic recordings in sick neonates are especially useful, since the behavioral repertoire of the neonate is somewhat restricted, with the result that different untoward events can produce comparable clinical pictures.

Although EEG machines are usually used for polygraphy in patients with epilepsy, they are not ideally suited to giving precise and detailed signals of other physiologic variables. Nevertheless, they may provide information for some parameters, which can be followed up using more appropriate apparatus.

It is possible to record simultaneously, using an EEG machine, the EEG, the electrocardiograph (ECG), the electromyograph (EMG), and the electro-oculograph (EOG). The ECG so obtained mainly gives details on heart rate, and allows ECG artefacts on the EEG trace to be recognized: detailed analysis of the ECG, itself, is not possible. Recording of the EMG with the EEG is discussed in Chapter 19f. The recording of eye movements (EOG) is essential in sleep studies per se, and in the staging of sleep during the investigation of epilepsy. The latter is particularly important when studying the neonate (Lombroso 1993).

Other variables which could be of interest are blood pressure, and respiration – respiratory rate, chest expansion and oxygen saturation. These need special monitors, which are of variable complexity; that for measurement of the respiratory rate is the simplest.

It is obligatory to ensure that the various recordings are time-locked. Simultaneous video recording should be arranged, in addition, if possible.

REFERENCE

Lombroso, CT. (1993) Neonatal EEG polygraphy in normal and abnormal newborns, in *Electroencephalography: Basic Principles, Clinical Applications and Related Fields*, (eds E. Niedermeyer and F. Lopes de Silva). Williams and Wilkins, Baltimore, pp. 803–75.

Epilepsy in Children. Edited by Sheila Wallace. Published in 1996 by Chapman & Hall, London. ISBN 0 412 56860 8

IMAGING: ANATOMIC AND FUNCTIONAL

20

Harry T. Chugani

In the past 10 years, the advent of various types of high-resolution tomographic neuro-imaging has had a significant impact on the diagnosis and management of epilepsy in children. **Anatomical imaging** obtained with X-ray computed tomography (CT) and magnetic resonance imaging (MRI) can readily detect gross anatomic abnormalities. In developing nations, anatomic abnormalities are detected in the majority of children with epilepsy, and, typically are associated with parasitic infections (Astiazaran *et al.*, 1993). In the more industrialized nations, however, these lesions are present in a relatively small proportion; although, with the influx of immigrants, the situation is changing somewhat. In this chapter discussion is based predominantly on studies performed in industrialized nations.

Since epilepsy is primarily a **functional** disturbance of the brain, **functional neuroimaging** modalities, such as positron emission tomography (PET) and single photon emission computed tomography (SPECT), are more sensitive than CT and MRI in detecting generalized and focal abnormalities. Furthermore, new probes for functional imaging in the epilepsies are being developed rapidly. These will provide important insight into the biochemistry and neuronal circuitry of seizures.

SKULL X-RAY

In general, skull X-rays are of limited value. In the acute setting of head trauma, skull films may be useful in diagnosing fractures associated with brain contusion and seizures.

Chronic conditions which include epilepsy as a manifestation may show calcification. Approximately 15–20% of brain tumors in children calcify; these include oligodendro-gliomata, astrocytomata, ependymomata, and craniopharyngomata. Various intrauterine infections, such as toxoplasmosis and cytomegalic inclusion disease, are often characterized by cerebral calcification. Probably, one of the commonest causes of cerebral calcification is tuberous sclerosis, in which the skull X-ray may show calcification along the walls of the ventricles, as well as in the cortical regions. Fahr's disease probably comprises several genetic disorders associated with basal ganglia calcification, choreoathetosis, and seizures. Both Down's syndrome and Cockayne's disease may reveal intracranial calcification, apparent on the skull X-ray, and associated with epilepsy.

Prior to the development of various CT techniques, the commonest procedure used to establish the diagnosis of Sturge–Weber syndrome was the skull X-ray, which demonstrated the classical tramtrack-like calcifications. Cerebral angiography in patients with Sturge–Weber syndrome revealed the vari-

Epilepsy in Children. Edited by Sheila Wallace. Published in 1996 by Chapman & Hall, London. ISBN 0 412 56860 8

able presence of arterial thromboses, absence of cortical veins, aberrant cerebral venous drainage and arteriovenous malformations, in addition to the characteristic leptomeningeal angioma commonly located in the posterior parietal distribution (Poser and Taveras, 1957; Bentson *et al.*, 1971).

CONVENTIONAL NUCLEAR MEDICINE TECHNIQUES

There has been minimal application of conventional nuclear medicine technology in the direct study of epilepsy. In some conditions in which epilepsy is a manifestation, brain scanning has been utilized for the purpose of elucidating the pathophysiology of the disorder rather than to evaluate the epilepsy. For example, Kuhl *et al.* (1972) performed ^{99m}Tc-pertechnetate brain scans on 14 patients with Sturge–Weber syndrome. They found the affected hemisphere to have a smaller but more radioactive image than the unaffected side. Calcified regions showed increased uptake of the tracer. At about the time that these findings were described, CT techniques became available, and quickly became the procedure of choice in Sturge–Weber syndrome.

COMPUTED TOMOGRAPHY

Cerebral imaging in patients with epilepsy became almost routine following the development and widespread availability of CT scanning. For the first time, it was possible to directly visualize the brain *in vivo*. Various pathologic entities causing epilepsy and previously detected only postmortem could now be diagnosed in the early stages. It was discovered that about half of large populations with epilepsy show some abnormality on the CT scan. Often, these are nonspecific atrophic changes, but sometimes neoplasms and porencephalies are detected (Gastaut and Gastaut, 1977). Epilepsies symptomatic of structural lesions are considered in Chapter 16.

PARTIAL EPILEPSY

The routine application of CT scanning in intractable partial epilepsy in search of a surgically treatable lesion has a disappointingly low yield. Among 98 children with chronic epilepsy, the greatest yield of CT abnormalities was in children with partial motor epilepsy, of whom 43% showed an abnormality; however, only 2% of these could be surgically treated (Bachman, Hodnes and Freeman, 1976). In another large study of 143 patients with chronic seizures, in whom previous neurodiagnostic evaluations had failed to disclose abnormalities that could justify surgical intervention, CT scans revealed focal lesions that could be treated with surgery in only four. Following resection, two subjects were seizure free and the other two showed significant improvement (Jabbari *et al.*, 1978).

Since mesial temporal sclerosis is a common pathologic finding in temporal lobe epilepsy, attempts have been made to detect sclerosis prior to surgery. Unfortunately, mesial temporal sclerosis is not readily detected by CT. The strategy developed by Wyler and Bolender (1983) was to use metrizamide-enhanced CT to demonstrate abnormalities of the mesial temporal structures in patients with intractable temporal lobe epilepsy; the findings correlated well with the electrographic identification of the epileptogenic temporal lobe.

Partial epilepsy resulting from brain injury can often be predicted from CT scans obtained in the acute stage. In one study of 219 head trauma patients, all 13 patients who later developed epilepsy had CT evidence of focal brain injury within 3 days of the traumatic event (D'Alessandro *et al.*, 1988).

SYNDROMES ASSOCIATED WITH EPILEPSY

Early characterization of the angiomatosis distribution in **Sturge–Weber syndrome** has been greatly aided by the advent of high-resolution anatomic neuroimaging modalities. CT has played an important diagnostic role because of its sensitivity in the detection of early calcification in the brain (Maki and Semba, 1979). In infants younger than about 1–2 years of age, CT scanning may show the affected hemisphere to be enlarged, with small arachnoid spaces and lateral ventricles. Following the administration of contrast medium, CT may reveal opacification of the angioma and adjacent regions of the hemisphere. The choroid plexus on the involved side is typically enlarged. In some cases, contrast infusion may reveal enhancement of the affected cerebral convolutions. Calcifications may also be seen within the angioma. As the disease progresses and the angioma is progressively excluded from the circulation, large areas of calcification may be seen on CT. This is accompanied by focal or generalized cerebral atrophy, presumably secondary to chronic ischemia.

When bilateral occipital corticosubcortical calcifications are present in the absence of cutaneous stigmata of Sturge–Weber syndrome in patients with epilepsy (Gobbi *et al.*, 1988), the diagnosis may be folate deficiency and celiac disease (Bye *et al.*, 1993). The calcifications are best shown with CT scanning.

Thirty-eight children with **Lennox–Gastaut syndrome** underwent CT scanning, and two were shown to have focal lesions that were amenable to surgical treatment; these consisted of tuberous sclerosis and temporal lobe astrocytoma (Zimmerman, Niedermeyer and Hodnes, 1977). In several other epilepsy syndromes of childhood, such as hemimegalencephaly and other gross malformations of the brain, CT continues to be useful in establishing the diagnosis early in the course of epilepsy.

MAGNETIC RESONANCE IMAGING

With the development of MRI, which has a relatively high spatial resolution, small and subtle lesions not seen with CT scanning can be detected. These include small sclerotic areas, tumors, vascular lesions, malformations, and focal atrophy. In the detection of heterotopic gray matter, which is often associated with epilepsy, MRI is clearly superior to CT and often plays an important role in the management of the child (Dunn *et al.*, 1986). Heterotopic gray matter appears as regions isointense with that of normal gray matter on T_1 and T_2-weighted images (Barkovich, Chuang and Norman, 1988; Smith *et al.*, 1988). In some cases, the abnormality of neuronal migration detected on MRI is generalized, resulting in a continuous band of heterotopic gray matter between the cerebral cortex and the lateral ventricles. This has been referred to as 'band heterotopias' and 'double cortex' (Barkovich, Jackson and Boyer, 1989; Palmini *et al.*, 1991a; Chapter 4a).

Even with the high spatial resolution and sensitivity of MRI, microdysgenesis, which has been reported in up to 42% of temporal lobe specimens, is typically not detected (Hardiman *et al.*, 1988). Also, caution must be taken in interpreting MRI studies performed during status epilepticus because of reports that transient abnormalities may occur during seizures, and resolve with repeated testing (Riela, Sims and Penny, 1991).

TEMPORAL LOBE EPILEPSY

Approximately 20% of patients with intractable temporal lobe epilepsy undergoing lobectomy are found to have gross structural lesions in the resected specimen. These lesions are now easily detected with MRI. For example, in 10 patients with cortical dysplasia and complex partial seizures who underwent temporal lobectomy, MRI showed clear abnormalities in five and blurring of the gray–white matter junction in another two. The remaining three patients had normal MRI studies (Kuzniecky *et al.*, 1991).

A further advantage of MRI over CT is that hippocampal (or mesial temporal) sclerosis,

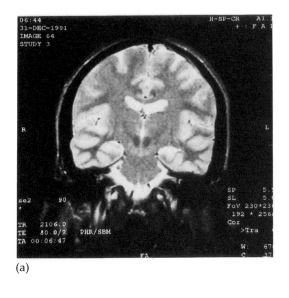

(a)

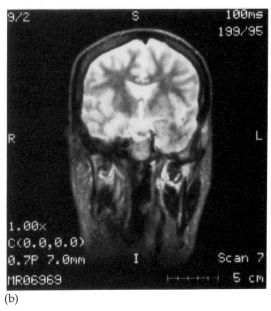

(b)

Fig. 20.1 MRI of mesial temporal sclerosis. (a) Coronal T_2 weighted section demonstrating asymmetry between the right and left temporal lobes, with the left side being smaller and having abnormal signal in the mesial aspect. (b) Coronal T_2 weighted section of another patient reveals greater temporal lobe asymmetry, with the right side being smaller and the presence of abnormal signal in the mesial aspect. (Courtesy of T. Slovis, MD, Children's Hospital of Michigan, Detroit.)

which is found in 60% of patients undergoing temporal lobectomy (Babb and Brown, 1987), can be directly visualized with MRI (Fig. 20.1). This has significantly diminished the need for invasive EEG techniques in the preoperative evaluation of patients with intractable temporal lobe epilepsy. The affected hippocampus appears atrophic and may also show increased signal intensity on T_2-weighted images (Jackson *et al.*, 1990; for review see Bronen, 1992). A retrospective analysis of pathology and MRI findings in 48 patients treated by temporal lobectomy showed that 34 had evidence of abnormal MRI signal preoperatively. All 12 structural lesions were detected by MRI. Severe gliosis was detected by MRI in 11 of 14 cases, whereas mild to moderate gliosis was detected in six of 12 cases (Kuzniecky *et al.*, 1987).

Berkovic *et al.* (1991) used coronal spin-echo images oriented perpendicularly to the long axis of the hippocampus in 10 patients with intractable temporal lobe epilepsy who had histories of prolonged childhood convulsions. All 10 subjects showed unilateral temporal lobe atrophy and increased signal on T_2-weighted images corresponding to EEG lateralization of epileptogenicity. Following temporal lobectomy in these 10 patients, eight became seizure free. Hippocampal tissue was available for examination in only three, and showed sclerosis. These investigators suggested that their patients may represent the subgroup of patients with temporal lobe epilepsy characterized by hippocampal sclerosis following prolonged childhood convulsions, and a favorable outcome following lobectomy (Falconer, 1974; Chapter 23d).

The relationship between early childhood prolonged febrile convulsions, decreased hippocampal volume on MRI, and mesial temporal sclerosis has been confirmed in more recent studies (Cendes *et al.*, 1993a, 1993b). In a prospective study of 34 patients who underwent temporal lobectomy, lateralized abnormalities were present on MRI in 25 subjects and usually predicted surgical success (82% predictive value) compared to patients with normal MRI studies (56% predictive value). Increased signal on T_2-weighted images and ipsilateral temporal horn enlargement also correlated with outcome in this study. Once again, a history of febrile convulsions associated with hippocampal atrophy indicated a particularly favorable surgical outcome (Kuzniecky *et al.*, 1993a). It is likely that the recent development of MRI T_2 relaxation mapping techniques will allow hippocampal sclerosis to be detected even earlier and more objectively (Jackson *et al.*, 1993).

The application of **quantitative** studies of hippocampal volume has further increased the sensitivity of MRI in detecting the abnormal temporal lobe in adults and older children with temporal lobe epilepsy (Jack *et al.*, 1990). In children with temporal lobe epilepsy, quantitative documentation of hippocampal atrophy was found in 63% of patients, with a sensitivity and specificity of 100% when mesial temporal sclerosis was present (Cascino *et al.*, 1992). Another study showed that the combined use of both amygdala and hippocampal volumetric measurements on MRI in patients with temporal lobe epilepsy allowed the abnormal temporal lobe, based on EEG, to be lateralized in 93% of cases, whereas the application of hippocampal measurements alone provided a lateralization in 87% of subjects in this series (Cendes *et al.*, 1993a).

The degree of hippocampal atrophy measured on MRI appears to reflect the severity of hippocampal sclerosis in the surgical specimen (Cascino *et al.*, 1991). In an analysis of MRI-derived hippocampal volume in 50 patients undergoing temporal lobectomy, Jack *et al.* (1992) found that patients with greater atrophy had a better postsurgical outcome.

The structural abnormalities evaluated by MRI in the hippocampus are associated with disturbances in memory and other neuropsychologic functions. In the study by Lencz *et al.* (1992), there was a significant correlation in patients with left temporal lobe epilepsy between left hippocampal volume and Wechsler logical memory percentage retention scores, and between left temporal lobe volume and verbal Selective Reminding Test scores. Hippocampal volume asymmetries and memory asymmetries revealed by the Wada test also appeared to show a significant correlation (Loring *et al.*, 1993).

OTHER PARTIAL EPILEPSIES

Gross brain malformations associated with epilepsy that is often very difficult to control medically have been detected with MRI (Fig. 20.2). Among 44 children with various intractable partial epilepsies, Kuzniecky *et al.* (1993b) found MRI abnormalities corresponding with EEG localization in 84%. Hippocampal sclerosis was present in 50% and tended to occur over the age of 12 years, whereas ganglioglial tumors tended to be seen in younger children. Neuronal migration errors (Chapter 4a) were seen in 25% of the children. In a study on much younger children with malignant partial epilepsy, Duchowny *et al.* (1990) found CT or MRI evidence of gross lesions in four of five infants less than 1 year of age who underwent focal resection.

Cortical dysplasia involving the rolandic region has been detected by MRI in several children who had no prior explanation for their focal cortical myoclonus and focal motor seizures. Surgical resection of the malformations resulted in considerable improvement

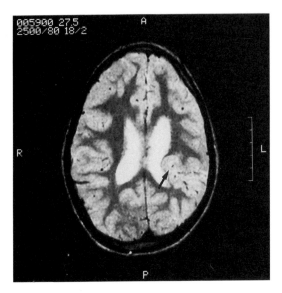

Fig. 20.2 Axial T$_2$-weighted MR image of a 5-year-old boy showing focal migration abnormality in the left parietotemporal region with gray matter (arrow) impinging on the ventricle. (Courtesy of T. Slovis, MD, Children's Hospital of Michigan, Detroit.)

of the neurologic symptoms (Kuzniecky *et al.*, 1988; Guerrini *et al.*, 1992a). Palmini *et al.* (1991b) in their report on 30 patients with partial epilepsy associated with localized areas of aberrant neuronal migration documented the superiority of MRI compared to CT in identifying the dysplastic lesions. Lesions involving the central region correlated with drop attacks, which were present in 27% of patients.

It is generally known that surgical treatment of frontal lobe epilepsy has been less rewarding than temporal lobe epilepsy. However, the likelihood of postoperative seizure control is higher when a lesion can be defined by MRI in the frontal lobe. For example, Cascino *et al.* (1992) reported that 67% of patients with frontal lobe lesions on MRI were seizure free following surgery, in contrast to 25% of those without apparent lesions.

SYNDROMES ASSOCIATED WITH EPILEPSY (see also Chapters 16, 17)

In general, MRI of patients with **Sturge–Weber syndrome** has shown similar findings to CT. Although CT better demonstrates the calcifications in Sturge–Weber syndrome, MRI is far superior to CT in demonstrating the vascular channels of the angioma. Furthermore, recent studies have indicated that gadolinium-enhanced MRI is extremely useful in accurately delineating the extent of the angiomatosis (Lipski *et al.*, 1990; Sperner *et al.*, 1990) even before the emergence of neurological abnormalities (Pascual-Castroviejo *et al.*, 1993). Jacoby *et al.* (1987) demonstrated accelerated myelination of the affected cerebral hemisphere in two infants (age 3 and 9 months) with Sturge–Weber syndrome. These investigators suggested that this seemingly paradoxical finding of a hypermyelinative state may be due to ischemia of brain tissue underlying the leptomeningeal angioma, and in that way, may be analogus to the myelin-rich lesions (status marmoratus) seen in neonatal hypoxic–ischemic insults.

In the syndrome of **gelastic seizures associated with hypothalamic hamartomata**, both the hypothalamic and frequent cortical abnormalities are best identified by MRI (Berkovic *et al.*, 1988), although the larger hamartomata may sometimes be detected by CT (Breningstall, 1985). Similarly, bilateral central rolandic and sylvian macrogyria in some patients with epilepsy, pseudobulbar palsy and mental retardation can be detected with CT but are most clearly imaged with MRI (Kuzniecky *et al.*, 1989; Aicardi, 1991; Guerrini *et al.*, 1992b). The affected cortex appears thick and symmetric, and surrounds a large sulcus. When atonic drop seizures become difficult to control in these patients, corpus callosotomy often provides relief.

The application of MRI and other neuroimaging modalities has led to a significant reduction in the cryptogenic cases of **West's**

syndrome (Chapter 11b), with an increasing number of patients being assigned to the symptomatic group. MRI studies on 46 children with West's syndrome revealed various abnormalities in 43, whereas CT showed abnormalities in 38 (van Bogaert *et al.*, 1993). Although many of the abnormalities were nonspecific and did not lead to any alteration in treatment, four of the five MRI abnormalities not detected by CT were focal lesions potentially treatable with surgery.

It is now recognized that MRI is highly efficient in characterizing the anatomic abnormalities in patients with **hemimegalencephaly**, which include not only a hypertrophied hemisphere, but also abnormal gyration and thickened cortex (Kalifa *et al.*, 1987). However, as will be discussed below, functional neuroimaging also plays an important role in this condition and provides information not obtained with MRI.

In **tuberous sclerosis**, several studies have shown that MRI is more sensitive than CT in the detection of cortical tubers (Fig. 20.3), and therefore may be useful in screening potentially affected family members (Roach, Williams and Laster, 1987; Nixon *et al.*, 1989). However, the periventricular nodules which tend to calcify are often easier to detect with CT than MRI (Inoue *et al.*, 1988). Cusmai *et al.* (1990) related MRI with EEG findings in 34 children with tuberous sclerosis; 26 had MRI evidence of large tubers which tended to correspond to EEG foci, with complete concordance in 10. Frontal lobe tubers were not likely to be associated with EEG foci until after age 2 years, when cortical function in this region has achieved some degree of maturity (Chugani and Phelps, 1986; Chugani, Phelps and Mazziotta, 1987a).

Although the neurocutaneous syndrome **hypomelanosis of Ito** continues to be poorly understood, MRI studies have shown that abnormal neuronal migration may be an important feature of the syndrome and can often be characterized prior to autopsy (Ardinger and Bell, 1986; Glover, Brett and Atherton, 1989). This brief account on the contribution of MRI in syndromes of infancy and childhood associated with epilepsy does not even begin to do justice to the many new findings that have directly resulted from MRI technology. With further improvements in MRI techniques, it is likely that a new level of understanding of these and other syndromes of infancy and childhood will be reached.

MAGNETIC RESONANCE SPECTROSCOPY

Although MRS technology has been available in the laboratory for some time, it has only been recently adapted and applied *in vivo*. The technique uses MRI equipment and even the same radiofrequency coils, but is different from MRI in that it produces spectra which describe measurements of cellular energetics and metabolites. Proton (^{1}H) spectroscopy allows relative determinations of brain lactate and various lipids, whereas ^{31}P MRS is useful in the study of local high-energy phosphate levels *in vivo*.

Both these techniques have been applied in the study of seizures and epilepsy. Woods and Chiu (1990) applied localized ^{1}H MRS in patients before and after electroconvulsive therapy. Findings included small increases in lactate following treatment, and a large increase in lipid signal believed to be due to activation of the phosphatidylinositol second messenger system as a result of the seizures.

^{1}H MRS has also been applied in the study of chronic focal encephalitis (Rasmussen's syndrome) (Chapters 7, 15b). Decreased signal from *N*-acetyl compounds, such as *N*-acetylaspartate, in the area of encephalitis may be a hallmark of neuronal loss in the region, but requires further evaluation. During epilepsia partialis continua in one of the children studied, the lactate signal was increased in the area of seizure focus (Matthews, Andermann and Arnold, 1990).

In patients with temporal lobe seizures, ^{31}P MRS has been used as another noninvasive test to lateralize the seizure focus. The

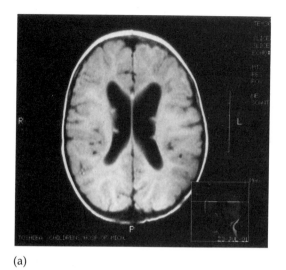

(a)

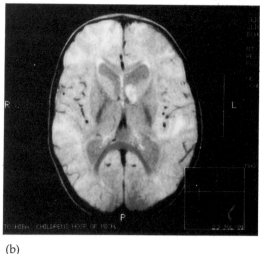

(b)

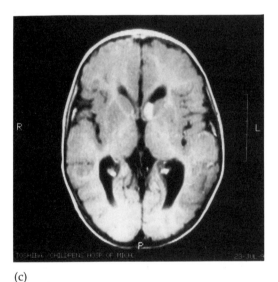

(c)

Fig. 20.3   MRI of a 1-year-old girl with tuberous sclerosis. (a) Nonenhanced axial image reveals subependymal tumors. No parenchymal lesions are seen in this section. (b) T_2-weighted axial image shows high signal intensity on the left with a giant cell astrocytoma in the region of the foramen of Monro. High signal intensity lesions are seen in the frontal and temporal areas suggestive of cortical tubers. (c) Contrast-enhanced axial T_1-weighted image shows the large giant cell astrocytoma with enhancement. Enhancement, however, does not necessarily indicate malignancy in this disease. (Courtesy of T. Slovis, MD, Children's Hospital of Michigan, Detroit.)

epileptogenic temporal lobe usually shows a decreased phosphocreatine/inorganic phosphate ratio compared both to controls and to the contralateral temporal lobe (Kuzniecky *et al.*, 1992). In all eight patients with temporal or frontal lobe epilepsy, ^{31}P MRS correctly lateralized the seizure focus, which showed increased alkalinity and inorganic phosphate and decreased phosphomonoesters (Hugg *et al.*, 1992). There is growing enthusiasm in applying MRS technology to the study of epilepsy, and it is hoped that important

neurochemical concepts of epileptogenesis and brain damage associated with epilepsy will be derived from such studies.

POSITRON EMISSION TOMOGRAPHY

(PET) is a noninvasive imaging method which can be used to measure local chemical functions in various body organs. The application of PET in the evaluation of children with epilepsy has had a significant impact on management, particularly when the epilepsy is refractory to pharmacotherapy and surgical intervention is being considered (see also Chapter 23d).

The success of epilepsy surgery is largely due to the identification of discrete epileptogenic foci that are lateralized to, or localized in, one hemisphere. In infants, particularly, the clinical and EEG features of seizures arising from a single focus are often difficult to differentiate from seizures that arise from multiple bilateral and diffuse foci. When the MRI fails to show a discrete lesion in intractable epilepsy, interictal and ictal scalp EEG localization is insufficient to permit proceeding to surgery and must, therefore, be confirmed by chronic intracranial EEG monitoring with depth or subdural electrodes. The noninvasive localization of the epileptic focus by PET with the tracer 2-deoxy-2[^{18}F]fluoro-D-glucose (FDG) eliminates the need for chronic invasive EEG monitoring in the majority of children undergoing epilepsy surgery. By fulfilling a similar role to the MRI, when the latter fails to show a lesion, PET provides a useful guide to the type of resection to be performed. Furthermore, PET can provide an assessment of the functional integrity of brain regions outside the epileptogenic area.

BASIC CONCEPTS OF PET METHODOLOGY

The PET technique employs a camera consisting of multiple pairs of oppositely situated detectors which are used to record the paired high energy (511 KeV) photons traveling in opposite directions as a result of positron decay (Hoffman and Phelps, 1986). Tracer kinetic models, which mathematically describe physiologic or biochemical reaction sequences of compounds labeled with positron-emitting isotopes, permit a characterization of the kinetics and the mathematic expression for calculating actual rates of the biologic process being studied (Huang and Phelps, 1986). The short half-life (minutes to hours) of the isotopes commonly used in PET, make it essential that the cyclotron used to generate these isotopes is situated either on-site or within 1–2 hours' driving distance from the PET scanning facility. The clinical and research applications of PET methodology have been steadily increasing, and over 300 substrates and drugs labeled with positron emitters are available for the study of various biologic functions *in vivo* (Fowler and Wolf, 1986). In the brain, PET has been applied in the study of local glucose and oxygen utilization, blood flow, protein synthesis, and neurotransmitter uptake and binding (Phelps and Mazziotta, 1985).

TEMPORAL LOBE EPILEPSY

In adults and children with temporal lobe epilepsy, studies performed with FDG-PET during the interictal period have identified areas of decreased glucose utilization (Fig. 20.4); these areas of 'hypometabolism' correspond anatomically with pathologic and depth electrode EEG localization of epileptogenic lesions (Engel *et al.*, 1982; Abou-Khalil *et al.*, 1987). Although ictal PET studies often reveal complex patterns of increased glucose metabolism, focal hypermetabolism may sometimes be seen on interictal PET scans in the presence of an active focal epileptiform discharge on the EEG (Chugani *et al.*, 1993a).

The sensitivity of PET in identifying the epileptic focus in patients with temporal lobe epilepsy is approximately the same as that in depth-electrode recording. However, PET is far less costly and is not associated with the morbidity and mortality of electrode implants. The application of FDG-PET in the presurgical evaluation of temporal lobe epilepsy patients has led to a significant reduction in the need for invasive EEG monitoring (Engel *et al.*, 1990; Theodore *et al.*, 1992). The sensitivity of FDG-PET may be further increased by activation procedures such as performance of a speech discrimination task during the tracer uptake period (Bromfield *et al.*, 1991), but these preliminary findings require further study and confirmation. On the other hand,

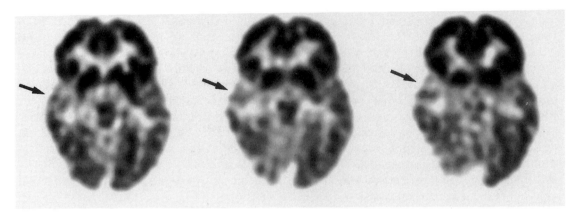

Fig. 20.4   PET scan of cerebral glucose metabolism of a 5-year-old boy with probable temporal lobe epilepsy, nonlateralizing interictal EEG, and a normal MRI. Glucose metabolic activity is decreased in the right temporal neocortex (arrows).

recent advances (reviewed earlier in this chapter) in analysis techniques of MRI have shown that **quantitative** MRI is very sensitive in detecting hippocampal atrophy in temporal lobe epilepsy, and will probably eliminate the need for invasive EEG monitoring in the majority of affected patients. Furthermore, with the greater availability of MRI compared to PET, it is likely that, in future, PET will be reserved only for those cases in which the MRI fails to provide the necessary localization.

The presence of temporal lobe hypometabolism may provide prognostic information about the success of temporal lobectomy. Radtke *et al.* (1993) found that both the degree and extent of temporal lobe hypometabolism correlated with a favorable surgical outcome. However, at least two other studies have not found any differences in outcome between patients who showed temporal lobe hypometabolism on PET and patients with a normal or nonlocalizing PET pattern (Engel, Babb and Phelps, 1987; Theodore *et al.*, 1990). An important recent finding relating temporal lobe hypometabolism to prognosis was that memory impairment, as determined by the intracarotid amobarbital procedure, was never present

contralateral to the side of hypometabolism, but was found ipsilateral to hypometabolism in as many as 65% of patients (Salanova *et al.*, 1992).

Attempts have been made, using FDG-PET, to distinguish between the metabolic patterns of seizure onset from mesial and lateral temporal lobe regions. One distinguishing feature is that, in patients with mesial gliosis, glucose metabolism in the entire temporal lobe was much lower than in patients who had lateral temporal onset of seizures, which were associated with only mild hypometabolism in the mesial temporal region (Hajek *et al.*, 1993).

EXTRATEMPORAL EPILEPSY

There are very few studies which have evaluated the use of FDG-PET in frontal lobe epilepsy occurring in older children and adults. The general experience with seizures of frontal lobe origin is that, in the absence of a discrete lesion or focal atrophy in the frontal lobe, the PET is usually normal. However, Swartz *et al.* (1989), who studied 22 patients with frontal lobe epilepsy, found 32% showed CT and 45% MRI abnormalities. Focal, regional or hemispheric hypometabolism was seen in 64% of patients, and correlated with electroclinical ictal localization. These findings have not been confirmed by other investigators.

When onset of frontal lobe seizures is in the neonatal period or in infancy, an underlying structural lesion is often present even when the MRI is normal. Under these circumstances, the FDG-PET can be useful in defining an area of hypometabolism which correlates both with the extent of microdysgenesis (Chugani *et al.*, 1988) and the area of epileptogenicity (Olson *et al.*, 1990).

INFANTILE SPASMS (see also Chapter 11b)

PET studies of cerebral glucose utilization have revolutionized the management of infants with intractable spasms and altered our concepts of their pathophysiology. Most infants diagnosed as having 'cryptogenic' spasms have focal cortical regions of decreased or increased glucose utilization on PET (Fig. 20.5). Focal ictal and/or interictal EEG abnormalities correspond to the PET focus in most of these cases (Chugani *et al.*, 1990). In infants with hypsarrythmia, these focal EEG abnormalities either precede or follow the presence of hypsarrythmia in the evolution of the infants' EEGs. When a single region of abnormal glucose utilization, corresponding to the EEG focus is apparent on PET and the seizures are intractable, surgical removal of the PET focus results not only in seizure control, but also in complete or partial reversal of the associated developmental delay. Of about 30 infants operated on at various centers thus far, about 75% are seizure free and most of the remainder are having far fewer seizures postoperatively. Most are developing much better, in contrast to the expectation of moderate to severe retardation based on their preoperative developmental decline. Neuropathologic examination of the resected tissue in the children who underwent surgery reveals that the epileptogenic zone is typically a previously unsus-

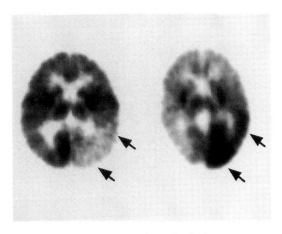

Fig. 20.5 PET images of cerebral glucose metabolism from two infants with intractable infantile spasms and normal MRI. The infant on the left (age 9 months) showed a focal area of hypometabolism involving the left occipital and temporal cortex (arrows). PET of the infant shown on the right (age 5 months) revealed hypermetabolism of the left occipital and temporal cortex (arrows). Scalp EEG showed epileptiform activity localized to the general region of the PET abnormality in each case. Both infants underwent surgical resection of the epileptogenic foci guided by PET and intraoperative corticography. Pathology revealed cortical dysplasia in both cases.

pected area of cortical dysplasia (Chugani *et al.*, 1990, 1993b).

Infantile spasms have been considered to be generalized seizures resulting from complex cortico-subcortical interactions. There has been considerable debate as to whether the spasms originate in the brainstem, basal ganglia, or cortex. PET studies have not only shown that cortical metabolic lesions are common in infants with spasms, but also that the lenticular nuclei and brainstem are often metabolically prominent (Fig. 20.6). Although the brainstem has been suspected of involvement in the generation of spasms, the lenticular nuclei findings are new and suggest that spasms result from focal or diffuse cortical abnormalities interacting with subcortical structures. Bilateral activation of the lenticular nuclei is consistent with the observation that infantile

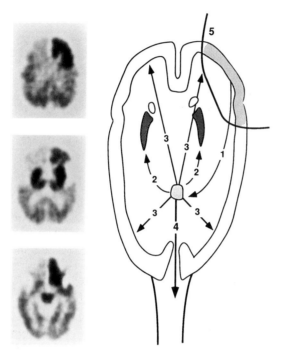

Fig. 20.6 The three PET images of cerebral glucose utilization on the left of the figure illustrate hypermetabolism of the left frontotemporal cortex, bilateral symmetric hypermetabolism of the lenticular nuclei, and the brainstem in a patient with intractable infantile spasms. On the right of the figure is a schematic diagram describing the proposed neuronal circuitry involved in the pathogenesis of infantile spasms: (1) noxious influence of abnormal cortical region on brainstem (raphe area); (2) raphe–striatal pathway, serotonergic (5HT$_{1D}$), under tonic control by corticosteroids; (3) generation of hypsarrhythmic pattern; (4) spinal cord propagation (direct or indirect) and lenticular nuclei involvement result in clinical infantile spasms; (5) surgical resection of primary cortical abnormality abolishes activation of circuitry.

spasms are clinically symmetric, even when focal cortical lesions are present. Thus, PET studies have significantly increased our understanding of the pathophysiology of infantile spasms. Based on these findings, the potential neuronal circuitry involved in the generation and propagation of infantile spasms has been proposed (Chugani *et al.*, 1992).

FURTHER CHILDHOOD EPILEPTIC AND OTHER SYNDROMES

PET scanning of cerebral glucose utilization has been applied in the study of a number of childhood epileptic syndromes other than infantile spasms. In children with **Lennox–Gastaut syndrome** (Chapter 12a), PET has provided a new classification based on metabolic anatomy. Four metabolic subtypes have been identified: unilateral focal, unilateral diffuse and bilateral diffuse hypometabolism, and normal patterns (Chugani *et al.*, 1987; Iinuma *et al.*, 1987; Theodore *et al.*, 1987). These glucose metabolic patterns may serve as a useful guide in determining the type of surgical intervention to be considered in those with uncontrolled seizures. Interestingly, there were no differences in glucose metabolic rates between PET studies performed during continuous slow spike-wave activity and studies in which there was minimal epileptiform activity on the EEG (Chugani *et al.*, 1987). This finding was confirmed in a later study on the effects of generalized spike and wave discharges on glucose metabolism (Ochs *et al.*, 1987).

In children and adults with advanced **Sturge–Weber syndrome** (Chapter 16), PET typically reveals widespread unilateral hypometabolism ipsilateral to the facial naevus in a distribution that extends beyond the abnormalities depicted on CT. In contrast, small infants (<1 year of age) with Sturge–Weber syndrome and recent seizure onset show a paradoxic pattern of increased glucose utilization in the cerebral cortex of the anatomically affected hemisphere, on interictal PET (Chugani, Mazziotta and Phelps, 1989). In Sturge–Weber syndrome patients with refractory epilepsy, PET has been useful both in guiding the extent of focal cortical resection (i.e. correlating better with intraoperative electrocorticography than CT or MRI) and in assessing candidacy for early hemispherectomy. Finally, PET provides not only a sensitive measure of the extent of early cerebral involvement in Sturge–Weber syndrome, but also a means of monitoring disease progression (Chugani and Dietrich, 1992).

Interictally, cortical tubers in **tuberous sclerosis** (Chapter 16) appear as hypometabolic areas on PET scanning (Szelies *et al.*, 1983), presumably due to the simplified dendritic arborization within tubers. When the PET study is performed ictally, the tuber is seen as a hypermetabolic zone. Some hypometabolic regions on PET do not correspond to abnormalities on CT and MR scans, and may either represent small tubers or be related to epileptogenic mechanisms.

Hemimegalencephaly is a rare developmental brain malformation characterized by congenital hypertrophy of one cerebral hemisphere and ipsilateral ventriculomegaly. When the epilepsy is medically uncontrolled, cerebral hemispherectomy is recommended. However, irrespective of seizure control postoperatively, hemimegalencephalic children, as a group, have a worse developmental outcome when compared to children who have had hemispherectomies for Sturge–Weber syndrome or chronic focal encephalitis of Rasmussen. PET studies of cerebral glucose metabolism have indicated that the worse developmental outcome in hemimegalencephaly is related to the presence of focal areas of cortical dysfunction in the remaining hemisphere, and that preoperative assessment with PET of the integrity of the less affected hemisphere may provide important prognostic information (Rintahaka *et al.*, 1993).

An FDG-PET study during sleep in three children with **acquired epileptic aphasia (Landau–Kleffner syndrome**; Chapter 13d) confirmed the general notion that this condition is heterogeneous. Metabolic disturbances consisting of hypermetabolism or hypometabolism were seen during sleep in the temporal lobes, and were right-sided, left-sided, or bilateral (Maquet *et al.*, 1990).

EFFECTS OF ANTICONVULSANTS ON CEREBRAL GLUCOSE UTILIZATION

PET with FDG has been used to evaluate the effects of a number of anticonvulsant drugs on regional cerebral glucose metabolism, in order to gain a better understanding of mechanisms of action and toxicity. Barbiturates such as **phenobarbitone** and **primidone** had a large effect on cerebral glucose metabolism in seven of eight cortical regions analyzed, with a mean reduction of 37% (Theodore *et al.*, 1986a). **Phenytoin** decreased overall cerebral glucose metabolism by 13%, with the parietal and frontal cortex showing significant reductions (Theodore *et al.*, 1986b). **Carbamazepine** caused a 12% mean reduction of cerebral glucose metabolism, with the most significant changes in bilateral superior frontal, left parietal, right superior temporal, right caudate, and left cerebellar regions (Theodore, Bromfield and Onorati, 1989). **Valproate** reduced global cerebral glucose metabolism by 22% and significantly lowered metabolic rates in 15 of 26 regions analyzed (Leiderman *et al.*, 1991). None of these studies examined the relationship between the effects on brain metabolism and neuropsychologic function.

NEUROTRANSMITTER RECEPTOR PET

As illustrated above, the application of FDG-PET in the study of epilepsy has been rewarding and has altered management in many instances. However, FDG is but one of many potential chemical probes that can be applied quantitatively with PET technology. Based on several preliminary studies, there is now considerable enthusiasm for the further development, and application of a number of neurotransmitter receptors believed to be important in mechanisms of epilepsy.

Opioid mechanisms in the brain are believed to play an important role in epilepsy, particularly postictal phenomena (Chugani *et al.*, 1984). The application of PET using ^{11}C-carfentanil, a ligand with high affinity for mu-opiate receptors, in patients with temporal lobe epilepsy has shown that opiate receptor binding is increased in the temporal neocortex ipsilateral to the seizure focus compared to the opposite side, and correlated directly with a decrease in glucose metabolism. No asymmetries of receptor binding were observed in mesial temporal structures. The authors suggested that the observed temporal neocortical increase may represent a tonic inhibition of epileptogenicity in surrounding structures (Frost *et al.*, 1988). Further studies from the same group have shown that increased ^{11}C-carfentanil binding in temporal neocortex is associated with decreased binding in the amygdala ipsilateral to the seizure focus. Moreover, when PET was performed with ^{11}C-diprenorphine, which binds not only to mu-opiate but also to kappa- and delta-opiate receptors, there were no significant differences in binding between the epileptic focus and the contralateral temporal lobe (Mayberg *et al.*, 1991).

Using ^{11}C-doxepin, an antidepressant with a high affinity for histamine H1 receptors, Iinuma and colleagues (1993) documented increased binding in the temporal neocortex ipsilateral to the epileptic focus in eight of nine patients with complex partial seizures of temporal or frontal lobe origin. Since histamine in the brain is involved in termination of seizures and may function as an endogenous anticonvulsant, the investigators postulated that the increased binding may represent a defensive mechanism counteracting the spread of epileptic discharges.

PET studies of the benzodiazepine receptor using the antagonist ^{11}C-Ro 15–1788 (flumazenil) have shown that patients with partial epilepsy have a significantly reduced binding in the epileptic focus (Savic *et al.*, 1988). This is in contrast to patients with generalized epilepsy, in whom no significant changes in binding could be demonstrated, compared to brain regions outside the epileptic focus in patients with partial epilepsy (Savic *et al.*, 1990). Whether there is an absolute decrease

in benzodiazepine receptor binding in generalized epilepsy compared to controls remains to be determined.

SINGLE PHOTON EMISSION COMPUTED TOMOGRAPHY

Single photon emission computed tomography (SPECT) is a noninvasive functional imaging technique that uses simpler and less expensive equipment than PET. It provides tomographic imaging through the use of either a single rapidly rotating gamma camera or multiple cameras to detect and reconstruct gamma ray emissions (Ell *et al.*, 1987). As a result of the longer half-life of SPECT isotopes compared to those used in PET, and the readily available equipment, SPECT is suited for even the smallest hospitals and clinics. The isotopes can be obtained commercially and can be stored on site. However, the spatial resolution of SPECT images is about half that achieved with PET, a distinction which is particularly relevant in pediatric studies. The localizing value of SPECT in children with epilepsy is usually limited to detecting the involved lobe. Furthermore, SPECT techniques are semiquantitative at best, whereas PET is fully quantitative.

In brain studies, SPECT has been used primarily to provide an index of cerebral blood flow. Radioactive probes developed for this purpose have included the iodoamines, xenon, and technetium-99m hexamethyl propylene amine oxime (^{99m}Tc-HMPAO). When ictal and postictal localization of seizure foci are desired, SPECT studies are particularly useful for several reasons. For example, the iodoamines freely pass through the blood–brain barrier and reach peak concentrations in the brain approximately 20 minutes following intravenous administration. The iodoamine HIPDM reaches 75% of its peak brain concentration at 2 minutes after injection. Scanning of the brain can be initiated at leisure after the brain uptake phase because the trapped agent remains relatively stable for at least 1 hour, and the isotopes used in SPECT have a rather long half-life (e.g. [123]I has a half-life of 13 hours). In contrast, because of the short half-life of PET isotopes (e.g. 108 minutes for ^{18}F and 20 minutes for ^{11}C), it is extremely difficult to achieve planned ictal and postictal PET studies. Furthermore, ictal PET studies with FDG typically include a prolonged postictal phase as well as the ictus to yield a summation of the two phases, and are therefore often difficult to interpret.

PARTIAL EPILEPSY

After the demonstrastion of interictal hypometabolism and ictal hypermetabolism in the seizure focus with PET technology, a number of investigators attempted to replicate these findings with SPECT determinations of cerebral perfusion. Magistretti *et al.* (1982) showed ictal hyperperfusion of the seizure focus in a single patient studied with ^{123}I-iodoamphetamine SPECT. Using [133]xenon-SPECT in 12 of 18 patients with epilepsy, Bonte *et al.* (1983) showed interictal focal hypoperfusion and enhanced flow to an active seizure focus. In a further study on 50 patients with partial seizures, the same group reported a significant correlation between the position of interictal SPECT hypoperfusion and the location of neuropsychologic deficits revealed by the Halstead–Reitan Battery (Homan *et al.*, 1989). The roles of interictal, ictal, and postictal SPECT studies in epilepsy have all been investigated in relation to clinical utility.

There have been many **interictal** SPECT studies (Fig. 20.7) performed on children. Using ^{123}I-iodoamphetamine and SPECT, Denays *et al.* (1988) evaluated 14 children with a variety of seizure types. Of the nine children who had normal CT scans, five had SPECT abnormalities including focal hypoperfusion, diffuse hemispheric hypoperfusion, multifocal and bilateral hypoperfusion, and focal hyperperfusion. In this study, children with normal SPECT scans had a better overall prognosis than those with

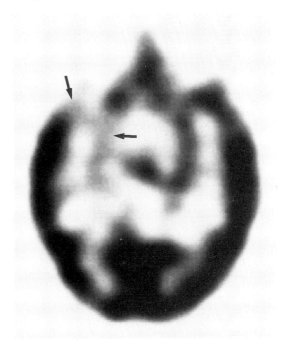

Fig. 20.7 Four-year-old girl with complex partial epilepsy. Transaxial view of interictal brain SPECT scan with ^{99m}Tc-HMPAO demonstrates decreased perfusion of anterior pole and mesial cortex of the right temporal lobe (arrows). (Courtesy of S. Kottamasu, MD, Children's Hospital of Michigan, Detroit.)

blood flow abnormalities. Also using ^{123}I-iodoamphetamine, Dietrich *et al.* (1991) reported that in 23 patients with complex partial seizures, SPECT revealed focal hypoperfusion in 21 cases, of whom 15 had good correspondence between SPECT and EEG foci. Four patients had multifocal SPECT abnormalities and two had discordance between SPECT and EEG localization. Ryvlin *et al.* (1992a) found that in temporal lobe epilepsy, ^{99m}Tc-HMPAO-SPECT hypoperfusion of the temporal lobe was more frequently seen when the MRI showed a nonspecific abnormality compared to when the MRI was normal. All 18 patients in this latter study had normal CT scans. In another ^{99m}Tc-HMPAO-SPECT study of 14 children with frequent seizures, the typical finding in 11 patients with partial secondary generalized seizures was a single hypoperfused area; three children with Lennox–Gastaut syndrome had multiple areas of hypoperfusion and a worse clinical outcome. SPECT was more sensitive than EEG, CT, or MRI in detecting abnormalities (Heiskala *et al.*, 1993).

Interictal SPECT has also been used in children with less malignant types of seizures. One such study showed that two children with complex febrile seizures among 19 presenting with febrile seizures had focal perfusion abnormalities on interictal SPECT using ^{99m}Tc-HMPAO. Of the 17 children who had simple febrile convulsions, nine also had focal perfusion abnormalities on SPECT. Abnormal perfusion typically involved frontotemporal regions, and was more often seen in children with EEG abnormalities and in those studied within 12 days of the seizure (Dierckx *et al.*, 1992).

Ictal SPECT appears to be more sensitive in detecting the epileptic focus than interictal studies in both temporal lobe and extratemporal epilepsy (Fig. 20.8). One group of investigators performed HIPDM-SPECT on 16 patients with refractory complex partial seizures; they were able to show the hyperperfused epileptic focus in 13 of 14 patients who had a unilateral temporal seizure onset. However, in two patients with bitemporal EEG foci, SPECT showed bilateral multifocal areas of increased blood flow which were difficult to interpret (Lee *et al.*, 1988). Ictal SPECT with ^{99m}Tc-HMPAO has proved to be useful in evaluating epilepsy with temporal and frontocentral onset, showing hyperperfusion which corresponded to EEG and structural localization in six of nine patients (Stefan *et al.*, 1990). In patients who exhibit ictal dystonia in one limb during a seizure, relative hyperperfusion of the basal ganglia contralateral to the side of dystonia was seen. Basal ganglia hyperperfusion was most marked if the tracer was injected during the dystonic episode (Newton *et al.*, 1992). Harvey *et al.*

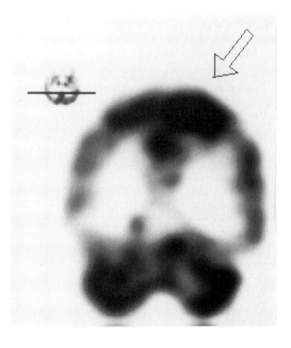

Fig. 20.8 Seven-year-old boy with intractable partial epilepsy. Coronal view of ictal brain SPECT following intravenous injection of ^{99m}Tc-HMPAO 3 minutes after seizure onset demonstrates a focus of intensely increased perfusion in the left high parietal cortex (arrow). (Courtesy of S. Kottamasu, MD, Children's Hospital of Michigan, Detroit.)

(1993) found that ictal studies were informative in 16 of 17 studies in 14 of 15 children with temporal lobe epilepsy, corresponding well with ictal EEG, MRI, and pathology. In contrast, temporal lobe hypoperfusion seen interictally often proved to be difficult to interpret because it tended to be less well localized and was sometimes bilateral.

Marks *et al.* (1992) found ictal ^{99m}Tc-HMPAO-SPECT to be a valuable tool in the localization of extratemporal epileptic foci. A well-circumscribed area of increased perfusion was the most common finding, and was particularly useful in patients with nonlocalizing ictal EEG. Similarly, in two children with focal cortical dysplasias in the frontal regions and nonlocalizing EEG, ictal ^{99m}Tc-

HMPAO-SPECT proved to be invaluable in providing the necessary localizing data to proceed to surgical resection (Kuzniecky *et al.*, 1993c).

Postictal SPECT studies have been found to be superior to interictal SPECT by some investigators (Rowe *et al.*, 1989). Of 78 seizures studied with HMPAO-SPECT in 51 patients with temporal lobe epilepsy, increased uptake, mainly in the anteromesial temporal region, was seen in 83% of patients during the first several minutes following the seizure. In 80% of studies, the mesial temporal hyperperfusion was accompanied by hypoperfusion in the lateral temporal cortex and other areas of the ipsilateral cortex corresponding to both the degree and the extent of postictal slow wave activity on the EEG. Such postictal hypoperfusion may last up to 20 minutes. As a result of postictal SPECT, the unilateral seizure focus could be localized correctly in 31 of 45 patients (Rowe *et al.*, 1991).

Other applications of SPECT in epilepsy have included the evaluation of the status of hemispheric blood flow during the Wada test. In one such study, Ryding *et al.* (1989) showed that the timing of ^{99m}Tc-HMPAO injection should be about 30 seconds after the onset of the barbiturate effect in order to best visualize the low-flow regions. Acute cerebellar hypoperfusion contralateral to the side of barbiturate injection was also detected, indicating a diaschisis phenomenon.

SYNDROMES ASSOCIATED WITH EPILEPSY

As in the case of PET, there have been many studies of the use of brain SPECT in various syndromes of infancy and childhood, some of which will be reviewed here. In two children with **hemimegalencephaly**, iofetamine-SPECT performed interictally showed a similar pattern of decreased perfusion in the malformed hemisphere (Konkol *et al.*, 1990), despite the very different EEG findings between the two patients, implying different prognoses, as suggested by Paladin *et al.* (1989).

Chiron *et al.* (1989) have studied patterns of interictal brain perfusion in children with **Sturge–Weber syndrome** using ^{133}xenon-SPECT. In 10 such patients, they found areas of decreased perfusion corresponding topographically to the CT scan abnormality. However, they documented focal hypoperfusion with SPECT in another three patients with no obvious focus on CT scan. The investigators suggested that focal hypoperfusion may have been the result of chronic ischemia and postictal mechanisms.

Focal areas of cortical hypoperfusion have been detected with ^{133}xenon-SPECT in patients with **West's syndrome** (Dulac *et al.*, 1987). In a further study, it was shown that mean cerebral blood flow decreased just after steroid treatment (Chiron *et al.*, 1993). In addition, areas of hypoperfusion appeared to be static in longitudinal studies, as had been shown with FDG-PET (Chugani *et al.*, 1990), whereas frontal regions of increased perfusion tended to diminish as the spasms became controlled. Yet another study showed that focal SPECT hypoperfusion in the parieto-occipital region is often associated with visual inattention at the time when the infants present with West's syndrome, and with long-term cognitive compromise (Jambaque *et al.*, 1993). This latter finding is of particular importance when focal cortical resection is being considered as a treatment option for intractable infantile spasms (Chugani *et al.*, 1990, 1993b).

NEURORECEPTOR STUDIES WITH SPECT

Compared to PET, there has been relatively little success in the development of suitable SPECT probes for the evaluation of neurotransmitter receptor abnormalities in epilepsy. In one study, muscarinic cholinergic receptor imaging with ^{123}I-iododexetimide and SPECT in four patients with complex partial seizures revealed decreased hippocampal binding by 40 ± 9% (mean ± SD), compared to the contralateral hippocampus (Muller-Gartner *et al.*, 1993).

COMPARISON OF CT, MRI, PET, AND SPECT

A number of studies have compared the ability of various imaging modalities to localize the area of epileptogenicity in the brain. For the most part, these comparative studies were performed on patients with refractory partial seizures who were being evaluated for surgical treatment.

In 35 patients with intractable complex partial seizures and nonfocal CT, Sperling *et al.* (1986) found lesions on MRI in seven patients; three of these also had FDG-PET studies, which were normal in all. Of the 18 patients with mesial temporal sclerosis on pathology, all had normal MRI, but 10 had temporal lobe hypometabolism. This study was conducted prior to the application of hippocampal volumetric measurements on MRI.

Among 20 children with partial epilepsy who had surgery, CT findings correlated with EEG foci in 14. MRI was more sensitive than CT and correlated with EEG foci in 13 out of 14 children who had the procedure performed. ^{99m}Tc-HmPAO-SPECT performed interictally showed cortical perfusion abnormalities that correlated with EEG foci in 14 of 20 children, whereas the combination of interictal and postictal SPECT studies detected the seizure focus in 16 of 20 (Adams *et al.*, 1992).

Latack *et al.* (1986) compared CT, MRI and FDG-PET in 50 patients with partial seizures, four of whom had surgery. Focal abnormalities were detected by CT in 13 and by MRI in 23 of the 50 patients. All of the 10 CT lesions were also detected by MRI. Only 14 patients were evaluated with FDG-PET; of these, metabolic asymmetries were present in 10 patients, seven of whom had a structural lesion on MRI.

The study of Ryvlin *et al.* (1992b) compared interictal FDG-PET with ^{99m}Tc-HMPAO-SPECT in temporal lobe epilepsy. In 20 patients with clear unilateral temporal lobe foci on EEG, MRI showed nonspecific abnormalities in the epileptogenic temporal lobe in 10, and was normal in the remaining 10. PET showed focal hypometabolism in eight and SPECT showed focal hypoperfusion in two of the 10 patients with normal MRI. Of the 10 subjects with abnormal MRI, PET showed hypometabolism in all, whereas SPECT detected hypoperfusion in nine.

A retrospective analysis on nine children with focal cortical dysplasia revealed MRI evidence of poor gray/white matter differentiation or pachygyria in six, interictal focal hypoperfusion with HmPAO-SPECT in four, and postictal SPECT hyperperfusion in two (Otsubo *et al.*, 1993).

The extent of epileptiform abnormalities determined with EEG generally exceeds that defined by MRI, and in some cases may even involve regions remote from the structural abnormality. Similarly, interictal PET glucose hypometabolism exceeds the extent of anatomic abnormalities on CT and MRI (Theodore *et al.*, 1986c). Nevertheless, it has been demonstrated that postoperative seizure control can usually be achieved with total resection of the lesion (Palmini *et al.*, 1991b; Awad *et al.*, 1991). Although there is some suggestion that high resolution functional neuroimaging with PET provides a good estimate of the epileptogenic zone in children with underlying microscopic structural abnormalities (Olson *et al.*, 1990), large studies comparing various imaging and electrographic modalities are not available.

CONCLUSION

In this chapter, it has been demonstrated that the evolution of various neuroimaging modalities has had a great impact on the diagnosis, treatment, and prognostic implications of epilepsy in infants and children. In many cases, imaging has led directly to new treatment options which were previously not considered. Of particular importance has been the development of MRI and functional neuroimaging techniques, which have opened up many research opportunities and led to increased surgical approaches for the child with intractable epilepsy. It should be emphasized that in most cases, anatomic and functional neuroimaging are complementary and should be carefully used together in the optimal management of the child with epilepsy.

REFERENCES

Abou-Khalil, B.W., Siegel, G.J., Sackellares, J.C. *et al.* (1987) Positron emission tomography studies of cerebral glucose metabolism in chronic partial epilepsy. *Annals of Neurology*, **22**, 480–6.

Adams, C., Hwang, P.A., Gilday, D.L. *et al.* (1992) Comparison of SPECT, EEG, CT, MRI, and pathology in partial epilepsy. *Pediatric Neurology*, **8**, 97–103.

Aicardi, J. (1991) The agyria–pachygyria complex: a spectrum of cortical malformations. *Brain and Development*, **13**, 1–8.

Ardinger, H.H. and Bell, W.E. (1986) Hypomelanosis of Ito: Wood's light and magnetic resonance imaging as diagnostic measures. *Archives of Neurology*, **43**, 848–50.

Astiazaran, A.G., Luna, N.L., Ruiz, M.G. and Suastegui, R. A. R. (1993) Neurocysticercosis in childhood: clinical and pharmacological features, in *New Trends in Pediatric Neurology* (eds N. Fejerman and N.A. Chamoles), Elsevier, Amsterdam, pp. 299–306.

Awad, I.A., Rosenfeld, J., Ahl, J. *et al.* (1991) Intractable epilepsy and structural lesions of the brain: mapping, resection strategies, and seizure outcome. *Epilepsia*, **32**, 179–86.

Babb, T.L. and Brown, W.J. (1987) Pathological findings in epilepsy, in *Surgical Treatment of the Epilepsies* (ed J. Engel, Jr), Raven, New York, pp. 511–40.

Bachman, D.S., Hodges, F.J. and Freeman, J.M. (1976) Computerized axial tomography in chronic seizure disorders of childhood. *Pediatrics*, **58**, 828–31.

Barkovich, A.J., Chuang, S.H. and Norman, D. (1988) MR of neuronal migration anomalies. *American Journal of Roentgenology*, **150**, 179–87.

Barkovich, A.J., Jackson, D.E. Jr and Boyer, R.S. (1989) Band heterotopias: a newly recognized neuronal migration anomaly. *Radiology*, **171**, 455–8.

Bentson, J.R., Wilson, G.H. and Newton, T.H. (1971) Cerebral venous drainage pattern of the Sturge–Weber syndrome. *Radiology*, **101**, 111–8.

Berkovic, S.F., Andermann, F., Melanson, D. *et al.* (1988) Hypothalamic hamartomas and ictal laughter: evolution of a characteristic epileptic syndrome and diagnostic value of magnetic resonance imaging. *Annals of Neurology*, **23**, 429–39.

Berkovic, S.F., Andermann, F., Olivier, A. *et al.* (1991) Hippocampal sclerosis in temporal lobe epilepsy demonstrated by magnetic resonance imaging. *Annals of Neurology*, **29**, 175–82.

Bonte, F.J., Stokely, E.M., Devous, M.D. *et al.* (1983) Single-photon tomographic study of regional cerebral blood flow in epilepsy: a preliminary report. *Archives of Neurology*, **40**, 267–270.

Breningstall, G.N. (1985) Gelastic seizures, precocious puberty, and hypothalamic hamartoma. *Neurology*, **35**, 1180–3.

Bromfield, E.B., Ludlow, C.L., Sedory, S. *et al.* (1991) Cerebral activation during speech discrimination in temporal lobe epilepsy. *Epilepsy Research*, **9**, 49–58.

Bronen, R.A. (1992) Epilepsy: the role of MR imaging. *American Journal of Roentgenology*, **159**, 1165–74.

Bye, A.M.E., Andermann, F., Robitaille, Y. *et al.* (1993) Cortical vascular abnormalities in the syndrome of celiac disease, epilepsy, bilateral occipital calcifications, and folate deficiency. *Annals of Neurology*, **34**, 399–403.

Cascino, G.D., Jack, C.R. Jr, Parisi, J.E. *et al.* (1991) MRI-based volume studies in temporal lobe epilepsy: pathological correlations. *Annals of Neurology*, **30**, 31–6.

Cascino, G.D., Jack, C.R. Jr, Parisi, J.E. *et al.* (1992) MRI in the presurgical evaluation of patients with frontal lobe epilepsy and children with temporal lobe epilepsy: pathologic correlation and prognostic importance. *Epilepsy Research*, **11**, 51–9.

Cendes, F., Andermann, F., Gloor, P. *et al.* (1993a) MRI volumetric measurement of amygdala and hippocampus in temporal lobe epilepsy. *Neurology*, **43**, 719–25.

Cendes, F., Andermann, F., Dubeau, F. *et al.* (1993b) Early childhood prolonged febrile convulsions, atrophy and sclerosis of mesial structures, and temporal lobe epilepsy: an MRI volumetric study. *Neurology*, **43**, 1083–7.

Chiron, C., Raynaud, C., Tzourio, N. *et al.* (1989) Regional cerebral blood flow by SPECT imaging in Sturge–Weber disease: an aid for diagnosis. *Journal of Neurology, Neurosurgery and Psychiatry*, **52**, 1402–9.

Chiron, C., Dulac, O., Bulteau, C. *et al.* (1993) Study of regional cerebral blood flow in West syndrome. *Epilepsia*, **34**, 707–15.

Chugani, H.T. and Dietrich, R.B. (1992) Sturge–Weber syndrome: recent developments in neuroimaging and surgical considerations, in *Fetal and Perinatal Neurology* (eds Y. Fukuyama, Y. Suzuki, S. Kamoshita and P. Casaer), Karger, Basel, pp. 187–96.

Chugani, H.T. and Phelps, M.E. (1986) Maturational changes in cerebral function in infants determined by [18]FDG positron emission tomography. *Science*, **231**, 840–3.

Chugani, H.T., Phelps, M.E. and Mazziotta, J.C. (1987) Positron emission tomography study of human brain functional development. *Annals of Neurology*, **22**, 487–97.

Chugani, H.T., Mazziotta, J.C. and Phelps, M.E. (1989) Sturge–Weber syndrome: a study of cerebral glucose utilization with positron emission tomography. *Journal of Pediatrics*, **114**, 244–53.

Chugani, H.T., Ackermann, R.F., Chugani, D.C. *et al.* (1984) Opioid-induced epileptogenic phenomena: anatomical, behavioral, and electroencephalographic features. *Annals of Neurology*, **15**, 361–8.

Chugani, H.T., Mazziotta, J.C., Engel, J. Jr and Phelps, M.E. (1987) The Lennox–Gastaut syndrome: metabolic subtypes determined by 2-deoxy-2[^{18}F]fluoro-D-glucose positron emission tomography. *Annals of Neurology*, **21**, 4–13.

Chugani, H.T., Shewmon, D.A., Peacock, W.J. *et al.* (1988) Surgical treatment of intractable neonatal-onset seizures: the role of positron emission tomography. *Neurology*, **38**, 1178–88.

Chugani, H.T., Shields, W.D., Shewmon, D.A., *et al.* (1990) Infantile spasms: I. PET identifies focal cortical dysgenesis in cryptogenic cases for surgical treatment. *Annals of Neurology*, **27**, 406–13.

Chugani, H.T., Shewmon, D.A., Sankar, R. *et al.* (1992) Infantile spasms: II. lenticular nuclei and brain stem activation on positron emission tomography. *Annals of Neurology*, **31**, 212–9.

Chugani, H.T., Shewmon, D.A., Khanna, S. *et al.* (1993a) Interictal and postictal focal hypermetabolism on positron emission tomography. *Pediatric Neurology*, **9**, 10–15.

Chugani, H.T., Shewmon, D.A., Shields, W.D. *et al.* (1993b) Surgery for intractable infantile spasms: neuroimaging perspectives. *Epilepsia* **34**, 764–71.

Cusmai, R., Chiron, C., Curatolo, P. *et al.* (1990) Topographic comparative study of magnetic resonance imaging and electroencephalography in 34 children with tuberous sclerosis. *Epilepsia*, **31**, 747–55.

D'Alessandro, R., Ferrara, R., Benassi, G. *et al.* (1988) Computed tomographic scans in post-traumatic epilepsy. *Archives of Neurology*, **45**, 42–3.

Denays, R., Rubinstein, M., Ham, H. *et al.* (1988) Single photon emission computed tomography in seizure disorders. *Archives of Disease in Childhood*, **63**, 1184–8.

Dierckx, R.A., Melis, K., Dom, L. *et al.* (1992) Technetium-99m hexamethylpropylene amine oxime single photon emission tomography in febrile convulsions. *European Journal of Nuclear Medicine*, **19**, 278–82.

Dietrich, M.E., Bergen, D., Smith, M.C. *et al.* (1991) Correlation of abnormalities of interictal *n*-isopropyl-*p*-iodoamphetamine single-photon emission tomography with focus of seizure onset in complex partial seizure disorders. *Epilepsia*, **32**, 187–94.

Duchowny, M.S., Resnick, T.J., Alvarez, L.A. and Morrison, G. (1990) Focal resection for malignant partial seizures in infancy. *Neurology*, **40**, 980–4.

Dulac, O., Chiron, C., Jambaque, I. *et al.* (1987) Infantile spasms. *Progress in Clinical Neuroscience*, **2**, 97–109.

Dunn, V., Mock, T., Bell, W.E. and Smith, W. (1986) Detection of heterotopic gray matter in children by magnetic resonance imaging. *Magnetic Resonance Imaging*, **4**, 33–9.

Ell, P.J., Jarritt, P.H., Costa, D.C. *et al.* (1987) Functional imaging of the brain. *Seminars in Nuclear Medicine*, **17**, 214–29.

Engel, J. Jr, Kuhl, D.E., Phelps, M.E. *et al.* (1982) Comparative localization of the epileptic foci in partial epilepsy by PCT and EEG. *Annals of Neurology*, **12**, 529–37.

Engel, J. Jr, Babb, T.L. and Phelps, M.E. (1987) Contributions of positron emission tomography to understanding mechanisms of epilepsy, in

Fundamental Mechanisms of Human Brain Function, (eds J.Engel, Jr, G.A. Ojemann, H.O. Luders and P.D. Williamson, Raven, New York, pp. 209–18.

Engel, J. Jr, Henry, T.R., Risinger, M.W. *et al.* (1990) Presurgical evaluation for partial epilepsy: relative contributions of chronic depth-electrode recordings versus FDG-PET and scalp-sphenoidal ictal EEG. *Neurology*, **40**, 1670–7.

Falconer, M.A. (1974) Mesial temporal (Ammon's horn) sclerosis as a common cause of epilepsy: aetiology, treatment and prevention. *Lancet*, **ii**, 767–70.

Fowler, J.S. and Wolf, A.P. (1986) Positron emitter-labeled compounds: priorities and problems, in *Positron Emission Tomography and Autoradiography: Principles and Applications for the Brain and Heart* (eds M.E. Phelps, J.C. Mazziotta and H.R. Schelbert), Raven, New York, pp. 391–450.

Frost, J.J., Mayberg, H.S., Fisher, R.S. *et al.* (1988) Mu-opiate receptors measured by positron emission tomography are increased in temporal lobe epilepsy. *Annals of Neurology*, **23**, 231–7.

Gastaut, H. and Gastaut, J.L. (1977) Computerized axial tomography in epilepsy, in *Epilepsy, the Eighth International Symposium* (ed. J.K. Penry), Raven Press, New York, pp. 5–15.

Glover, M.T., Brett, E.M. and Atherton, D.J. (1989) Hypomelanosis of Ito: spectrum of the disease. *Journal of Pediatrics*, **115**, 75–80.

Gobbi, G., Sorrenti, G., Santucci, M. *et al.* (1988) Epilepsy with bilateral occipital calcifications: a benign onset with progressive severity. *Neurology*, **38**, 913–20.

Guerrini, R., Dravet, C., Raybaud, C. *et al.* (1992a) Epilepsy and focal gyral anomalies detected by MRI: electroclinico-morphological correlations and follow-up. *Developmental Medicine and Child Neurology*, **34**, 706–18.

Guerrini, R., Dravet, C., Raybaud, C. *et al.* (1992b) Neurological findings and seizure outcome in children with bilateral opercular macrogyric-like changes detected by MRI. *Developmental Medicine and Child Neurology*, **34**, 694–705.

Hajek, M., Antonini, A., Leenders, K.L. and Wieser, H.G. (1993) Mesiobasal versus lateral temporal lobe epilepsy: metabolic differences in the temporal lobe shown by interictal ^{18}F-FDG positron emission tomography. *Neurology*, **43**, 79–86.

Hardiman, O., Burke, T., Phillips, J. *et al.* (1988) Microdysgenesis in resected temporal neo-cortex: incidence and clinical significance in focal epilepsy. *Neurology*, **38**, 1041–7.

Harvey, A.S., Bowe, J.M., Hopkins, I.J. *et al.* (1993) Ictal ^{99m}Tc-HMPAO single photon emission computed tomography in children with temporal lobe epilepsy. *Epilepsia*, **34**, 869–77.

Heiskala, H., Launes, J., Pihko, H. *et al.* (1993) Brain perfusion SPECT in children with frequent fits. *Brain and Development*, **15**, 214–8.

Hoffman, E.J. and Phelps, M.E. (1986) Positron emission tomography: principles and quantitation, in *Positron Emission Tomography and Autoradiography: Principles and Applications for the Brain and Heart* (eds M.E. Phelps, J.C. Mazziotta and H.R. Schelbert), Raven, New York, pp. 237–86.

Homan, R.W., Paulman, R.G., Devous, M.D. *et al.* (1989) Cognitive function and regional cerebral blood flow in partial seizures. *Archives of Neurology*, **46**, 964–70.

Huang, S.C. and Phelps, M.E. (1986) Principles of tracer kinetic modeling in positron emission tomography and autoradiography, in *Positron Emission Tomography and Autoradiography: Principles and Applications for the Brain and Heart* (eds M.E. Phelps, J.C. Mazziotta and H.R. Schelbert), Raven, New York, pp. 287–346.

Hugg, J.W., Laxer, K.D., Matson, G.B. *et al.* (1992) Lateralization of human focal epilepsy by ^{31}P magnetic resonance spectroscopic imaging. *Neurology*, **42**, 2011–8.

Iinuma, K., Yanai, K., Yanagisawa, T. *et al.* (1987) Cerebral glucose metabolism in five patients with Lennox–Gastaut syndrome. *Pediatric Neurology*, **3**, 12–8.

Iinuma, K., Yokoyama, H., Otsuki, T. *et al.* (1993) Histamine H_1 receptors in complex partial seizures. *Lancet*, **341**, 238.

Inoue, Y., Nakajima, S., Fukuda, T. *et al.* (1988) Magnetic resonance images of tuberous sclerosis: further observations and clinical correlations. *Neuroradiology*, **30**, 379–84.

Jabbari, B., Huott, A.D., DiChiro, G. *et al.* (1978) Surgically correctable lesions detected by CT in 143 patients with chronic epilepsy. *Surgical Neurology*, **10**, 319–22.

Jack, C.R. Jr, Sharbrough, F.W., Twomey, C.K. *et al.* (1990) Temporal lobe seizures: lateralization with MR volume measurements of hippocampal formation. *Radiology*, **175**, 423–9.

Jack, C.R. Jr, Sharbrough, F.W., Cascino, G.D. *et al.* (1992) Magnetic resonance imaging-based hippocampal volumetry: correlation with outcome after temporal lobectomy. *Annals of Neurology*, **31**, 138–46.

Jackson, G.D., Berkovic, S.F., Tress, B.M. *et al.* (1990) Hippocampal sclerosis can be reliably detected by magnetic resonance imaging. *Neurology*, **40**, 1869–75.

Jackson, G.D., Connelly, A., Duncan, J.S. *et al.* (1993) Detection of hippocampal pathology in intractable partial epilepsy: increased sensitivity with quantitative magnetic resonance T_2 relaxometry. *Neurology*, **43**, 1793–9.

Jacoby, C., Yuh, W., Afifi, A. *et al.* (1987) Accelerated myelination in early Sturge–Weber syndrome demonstrated by MR imaging. *Journal of Computer Assisted Tomography*, **11**, 226–31.

Jambaque, I., Chiron, C., Dulac, O. *et al.* (1993) Visual inattention in West syndrome: a neuropsychological and neurofunctional imaging study. *Epilepsia*, **34**, 692–700.

Kalifa, G.L., Chiron, C., Sellier, N. *et al.* (1987) Hemimegalencephaly: MR imaging in five children. *Radiology*, **165**, 29–33.

Konkol, R.J., Maister, B.H., Wells, R.G. and Sty, J.R. (1990) Hemimegalencephaly: clinical, EEG, neuroimaging, and IMP-SPECT correlation. *Pediatric Neurology*, **6**, 414–18.

Kuhl, D.E., Bevilacqua, J.E., Mishkin, M.M. and Sanders, T.P. (1972) The brain scan in Sturge–Weber syndrome. *Radiology*, **103**, 621–6.

Kuzniecky, R., de la Sayette, V., Ethier, R. *et al.* (1987) Magnetic resonance imaging in temporal lobe epilepsy: pathological correlations. *Annals of Neurology*, **22**, 341–7.

Kuzniecky, R., Berkovic, S., Andermann, F. *et al.* (1988) Focal cortical myoclonus and rolandic cortical dysplasia: clarification by magnetic resonance imaging. *Annals of Neurology*, **23**, 317–25.

Kuzniecky, R., Andermann, F., Tampieri, D. *et al.* (1989) Bilateral central macrogyria: epilepsy, pseudobulbar palsy, and mental retardation – a recognizable neuronal migration disorder. *Annals of Neurology*, **25**, 547–54.

Kuzniecky, R., Garcia, J.H., Faught, E. and Morawetz, R.B. (1991) Cortical dysplasia in temporal lobe epilepsy: magnetic resonance imaging correlations. *Annals of Neurology*, **29**, 293–8.

Kuzniecky, R., Elgavish, G.A., Hetherington, H.P. *et al.* (1992) *In vivo* ^{31}P nuclear magnetic resonance spectroscopy of human temporal lobe epilepsy. *Neurology*, **42**, 1586–90.

Kuzniecky, R., Burgard, S., Faught, E. *et al.*

(1993a) Predictive value of magnetic resonance imaging in temporal lobe epilepsy surgery. *Archives of Neurology*, **50**, 65–9.

Kuzniecky, R., Murro, A., King, D. *et al.* (1993b) Magnetic resonance imaging in childhood intractable partial epilepsies: pathologic correlations. *Neurology*, **43**, 681–7.

Kuzniecky, R., Mountz, J.M., Wheatley, G. and Morawetz, R. (1993c) Ictal single-photon emission computed tomography demonstrates localized epileptogenesis in cortical dysplasia. *Annals of Neurology*, **34**, 627–31.

Latack, J.T., Abou-Khalil, B.W., Siegel, G.J. *et al.* (1986) Patients with partial seizures: evaluation by MR, CT, and PET imaging. *Radiology*, **159**, 159–63.

Lee, B.I., Markand, O.N., Wellman, H.N., *et al.* (1988) HIPDM-SPECT in patients with medically intractable complex partial seizures: ictal study. *Archives of Neurology*, **45**, 397–402.

Leiderman, D.B., Balish, M., Bromfield, E.B. and Theodore, W.H. (1991) Effect of valproate on human cerebral glucose metabolism. *Epilepsia*, **32**, 417–22.

Lencz, T., McCarthy, G., Bronen, R.A. *et al.* (1992) Quantitative magnetic resonance imaging in temporal lobe epilepsy: relationship to neuropathology and neuropsychological function. *Annals of Neurology*, **31**, 629–37.

Lipski, S., Brunelle, F., Aicardi, J. *et al.* (1990) Gd-DOTA-enhanced MR imaging in two cases of Sturge–Weber syndrome. *American Journal of Neuroradiology*, **11**, 690–2.

Loring, D.W., Murro, A.M., Meador, K.J. *et al.* (1993) Wada memory testing and hippocampal volume measurements in the evaluation for temporal lobectomy. *Neurology*, **43**, 1789–93.

Magistretti, P., Uren, R., Blume, H. *et al.* (1982) Delineation of epileptic focus by single photon emission tomography. *European Journal of Nuclear Medicine*, **7**, 484–5.

Maki, Y. and Semba, A. (1979) Computed tomography of Sturge–Weber disease. *Childs Nervous System*, **5**, 51–61.

Maquet, P., Hirsch, E., Dive, D. *et al.* (1990) Cerebral glucose utilization during sleep in Landau–Kleffner syndrome: a PET study. *Epilepsia*, **31**, 778–3.

Marks, D.A., Katz, A., Hoffer, P. and Spencer, S.S. (1992) Localization of extratemporal epileptic foci during ictal single photon emission computed tomography. *Annals of Neurology*, **31**, 250–5.

Matthews, P.M., Andermann, F. and Arnold, D.L. (1990) A proton magnetic resonance spectroscopy study of focal epilepsy in humans. *Neurology*, **40**, 985–9.

Mayberg, H.S., Sadzot, B., Meltzer, C.C. *et al.* (1991) Quantification of mu and non-mu opiate receptors in temporal lobe epilepsy using positron emission tomography. *Annals of Neurology*, **30**, 3–11.

Muller-Gartner, H.W., Mayberg, H.S., Fisher, R.S. *et al.* (1993) Decreased hippocampal muscarinic cholinergic receptor binding measured by ^{123}I-iododexetimide and single-photon emission computed tomography in epilepsy. *Annals of Neurology*, **34**, 235–8.

Newton, M.R., Berkovic, S.F., Austin, M.C. *et al.* (1992) Dystonia, clinical lateralization, and regional blood flow changes in temporal lobe seizures. *Neurology*, **42**, 371–7.

Nixon, J.R., Houser, O.W., Gomez, M.R. and Okazaki, H. (1989) Cerebral tuberous sclerosis: MR imaging. *Radiology*, **170**, 869–73.

Ochs, R.F., Gloor, P., Tyler, J.L. *et al.* (1987) Effect of generalized spike-and-wave discharge on glucose metabolism measured by positron emission tomography. *Annals of Neurology*, **21**, 458–64.

Olson, D.M., Chugani, H.T., Shewmon, D.A. *et al.* (1990) Electrocorticographic confirmation of focal positron emission tomographic abnormalities in children with intractable epilepsy. *Epilepsia*, **31**, 731–9.

Otsubo, H., Hwang, P.A., Jay, V. *et al.* (1993) Focal cortical dysplasia in children with localization-related epilepsy: EEG, MRI, and SPECT findings. *Pediatric Neurology* **9**, 101–7.

Paladin, F., Chiron, C., Dulac, O. *et al.* (1989) Electroencephalographic aspects of hemimegalencephaly. *Developmental Medicine and Child Neurology*, **31**, 377–83.

Palmini, A., Andermann, F., Aicardi, J. *et al.* (1991a) Diffuse cortical dysplasia, or the 'double cortex' syndrome: the clinical and epileptic spectrum in 10 patients. *Neurology*, **41**, 1656–62.

Palmini, A., Andermann, F., Olivier, A. *et al.* (1991b) Focal neuronal migration disorders and intractable partial epilepsy: a study of 30 patients. *Annals of Neurology*, **30**, 741–49.

Pascual-Castroviejo, I., Diaz-Gonzalez, C., Garcia-Melian, R.M. *et al.* (1993) Sturge–Weber syndrome: study of 40 patients. *Pediatric Neurology*, **9**, 283–8.

Phelps, M.E. and Mazziotta, J.C. (1985) Positron emission tomography: human brain function and biochemistry. *Science*, **228**, 799–809.

Poser, C.M. and Taveras, J.M. (1957) Cerebral angiography in encephalotrigeminal angiomatosis. *Radiology*, **68**, 327–36.

Radtke, R.A., Hanson, M.W., Hoffman, J.M. *et al.* (1993) Temporal lobe hypometabolism on PET: predictor of seizure control after temporal lobectomy. *Neurology*, **43**, 1088–92.

Riela, A.R., Sires, B.P. and Penry, J.K. (1991) Transient magnetic resonance imaging abnormalities during partial status epilepticus. *Journal of Child Neurology*, **6**, 143–5.

Rintahaka, P.J., Chugani, H.T., Messa, C. *et al.* (1993) Hemimegalencephaly: evaluation with positron emission tomography. *Pediatric Neurology*, **9**, 21–8.

Roach, E.S., Williams, D.P. and Laster, D.W. (1987) Magnetic resonance imaging in tuberous sclerosis. *Archives of Neurology*, **44**, 301–3.

Rowe, C.C., Berkovic, S.F., Sia, S.T.B. *et al.* (1989) Localization of epileptic foci with postictal single photon emission computed tomography. *Annals of Neurology*, **26**, 660–8.

Rowe, C.C., Berkovic, S.F., Austin, M.C. *et al.* (1991) Patterns of postictal blood flow in temporal lobe epilepsy: qualitative and quantitative analysis. *Neurology*, **41**, 1096–103.

Ryding, E., Sjoholm, H., Skeidsvoll, H. *et al.* (1989) Delayed decrease in hemispheric cerebral blood flow during WADA test demonstrated by ^{99m}Tc-HMPAO single photon emission computed tomography. *Acta Neurologica Scandinavica*, **80**, 248–54.

Ryvlin, P., Garcia-Larrea, L., Philippon, B. *et al.* (1992a) High signal intensity on T_2-weighted MRI correlates with hypoperfusion in temporal lobe epilepsy. *Epilepsia*, **33**, 28–35.

Ryvlin, P., Philippon, B., Cinotti, L. *et al.* (1992b) Functional neuroimaging strategy in temporal lobe epilepsy: a comparative study of ^{18}FDG-PET and ^{99m}Tc-HMPAO-SPECT. *Annals of Neurology*, **31**, 650–6.

Salanova, V., Morris, H.H., Rehm, P. *et al.* (1992) Comparison of the intracarotid amobarbital procedure and interictal cerebral 18-fluorodeoxyglucose positron emission tomography scans in refractory temporal lobe epilepsy. *Epilepsia*, **33**, 635–8.

Savic, I., Persson, A., Roland, P. *et al.* (1988) *In vivo* demonstration of BZ receptor binding in human epileptic foci. *Lancet*, **ii**, 863–6.

Savic, I., Widen, L., Thorell, J.O. *et al.* (1990) Cortical benzodiazepine receptor binding in patients with generalized and partial epilepsy. *Epilepsia*, **31**, 724–30.

Smith, A.S., Weinstein, M.A., Quencer, R.M. *et al.* (1988) Association of heterotopic gray matter with seizures: MR imaging. *Radiology*, **168**, 195–8.

Sperling, M.R., Wilson, G., Engel, J. Jr, *et al.* (1986) Magnetic resonance imaging in intractable partial epilepsy: correlative studies. *Annals of Neurology*, **20**, 57–62.

Sperner, J., Schmauser, I., Bittner, R. *et al.* (1990) MR-imaging findings in children with Sturge–Weber syndrome. *Neuropediatrics*, **21**, 146–52.

Stefan, H., Baner, J., Feistel, H. *et al.* (1990) Regional cerebral blood flow during focal seizures of temporal and frontocentral onset. *Annals of Neurology*, **27**, 162–6.

Swartz, B.E., Halgren, E., Delgado-Escueta, A.V. *et al.* (1989) Neuroimaging in patients with seizures of probable frontal lobe origin. *Epilepsia*, **30**, 547–58.

Szelies, B., Herholz, K., Heiss, W.D. *et al.* (1983) Hypometabolic cortical lesions in tuberous sclerosis with epilepsy: demonstration by positron emission tomography. *Journal of Computer Assisted Tomography*, **7**, 946–53.

Theodore, W.H., Bromfield, E. and Onorati, L. (1989) The effect of carbamazepine on cerebral glucose metabolism. *Annals of Neurology*, **25**, 516–20.

Theodore, W.H., DiChiro, G., Margolin, R. *et al.* (1986a) Barbiturates reduce human cerebral glucose metabolism. *Neurology*, **736**, 60–4.

Theodore, W.H., Bairamian, D., Newmark, M.E. *et al.* (1986b) Effect of phenytoin on human cerebral glucose metabolism. *Journal of Cerebral Blood Flow and Metabolism*, **6**, 315–20.

Theodore, W.H., Holmes, M.D., Dorwart, R.H. *et al.* (1986c) Complex partial seizures: cerebral structure and cerebral function. *Epilepsia*, **27**, 576–82.

Theodore, W.H., Rose, D., Patronas, N. *et al.* (1987) Cerebral glucose metabolism in the Lennox–Gastaut syndrome. *Annals of Neurology*, **21**, 14–21.

Theodore, W.H., Katz, D., Kufta, C. *et al.* (1990) Pathology of temporal lobe foci: correlation with CT, MRI and PET. *Neurology*, **40**, 797–803.

Theodore, W.H., Sato, S., Kufta, C. *et al.* (1992) Temporal lobectomy for uncontrolled seizures: the role of positron emission tomography. *Annals of Neurology*, **32**, 789–94.

van Bogaert, P., Chiron, C., Adamsbaum, C. *et al.* (1993) Value of magnetic resonance imaging in West syndrome of unknown etiology. *Epilepsia*, **34**, 701–6.

Woods, B.T. and Chiu, T.M. (1990) *In vivo* ^{1}H spectroscopy of the human brain following electroconvulsive therapy. *Annals of Neurology*, **28**, 745–9.

Wyler, A.R. and Bolender, N.F. (1983) Preoperative CT diagnosis of mesial temporal sclerosis for surgical treatment of epilepsy. *Annals of Neurology*, **13**, 59–64.

Zimmerman, A.W., Niedermeyer, E. and Hodges, F.J. (1977) Lennox–Gastaut syndrome and computerized axial tomography findings. *Epilepsia*, **18**, 463–4.

HEMATOLOGIC, MICROBIOLOGIC AND BIOCHEMICAL INVESTIGATIONS

21

Frances M. Gibbon, Chaniyil Ramesh and Sheila J. Wallace

Investigation is relevant in three main areas: the seizures themselves, treatment, and etiology. Many of those tests appropriate to biochemical and microbiologic areas are considered in Chapter 4c and 4d, respectively, and for children with febrile seizures in Chapter 10.

HEMATOLOGIC INVESTIGATIONS

SEIZURES

No hematologic changes occur in association with brief seizures. Once status epilepticus reaches the phase of decompensation, leukocytosis and a consumptive coagulopathy with low platelet levels can be found.

ANTIEPILEPTIC DRUG THERAPY

The adverse hematologic effects of individual antiepileptic drugs (AEDs) are listed in more detail in Chapter 22. Blood dyscrasias have been reported in association with the use of all AED, but there is not always a clear relationship to individual drugs. However, in particular, aplastic anemia has been associated with felbamate; megaloblastic anemia with phenytoin and barbiturates; leukopenia, reversible and often cyclic, with carbamazepine (irreversible agranulocytosis occurs in an infinitesimal proportion of patients on carbamazepine); and thrombocytopenia with valproate.

Screening of asymptomatic children with epilepsy for hematologic changes is not worthwhile (Camfield *et al.*, 1986).

In addition to alterations in the blood cells, systemic lupus erythematosus has occurred in association with phenytoin, ethosuximide, and carbamazepine.

ETIOLOGY

Since seizures can be symptomatic of any systemic disorder which might affect the brain, it is relevant to consider very briefly investigations which could help to establish the diagnosis in primary hematologic or vasculitic illnesses. These are listed in Tables 21.1 and 21.2.

For conditions where the blood cells themselves are involved, either stroke or hemorrhage are likely to accompany or precede seizures. Neurological events occur in about 6–8% of patients with sickle cell disease, and seizures are long-term problems in approximately 50% of those affected (Powars *et al.*, 1978). Seizures can occur in association with acute intracerebral hemorrhage secondary to coagulopathies or thrombocytopenia, either primary or secondary to other blood disorders. Very rarely, chronic childhood leukemias, in themselves very uncommon, may present with seizures symptomatic of leukemic deposits in the brain or adjacent meninges.

Epilepsy in Children. Edited by Sheila Wallace. Published in 1996 by Chapman & Hall, London. ISBN 0 412 56860 8

Table 21.1 Hematologic disorders

Disorder	Additional major neurologic features	Investigations
Sickle cell anemia	Stroke	Hemoglobin electrophoresis
Chronic leukemias	Raised intracranial pressure due to leukemic deposits Meningism	Blood count, marrow examination
Acute leukemias	Intracranial hemorrhage Meningism	Blood count, marrow examination
Idiopathic thrombocytopenia	Intracranial hemorrhage	Platelet count, marrow
Clotting factor deficiencies	Intracranial hemorrhage	Coagulation screen

Table 21.2 Vasculitic disorders

Disorder	Additional neurologic features	Investigations
Hemolytic uremic syndrome	Acute encephalopathy	Typical red cell and platelet dysfunction
Henoch–Schönlein purpura	Subacute encephalopathy	Blood count, renal and skin biopsies
Systemic lupus erythematosus (SLE)	Cerebrovascular occlusion or intracranial hemorrhage	Antinuclear, anti-DNA and antineuronal antibodies. IgG cardiolipin antibody
Polyarteritis nodosa	As for SLE	Skin, muscle or renal biopsy Antinuclear cytoplasmic antibodies
Kawasaki's disease	Acute encephalopathy Stroke	Cardiac imaging (coronary artery aneurysms)

In vasculitic diseases, seizures are either part of an encephalopathy or symptomatic of vascular occlusion or hemorrhage. Seizures occur in approximately 30–40% of children with the hemolytic-uremic syndrome (Sheth, Swick and Haworth, 1986). They are usually generalized but can be partial, motor; they may be presenting features. Microangiopathic hemolytic anemia and red blood cell fragmentation, and thrombocytopenia with abnormal platelet function, i.e. reduced aggregation with adenosine diphosphate and collagen, are typical. Seizures are features of the acute phase of Henoch–Schönlein purpura in up to 4% of cases (Belman *et al.*, 1985). Leukocytosis and thrombocytosis may occur. Skin and renal biopsies show leukocytoclastic vasculitis with IgA deposition. Between 15 and 20% of young patients with systemic lupus erythematosus (SLE) have seizures. These can be generalized or partial (Steinberg and Frank, 1993). The seizures

may be presenting features, but are commoner as the disease progresses. Although tests helpful in the diagnosis of SLE are listed in Table 21.2, none is diagnostic. If seizures occur in polyarteritis nodosa, they tend to be manifest late in the disease. Focal necrosis of the walls of small- and medium-size arteries is found in biopsy material. Kawasaki's disease presents acutely, in young children, with fever, a maculopapular rash, cervical lymphadenopathy, and conjunctivitis. Although encephalopathy can occur, the main manifestations are cardiac, including myocardial infarction, arrhythmias and coronary aneurysms; thus, the crucial investigation is imaging of the cardiac vasculature.

MICROBIOLOGIC INVESTIGATIONS

The only occasions on which microbiologic investigations may be relevant to the epilepsy or its treatment arise when AED therapy has

Table 21.3 Investigation of child with acute infectious disorders and seizures (see also Chapter 4d)

All children:
Full blood count
Blood culture
Urinary microscopy and culture
Blood viral titers
Fecal culture and microscopy

In children with meningism, prolonged, repeated or lateralized seizures, failure to return to alertness in the expected time, purpuric rash, aged less than 18 months:
Lumbar puncture with examination of CSF: glucose and protein levels, organisms, cells and culture. Rapid diagnostic techniques include countercurrent immunoelectrophoresis, latex agglutination for *Hemophilus influenzae*, pneumococcus and meningococcus groups A, C, D, and W135 (but not group B). Herpes DNA by PCR if herpes simplex encephalitis suspected

In tropical countries:
Look for eosinophilia – hydatid, cysticercosis
ELISA – hydatid, schistosomiasis
Indirect hemagglutination titer: cysticercosis
Examine CSF for trophozoites (amebic meningoencephalitis)
Examine blood film for malaria

For further details of diagnostic tests in infection, see Lambert (1991).

led to alterations in the numbers or effectiveness of leukocytes or immunoglobulins, with a consequent increase in liability to infection.

ETIOLOGY

The roles of infections and postinfective causes are considered in Chapter 4d; and for febrile seizures, specifically, in Chapter 10. It is important to recognize that bacterial, viral, fungal, and parasitic diseases may all be associated with seizures, either acutely or chronically.

The investigations appropriate when a child presents with an acute illness complicated by seizures and a fever are listed in Table 21.3. When seizures are associated with a more chronic and intermittently febrile illness, investigations to identify microbiologic agents which may be responsible are indicated in Table 21.4.

Cerebral abscesses may present with seizures. Most of the organisms involved are anaerobes. A definitive bacterial diagnosis may be made by aspiration of the abscess, but blood culture, particularly when an abscess is secondary to septic emboli from subacute bacterial endocarditis, can be useful. If a cerebral abscess is suspected, it is dangerous to perform a lumbar puncture: CT or NMR scans should be examined first.

It can be difficult to get direct information on organisms when seizures are secondary to scarring from previous infections or to chronic encapsulated lesions. Often serologic or cerebrospinal fluid titers or neuroimaging, are the most helpful approaches. Appropriate tests are listed in Table 21.5. Some infections with chronic implications can be acquired prenatally, e.g. toxoplasmosis.

HIV infection deserves a special note. When acquired prenatally, no specific neurologic disorder may be present initially, but poor thriving and somewhat delayed overall development are usual. Opportunistic infection, particularly with toxoplasma, cryptococcus and/or tuberculosis, resulting in brain abscesses should be alerting factors for a search for immunodeficiency and the virus itself.

Table 21.4   Investigation if subacute or relapsing infective disease suspected (see Lambert 1991; Chapter 4d)

Blood culture:
Examine for organisms likely to cause subacute infection: e.g. *Listeria, Borrelia,* fungi

CSF microscopy and culture for:
Listeria, Actinomyces, Nocardia, Borrelia
Mycobacterium tuberculosis
Fungi . . . take large volume of CSF

Chest X-ray:
Tuberculosis
Fungal diseases

CT head scan:
Chronic meningitides
Tuberculosis
Lyme disease
Fungal diseases

CSF antibodies:
ELISA – tuberculosis
Latex particle agglutination – tuberculosis
Borrelia burgdorferi

Skin and mucous membrane scrapings:
Fungal diseases

Serology:
Some fungal diseases

Aspiration of abscess:
Microscopy and culture for all types of organisms possibly causative

Table 21.5   Investigation of chronic infection as a cause of seizures (see also Chapter 4d)

Blood count:
Eosinophilia – variably present in hydatid cysticercosis

Serologic titers:
Toxoplasmosis, cytomegalovirus, rubella, measles
Some fungal diseases
Toxocariasis
Hydatid
HIV

CT head scan:
Cysticercosis (elliptiform calcifications or calcified scolices)
Toxoplasmosis
Hydatid

ELISA in CSF:
Cysticercosis

Complement fixation antibody titer to measles:
Subacute sclerosing panencephalitis

BIOCHEMICAL INVESTIGATIONS

SEIZURES

Brief seizures do not cause biochemical abnormalities in the blood or CSF. Attacks of longer than 30 minutes' duration are associated with increased CSF lactate levels, but this is not an investigation which would be done at this time for diagnostic or therapeutic reasons. In tonic-clonic status epilepticus, once the stage of decompensation is reached the following changes occur: hypoglycemia, hyponatremia, hypo- or hyperkalemia, metabolic and respiratory acidosis, hepatic and renal dysfunction, and rhabdomyolysis and myoglobinuria (Chapter 18; Shorvon, 1994). Clearly, where tonic-clonic status epilepticus is proving difficult to control, it is important to monitor the plasma glucose, electrolytes, acid–base status, liver and renal function, and the creatine kinase.

ANTIEPILEPTIC DRUG THERAPY

The possible adverse effects of individual drugs are given in Chapter 22. Hepatotoxicity has been reported in association with valproate, carbamazepine, and felbamate. Monitoring of liver function tests in symptomless children is not considered useful for those on carbamazepine or valproate (Camfield *et al.*, 1986), but the situation is less clear in relation to felbamate, now available only in the USA, and then only for extremely resistant cases. Valproate may cause hyperammonemia, which is probably significant only in those children with underlying metabolic disorders, particularly Alper's disease. Nevertheless, any young child with neurologic handicaps and severe seizures who becomes drowsy or comatose when placed on valproate should have the blood ammonia and other liver function tests examined urgently.

Table 21.6 Biochemical investigation of seizures (see also Chapter 4c)

	Neonates	Older infants and children
Blood		
Glucose	+	+
Amino acids	+	+
Ammonia	+	+
Uric acid	+	+
Very long chain fatty acids	+	+
Lactate		+
Free carnitine		+
Lysosomal enzymes		+
Biotinidase		+
Mitochondrial DNA		+
Copper		+
CSF		
Glucose	+	+
Lactate	+	+
Amino acids	+	+
Gamma-amino-butyric acid	+	
Biogenic amines		+
Urine		
Glucose	+	+
Amino acids	+	+
Organic acids	+	+
Lactate		+
Sulfite, purines	+	+
Bile acids	+	

Enzyme assays may be done in skin fibroblasts, platelets, liver and muscle in specific disorders.
+ = Appropriate in this age group.

Monitoring of plasma levels of AED is discussed in Chapter 22.

ETIOLOGY

Disorders of metabolism in which epilepsy presents early and plays an important role in the diagnostic process, is manifest as a specific syndrome, or proves particularly difficult to control are considered in Chapter 4c. A brief resumé of the tests which should be considered is given in Table 21.6. Obviously, not all investigations are necessary in all patients. Reference to Chapter 4c will give appropriate guidance. Biochemical tests should be considered in the context of other investigations (Wallace, 1994).

Progressive myoclonus epilepsies are those most likely to be associated with definable metabolic disorders (Chapter 15a). Often the signs associated with seizures will give clues to the most appropriate investigations. Where such signs are not elicited, a full metabolic screen should be performed, since phenotypes do not always fit with previous descriptions, particularly early in the evolution of the condition. The diagnosis of conditions such as the ceroid lipofuscinoses, neuraxonal dystrophy, Alper's disease and Hallervorden–Spatz disease requires tissue examination.

CONCLUSIONS

Laboratory investigation of the child with epilepsy can be planned appropriately only when the history and other physical findings are taken into account. Neuroimaging can help to direct both microbiologic and biochemical tests, since there are specific findings in some infective disorders and in some diseases which are associated with cerebral degeneration.

REFERENCES

Belman, A.L., Leicher, C.R., Moshé, S.L. and Mezey, A.P. (1985) Neurological manifestations of Schoenlein–Henoch purpura; report of three cases and review of the literature. *Pediatrics*, **75**, 687–92.

Camfield, C.S., Camfield, P.C., Smyth, R.N., and Tibbles, T.A.R. (1986) Asymptomatic children with epilepsy: little benefit from screening for anticonvulsant induced liver, blood or renal damage. *Neurology*, **36**, 834–41.

Lambert, H.P. (1991) *Infections of the Nervous System*, Edward Arnold, London.

Powars, D., Wilson, B., Imbus, C. *et al.* (1978). The natural history of stroke in sickle cell disease. *American Journal of Medicine*, **65**, 461–71.

Sheth, K., Swick, H.M. and Haworth, N. (1986) Neurological involvement in hemolytic uremic syndrome. *Annals of Neurology*, **19**, 90–3.

Shorvon, S. (1994) *Status Epilepticus: Its Clinical Features and Treatment in Children and Adults,* Cambridge University Press, Cambridge.

Steinberg, A. and Frank, Y. (1993) Neurological manifestations of rheumatic diseases, *Neuro-logical Manifestations of Systemic Diseases in Children.* Raven Press, New York.

Wallace, S.J. (1994) Neurology, in *Investigations in Paediatrics* (ed. D.P. Addy), W.B. Saunders, London, pp. 135–48.

PHARMACOLOGY AND PHARMACOKINETICS OF ANTIEPILEPTIC DRUGS

22

Alan Richens

INTRODUCTION

A knowledge of the pharmacokinetics of antiepileptic drugs in children is essential if these therapeutic agents are to be used effectively. A major difference between adults and children in drug handling is the rate at which drugs are metabolized. Children break down drugs at a much faster rate than adults because metabolic rate is inversely proportional to body surface area. This difference gradually diminishes until puberty is reached, at which time the adolescent metabolizes drugs at the same rate as an adult. Various other differences in pharmacokinetics have been identified and these will

be discussed first. For a general review the reader is referred to Morselli (1977, 1983). Table 22.1 summarizes some of the pharmacokinetic factors involved.

PHARMACOKINETICS IN CHILDREN

ABSORPTION

In neonates, the absorption of drugs from the gastrointestinal tract is sometimes slow and unpredictable. This is particularly so for relatively insoluble drugs such as phenytoin and carbamazepine, whose bioavailability in the neonate may be poor. This may be related

Table 22.1 Summary of physiologic variables affecting drug disposition in neonates, infants and children compared with adults

	Neonates	*Infants and children*
Absorption		
Oral	Slow and unpredictable	Increased
IM	Variable	Increased
Rectal	Very efficient	Efficient
Plasma protein binding	Reduced for all drugs	As adults for acidic drugs (e.g. phenytoin, valproate)
Metabolism	Slow, particularly in premature neonates	Increased, gradually falling to adult rates at puberty
Renal excretion	May be reduced for acidic drugs (e.g. phenobarbitone)	Comparable to adults from 6 months

Epilepsy in Children. Edited by Sheila Wallace. Published in 1996 by Chapman & Hall, London. ISBN 0 412 56860 8

partly to the lack of acid production by the stomach. Gastric pH is neutral during the first 10–15 days of life and does not fall to adult values until about 2 years of age (Rane and Wilson, 1976). Gastric emptying is also slow and erratic for the first 6–8 months of life (Cavell, 1979). For example, phenobarbitone absorption is both delayed and incomplete in neonates up to the age of 15 days (Wallin, Jalling and Boréus, 1974). During postnatal development the absorptive processes rapidly mature, so that oral bioavailability of phenobarbitone and other antiepileptic drugs in infants and children is often greater than in adults.

The rate of absorption of many drugs is dependent to some degree on the formulation administered. Liquid formulations or chewable tablets tend to be absorbed more rapidly because dissolution of a capsule or tablet coating is not a rate-limiting step. Modified-release formulations, such as enteric-coated tablets, or extended-release preparations are specifically designed to control the rate of absorption.

The rectal route of administration can provide a useful alternative when oral administration is not possible, such as in a convulsing child. Lipid-soluble drugs such as diazepam are remarkably rapidly absorbed from the rectum, and anticonvulsant plasma concentrations of the drug can be reached within a few minutes. Rectal absorption of diazepam from suppositories is slower than with liquid formulations (Knudsen, 1977), and several manufacturers offer preparations which are convenient for use by parents or professional staff.

In emergency situations, such as prolonged febrile seizures (Chapter 10) or status epilepticus (Chapter 18), immediate and effective therapy is required. Drug absorption from intramuscular sites is generally too slow for emergency use and therefore the intravenous route is to be preferred. However, intramuscular injection may be useful when a child is unable to take a medicine orally or when gastrointestinal absorption is inefficient, such as with phenobarbitone in neonates (Perucca and Richens, 1985). Intramuscular phenytoin and diazepam tend to be absorbed slowly and erratically, and can cause local muscle damage and pain (Wilensky and Lowden, 1973), but midazolam, a water-soluble benzodiazepine, is absorbed rapidly and efficiently (Heizmann, Eckert and Ziegler, 1983).

DISTRIBUTION AND PROTEIN BINDING

The plasma protein binding of acidic drugs such as phenytoin and valproate is significantly lower in the neonate than at later ages. Premature infants in particular show markedly reduced binding. This is due to a combination of factors, including a persistence of fetal albumin which is less able to bind drugs, a relatively low total protein content in plasma, and the displacing effects of high circulating levels of bilirubin and free fatty acids (Krasner, Giacoia and Yaffe, 1973).

The net effect of reduced plasma protein binding is to lower the total concentration of drug in plasma because less is carried by proteins. Measuring the total drug level will therefore give a falsely low estimate of the drug's pharmacologic effect. The latter is related to the free drug level, i.e. the concentration of drug dissolved in plasma water, and this is independent of the amount carried by plasma proteins (Perucca and Richens, 1985).

With drug level monitoring, it is normally the total concentration which is measured, but when binding is known to be altered the free level can be measured in order to give a more accurate estimate of the amount of drug available for a therapeutic effect. This can be done by ultrafiltration of a plasma sample or, for some drugs such as phenytoin and carbamazepine, by measuring the concentration in saliva. The salivary glands act as a filter, allowing only free drug to diffuse into the saliva. Unfortunately, the partitioning of some drugs into saliva is dependent on saliva pH and therefore monitoring them in this way is unreliable (e.g. phenobarbitone, valproate).

The distribution of drugs in the neonate and infant differs from the older child and adult in that the brain and liver make up a larger proportion of body weight. Animal studies have shown that greater amounts of protein-bound drugs cross the blood–brain barrier in neonates than in adults, possibly as a result of changes in cerebral blood flow and capillary transit time (Cornford *et al.*, 1983). The clinical significance of these observations is uncertain.

ELIMINATION

Drugs are eliminated from the body by renal clearance of the unchanged drug or by metabolism in the liver followed by renal clearance of the metabolites. In general, antiepileptic drugs are highly lipid soluble because they have to cross the lipid blood–brain barrier before they can act. Drugs of this nature tend not to be renally eliminated because they diffuse back into the plasma as they pass down the renal tubules. Conversion into water-soluble metabolites in the liver is therefore necessary before they can be excreted in the urine. Phenytoin, carbamazepine, and valproate are all examples of anticonvulsant drugs that require biotransformation in the liver before they can be renally eliminated. There are two new drugs, however, which are exceptions to this general rule. Both vigabatrin and gabapentin are readily eliminated unchanged by the kidneys and very little metabolism occurs.

In neonates, drug-metabolizing enzyme activity may be immature, particularly in those born prematurely (Perucca, 1987), and this results in a slow elimination of drugs which require metabolism. In neonates born to mothers taking enzyme-inducing antiepileptic drugs (phenytoin, phenobarbitone, primidone, and carbamazepine), stimulation of the hepatic microsomal enzymes occurs because the drugs readily cross the placental barrier and enter the fetal circulation (Nau *et al.*, 1982).

Drug-metabolizing enzyme activity soon matures after birth, so that the neonate's capacity to hydroxylate and conjugate drugs enables antiepileptic drugs to be cleared efficiently. Compared with adults, infants are fast metabolizers, achieving rates of two to six times the adult rate during the first 6 months of life (Morselli, Franco-Morselli and Bossi, 1980). Thereafter, as the infant grows the rate of drug metabolism decreases to around twice the adult rate at the age of 6 years. At puberty, adult metabolism patterns are adopted.

These changes have important practical implications. The wide variation in rates of metabolism in children make it difficult to individualize the dose. Larger doses relative to body weight are required in children compared with adults, and the shorter elimination half-lives which they show demand more frequent dosing in order to maintain a steady-state plasma level. The value of drug level monitoring is probably greater in pediatric practice than in the management of adult patients if optimum responses to drug therapy are to be achieved.

When renal excretion is the major route of drug elimination, variability is less of a problem. However, the neonatal kidney is functionally and anatomically immature, and only at the age of 6–10 months is full renal function developed (Rane and Wilson, 1976). Thereafter, renal clearance of drugs seems to be comparable to that observed in adults.

PLASMA ELIMINATION HALF-LIFE

The plasma elimination half-life of a drug is determined by two factors, the rate of clearance (whether renal or hepatic) and the volume of distribution (i.e. the size of the drug pool in the body). Although the latter probably shows differences between children and adults, the most important distinguishing factor is the clearance rate. Excluding the neonate, children generally have shorter drug half-lives than adults, particularly for anticonvulsants that are metabolized in the liver. The elimination half-life usually determines the duration of action of a drug, although there are exceptions such as vigabatrin. This drug has a long pharmacodynamic half-life because it irreversibly inhibits the enzyme GABA-transaminase, and the enzyme has to be resynthesized, a process which takes several days. The short elimination half-life of vigabatrin is therefore of no clinical relevance.

In addition to determining the duration of action of a drug, the elimination half-life is the principle factor influencing the time taken to achieve a steady-state plasma concentration. For practical purposes a steady state is reached at five times the half-life value. A child put on phenobarbitone may have a half-life of 60 hours and require 12–13 days to reach steady state, whereas an adult with a half-life twice as long will require 2–3 weeks. The pharmacokinetics of the standard antiepileptic drugs in children have been reviewed by Morrow and Richens (1989).

INDIVIDUAL ANTIEPILEPTIC DRUGS

VALPROIC ACID

For a general review of valproic acid the reader is referred to Davis, Peters and McTavish (1994).

This drug is usually marketed either as the free acid or as the sodium salt, although some formulations combine both substances. Liquid or plain solid dose formulations tend to be irritant to the stomach, and therefore enteric-coated formulations are widely used. Controlled-release tablets have been introduced in a number of countries, although the advantage of this dosage form is open to question (see below).

Mode of action

Despite many attempts to define the mode of action of valproic acid, the mechanisms by which it has an antiepileptic effect are still largely undefined (Löscher, 1993). Originally, it was thought to be a GABA-transaminase inhibitor, but this is now known to occur only at concentrations that are not achieved with therapeutic doses. Nevertheless, it appears to increase GABA transmission by some other, as yet unidentified, mechanism. Hyperpolarization of neurons occurs, possibly by opening of potassium channels. The 2-en metabolite of valproic acid is pharmacologically active. It is probable that this metabolite and the parent drug have more than one site of action, accounting for the broad spectrum of activity of valproic acid. All seizure types in man are suppressed by the drug.

Pharmacokinetics

Table 22.2 summarizes the pharmacokinetics of valproic acid. The drug is rapidly absorbed following oral administration in infants and children and has a high bioavailability, but in

Table 22.2 Summary of pharmacokinetic data for valproic acid in children

Range of daily maintenance dose	10–40 mg/kg/day
Minimum dose frequency	Once daily
Time to peak plasma level	1–3 h (liquid and solid formulations) 2–6 h (enteric coated)
Percentage bound to plasma proteins	90% (less in neonates)
Main route of elimination	Hepatic metabolism
Major metabolite	β and ω oxidation products (some active)
Elimination half-life	10–70 h (neonates) 5–15 h (infants and children) 9–21 h (adults)

neonates the oral absorption is less satisfactory. Peak plasma concentrations occur within 1–3 hours following administration of liquid or solid dose oral formulations, with the exception of enteric-coated tablets which do not release their drug content until they reach the neutral environment of the duodenum. Controlled-release formulations (e.g. Epilim Chrono) result in a smoother plasma concentration time profile with once-daily dosing than can be achieved by dosing twice daily with enteric-coated tablets.

Valproic acid is extensively bound to plasma proteins but this is reduced in neonates by the various factors outlined earlier. Free fatty acids (FFAs) compete with valproic acid for plasma protein binding sites. As FFAs show considerable diurnal fluctuation, the amount of valproic acid bound in plasma varies in a reciprocal fashion, leading in turn to variation in the total plasma drug concentration. The percentage of valproic acid bound decreases as the plasma concentration rises, indicating saturation of binding sites (Herngren, Lundberg and Nergårdh, 1991).

Valproic acid has a relatively low apparent volume of distribution (about 0.15 l/kg), indicating that the drug is confined principally to the plasma and extracellular fluid.

Neonates metabolize valproic acid poorly, but in infancy the rate of metabolism increases to exceed slightly the rate in adults, giving elimination half-life values in infants and children which are less than in adults. By the age of 10 years adult values are reached. Enzyme-inducing drugs administered concurrently increase the clearance of valproic acid, shortening the half-life further (Hall *et al.*, 1985; Cloyd *et al.*, 1993).

Valproic acid is metabolized in the liver to various oxidation products and a glucuronide conjugate. A 2-en metabolite has anticonvulsant activity and a 4-en metabolite possibly contributes to the drug's hepatotoxic effect.

Drug interactions (Brodie, 1992)

As has already been mentioned, drugs which induce liver enzymes, such as phenytoin, carbamazepine, phenobarbitone, and primidone, stimulate the breakdown of valproic acid and this results in lower plasma concentrations of the drug. Higher doses of valproic acid may be necessary when used together with one of these drugs (Cloyd *et al.*, 1993). On the other hand, the new antiepileptic drug felbamate (no longer available), inhibits the metabolism of valproic acid, reducing its clearance by up to 50% (Wagner *et al.*, 1991).

Valproic acid is itself a potential inhibitor of drug metabolism. The effect is usually relatively small but a marked interaction occurs with lamotrigine, such that the elimination half-life of this drug may be doubled by concurrent valproic acid therapy. The dose of lamotrigine should be reduced by one-half when it is used under these circumstances (Yuen *et al.*, 1992).

Plasma levels of phenobarbitone increase in children on addition of valproic acid (Suganuma *et al.*, 1981), causing sedation. Although valproic acid inhibits phenytoin metabolism, causing a slight increase in the free plasma concentration, this is masked by a fall in total plasma concentration as a result of displacement of phenytoin from plasma protein binding sites. Valproic acid inhibits the clearance of the epoxide metabolite of carbamazepine, leading to an increase in its plasma level, but usually the level of the parent drug is unaffected. A related drug (valpromide), however, has a much more potent effect (Pisani *et al.*, 1986). Other drugs whose metabolism is inhibited by valproic acid include ethosuximide and felbamate.

Monitoring plasma levels

Plasma valproic acid levels fluctuate widely throughout the day as a result of three factors: rapid absorption, a short half-life, and variable plasma protein binding due to variations in circulating free fatty acid levels.

Table 22.3 Adverse effects of valproic acid (Davis, Peters and McTavish, 1994)

Adverse effect	Approximate incidence (%)
Dose related	
Gastrointestinal upsets (direct irritant effect)	5–10 (depends upon formulation)
Weight gain	5
Fine tremor	10
Drowsiness and ataxia	10
Hyperkinesia	5
Transient asymptomatic elevation of liver enzyme activity	10
Hair loss	5
Less obviously dose related	
Hyperammonemia (occasionally symptomatic)	20–40
Hepatotoxicity	0.01
Thrombocytopenia	1
Teratogenicity (spina bifida)	1–2

These probably explain why it has been difficult to demonstrate a relationship between drug level and therapeutic effect. It is possible also that valproic acid has a more constant pharmacologic action than is predicted by fluctuations in plasma level. Under these circumstances the case for monitoring drug levels regularly is poor. In neonates or infants, in whom the drug's pharmacokinetics are poorly predictable, there may be a stronger case. Noncompliance can also be detected if no drug is found in the plasma of a child who is supposed to be taking a therapeutic dose. The usually quoted therapeutic range is 350–700 μmol/l (50–100 mg/l), although the supporting evidence is poor.

Adverse effects

Serious adverse reactions to valproic acid are rare (Table 22.3). A fatal hepatotoxic reaction was reported to occur in about one in 10 000 cases (Dreifuss *et al.*, 1987), with high risk factors being: multiple drug therapy, age 2 years or less, presence of genetic metabolic disorder, severe epilepsy, mental handicap, or other associated hereditary pathology. However, hepatotoxicity is now very rare (one in 50 000 cases), presumably due to recognition of risk factors (Dreifuss *et al.*, 1989). Routine monitoring of liver function tests is not indicated.

Hyperammonemia is frequently found in children receiving valproic acid. This is caused either by an increase in renal production of ammonia (Matsuda, Ontani and Ninomiya, 1986) or inhibition of hepatic urea synthesis (Hjelm *et al.*, 1986). Only rarely does the ammonia concentration rise to levels that cause symptoms (Murphy and Marquard, 1982).

Valproic acid is generally well tolerated (Dulac *et al.*, 1986; Herranz, Armigo and Arteaga, 1988). The most common adverse reactions are listed in Table 22.3. Skin rashes occur very rarely with valproic acid.

CARBAMAZEPINE

Carbamazepine is marketed as liquid formulations, chewable tablets, plain tablets, and controlled-release formulations. The latter allow twice-daily administration.

Mode of action

Carbamazepine reduces high-frequency repetitive firing in neurons by blocking sodium channels in a use-and-frequency-dependent manner. It also decreases sodium and calcium fluxes through NMDA-type glutamate excitatory receptors. There is no evidence that carbamazepine influences GABA-mediated inhibition. Carbamazepine is effective against partial and secondarily generalized tonic-clonic seizures, but ineffective in absences or myoclonus. It therefore has a limited role in idiopathic generalized epilepsies.

Table 22.4 Summary of pharmacokinetic data for carbamazepine in children

Range of daily maintenance dose	10–30 mg/kg/day
Minimum dose frequency	Twice daily
Time to peak plasma level	2–6 h (plain tablets)
Percentage bound to plasma proteins	75%
Main route of elimination	Hepatic metabolism
Major metabolite	10,11-epoxide (active)
Elimination half-life	8–35 h (neonates) 3–15 h (infants and children) 10–30 h (adults)

Pharmacokinetics

A summary of pharmacokinetic data for carbamazepine is given in Table 22.4 Carbamazepine is poorly water soluble and is absorbed relatively slowly and erratically following oral administration. Infants and children absorb the drug faster than adults (Morselli, 1983). Absorption can be sufficiently rapid to produce adverse effects such as dizziness and diplopia, coinciding with the time of peak absorption.

Carbamazepine is highly lipid soluble and distributes extensively to the tissues, giving an apparent volume of distribution of about 1.5 l/kg, i.e. ten times as great as valproic acid. Plasma protein binding is less extensive however, and binding interactions are not important. The concentration of carbamazepine in saliva reflects closely the unbound drug in plasma, i.e. about 25% of the total plasma level, and can therefore be used for drug level monitoring when venepuncture is difficult or undesirable (Chambers *et al.*, 1977).

Carbamazepine is metabolized mainly to carbamazepine 10,11-epoxide which is pharmacologically active (Bertilsson and Tomson, 1986). In adults, the plasma concentration of this metabolite is low, but in infants and children, who metabolize carbamazepine much more quickly, it can reach the concentration of the parent drug. When account is taken of this lower plasma protein binding (about 50% compared with 75% for the parent drug), it may contribute substantially to the therapeutic effect.

Carbamazepine induces its own metabolism (autoinduction), so that the rate of metabolism increases over the first 4 weeks of administration. This causes the plasma level to drift downwards and the elimination half-life effectively shortens, leading to more fluctuation in the plasma level. Its metabolism is also stimulated by other enzyme-inducing antiepileptic drugs.

The short plasma half-life in children requires at least two daily doses of the drug and, in infants, preferably more if liquid formulations or plain tablets are used. Extended-release tablets effectively smooth out the peaks and troughs, although their bioavailability may be slightly less.

Drug interactions (Brodie, 1992)

As mentioned above, the metabolism of carbamazepine to its epoxide metabolite is stimulated by enzyme-inducing drugs. This increases the ratio of epoxide to parent drug. The epoxide probably has less anticonvulsant activity than carbamazepine, consequently the overall efficacy is reduced. Conversely, valproic acid and valpromide inhibit carbamazepine metabolism (p. 517). Lamotrigine, cimetidine, erythromycin, propoxyphene, and verapamil can do likewise.

Carbamazepine itself is an enzyme inducer and, apart from stimulating its own breakdown, it can lower the plasma levels of other antiepileptic drugs which undergo hepatic metabolism, particularly valproic acid and lamotrigine. It also reduces the effectiveness of drugs used for other purposes, such as corticosteroid hormones (Bartoszek, Brenner and Szefler, 1987), vitamin D, and warfarin.

Monitoring plasma levels

A relationship between plasma concentration and efficacy has been demonstrated for carbamazepine in children (Sillanpää *et al.*, 1979). In view of the wide variation in rates of metabolism, monitoring carbamazepine levels is helpful in pediatric practice. Some argue that the epoxide level should be measured also because it is particularly high in children (Schoemen *et al.*, 1984), but insufficient evidence is available for interpreting the results. Carbamazepine appears to cause fewer adverse reactions in children than in adults, although the possibility of unrecognized hyponatremia and water intoxication need to be borne in mind and are reasons for monitoring levels. The most widely quoted range of plasma levels is 20–40 µmol/l (5–10 mg/l).

Adverse effects

These are listed in Table 22.5. About 10% of children started on carbamazepine develop an allergic reaction comprising a skin rash

Table 22.5 Adverse effects of carbamazepine

Adverse effect	Approximate incidence (%)
Dose related	
CNS effects (dizziness, blurred vision, diplopia, ataxia)	5–10
Reduced psychomotor performance	5–10
Dyskinesia, asterixis	0–1
Nausea, vomiting	5
Hyponatremia	1
Benign elevation of alkaline phosphatase and gamma glutamyl transferase	50
Less obviously dose related	
Skin rashes, allergy	10
Hepatitis (hypersensitivity)	0.1
Reversible leukopenia	5
Irreversible agranulocytosis	0.0005
Teratogenicity (craniofacial defects, spina bifida)	1

and other manifestations of hypersensitivity. There is evidence that this reaction may be more common with a high starting plasma concentration (Chadwick *et al.*, 1984).

Agranulocytosis is an exceedingly rare adverse effect of carbamazepine (about one in 200 000 patients/year). Mild, reversible leukopenia, however, is relatively common – about 10 000 times more so. Monitoring hematologic function by white cell counts picks up large numbers of benign leukopenias, but there is no evidence that it anticipates the onset of agranulocytosis. Regular blood counts on starting carbamazepine therapy are not indicated.

PHENYTOIN

Phenytoin is marketed in a variety of oral formulations: liquids, capsules, tablets, chewable tablets. Most contain the sodium salt, but some contain phenytoin acid. In the latter, the dose may be greater than the sodium salt equivalent because the molecular weight of the acid is less than the sodium salt. For example, Epanutin Infatabs contain 50 mg of phenytoin acid, while the equivalent size of tablets or capsules contains 50 mg of the sodium salt, which is equivalent to about 46 mg of the acid. Although this difference is small, it may be sufficient to precipitate phenytoin intoxication when a change is made from sodium salt preparations to Epanutin Infatabs, because phenytoin undergoes saturable metabolism.

Mode of action

Phenytoin has many actions in neuronal systems, but its ability to block sodium channels is probably its most important anticonvulsant action (Macdonald and Meldrum, 1989). This blockade is use-and-frequency dependent, i.e. the more frequently the sodium channels open the greater the degree of blockade. This action has a number of consequences but probably the most import-

Table 22.6 Summary of pharmacokinetic data for phenytoin in children

Range of daily maintenance dose	5–15 mg/kg/day
Minimum dose frequency	Once daily
Time to peak plasma level	4–12 h (oral)
Percentage bound to plasma proteins	85–90% (less in neonate)
Main route of elimination	Hepatic metabolism
Major metabolite	5-(*p*-hydroxyphenyl)-5-phenylhydantoin (inactive)
Elimination half-life (at therapeutic plasma concentrations)	10–20 h (longer in neonates) 10–50 h (adults)

ant is a decrease in the rate of recovery of sodium channels following repetitive firing.

Pharmacokinetics

The main pharmacokinetic properties of phenytoin are summarized in Table 22.6 (for review see Richens, 1979). Phenytoin is poorly soluble in water and the surface area presented by the particles in an oral formulation is a major factor determining rate and extent of absorption. There have been a number of instances of poor bioavailability with different formulations of the drug, but the factors involved are now well understood and most marketed formulations of the sodium salt are bioequivalent. Enteral feeding in children can markedly reduce phenytoin absorption by the oral route, and it may therefore be necessary to give the drug intravenously (O'Hagan and Wallace, 1994). Parenteral preparations of phenytoin should not be given intramuscularly because crystals of drug precipitate in the muscle, causing damage and being very slowly absorbed (Wilder and Ramsay, 1976). If parenteral administration is necessary, for example in treating status epilepticus, it should be given slowly intravenously, under ECG control.

Phenytoin is about 90% bound to plasma proteins. Binding is reduced in conditions which cause hypoalbuminemia (i.e. hepatic and renal disease, pregnancy), in neonates and by concurrent administration of valproic acid, which competes with its binding sites. The concentration of the drug in saliva and CSF reflects the unbound plasma concentration. Phenytoin penetrates rapidly into the brain when loading doses are given for the treatment of status epilepticus.

Phenytoin is metabolized in the liver to a hydroxy-metabolite which is pharmacologically inactive and is excreted in the urine. The rate of metabolism is faster in infants and young children than in the adult (Blain *et al.* 1981). The enzyme responsible for this conversion is saturable within the therapeutic range of plasma concentrations, and therefore the increase in steady-state plasma level resulting from a dose increment is greater than is predicted by first-order kinetics. Increases in dose must take this into account if toxicity is to be avoided. Variable compliance can cause marked changes in plasma concentration. Saturation kinetics also makes phenytoin very susceptible to drug interactions.

The plasma half-life of phenytoin is dependent upon the degree of saturation of the hydroxylase enzyme. At low plasma phenytoin concentrations the half-life is short, but it progressively lengthens as the concentration rises. Fluctuations in the plasma level lessen as the steady-state concentration rises.

Drug interactions

Phenytoin metabolism is inducible by carbamazepine but less so by phenobarbitone. Conversely, it is inhibited by various drugs including valproic acid, felbamate, propoxyphene, chloramphenicol, isoniazid, cimetidine, omeprazole, and amiodarone. As mentioned earlier, valproic acid displaces phenytoin from albumin binding sites as well as inhibiting its metabolism. The net effect is an increase in free drug concentration but a reduction in the total plasma level.

Phenytoin is itself an enzyme inducer and, like carbamazepine, it can stimulate the breakdown of other hepatically metabolized antiepileptic drugs (carbamazepine, valproic acid, benzodiazepines, lamotrigine, and felbamate) as well as various other drugs such as corticosteroids (Bartoszck, Brenner and Szefler, 1987), vitamin D, and folic acid.

Plasma level monitoring

Monitoring phenytoin levels is essential if individualization of the dose is to be achieved and toxicity avoided. The reason is that, in addition to saturation kinetics, phenytoin shows wide variation in rates of metabolism between children and it is not possible to achieve a satisfactory therapeutic level without monitoring. Circumstances causing altered binding need to be borne in mind. If necessary the free level can be measured by ultrafiltration of a plasma sample or by using saliva. The therapeutic range of plasma concentrations is usually quoted as 40–80 μmol/l (10–20 mg/l); free concentrations are in the range of 4–8 μmol/l (1–2 mg/l).

Adverse effects

The main adverse effects caused by phenytoin are given in Table 22.7. Cerebellar signs of intoxication occur almost universally if the plasma level rises high enough. Although folate levels frequently fall (probably by hepatic enzyme induction), hematologic abnormalities only occur rarely. Skin rashes appear to be more common in children when large loading doses of phenytoin are given (Wilson, Hojer and Rane, 1976). The frequency with which phenytoin causes adverse reactions, together with its difficult pharmacokinetics, make it no longer a drug of first choice in epilepsy.

Table 22.7 Adverse effects of phenytoin

Adverse effect	Approximate incidence (%)
Dose related	
Nystagmus, ataxia, dysarthria, sedation	Almost inevitable with high enough plasma level
Cognitive dysfunction	20
Dyskinesias	0.1
Peripheral neuropathy	1
Low folate level	5
Megaloblastic anemia	0.1
Osteomalacia	0.05
Gingival hyperplasia	30
Less obviously dose related	
Skin rashes	5
Systemic hypersensitivity	1
Coarse facies, hirsutism	10
Lymphadenopathy	0.1
Systemic lupus erythematosus	0.1
Teratogenicity (especially cleft lip/palate and cardiovascular malformation)	5
Neonatal vitamin K deficiency	1

PHENOBARBITONE AND PRIMIDONE

These drugs will be dealt with briefly because they are now seldom used in treating children with epilepsy in developed countries, but remain important where the overall economic level is poor. Primidone is metabolized mainly to phenobarbitone and this metabolite accounts for most of its therapeutic effects. However, unchanged primidone and a second metabolite, phenylethylmalonamide, probably contribute. In particular, the parent drug is responsible for the acute intolerance so frequently seen on starting primidone therapy.

Mode of action

Phenobarbitone enhances GABA inhibitory neurotransmission by acting on a receptor site linked to the postsynaptic chloride chan-

Table 22.8 Summary of pharmacokinetic data for phenobarbitone in children

Range of daily maintenance dose	2–6 mg/kg/day
Minimum dose frequency	Once daily
Time to peak plasma level	1–6 h
Percentage bound to plasma proteins	45%
Main route of elimination	Hepatic metabolism + renal elimination
Major metabolite	*p*-hydroxyphenobarbitone
Elimination half-life	60–400 h (neonates) 40–80 h (infants and children) 50–160 h (adults)

Table 22.9 Summary of pharmacokinetic data for primidone in children

Range of daily maintenance dose	15–30 mg/kg/day
Minimum dose frequency	Twice daily
Time to peak plasma level	2–5 h
Percentage bound to plasma proteins	Less than 20%
Main route of elimination	Hepatic metabolism
Major metabolite	Phenobarbitone (active) Phenylethylmalonamide (inactive)
Elimination half-life	10–35 h (neonates) 4–15 h (infants and children) 4–15 h (adults)

nel. It prolongs the opening time of these channels, allowing more negatively charged chloride ions to enter the neuron, resulting in hyperpolarization of its membrane.

Pharmacokinetics (Tables 22.8, 22.9)

Although phenobarbitone is absorbed poorly following oral administration in neonates, it is slowly but completely absorbed in infants and children (Jalling, 1976). It is approximately 45% bound to plasma proteins and distributes to the brain relatively slowly. The conversion of primidone to phenobarbitone is initially relatively slow, but the pathway involved becomes induced with chronic treatment.

Phenobarbitone is partly excreted unchanged (about 25%), the rest being metabolized to parahydroxyphenobarbitone, which is inactive. The rate of metabolism is relatively slow, giving an elimination half-life which is compatible with once-daily administration. It is preferable to give primidone more frequently because single large doses can produce high levels of the unchanged drug in the plasma, and increase the likelihood of intolerance.

Drug interactions

Like phenytoin and carbamazepine, phenobarbitone can induce the metabolism of other drugs. Valproic acid can inhibit the metabolism of phenobarbitone, increasing its plasma level by 25–50%.

Plasma level monitoring

Monitoring phenobarbitone levels is relatively unhelpful because tolerance to the drug occurs, making it difficult to identify a therapeutic range. Dosage titration should be judged by efficacy and adverse effects. There is no indication for measuring unchanged primidone.

Adverse effects

These are listed in Table 22.10. The frequency with which behavioral disturbances and hyperkinesia occur in children make phenobarbitone and primidone drugs to be avoided unless others fail. There is concern about the effect of phenobarbitone on learning in children (Vining *et al.*, 1987).

Table 22.10 Adverse effects of phenobarbitone and primidone

Adverse effect	Approximate incidence
Dose related	
Behavioral disturbances } Hyperkinesia } Impaired learning }	20–40%
Sedation, nystagmus, ataxia, dysarthria }	Inevitable with high doses
Acute intolerance (primidone only)	Very common, unless very small starting dose used
Tolerance, withdrawal seizures	Usual
Vitamin deficiencies (folate, D, and K)	Uncommon
Less obviously dose related	
Skin rash	2%
Teratogenicity	5%

Table 22.11 Summary of pharmacokinetic data for diazepam in children

Size of single dose	0.5–1.0 mg/kg
Time to peak plasma level	0.5–1.5 h (oral) 10–30 min (rectal)
Percentage bound to plasma proteins	97% (less in neonate)
Main route of elimination	Hepatic metabolism
Major metabolite	N-desmethyldiazepam (active)
Elimination half-life	18–100 h (neonates) 8–30 h (infants and children) 20–60 h (adults)

Table 22.12 Summary of pharmacokinetic data for clonazepam in children

Range of daily maintenance dose	0.05–0.15 mg/kg/day
Minimum dose frequency	Once daily
Time to peak plasma level	1–2 h
Percentage bound to plasma proteins	85%
Main route of elimination	Hepatic metabolism
Major metabolite	7-aminoclonazepam (inactive)
Elimination half-life	20–45 h (neonates) 20–30 h (infants and children) 20–60 h (adults)

BENZODIAZEPINE DRUGS

Only diazepam and clonazepam will be dealt with here, the first because it is one of the most highly lipid soluble and fast acting of the benzodiazepine drugs, invaluable in the acute treatment of seizures, and the second because it is one of the most widely used of benzodiazepines for chronic therapy.

Mode of action

The benzodiazepine drugs act on the alpha subunit of the $GABA_A/Cl^-$ ionophore complex and in so doing they facilitate inhibitory transmission leading to hyperpolarization of the postsynaptic neuron.

Pharmacokinetics (Tables 22.11, 22.12)

Both diazepam and clonazepam are rapidly absorbed orally because they are highly lipid soluble. Peak plasma levels occur within 1 hour if taken on an empty stomach, but absorption is slowed if they are taken after a meal. Diazepam is also used rectally and it is

rapidly absorbed from this site if given in a liquid formulation, peak plasma levels occurring within 10–20 minutes (Langslet *et al.*, 1978). If given intramuscularly it is slowly absorbed because it crystallizes in the muscles. If speed of action is required, e.g. in status epilepticus, it should be given intravenously.

Both drugs enter the brain very rapidly; when given intravenously, diazepam stops seizures within 1–2 minutes. It concentrates initially in organs with a high blood flow, such as the brain, and subsequently redistributes to muscle and fat. It is this which determines the duration of action after an intravenous bolus dose. This can be measured by the distribution (α) half-life which precedes the elimination (β) half-life. The former is short (minutes), whereas the latter is long (hours). Infused diazepam accumulates and its effects wear off slowly because elimination rather than redistribution determines the duration of action in this situation.

Diazepam is metabolized to an active metabolite *N*-desmethyldiazepam which is eliminated more slowly than the parent drug. Clonazepam does not have active metabolites.

Drug interactions

The metabolism of both drugs is enhanced by enzyme-inducing drugs, resulting in shortened half-lives and lower steady-state plasma levels. For diazepam, this involves both the parent drug and active metabolite, so the effect of the drug is reduced. Conversely, cimetidine inhibits diazepam metabolism. Valproic acid displaces diazepam from plasma protein binding sites and may also inhibit its metabolism, thereby increasing the free concentration and pharmacologic effect (Dhillon and Richens, 1982). Benzodiazepines have little if any effect on the metabolism of other drugs.

Plasma level monitoring

A correlation between plasma level and effect has been shown with acute effects of benzodiazepine drugs on the brain, but not with chronic effects such as their antiepileptic action. This is presumably partly the result of the development of tolerance. There is no rationale for monitoring the plasma concentration of any benzodiazepine drug given for epilepsy.

Table 22.13 Adverse effects with benzodiazepine drugs

Adverse effect	Approximate incidence
Dose related	
Sedation, diplopia, ataxia, dysarthria	Inevitable, with high enough dose
Hypotension, respiratory arrest	After large IV doses
Muscle hypotonicity in neonate born to mother on benzodiazepine	
Tolerance, withdrawal seizures	Usual

Adverse effects

These are listed in Table 22.13. Apart from dose-related CNS adverse effects, benzodiazepine drugs are well tolerated. Idiosyncratic adverse effects do not occur.

ETHOSUXIMIDE

Ethosuximide is useful only in absence seizures and myoclonus. It is the most widely used of the succinimide drugs.

Mode of action

Ethosuximide has been shown to block T-calcium channel activation in neurons. These channels are involved in the control of neuronal activity rather than in transmitter release. This action is thought to account for ethosuximide's antiabsence activity (Coulter, Huguenard and Prince, 1989).

Pharmacokinetics

These are summarized in Table 22.14. Ethosuximide is absorbed rapidly and completely (Buchanan, Kinkel and Smith, 1973). It is not bound to plasma proteins and is metabolized into inactive hydroxylated metabolites. Its plasma half-life is long enough for once-daily administration, even in children, but large

Table 22.14 Summary of pharmacokinetic data for ethosuximide in children

Range of daily maintenance dose	10–15 mg/kg/day
Minimum dose frequency	Once daily
Time to peak plasma level	1–4 h
Percentage bound to plasma proteins	Negligible
Main route of elimination	Hepatic metabolism
Major metabolites	Hydroxymetabolites (inactive)
Elimination half-life	35–60 h (neonates) 20–50 h (infants and children) 40–70 h (adults)

single doses can cause gastrointestinal adverse effects.

Drug interactions

Enzyme-inducing drugs accelerate the metabolism of ethosuximide, necessitating higher doses. On the other hand, valproic acid may cause a slight inhibition of its metabolism. Ethosuximide does not affect the metabolism of other drugs.

Plasma level monitoring

As ethosuximide is used largely for treating absence seizures, clinical and EEG monitoring give a good indication of its therapeutic effect, making plasma level monitoring unimportant. A therapeutic range of 350–700 µmol/l (50–100 mg/l) has been defined (Sherwin, Robb and Lechter, 1973).

Adverse effects

These are listed in Table 22.15. Dose-related gastrointestinal symptoms are the commonest problem.

Table 22.15   Adverse effects with ethosuximide

Adverse effect	Approximate incidence (%)
Dose related	
Nausea, abdominal discomfort, hiccups	20
Drowsiness, headache	10
Less obviously dose related	
Behavioral and psychologic effects	10
Skin rashes	2
Systemic lupus erythematosus	0.01

VIGABATRIN

The chemical name of vigabatrin is gamma-vinyl-GABA, indicating its similarity with the naturally occurring inhibitory transmitter GABA. It is a racemic mixture of a pharmacologically active S(+)-enantiomer and an inactive R(−)-enantiomer.

Mode of action

Vigabatrin irreversibly inhibits the enzyme GABA-transaminase, which is responsible for the degradation of GABA at inhibitory synapses (Metcalf, 1979). It forms a stable intermediate and the enzyme has to be resynthesized for transmission to return to normal. It causes an increase in GABA-mediated neuronal inhibition.

Pharmacokinetics

These are summarized in Table 22.16 and are reviewed by Rey, Pons and Olive (1992). Vigabatrin is absorbed readily from the gastrointestinal tract but the peak plasma concentration of the S(+)-enantiomer is about one-half the concentration of the R(−)-enantiomer (Rey *et al.*, 1990). It is eliminated from the body entirely by renal clearance of the unchanged drug. Its plasma half-life is relatively short but correlates with the duration of action, which lasts several days because of its irreversible effect on GABA-transaminase.

Table 22.16 Summary of pharmacokinetic data for vigabatrin in children

Range of daily maintenance doses	50–80 mg/kg/day
Minimum dose frequency	Once daily
Time to peak plasma level	1–2 h
Percentage bound to plasma proteins	Nil
Main route of elimination	Renal elimination
Major metabolite	Nil
Elimination half-life	4–7 h (infants and children) 5–7 h (adults)

Drug interactions

Vigabatrin causes a small fall in plasma phenytoin levels by an unidentified mechanism, but otherwise, no significant interactions occur.

Plasma level monitoring

There is no relationship between plasma vigabatrin levels and its pharmacological effects because of the dissociation between its pharmacokinetic and pharmacodynamic half-lives. Measuring vigabatrin levels is therefore unhelpful.

Adverse effects

Experience in children is relatively limited. Mild CNS effects such as somnolence, fatigue, irritability, dizziness, and headache occur in adults. In children, hyperactivity can be a problem. Psychosis is a rare adverse effect but has not been reported in children. Skin rashes do not occur.

LAMOTRIGINE

This was developed in a search for folate antagonists which have antiepileptic activity.

However, its mode of action in epilepsy is by a different mechanism.

Mode of action

Lamotrigine inhibits the release of the excitatory neurotransmitter glutamate by a blocking effect on fast sodium channels in presynaptic terminals (Leach, Marden and Miller, 1986).

Pharmacokinetics

Little information has been published on the pharmacokinetics of lamotrigine in children (Goa, Ross and Chrisp, 1993). What is available indicates that children metabolize the drug more rapidly than adults, giving a plasma half-life that may require twice daily administration (Table 22.17). The half-life is highly dependent upon comedication. Enzyme inducers (carbamazepine, phenytoin, phenobarbitone, and primidone) shorten the half-life and valproic acid lengthens it by inhibition of its metabolism. The latter effect may double the half-life and require a starting and maintenance dose which is half that when it is used in monotherapy. The manufacturer's prescribing information allows for this.

Drug interactions

Apart from the effects of other drugs on lamotrigine metabolism described above, there are no significant interactions. Lamotrigine does not alter the kinetics of other antiepileptic drugs but it may precipitate diplopia and dizziness when added to carbamazepine therapy, probably by a pharmacodynamic interaction.

Plasma level monitoring

There is insufficient information available to know whether monitoring lamotrigine levels will be helpful.

Table 22.17 Summary of pharmacokinetic data for lamotrigine in children

Range of daily maintenance dose	Enzyme induced	7–15 mg/kg/day (infants and children)
	Monotherapy Valproate comedication:	5–10 mg/kg/day (infants and children) 1–2 mg/kg/day (infants) 2–4 mg/kg/day (children)
Minimum dose frequency	Twice daily	
Time to peak plasma level	2–3 h	
Percentage bound to plasma proteins	55%	
Main route of elimination	Hepatic metabolism	
Major metabolite	Glucuronide (inactive)	
Elimination half-life (see text)	5–30 h (infants and children) 15–90 h (adults)	

Adverse effects

Skin rashes, usually mild and reversible, occur in about 5% of patients, but the incidence is related to the size of the starting dose. A low dose is less likely to cause a rash (Goa, Ross and Chrisp, 1993). Agitation, ataxia, and drowsiness have been reported in children. Other mild CNS effects such as dizziness, diplopia, and blurred vision have occurred in adults.

GABAPENTIN

There is little information available on the use of gabapentin in children. Experience in adults has been reviewed by Foot and Wallace (1991). Gabapentin is an analog of GABA but it does not have GABA agonist actions. It binds to a peptide binding site on neuronal membranes which is thought to be linked to an amino acid transport mechanism (Suman-Chauhan *et al.*, 1993). The relevance of this is uncertain.

The pharmacokinetics of gabapentin are summarized in Table 22.18 but little information is available in children. There is evidence of saturable absorption from the gut in adults; the significance of this in children is not known. It is renally eliminated and therefore its clearance is reduced by impaired

Table 22.18 Summary of pharmacokinetic data for gabapentin in children

Range of daily maintenance dose	20–40 mg/kg/day
Minimum dose frequency	Three times daily
Time to peak plasma level	2–3 h
Percentage bound to plasma proteins	Nil
Main route of elimination	Renal elimination
Major metabolite	Nil
Elimination half-life	5–7 h (infants and children) 5–7 h (adults)

renal function. It has a short plasma half-life and therefore requires at least three doses per day. No clinically important drug interactions have been described. Mild CNS adverse effects such as drowsiness, fatigue, and dizziness have been reported in adults.

FELBAMATE

This drug is chemically related to meprobamate, which is now a little used tranquillizer. Felbamate has undergone trials in Lennox–Gastaut syndrome in children (Felbamate

Table 22.19 Summary of pharmacokinetic data for oxcarbazepine in children

Range of daily maintenance dose	20–50 mg/kg/day
Minimum dose frequency	Twice daily
Time to peak plasma level*	2–6 h
Percentage bound to plasma proteins*	50%
Main route of elimination	Rapid hepatic metabolism to active metabolite
Major metabolite	10,11-dihydro-10-hydroxy-carbamazepine (DHC) (active)
Elimination half-life*	10–13 h (adults) Shorter in children

*Data given are for the active metabolite, DHC.

Study Group, 1993). Its mode of action is unknown, but there is evidence that it acts as an antagonist at glycine recognition sites on the NMDA glutamate receptor (McCabe *et al.*, 1993). Glycine is known to enhance excitatory transmission at these receptors.

Felbamate is rapidly absorbed and largely metabolized in the liver. Its plasma half-life is probably shorter in children than in adults, and requires twice daily administration. It inhibits the metabolism of phenytoin and valproic acid, causing a rise in their plasma levels, but it lowers carbamazepine concentration, presumably by hepatic enzyme induction. It causes frequent gastrointestinal adverse effects (nausea, vomiting) and CNS intolerance (dizziness, dysphasia, headaches). Unacceptable incidences of aplastic anemia and hepatic failure led to its withdrawal in 1994.

OXCARBAZEPINE

This is an analog of carbamazepine which is essentially a prodrug, being rapidly metabolized in the liver to its 10-hydroxy-derivative (DHC) which mediates the drug's pharmacologic effects (Table 22.19) (Klosterskov Jensen,

Gram and Schmutz, 1991). It is presumed to act in a similar way to carbamazepine, i.e. by blocking sodium channels in the neuronal membrane. It probably has the same indications as carbamazepine but it is less likely to cause skin rashes. Only about one-quarter of patients who develop a rash with carbamazepine show cross-allergy with oxcarbazepine. Otherwise, the range of adverse effects appears to be similar to carbamazepine. There is little information available on the use of this drug in children.

REFERENCES

Bartoszek, M., Brenner, A.M. and Szefler, S.J. (1987) Prednisolone and methylprednisolone kinetics in children receiving anticonvulsant therapy. *Clinical Pharmacology and Therapeutics*, **42**, 424–32.

Bertilsson, L. and Tomson, T. (1986) Clinical pharmacokinetics and pharmacological effects of carbamazepine and carbamazepine 10,11-epoxide: an update. *Clinical Pharmacokinetics*, **11**, 177–98.

Blain, P.G., Mucklow, J.C., Bacon, C.J. *et al.* (1981) Pharmacokinetics of phenytoin in children. *British Journal of Clinical Pharmacology*, **12**, 659–61.

Brodie, M.J. (1992) Drug interactions in epilepsy. *Epilepsia*, **33** (suppl. 1) S13–22.

Buchanan, R.A., Kinkel, A.W. and Smith, T.C. (1973) The absorption and excretion of ethosuximide. *International Journal of Clinical Pharmacology and New Drugs*, **7**, 213–18.

Cavell, B. (1979) Gastric emptying in preterm infants. *Acta Paediatrica Scandinavica*, **68**, 725–30.

Chadwick, D., Shaw, M.D.M., Foy, P. *et al.* (1984) Serum anticonvulsant concentrations and the risk of drug induced skin eruptions. *Journal of Neurology, Neurosurgery and Psychiatry*, **47**, 642–4.

Chambers, R.E., Homeida, M., Hunter, K.R. *et al.* (1977) Salivary carbamazepine concentrations. *Lancet*, **i**, 656–7.

Cloyd, J.C., Fischer, J.H., Kriel, R.L. *et al.* (1993) Valproic acid pharmacokinetics in children. IV. Effects of age and antiepileptic drugs on protein binding and intrinsic clearance. *Clinical Pharmacology and Therapeutics*, **53**, 22–9.

Cornford, E.M., Partridge, W.M., Braun, L.D. *et al.* (1983) Increased blood–brain barrier transport of protein bound anticonvulsant drugs in the newborn. *Journal of Cerebral Blood Flow and Metabolism*, **3**, 280–6.

Coulter, D.A., Huguenard, J.R. and Prince, D.A. (1989) Characterization of ethosuximide reduction of low threshold calcium current in thalamic neurones. *Annals of Neurology*, **25**, 482–93.

Davis, R., Peters, D.H. and McTavish, D. (1994) Valproic acid. A reappraisal of its pharmacological properties and clinical efficacy in epilepsy. *Drugs*, **47**, 332–72.

Dhillon, S. and Richens, A. (1982) Valproic acid and diazepam interaction in *vivo*. *British Journal of Clinical Pharmacology*, **13**, 553–60.

Dreifuss, F.E., Santilli, N., Langer, D.H. *et al.* (1987) Valproic acid hepatic fatalities: a retrospective review. *Neurology*, **37**, 379–85.

Dreifuss, F.E., Langer, D.H., Moline, K.A. *et al.* (1989) Valproic acid hepatic fatalities II: US experience since 1984. *Neurology*, **39**, 201–7.

Dulac, O., Stern, D., Rey, E. *et al.* (1986) Sodium valproate monotherapy in childhood epilepsy. *Brain and Development*, **8**, 47–52.

Felbamate Study Group (1993) Efficacy of felbamate in childhood epileptic encephalopathy (Lennox–Gastaut syndrome). *New England Journal of Medicine*, **328**, 29–33.

Foot, M. and Wallace, J. (1991) Gabapentin, in *New Antiepileptic Drugs* (eds F. Pisani, E. Perucca, G. Avanzini and A. Richens), Elsevier, Amsterdam, pp. 109–14.

Goa, K.L., Ross, S.R. and Chrisp, P. (1993) Lamotrigine. A review of its pharmacological properties and clinical efficacy in epilepsy. *Drugs*, **46**, 152–76.

Hall, K., Otten, N., Johnston, B. *et al.* (1985) A multivariable analysis of factors governing steady-state pharmacokinetics of valproic acid in 52 young epileptics. *Journal of Clinical Pharmacology*, **25**, 261–8.

Heizmann, P., Eckert, M. and Ziegler, G. (1983) Pharmacokinetics and bioavailability of midazolam in man. *British Journal of Clinical Pharmacology*, **16**, 43S–9S.

Herngren, L., Lundberg, B, and Nergårdh, A. (1991) Pharmacokinetics of total and free valproic acid during monotherapy in infants. *Journal of Neurology*, **238**, 315–19.

Herranz, J.L., Armigo, J.A. and Arteaga, R. (1988) Clinical side effects of phenobarbital, primidone, phenytoin, carbamazepine, and valproate during monotherapy in children. *Epilepsia*, **29**, 794–804.

Hjelm, M., Oberholzer, V., Seakins, J., Thomas, S. and Kay, J.D.S. (1986) Valproate-induced inhibition of urea synthesis and hyperammonaemia in healthy subjects. *Lancet*, **ii**, 859.

Jalling, B. (1976) Plasma and CSF concentrations of phenobarbital in infants given single doses. *Developmental Medicine and Child Neurology*, **16**, 781–93.

Klosterskov Jensen, P., Gram, L. and Schmutz, M. (1991) Oxcarbazepine, in *New Antiepileptic Drugs* (eds F. Pisani, E. Perucca, G. Avanzini and A. Richens), Elsevier, Amsterdam, pp. 135–40.

Knudsen, F.U. (1977) Plasma diazepam in infants after rectal administration in solution and by suppository. *Acta Paediatrica Scandinavica*, **66**, 563–7.

Krasner, J., Giacoia, G.P. and Yaffe, S.J. (1973) Drug protein binding in the newborn infant. *Annals of the New York Academy of Sciences*, **226**, 101–14.

Langslet, A., Meberg, A., Bredesen, J.E. *et al.* (1978) Plasma concentrations of diazepam and N-desmethyl-diazepam in newborn infants after intravenous, intramuscular, rectal and oral administration. *Acta Paediatrica Scandinavica*, **67**, 699–704.

Leach, M.J., Marden, C.M., and Miller, A.A. (1986) Pharmacological studies in lamotrigine, a novel potential antiepileptic drug. II. Neurochemical studies on the mechanism of action. *Epilepsia*, **27**, 490–7.

Löscher, W. (1993) Effects of the antiepileptic drug valproate on metabolism and function of inhibitory excitatory amino acids in the brain. *Neurochemical Research*, **18**, 485–502.

Macdonald, R.L., and Meldrum, B.S. (1989) Principles of antiepileptic drug action, in *Antiepileptic Drugs* (eds. R. Levy, R. Mattson, B. Meldrum *et al.*) Raven, New York, pp. 59–83.

McCabe, R.T., Wasterlain, C.G., Kucharczyk, N. *et al.* (1993) Evidence for anticonvulsant and neuroprotectant action of felbamate mediated by strychnine-insensitive glycine receptors. *Journal of Pharmacology and Experimental Therapeutics*, **264**, 1248–52.

Matsuda, I., Ohtani, Y. and Ninomiya, N. (1986) Renal handling of carnitine in children with carnitine deficiency and hyperammonaemia associated with valproate therapy. *Journal of Pediatrics*, **109**, 131–4.

Metcalf, B.W. (1979) Inhibitors of GABA metabolism. *Biochemical Pharmacology*, **28**, 1705–12.

Morrow, J.I. and Richens, A. (1989) Disposition of anticonvulsants in childhood. *Clinical Pharmacokinetics*, **17**, (suppl. 1) 89–104.

Morselli, P. L. (ed.) (1977) *Drug Disposition During Development*, Spectrum, New York.

Morselli, P.L. (1983) Development of physiological variables important for drug kinetics, in *Antiepileptic Drug Therapy in Paediatrics* (eds P.L., Morselli, C.E. Pippenger and J.K. Penry), Raven, New York, pp. 1–12.

Morselli, P.L., Franco-Morselli, R. and Bossi, L. (1980) Clinical pharmacokinetics in newborns and infants. *Clinical Pharmacokinetics*, **5**, 485–527.

Murphy, J.V. and Marquard, K. (1982) Asymptomatic hyperammonaemia in patients receiving valproic acid. *Archives of Neurology*, **39**, 591–2.

Nau, H., Kuhnz, W., Egger, H.J. *et al.* (1982) Anticonvulsants during pregnancy and lactation. Transplacental transfer, maternal and neonatal pharmacokinetics. *Clinical Pharmacokinetics*, **7**, 508–63.

O'Hagan, M. and Wallace, S.J. (1994) Enteral formula feeds interfere with phenytoin absorption. *Brain and Development*, **16**, 165–7.

Perucca, E. (1987) Drug metabolism in pregnancy, infancy and childhood. *Pharmacology and Therapeutics*, **34**, 129–43.

Perucca, E. and Richens, A. (1985) Clinical pharmacokinetics of antiepileptic drugs, in *Antiepileptic Drugs: Handbook of Experimental Pharmacology*, vol. 74 (eds D. Janz and H.H. Frey), Springer Verlag, Berlin, pp. 661–723.

Pisani, F., Fazio, A., Oteri, G. *et al.* (1986) Sodium valproate and valpromide: differential interactions with carbamazepine in epileptic patients. *Epilepsia*, **27**, 548–52.

Rane, A. and Wilson, J.T. (1976) Clinical pharmacokinetics in infants and children. *Clinical Pharmacokinetics*, **1**, 2–24.

Rey, E., Pons, G. and Olive, G. (1992) Vigabatrin. Clinical pharmacokinetics. *Clinical Pharmacokinetics*, **24**, 267–78.

Rey, E., Pons, G., Richard, M.O. *et al.* (1990) Pharmacokinetics of the individual enantiomers of vigabatrin (γvinyl GABA) in epileptic children. *British Journal of Clinical Pharmacology*, **30**, 253–7.

Richens, A. (1979) Clinical pharmacokinetics of phenytoin. *Clinical Pharmacokinetics*, **4**, 153–69.

Schoeman, J.F., Elyas, A.A., Brett, E.M. *et al.* (1984) Altered ratio of carbamazepine-10,11-epoxide/carbamazepine in plasma of children: evidence of anticonvulsant drug interaction. *Developmental Medicine and Child Neurology*, **26**, 749–55.

Sherwin, A.L., Robb, J.P. and Lechter, M. (1973) Improved control of epilepsy by monitoring plasma ethosuximide. *Archives of Neurology*, **28**, 178–81.

Sillanpää, M., Pynnönen, S., Laippala, P. *et al.* (1979) Carbamazepine in the treatment of partial epileptic seizures in infants and young children: a preliminary study. *Epilepsia*, **20**, 563.

Suganuma, T., Ishizaki, T., Chiba, K. *et al.* (1981) The effect of concurrent administration of valproate sodium on phenobarbital plasma concentration/dosage ratio in pediatric patients. *Journal of Pediatrics*, **99**, 314–7.

Suman-Chauhan, N., Webdale, L., Hill, D.R. *et al.* (1993) Characterisation of [³H] gabapentin binding to a novel site in rat brain: homogenate binding studies. *European Journal of Pharmacology – Molecular Pharmacology Section*, **244**, 293–301.

Vining, E.P.G., Mellits, E.D., Dorsen, M.M. *et al.* (1987) Psychologic and behavioural effects of antiepileptic drugs in children: a double-blind comparison between phenobarbital and valproic acid. *Pediatrics*, **80**, 165–74.

Wagner, M.L., Graves, N.M., Leppik, I.E. *et al.* (1991) The effect of felbamate on valproate disposition. *Epilepsia*, **32**, 15.

Wallin, A., Jalling, B. and Boréus, L.O. (1974) Plasma concentrations of phenobarbital in the neonate during prophylaxis for neonatal hyperbilirubinaemia. *Journal of Pediatrics*, **85**, 392–7.

Wilder, B.J. and Ramsay, R.E. (1976) Oral and intramuscular phenytoin. *Clinical Pharmacology and Therapeutics*, **19**, 360–4.

Wilensky, A.J. and Lowden, J.A. (1973) Inadequate serum levels after intramuscular administration of diphenylhydantoin. *Neurology*, **23**, 318–24.

Wilson, J.T., Hojer, B. and Rane, A. (1976) Loading and conventional dose therapy with phenytoin in children: kinetic profile of parent drug and main metabolite in plasma. *Clinical Pharmacology and Therapeutics*, **20**, 48.

Yuen, A.W.C., Land, G., Weatherley, B.C. *et al.* (1992) Sodium valproate acutely inhibits lamotrigine metabolism. *British Journal of Clinical Pharmacology*, **33**, 511–3.

Blaise F.D. Bourgeois

PHENOBARBITONE

Despite the fact that phenobarbitone has been in clinical use since 1912, it is still considered to be one of the major antiepileptic drugs. Its known sedative and behavioral side-effects are often outweighed by the fact that it is otherwise relatively safe, effective, and easy to administer. The use of phenobarbitone has remained particularly common in the pediatric age range, major reasons being its convenient pharmacokinetics and relatively low cost. When compared with other major drugs such as phenytoin, carbamazepine, and valproate, phenobarbitone has certain advantages. The potential cardiovascular problems of phenytoin, such as bradyarrhythmia and hypotension, necessitate cautious intravenous administration, and the nonlinear kinetics of phenytoin can make dosage adjustments particularly difficult in children. Carbamazepine cannot be administered parenterally, and its very short half-life in children causes wide fluctuations of the levels, necessitating frequent administration. Valproate is associated with a risk of hepatotoxicity which is inversely related to age (Dreifuss *et al.*, 1989). Also, there is no evidence that valproate is effective parenterally in the acute treatment of convulsive seizures.

The indications for phenobarbitone in the treatment of epilepsy in the pediatric age range are summarized in Table 23a.1. In the treatment of partial seizures in children, phenobarbitone was found to be as effective

Table 23a.1 Indications for phenobarbitone in the treatment of epilepsy in children

Generalized tonic-clonic seizures
Simple and complex partial seizures
Generalized convulsive and simple or complex
  partial status epilepticus
Neonatal seizures
Juvenile myoclonic epilepsy
Prophylaxis of febrile seizures

as carbamazepine for up to 1 year (Mitchell and Chavez, 1987). This is in good agreement with the large-scale controlled comparison of phenytoin, carbamazepine, phenobarbitone, and primidone in adults (Mattson *et al.*, 1985). Phenobarbitone can be effective in the treatment of generalized myoclonic seizures in general, and in the treatment of juvenile myoclonic epilepsy (Chapter 14b) in particular (Resor and Resor, 1990), but valproate is now the preferred drug for this form of epilepsy. In the treatment of convulsive status epilepticus (Chapter 18), phenobarbitone remains a major drug. It is usually administered after a benzodiazepine and phenytoin, and it was found to be as effective as diazepam and phenytoin (Shaner *et al.*, 1988). The intravenous loading dose of phenobarbitone in the treatment of status epilepticus varies between 10 and 30 mg/kg, and a dose of 15–20 mg/kg is most commonly used. Very high doses of phenobarbitone have been recommended in the treatment of refractory status epilepticus in children (Crawford *et al.*, 1988). This approach controlled seizures

Epilepsy in Children. Edited by Sheila Wallace. Published in 1996 by Chapman & Hall, London. ISBN 0 412 56860 8

when no limits were imposed in relation to the maximal dose, and serum levels of 70–344 mg/l were reached. In this series, most patients were initially intubated, but recovered good spontaneous respiration despite persistently high phenobarbitone levels; hypotension was uncommon. Mainly for the reasons outlined above, phenobarbitone remains a drug of first choice in newborns with seizures. The initial loading dose of 15–20 mg/kg is similar to the dose used in children and adults, and the maintenance dose is 3–4 mg/kg/day. An efficacy rate of 85% against various neonatal seizures was achieved with high loading doses of up to 40 mg/kg (Gal *et al.*, 1982).

Phenobarbitone has been the most widely used drug in the chronic prophylaxis of febrile seizures (Chapter 10). Efficacy in preventing recurrences could be demonstrated at levels above 15 mg/l (Wolf and Forsythe, 1978). However, chronic prophylactic treatment of febrile seizures with phenobarbitone is now more the exception than the rule. There are several reasons for this: a better understanding of the benign nature of simple febrile seizures, the demonstration of the efficacy of intermittent short-term diazepam therapy (Knudsen, 1985) and, finally, reservations about the efficacy of phenobarbitone prophylaxis, as well as the possible detrimental effect on the IQ (Farwell *et al.*, 1990; McKinlay and Newton, 1989). Failure of prophylaxis was often associated with noncompliance with the regimen and subtherapeutic levels at the time of the seizure recurrences.

The daily maintenance dose of phenobarbitone in children varies between 2 and 8 mg/kg, and is roughly inversely proportional to the child's age. Because of the long elimination half-life and slow accumulation of phenobarbitone, the full maintenance dose can be given on the first day. After chronic administration, discontinuation of phenobarbitone should always be gradual over several weeks. Barbiturates and benzo-

diazepines are the antiepileptic drugs most commonly associated with withdrawal seizures upon rapid discontinuation.

PHENYTOIN

Phenytoin has remained a major antiepileptic drug since its introduction into clinical use in 1938. Worldwide it is still one of the most commonly used antiepileptic drugs. It has a range of efficacy that is similar to phenobarbitone, with the exception of the prophylaxis of febrile seizures, for which it has no proven efficacy. Phenytoin can be administered intravenously and has been used in every age group. It is not sedating and causes little or no respiratory depression. Phenytoin distinguishes itself from all other currently used antiepileptic drugs by its nonlinear elimination kinetics, resulting in a disproportionate increase in steady-state serum levels as the maintenance dose is increased. In addition, the elimination kinetics vary as a function of age.

As shown in Table 23a.2, phenytoin can be useful in the treatment of generalized tonic-clonic seizures, simple and complex partial seizures, generalized convulsive status epilepticus, simple or complex partial status epilepticus, and neonatal seizures. Phenytoin cannot be recommended for the treatment of infantile spasms (Chapter 11b), the Lennox–Gastaut syndrome (Chapter 12a) and related syndromes, or absence seizures. In the treatment of partial and secondarily generalized seizures, controlled studies in adults have shown no substantial difference in efficacy between carbamazepine, phenobarbital,

Table 23a.2 Indications for phenytoin in the treatment of epilepsy in children

Generalized tonic-clonic seizures
Simple and complex partial seizures
Generalized convulsive and simple or complex
  partial status epilepticus
Neonatal seizures

phenytoin, primidone, and valproate (Mattson *et al.*, 1985, 1992). Comparable comprehensive studies have not been carried out in children, but the available evidence in children tends to corroborate the findings in adults.

Phenytoin is an essential drug in the treatment of status epilepticus (Chapter 18) at any age. Although benzodiazepines, because of their very rapid onset of action, are given as the first drug to interrupt status epilepticus, their duration of action is relatively short. Phenytoin is the drug of choice for subsequent protection against recurrences: it is effective, it can be given intravenously and, unlike phenobarbitone, it does not exacerbate the respiratory depression caused by the benzodiazepines. The dose for intravenous phenytoin in the treatment of status is the same in children as in adults, i.e. 15–20 mg/kg. In order to avoid bradyarrhythmia and hypotension, phenytoin needs to be administered slowly. The recommended rate is ≤50 mg/min in adolescents and adults. In children, the maximal rate is 3 mg/kg/min, which is about one-seventh to one fifth of the initial bolus per minute. Further doses can be given subsequently if needed, up to a total of 30 mg/kg. However, it has been suggested that these additional doses should be guided by plasma level monitoring (Richard *et al.*, 1993). Phenytoin is a useful drug in the treatment of seizures and status epilepticus also during the neonatal period (Chapter 9). Usually, it is administered after phenobarbitone has failed (Painter *et al.*, 1981). Although the volume of distribution of phenytoin is slightly larger in newborns than in older children and adults (about 1.0 l/kg versus 0.8 l/kg), the initial intravenous loading dose of phenytoin in newborns is also 15–20 mg/kg. Additional loading doses can be given on the basis of serum level determinations.

The chronic maintenance dose of phenytoin is quite variable and age-dependent. In recognition of the nonlinear kinetics, it is advisable to titrate the dose upward, with progressively smaller increments in daily doses. The initial dose should be about 5 mg/kg/day in older children and 8 mg/kg/day in young infants. Serum levels should be determined 1–3 weeks after any dosage adjustment. Dosage increases will invariably result in disproportionately larger increases in the steady-state serum level. The nonlinear kinetics of phenytoin initially described in adults were also demonstrated in children of any age (Dodson, 1980), including in newborns (Bourgeois and Dodson, 1983). In certain individuals, this can lead to very labile levels in the therapeutic range, dosage increases of 10–20% being associated with increases in steady-state levels of 50–100%. In such patients, changing from a preparation of sodium phenytoin, which contains 92% phenytoin, to a preparation of phenytoin base may cause a substantial increase in concentration. In newborns, the elimination of phenytoin is initially slow, but there is a rapid acceleration during the first month of life (Bourgeois and Dodson, 1983). Consequently, the elimination kinetics of phenytoin in infants less than 1 year old are faster than at any other age (Dodson, 1982). Accordingly, in older newborns and young infants, daily maintenance doses of phenytoin as high as 20 mg/kg may be required to maintain good therapeutic levels.

VALPROATE

The introduction of valproate (or valproic acid) has had a major impact on the drug treatment of epilepsy, and particularly of epilepsy in the pediatric age range. Valproate distinguishes itself from all previously introduced antiepileptic drugs in terms of its spectrum of efficacy. Its efficacy against a range of generalized seizures as well as against partial seizures is shared by no other drug. Valproate is not sedative and it causes less cognitive or behavioral effects than phenobarbitone.

The indications for valproate in the treat-

Table 23a.3 Indications for valproate in the treatment of epilepsy in children

Absences
Myoclonic seizures
Generalized tonic-clonic seizures
Juvenile myoclonic epilepsy
Lennox–Gastaut syndrome
Infantile spasms
Simple and complex partial seizures

ment of epilepsy are summarized in Table 23a.3. The initial primary indication was the treatment of absence seizures (Chapter 13a). The administration of valproate reduces the frequency and duration of spike-and-wave discharges in patients with typical and atypical absences (Maheshwari and Jeavons, 1975; Braathen *et al.*, 1988). The duration of spike-and-wave discharges was reduced in 21 of 25 patients with absence seizures treated for 10 weeks, and the reduction was by more than 75% in 11 of these patients (Villareal *et al.*, 1978). In terms of efficacy against absence seizures, valproate and ethosuximide were found to be equally effective in two independent comparison studies (Callaghan *et al.*, 1982; Sato *et al.*, 1982). Complete control of simple absence seizures is usually achieved with valproate therapy in at least 80% of the patients (Henriksen and Johannessen, 1982; Bourgeois *et al.*, 1987). The response appears to be particularly favorable when absence seizures do not occur in combination with another seizure type. In an open evaluation of 25 patients, valproate has also been shown to be very effective in preventing the recurrence of absence status (Berkovic *et al.*, 1989).

Valproate is also effective in generalized convulsive seizures. In the control of generalized tonic-clonic seizures, valproate is comparable to the other major antiepileptic drugs (Spitz and Deasy, 1991; Ramsey *et al.*, 1992). Such seizures were completely controlled by the addition of valproate in 14 of 42 children with intractable epilepsy (Henriksen and Johannessen, 1982). When used as monotherapy, in children with generalized tonic-clonic seizures, valproate was associated with an excellent outcome (Dulac *et al.*, 1986).

Valproate is currently one of the most effective drugs for myoclonic seizures, particularly those seen with primary or idiopathic generalized epilepsies. In a group of patients with myoclonic epilepsy of adolescence, many of whom had not responded to previous medications, 17 of 22 were fully controlled (Covanis, Gupta and Jeavons, 1982). Epilepsy with photosensitivity shows a good response to valproate, regardless of the associated seizure type, such as tonic-clonic, absence or myoclonic seizures (Jeavons, Bishop and Harding, 1986). The role of valproate as the drug of choice in the treatment of juvenile myoclonic epilepsy (Chapter 14b) is supported by several other reports (Delgado-Escueta and Enrile-Bacsal, 1984; Resor and Resor, 1990). Benign myoclonic epilepsy of infancy (Chapter 11d) is another form of idiopathic generalized epilepsy with myoclonic seizures which seems to respond quite well to valproate (Dulac *et al.*, 1986). Successful treatment with valproate in combination with clonazepam has been reported for tonic-clonic and myoclonic seizures in patients with severe progressive myoclonic epilepsy (Chapter 15a) (Iivainen and Himberg, 1982).

Another aspect of valproate therapy specific to the pediatric age range is its use in the treatment of the Lennox–Gastaut syndrome (Chapter 12a), and related forms of epilepsy, including infantile spasms (Chapter 11b). Among 38 patients with 'myoclonic astatic epilepsy', the addition of valproate led to a 50–80% improvement in one-third of the group, and seven patients were fully controlled (Covanis, Gupta and Jeavons, 1982). Nine of 39 children with 'atonic seizures' are reported free of seizures after the addition of valproate (Henriksen and Johannessen, 1982). The role of valproate in the prevention of infantile spasms is more difficult to assess, because the available information is based either on small series of patients, or on the combination of valproate with ACTH. In two studies, the efficacy of valproate has been assessed in the absence of ACTH. Bachman (1982) treated 19 infants with infantile spasms with either valproate or ACTH as a first drug. Eight patients experienced good control with valproate (20–60 mg/kg/day) as the first drug, and did not require ACTH. Patients with failure on either ACTH or valproate as the first treatment were switched to the other regimen. The outcome suggested a slightly better response to ACTH, but side-effects were more frequent and more severe with ACTH. The other study was carried out in 18 infants who received 20 mg/kg/day of valproate as their first treatment for infantile spasms (Pavone *et al.*, 1981). The short-term response was judged to be good to excellent in 12 patients. The response was considered similar to the authors' experience with ACTH or steroids, but with fewer side-effects.

Much less information is available on the efficacy of valproate against simple and complex partial seizures, and most has been obtained in adult patients. Among 13 children with uncontrolled simple partial seizures, one was controlled by the addition of valproate, and six experienced a seizure reduction of more than 50% (Henriksen and Johannessen, 1982). In the same study, four of 19 children with complex partial seizures became seizure free after the addition of valproate and the seizure frequency was reduced by at least 50% in 10. Valproate monotherapy was compared with carbamazepine monotherapy in a randomized, multicenter, double-blind trial in 480 adult patients with complex partial or secondarily generalized tonic-clonic seizures (Mattson *et al.*, 1992). Carbamazepine and valproate were equally effective against secondarily generalized seizures, with a similar composite score of efficacy and toxicity. Against complex partial seizures, four out of five efficacy parameters indicated slightly higher effect-

iveness for carbamazepine, which also had a higher composite score of efficacy and toxicity.

Valproate has been shown to be clearly effective in preventing the recurrence of febrile seizures. However, based on risk versus benefit considerations as well as on the alternative of using intermittent diazepam during febrile episodes, valproate cannot be recommended for this indication. Intermittent diazepam appears to be as effective as valproate (Lee, Taudorf, and Hvorslev, 1986). Neonates with seizures have also been successfully treated with valproate. It was administered orally as syrup in six newborns refractory to high levels of phenobarbitone (Gal *et al.*, 1988). In this series, seizure control was achieved in five of the six patients. The maintenance dose was 5–10 mg/kg/day, following a loading dose of 20–25 mg/kg.

Valproate therapy is usually initiated at a daily dose of 15 mg/kg. Subsequently, the dose can be increased at weekly intervals by 5 mg/kg/day, as necessary and as tolerated. The final maintenance dose of valproate can vary widely as a function of comedication, seizure type, and age. With valproate monotherapy, levels within the recommended therapeutic range and a satisfactory clinical response are usually achieved with doses between 10 and 20 mg/kg/day (Henriksen and Johannessen, 1982; Bourgeois *et al.*, 1987). Combination therapy with inducing drugs such as phenytoin, carbamazepine, phenobarbitone, and primidone invariably increases the dosage requirements to 30 mg/kg/day and above. Age-dependent kinetics may also increase the dosage requirements in children (Covanis, Gupta and Jeavons, 1982). Due to a combination of age-dependent kinetics and pharmacokinetic interactions, valproate levels within the therapeutic range can sometimes not be achieved in children on comedication, even at valproate doses above 100 mg/kg/day (Henriksen and Johannessen, 1982). The optimal dose or serum level of valproate can also vary as a function of the seizure type (Lundberg, Nergardh and Boreus, 1982), idiopathic generalized seizures usually being controlled at lower levels than partial seizures.

CARBAMAZEPINE

Carbamazepine is clearly one of the four drugs that have dominated the medical treatment of epilepsy until recently, the other three drugs being phenytoin, valproate and phenobarbital. The clinical efficacy and spectrum of action of carbamazepine is similar to that of phenytoin, but carbamazepine is not available for parenteral administration. This precludes its use in the treatment of status epilepticus and markedly reduces its usefulness in the treatment of neonatal seizures. The important role of carbamazepine is therefore in the treatment of simple and complex partial seizures and of primarily or secondarily generalized tonic-clonic seizures. Carbamazepine is ineffective against absence seizures and febrile seizures. It causes little or no sedation and has fewer cognitive or behavioral effects than phenobarbitone.

In the treatment of partial seizures, carbamazepine is at least as effective as any other major antiepileptic drug. Major controlled trials were carried out in adults (Mattson *et al.*, 1985, 1992). In these trials, carbamazepine was found to be as effective as phenytoin, phenobarbitone, primidone, and valproate. Carbamazepine was possibly more effective than any of the four other drugs against partial seizures without secondary generalization. When composite scores of efficacy and toxicity were analyzed against partial seizures with or without secondary generalization, carbamazepine and phenytoin scored higher than the other three drugs (Mattson *et al.*, 1985, 1992). Similar controlled trials focusing on partial seizures were not conducted in children, and it is therefore difficult to compare the efficacy of carbamazepine in children with the efficacy in adults. The outcome of carbamazepine monotherapy

was analyzed in a group of 90 children with partial or generalized tonic-clonic seizures with or without focal paroxysms on the EEG (Okuno *et al.*, 1989). Complete seizure control for at least 3 years was achieved in 74%. The prognosis was poorer for patients with partial seizures with secondary generalization. These results do not differ from those obtained in adults, and do not suggest that carbamazepine is less effective in children. A comparison between carbamazepine and phenobarbitone for the treatment of partial seizures in children revealed no difference in efficacy (Mitchell and Chavez, 1987).

In terms of side-effects, carbamazepine certainly seems to be well tolerated in children. In a comparative study of monotherapy with phenobarbitone, primidone, phenytoin, carbamazepine, and valproate, the rate of side-effects was the same for carbamazepine and valproate, and higher for phenytoin and phenobarbitone (Herranz, Armijo and Arteaga, 1988). Serious side-effects requiring discontinuation of the drug were least common with carbamazepine. Among the five drugs, carbamazepine was ranked by the authors as the best tolerated. Carbamazepine has little or no role in the treatment of primary (i.e. idiopathic/familial) generalized epilepsies or secondary generalized epilepsies (such as the Lennox-Gastaut syndrome). In children with the Lennox-Gastaut syndrome (Chapter 12a), or similar types of epilepsies, carbamazepine can exacerbate certain seizures such as myoclonic and drop attacks (Snead and Hosey, 1985).

The daily maintenance dose of carbamazepine that will achieve therapeutic levels is quite variable, and almost always higher in children than in adults. Children eliminate carbamazepine faster than adults and have a larger volume of distribution. In addition, comedication with phenytoin or phenobarbital further accelerates the elimination of carbamazepine. The initial maintenance dose of carbamazepine should always be relatively low, in children 5–10 mg/kg/day. There are two reasons for the low initial dose. First, side-effects often occur during the first days of treatment at serum levels that are well tolerated later in the course of treatment. Secondly, carbamazepine accelerates its own elimination rate through hepatic enzyme induction, a phenomenon called autoinduction. The maintenance dose of carbamazepine can be increased by 5–10 mg/kg/day at weekly intervals, and final maintenance doses of 30 mg/kg/day or more are not unusual in children, especially during combination therapy.

ETHOSUXIMIDE

Ethosuximide has been in clinical use for the treatment of absence seizures since 1960. It is still a drug of first choice in patients who have absence seizures only. Although its gastrointestinal side-effects may be bothersome, it is practically free of serious side-effects. Ethosuximide is highly effective against the 'typical absences' (as opposed to 'atypical absences') seen in primary generalized epilepsies such as childhood absence epilepsy (Chapter 13a). Complete seizure control is achieved in approximately 80% of the patients. With seizure control, a concomitant disappearance of spike-and-wave paroxysms in the EEG is the rule. Without a normalization of the EEG, full therapeutic success is questionable. It is a common observation that absence seizures that occur as the sole seizure type in a patient are more likely to be fully controlled by medication than if they occur in conjunction with another seizure type (Sato, Dreifuss and Penry, 1976). The therapeutic results with ethosuximide are also better against typical than against atypical absences.

The efficacy of ethosuximide in the control of absence seizures is similar to that of valproate. In two independent studies, a controlled comparison of the two drugs revealed a similar percentage of patients who became seizure-free (Callaghan *et al.*, 1982; Sato *et al.*, 1982). Valproate and ethosuximide

may have a beneficial synergistic interaction. A group of patients with absence seizures that had not been controlled by adequate trials of ethosuximide alone, or valproate alone, became free of seizures on a combination of ethosuximide and valproate (Rowan *et al.*, 1983). Although there is no clear evidence that ethosuximide alone is effective against any other seizure type besides absences, its use as adjunctive therapy may be effective against myoclonic seizures and against falling spells (Snead, 1987; Snead and Hosey, 1987).

Therapy with ethosuximide in children can be initiated at a dose of about 10 mg/kg/day. The dose can be titrated up at intervals of 5–7 days as necessary and as tolerated, up to a dose of approximately 30–40 mg/kg/day. This should be given preferably with or after meals in three divided doses, in order to minimize the occurrence of gastrointestinal side-effects.

PRIMIDONE

Primidone remains one of the major antiepileptic drugs. However, it is not a drug of first choice. There are two reasons for this: first, it has neurologic side-effects similar to phenobarbitone and, second, there has never been a clear demonstration that treatment with primidone truly differs from treatment with phenobarbitone in clinical practice. Primidone is converted *in vivo* to phenobarbitone, which accumulates significantly during chronic therapy. Therefore, primidone may only represent a phenobarbitone prodrug. Although primidone therapy is often referred to as a barbiturate therapy, primidone itself is not a barbiturate in the true sense. The pyrimidine ring of primidone lacks one of the three carbonyl groups that characterize the barbituric acid molecule. Independent seizure protection by primidone has been demonstrated repeatedly in animal models, but the actual contribution of primidone to the overall therapeutic effect during chronic therapy in humans is very difficult to ascertain. It is

Table 23a.4 Indications for primidone in the treatment of epilepsy in children

Generalized tonic-clonic seizures
Simple and complex partial seizures
Neonatal seizures
Juvenile myoclonic epilepsy
Prophylaxis of febrile seizures

unlikely that the other active metabolite of primidone, phenylethylmalonamide (PEMA), contributes in any way to the clinical effect (Bourgeois, Dodson and Ferrendelli, 1983a, 1983b).

Indications for primidone are similar to those for phenobarbitone (Table 23a.4). However, primidone is not available for parenteral administration and is not used in the acute treatment of status epilepticus. Primidone and phenobarbitone have been compared in several clinical studies. They were found to be equally effective in most of them (White, Pott and Norton, 1966; Oleson and Dam, 1967). In one cross-over study in patients with generalized tonic-clonic seizures, primidone was found to be slightly more effective than phenobarbitone in the presence of similar phenobarbitone levels before and after the cross-over (Oxley *et al.*, 1980). Primidone was compared with phenytoin, carbamazepine, and phenobarbitone in a large controlled study in patients with partial and secondarily generalized seizures (Mattson *et al.*, 1985). The four drugs were found to be similarly effective, but treatment failures occurred more often with primidone because of more pronounced side-effects during the early phases of the study. Primidone is also effective in the treatment of juvenile myoclonic epilepsy (Chapter 14b) (Delgado-Escueta and Enrile-Bacsal, 1984; Resor and Resor, 1990). However, valproic acid is now the drug of choice in this type of epilepsy. Primidone has been evaluated as adjunctive therapy in newborns with seizures (Powell, Painter and Pippenger, 1984). In 24 patients who had persistent seizures despite treatment with

both phenytoin and phenobarbitone, primidone was administered orally at an initial loading dose of 15–25 mg/kg, followed by a maintenance dose ranging from 12 to 20 mg/kg/day. Seizure control was achieved in 13 infants. Monitoring of phenobarbitone levels before and after discontinuation of phenobarbitone therapy suggested that newborns cannot convert primidone to phenobarbitone. Similar conclusions were reached in another independent study, both in terms of efficacy and in relation to the limited conversion of primidone to phenobarbitone in neonates and young infants (Sapin, Rivello and Grover, 1988).

When primidone is prescribed, it appears to be more rational to prescribe it as monotherapy or in combination with a noninducing drug such as valproate or a benzodiazepine. The primidone : phenobarbitone concentration ratio will be shifted in favor of phenobarbitone by an inducing drug, and this will tend to obliterate any possible difference between prescribing primidone and prescribing phenobarbitone. For the same reason, prescribing primidone and phenobarbitone together does not appear to have a rational basis. More than most other antiepileptic drugs, primidone must be introduced slowly, with a low initial dose. The initial doses may cause transient dizziness, drowsiness, and nausea. The initial dose may have to be as low as 62.5–125 mg in adults (1–2 mg/kg in children) at bedtime, with dosage increases at intervals of 3 days. The final dose is about 10–20 mg/kg/day. Compared to other major antiepileptic drugs, primidone appears to be tolerated better in children than in adults (Herranz, Armijo and Arteaga, 1988). In the presence of an inducing drug such as phenytoin or carbamazepine, steady-state phenobarbitone levels will be higher at any given dose of primidone, because of accelerated synthesis of phenobarbitone. Thus, higher primidone maintenance doses are usually tolerated when primidone is not administered with an inducing drug.

VIGABATRIN

Vigabatrin, or gamma-vinyl GABA, belongs to the new generation of antiepileptic drugs. The clinical experience with this drug is not as extensive as with the drugs discussed so far. However, it has been the object of a remarkable number of controlled studies in adults and in children, and it has been marketed first in European countries. Vigabatrin appears to be mainly effective against partial seizures. Controlled studies in adults have clearly demonstrated that vigabatrin reduces the frequency of complex partial seizures (Rimmer and Richens, 1984; Gram, Klosterkov and Dam, 1985; Tassinari *et al.*, 1987). In general, little benefit could be demonstrated against other seizure types (Tassinari *et al.*, 1987).

Several uncontrolled and controlled trials of vigabatrin in children have been reported. Experience in children has been the subject of two reviews (Gram, Sabers and Dulac, 1992; Appleton, 1993). In an open, noncontrolled add-on multicenter study, 135 children with partial seizures, generalized seizures, Lennox–Gastaut and West's syndrome were enrolled (Livingston *et al.*, 1989). Their ages ranged from 2 months to 12 years (mean 7.1 years). The average dose of vigabatrin was 87 mg/kg/day. A seizure reduction of at least 50% was observed in 38% of the patients. The best results were achieved against partial seizures. The most frequent side-effects were agitation and insomnia. In an add-on, single-blind, placebo-controlled 16-week trial, vigabatrin was given to 61 children with various seizure types (Luna *et al.*, 1989). Significant results were seen only in patients with cryptogenic partial seizures. The main side-effect was agitation. In a study of 16 children with refractory epilepsy, a fixed dose of vigabatrin was administered for 2 months, following 1 month of single-blind add-on

placebo (Arteaga *et al.*, 1992). The average seizure frequency was reduced from 51.4 to 22.3 per month. The great majority of these children had partial seizures. However, the efficacy of vigabatrin in children does not seem to be limited to partial seizures. An add-on open study was carried out in a total of 70 patients with infantile spasms (Chiron *et al.*, 1991; Chapter 11b). In a subgroup, a 2–4-week single-blind placebo phase was included. A seizure reduction of at least 50% was seen in 68% of the patients, and 43% became seizure free. In this study, vigabatrin appeared to be particularly effective in patients with tuberous sclerosis. In this subgroup, a 50% reduction or better was achieved in 86%, and 71% of these patients became seizure free. Like several other antiepileptic drugs, vigabatrin may at times exacerbate seizures. In a review of 194 children, this occurred in 10% of the patients. This exacerbation was clearly related to the type of epilepsy syndrome, and occurred predominantly among patients with non-progressive myoclonic epilepsy and the Lennox–Gastaut syndrome (Lortie *et al.*, 1993).

The recommended dose of vigabatrin in children is usually 40–85 mg/kg/day, but higher doses have been used and well tolerated. In the open study of Livingston *et al.* (1989), the average dose was 87 mg/kg/day, with a range of 27–600 mg/kg/day. Doses of 100–200 mg/kg/day are recommended in infants treated for infantile spasms.

LAMOTRIGINE

Lamotrigine belongs to the new generation of antiepileptic drugs that have been extensively tested in patients. It was first released in European countries. The first tests were in adults with refractory partial seizures. Twenty-one adults completed a double-blind, placebo-controlled cross-over trial

(Jawad *et al.*, 1989). Compared with placebo, lamotrigine significantly reduced the frequency of total seizures, partial seizures, and secondarily generalized seizures. In a similar trial, only 11 of 62 patients experienced a 50% or greater seizure reduction (Smith *et al.* 1993). The dose-response was assessed in 216 adults with partial seizures undergoing a placebo-controlled parallel-group trial with two lamotrigine groups: 300 mg/day and 500 mg/day (Matsuo *et al.* 1993). A seizure reduction of 50% or more was achieved in one-fifth of the 300 mg group and in one-third of the 500 mg group. Compared to placebo, the reduction in seizure frequency was significant only in the 500 mg group.

The experience with lamotrigine in children is derived from open studies only. Five children with frequent atypical absence seizures were treated in an open fashion (Betts, Pigott and Grace, 1989). All showed a dramatic response to lamotrigine, which was sustained. There was at least a 95% reduction in seizure frequency. Recurrent episodes of nonconvulsive status epilepticus were prevented in two of the patients. Lamotrigine was tested in an open-label add-on trial in 15 children aged 5–11 years with various types of seizures (Wallace, 1990). A moderate to marked improvement was seen in eight of 15 children, with a reduction in myoclonic seizures, myoclonic absences, atonic and tonic seizures. The efficacy of lamotrigine in the treatment of patients with the Lennox–Gastaut syndrome has been evaluated in at least two studies. In a group of 13 patients with this syndrome, an average dose of lamotrigine of 223 mg/day was administered in an open add-on fashion (Ollèr, Russi and Oller Daurella, 1991). Their ages ranged from 5.5 to 27 years (mean 15.9 years). Five patients were seizure free during a follow-up of 2–26 months, and one of the seizure types was controlled in three. In another open add-on study in 11 patients with the Lennox–Gastaut syndrome (Timmings and Richens, 1992), lamotrigine was titrated up to 400 mg/day. After 3 months, a seizure reduction of 50% or more was observed in 10 patients, one of whom became seizure free.

The appropriate dosage of lamotrigine varies as a function of comedication. Valproate inhibits the metabolism of lamotrigine and thus decreases the dosage requirements. In infants and children on valproate, the initial dose should be 0.2 mg/kg/day, with a final maintenance dose of 1–5 mg/kg/day. If taking other antiepileptic drugs, infants and children can start taking lamotrigine at 2 mg/kg/day, with subsequent increases to 5–15 mg/kg/day.

CLONAZEPAM

Of the benzodiazepines, clonazepam is the one most widely used in the chronic treatment of epilepsy. Clonazepam typifies the advantages and disadvantages of benzodiazepines. Benzodiazepines have several advantages. They have a very rapid onset of action; can be administered orally, rectally, intramuscularly, and intravenously; have a wide spectrum of efficacy, and have been shown to have some protective effect against every type of seizure. They cause no significant pharmacokinetic interactions with other antiepileptic drugs. Finally, they have virtually no systemic or serious side-effects. Unfortunately, benzodiazepines have two major disadvantages: they have sedative and behavioral side-effects, particularly in children, and they produce tolerance. The duration of their efficacy is limited in time in a relatively high percentage of patients. Also, despite their wide spectrum of efficacy, they are often less effective than the more specific antiepileptic drugs against any seizure type. Benzodiazepines must be tapered carefully after chronic use because of the risks of withdrawal seizures. Based on this profile, benzodiazepines are particularly useful for the acute and intermittent treatment of epilepsy, in situations such as status epilepticus (see Chapter 18), intermittent prophylaxis of febrile seizures (Chapter 10), periodic seizure clusters, and catamenial epilepsy.

Clonazepam is rarely used in monotherapy. In children, it is most likely to be used as an adjunct in the treatment of the Lennox–Gastaut syndrome (and related epilepsies) (Chapter 12), and of absence seizures (Chapter 13a). It is also used as a secondary drug against infantile spasms and myoclonic seizures, in general. Clonazepam is highly effective against absence seizures, at least initially (Dreifuss *et al.*, 1975; Mikkelsen *et al.*, 1976). Like ethosuximide, clonazepam can be particularly useful in combination with valproate, against absences, as well as against complex partial seizures (Mireles and Leppik, 1985). However these favorable results are offset by side-effects and tolerance to the antiepileptic effect. Quite favorable results of clonazepam monotherapy in children were reported by Ishikawa *et al.* (1985); they treated 60 children between the ages of 1 month and 14 years, excluding those with infantile spasms. According to the authors, seizure control was achieved in 77% of the patients, with side-effects such as drowsiness and ataxia in 5% only. Among responders, the average dose was 0.09 mg/kg/day in infants, and 0.06 mg/kg/day in older children.

The Lennox–Gastaut syndrome and related epilepsies of childhood (Chapter 12) probably represent the most common indication for the chronic use of clonazepam. The atypical absences, myoclonic seizures, and falling spells can be reduced (Vassella *et al.*, 1973). Although valproate is now used preferentially, the combination of valproate and clonazepam can be of additional benefit (Mireles and Leppik, 1985). For infantile spasms, clonazepam is certainly not considered to be a drug of choice, but a favorable response has been documented (Vassella *et al.*, 1973). Clonazepam has also been used successfully in the treatment of epilepsies with myoclonus as the predominant seizure type. Patients with severe progressive myoclonus epilepsy (Chapter 15a) can improve with a combination of clonazepam and valproate (Iivainen and Himberg, 1982). Clonazepam is also undoubtedly effective in controlling the myoclonic seizures occurring in patients with juvenile myoclonic epilepsy (Chapter 14b). However, it seems to be ineffective against the generalized tonic-clonic seizures that these patients often experience. In one series, injuries from generalized tonic-clonic seizures were more frequent when the myoclonic seizures were controlled by monotherapy with clonazepam (Obeid and Panayiotopoulos, 1989).

Like other benzodiazepines, clonazepam has been used successfully in the treatment of different forms of status epilepticus in children (Congdon and Forsythe, 1980). However, in certain countries such as the USA, clonazepam is not available for parenteral use. In patients with the Lennox–Gastaut syndrome who are in myoclonic or nonconvulsive status, clonazepam can induce a generalized tonic state (Bittencourt and Richens, 1981). This effect can be seen with other benzodiazepines, such as diazepam. Intravenous clonazepam has also been tried in 18 neonates with frequent seizures refractory to phenobarbitone (Andre *et al.*, 1986). The clearance of the drug was 50–70% less than in adults and older children. Excellent results were achieved in seven out of eight newborns who received 0.1 mg/kg. Results were less encouraging in the patients who received 0.2 mg/kg, suggesting an optimal response at the lower dose with a detrimental effect beyond a certain level.

It is important to initiate therapy with clonazepam slowly, using initial doses of 0.01–0.03 mg/kg/day. Dosage increases should be carried out at intervals of 1 week or more, titrating the dose as necessary and as tolerated up to approximately 0.2–0.3 mg/kg/day. Children require higher doses than adults on a mg/kg basis, and the maintenance dose should be divided into three daily doses. In an attempt to avoid the development of tolerance with chronic use, administration of clonazepam on alternate days has been studied, with improvement in seizure control in some patients (Sher, 1985). In the treatment of status epilepticus, parenteral doses in children are usually 1–2 mg, up to a total of 4 mg.

NITRAZEPAM

The statements made about benzodiazepines in the discussion on clonazepam also apply to nitrazepam. Unlike clonazepam, which has a relatively broad use in the treatment of epilepsy, nitrazepam has been used more restrictively, mainly for infantile spasms with hypsarrhythmia and in children with the Lennox–Gastaut and related syndromes (Chapter 12). Nitrazepam was compared with ACTH against infantile spasms in a randomized controlled study (Dreifuss *et al.*, 1986). A 75–100% seizure reduction could be achieved in 57% of the patients treated with ACTH and in 52% of the patients treated with nitrazepam.

The maintenance dose of nitrazepam varies between 0.25 and 3 mg/kg/day, the higher doses being used predominantly in infants. Average doses are 1 mg/kg/day in children and 0.5 mg/kg/day in adolescents and adults. The initial dose should be lower than the maintenance dose. The development of tolerance occurs, as with other benzodiazepines. Side-effects are also similar, but nitrazepam seems to more specifically cause drooling and aspiration, which may be responsible for cases of pneumonia and possibly death (Wyllie *et al.*, 1986; Murphy *et al.*, 1987).

CLOBAZAM

Clobazam differs structurally from all other commonly used benzodiazepines. Based on the different position of one nitrogen in one of the rings, it is a 1,5-benzodiazepine, as opposed to a 1,4-benzodiazepine. With the possible exception of milder side-effects, clobazam appears to have a similar spectrum of efficacy and to be associated with the same development of tolerance as other benzodiazepines (approximately 50% of the patients). In the countries where it is marketed, clobazam is now one of the favorite benzodiazepines in the treatment of epilepsy, particularly as adjunctive therapy of partial seizures (Robertson, 1986). In a placebo-controlled cross-over study in 26 institutionalized patients with refractory epilepsy, clobazam was associated with a highly significant decrease in seizure frequency, with full control in three patients (Allen *et al.*, 1983). The effect on partial seizures was particularly evident, but the long-term follow-up was disappointing. Of the 26 responders, 20 (77%) developed tolerance to the antiepileptic effect after a median interval of 3.5 months (Allen *et al.*, 1985). Good initial results with clobazam were also obtained in monotherapy in children with various types of seizures (Dulac *et al.*, 1983). In 25 children treated for an average duration of 9 months, the results were considered satisfactory in 11 patients, and six patients experienced a seizure reduction of 75%. The authors considered clobazam particularly effective in benign partial epilepsy. In a more recent double-blind placebo-controlled study of clobazam in children with generalized and partial seizures, 52% of the patients on clobazam had a greater than 50% reduction in their seizure frequency (Keene, Whiting and Humphreys, 1990). Clobazam can be successful in the intermittent treatment of catamenial epilepsy (Feely and Gibson, 1984).

The maintenance dose is usually between 0.5 and 1 mg/kg/day. Side-effects are more likely at total daily doses of more than 30 mg/day, without clear evidence of improved effectiveness. Clobazam is not available for parenteral use but can be administered rectally in semiacute situations at doses of 20–30 mg.

ADRENOCORTICOTROPHIC HORMONE AND STEROIDS

Adrenocorticotropic hormone (ACTH) differs from all other antiepileptic drugs in that its use is limited to one or two indications, for the purpose of achieving a cure, rather than as chronic prophylaxis. ACTH established itself as the treatment of choice for infantile spasms with hypsarrhythmia (West's syndrome; Chapter 11b). When effective, it not only controls the infantile spasms, but it also normalizes the EEG. Less commonly, ACTH is used in children with refractory epilepsies such as the Lennox–Gastaut and related syndromes (Chapter 12). The indications for steroids in the treatment of epilepsy are the same as for ACTH. There are ongoing controversies as to whether ACTH is superior to steroids; whether ACTH should be used as soon as a diagnosis of West's syndrome is made; and, what represents the optimal dose and treatment duration with ACTH. In general, one-half to two-thirds of patients with infantile spasms will benefit significantly from either ACTH or steroid therapy. In a double-blind study, the patients were randomized to either prednisone 2 mg/kg/day or ACTH 20 U/day, with a corresponding oral or intramuscular placebo (Hrachovy *et al.*, 1983). No difference in efficacy was found between ACTH and steroids. The success rate was not related to the duration of the epilepsy before the onset of treatment. In contrast, Lombroso (1983) concluded that the long-term outcome was better with ACTH than with prednisone in patients with cryptogenic infantile spasms. In this, as well as in another report (Singer, Rabe and Haller, 1980), better results were obtained when ACTH therapy was initiated within the first month following the onset of spasms. Various initial doses and rates of tapering have been recommended. The initial daily dose usually lies between 110 (Lombroso, 1983) and 150 (Snead *et al.*, 1989) units per m² body surface. In an open study, Snead *et al.* achieved better seizure control with ACTH at 150 U/m²/day than with prednisone 2 mg/kg/day (90% versus 40% of patients).

The initial dose of ACTH is given intramuscularly in two divided doses for 1–3 weeks. The dose is then reduced gradually and the total duration of treatment may vary from 3 weeks to 3 months. For example, the regimen advocated by Snead *et al.* (1989) starts with 75 U/m²/day twice daily for 1 week, followed by 75 U/m²/day once daily for 1 week, then 75 U/m²/day every other day during the third week. The dose is then tapered over the ensuing 9 weeks. Based on the age of occurrence of infantile spasms, the body surface of the patients is usually between one-third and one-half m². Thus, the initial dose would be approximately 25–40 U twice daily. Therapy with ACTH is best started in the hospital. This will allow monitoring of blood glucose and blood pressure carefully, as well as to teaching the parents to inject ACTH and to check for glycosuria. After discharge, blood pressure should be measured first daily, then every 2–3 days.

Although it was found to be less effective in certain studies, prednisone therapy may have less serious side-effects and requires no initial hospitalization. Steroids and ACTH are by no means harmless. A serious infection is the main concern, in addition to hypertension, hyperglycemia with glucosuria, and congestive heart failure.

FELBAMATE

Felbamate was first released in North America in 1993, as the first new antiepileptic drug in 15 years. As a dicarbamate, felbamate resembles meprobamate, but it does not share its sedative or tranquillizing properties. Although it was found to have various effects on inhibitory and excitatory systems, the precise antiepileptic mechanism of action of felbamate has not been established. In experimental seizure models, felbamate has a wide spectrum of activity, being effective against seizures elicited both by maximal electroshock and by systemically administered chemical convulsants. It was also found to have very low toxicity, in particular neurotoxicity, in animal models. The clinical development of felbamate has differed from the classic development models. It was submitted to innovative and unconventional trials in adults, and it was also the first drug to be tested in a placebo-controlled trial in children with the Lennox–Gastaut syndrome (Felbamate Study Group in Lennox–Gastaut Syndrome, 1993). Unfortunately, unacceptable numbers of patients treated with felbamate developed aplastic anemia and/or hepatic failure.

GABAPENTIN

Gabapentin was released very recently. Thus, clinical experience is still limited. Despite its similarity with the inhibitory neurotransmitter GABA, the mechanism of action of gabapentin does not seem to be related to activation of GABA-mediated processes or to an increase in the concentration of GABA. Gabapentin has pharmacokinetic properties that are clinically desirable: being entirely eliminated by the kidneys, it is neither the cause nor the object of pharmacokinetic interactions. Due to its lack of binding to plasma proteins, there are also no interactions related to displacement.

So far, the clinical efficacy of gabapentin has been demonstrated in the treatment of partial epilepsy in adults (UK Gabapentin Study Group, 1990; US Gabapentin Study Group No. 5, 1993). Somnolence, dizziness, ataxia, and fatigue were the most common side-effects. Results of studies of gabapentin in the treatment of partial seizures in patients below the age of 16 years are not available at this time. However, a double-blind, placebo-controlled study in new-onset absence seizures (Chapter 13a) performed in 33 children demonstrated no efficacy of gabapentin against absences (Leiderman, Garofalo and LaMoreaux, 1993).

No dosage recommendations for children have been provided. In the study of gabapentin in absence seizures in children, doses of 15–20 mg/kg/day were administered. There is no need to monitor serum levels of gabapentin; no therapeutic range has been recommended.

TIAGABINE

Tiagabine is still in a relatively early phase of development, and has not been released in any country at the present time. Structurally, it is nipecotic acid linked to a lipophilic moiety that allows it to cross the blood–brain barrier. Nipecotic acid inhibits uptake of GABA into glia, thus increasing synaptic GABA concentration. So far, tiagabine trials have included only adults with partial seizures. Significant efficacy, compared to placebo, was demonstrated at doses of 32 mg/day and above. Tiagabine does not seem to affect the levels of other antiepileptic drugs, but carbamazepine, phenytoin, and primidone markedly shorten the elimination half-life of tiagabine. Also, valproate increases the free fraction of tiagabine. No trials of tiagabine in children have been completed at this time.

VITAMIN B6

The use of vitamin B6, or pyridoxine, in the treatment of epilepsy has not been limited to cases of pyridoxine deficiency or dependency (Chapter 4c). The link between pyridoxine and epilepsy is most likely based on the fact that pyridoxine is an essential part of a coenzyme responsible for the synthesis of the inhibitory neurotransmitter GABA. Pyridoxine dependency, an autosomal recessive inborn error of metabolism, does not have characteristic clinical features and it should be considered in any child with refractory seizures up to the age of 2 years, including those with infantile spasms (Mikati *et al.*, 1991). Most commonly, pyridoxine dependency presents with intractable seizures during the neonatal period. The diagnosis can be established by administering 50–100 mg of pyridoxine intravenously during a flurry of seizures, if possible while recording the EEG. If there is a good response within minutes to hours, this should be followed by a maintenance dose of pyridoxine of 50–100 mg/day orally. The use of very high doses of pyridoxine (200–400 mg/kg/day) in patients with infantile spasms has been the subject of several reports. In a recent pilot study, 17 children with recently diagnosed infantile spasms (Chapter 11b) received pyridoxine 300 mg/kg/day orally as their initial treatment (Pietz *et al.*, 1993). Five responded to pyridoxine within 2 weeks and were seizure free within 4 weeks. Besides gastrointestinal side-effects, which improved with dosage reduction, there were no serious adverse reactions. Considering the potentially serious side-effects of ACTH, steroids, and valproate in this age group, pyridoxine is an attractive alternative. In a group of 18 patients, pyridoxine at lower doses (40–50 mg/kg/day) was combined with low doses of ACTH (0.4 units/kg/day). The success rate was similar to that achieved with high doses of ACTH (Takuma, Seki and Hirai, 1990).

REFERENCES

Allen, J.W., Jawad, S., Oxley, J. and Trimble, M. (1985) Development of tolerance to anticonvulsant effect of clobazam. *Journal of Neurology, Neurosurgery and Psychiatry*, **48**, 284–5.

Allen, J.W., Oxley, J., Robertson, M. *et al.* (1983) Clobazam as adjunctive treatment in refractory epilepsy. *British Medical Journal*, **286**, 1246–7.

André, M., Boutroy, M.J., Dubruc, C. *et al.* (1986) Clonazepam pharmacokinetics and therapeutic efficacy in neonatal seizures. *European Journal of Clinical Pharmacology*, **30**, 585–9.

Appleton, R.E. (1993) The role of vigabatrin in the management of infantile epileptic syndromes. *Neurology*, **43**(suppl. 5), S21–3.

Arteaga, R., Herranz, J.L., Valdizan, E.M. and Armijo, J.A. (1992) γ-vinyl GABA (vigabatrin): relationship between dosage, plasma concentration, platelet GABA-transaminase inhibition, and seizure reduction in epileptic children. *Epilepsia*, **33**, 923–31.

Bachman, D.S. (1982) Use of valproic acid in treatment of infantile spasms. *Archives of Neurology*, **39**, 49–52.

Berkovic, S.F., Andermann, F., Guberman, A. *et al.* (1989) Valproate prevents the recurrence of absence status. *Neurology*, **39**, 1294–7.

Betts, T., Pigott, C. and Grace, E. (1989) Good response of atypical generalised absences to lamotrigine. Cited in Richens, A. and Yuen, A.W. C. (1991) Overview of the clinical efficacy of lamotrigine. *Epilepsia*, **32**(suppl.2), S13–6.

Bittencourt, P.R.M. and Richens, A. (1981) Anticonvulsant-induced status epilepticus in Lennox–Gastaut syndrome. *Epilepsia*, **22**, 129–34.

Bourgeois, B.F.D. and Dodson, W.E. (1983) Phenytoin elimination in newborns. *Neurology*, **33**, 173–8.

Bourgeois, B.F.D., Dodson, W. E. and Ferrendelli, J.A. (1983a) Primidone, phenobarbital and PEMA: I. Seizure protection, neurotoxicity and therapeutic index of individual compounds in mice. *Neurology*, **33**, 283–90.

Bourgeois, B.F.D., Dodson, W.E. and Ferrendelli, J.A. (1983b) Primidone, phenobarbital and PEMA: II. Seizure protection, neurotoxicity and therapeutic index of varying combinations in mice. *Neurology*, **33**, 291–5.

Bourgeois, B., Beaumanoir, A., Blajev, B. *et al.* (1987) Monotherapy with valproate in primary generalized epilepsies. *Epilepsia*, **28**(suppl. 2), S8–11.

Braathen, G., Theorell, K., Persson, A. and Rane, A. (1988) Valproate in the treatment of absence epilepsy in children: a study of dose–response relationships. *Epilepsia*, **29**, 548–52.

Callaghan, N., O'Hare, J., O'Driscoll, D. *et al.* (1982) Comparative study of ethosuximide and sodium valproate in the treatment of typical absence seizures (petit mal). *Developmental Medicine and Child Neurology*, **24**, 830–6.

Chiron, C., Dulac, O., Beaumont, D., *et al.* (1991) Therapeutic trial of vigabatrin in infantile spasms. *Journal of Child Neurology*, **6** (suppl. 2), 2S52–9.

Congdon, P.J. and Forsythe, W.I. (1980) Intravenous clonazepam in the treatment of status epilepticus in children. *Epilepsia*, **21**, 97–102.

Covanis, A., Gupta, A.K. and Jeavons, P.M. (1982) Sodium valproate: monotherapy and polytherapy. *Epilepsia*, **23**, 693–720.

Crawford, T.O., Mitchell, W.G., Fishman, L.S. and Snodgrass, S.R. (1988) Very-high-dose phenobarbital for refractory status epilepticus in children. *Neurology*, **38**, 1035–40.

Delgado-Escueta, A.V. and Enrile-Bacsal, F. (1984) Juvenile myoclonic epilepsy of Janz. *Neurology*, **34**, 285–94.

Dodson, W.E. (1980) Phenytoin elimination in childhood: effect of concentration dependent kinetics. *Neurology*, **30**, 196–9.

Dodson, W.E. (1982) The nonlinear kinetics of phenytoin in children. *Neurology*, **32**, 42–8.

Dreifuss, F.E., Penry, J.K., Rose, S.W. *et al.* (1975) Serum clonazepam concentrations in children with absence seizures. *Neurology*, **23**, 255–8.

Dreifuss, F., Farwell J., Holmes G. *et al.* (1986) Infantile spasms. Comparative trial of nitrazepam and corticotropin. *Archives of Neurology*, **43**, 1107–10

Dreifuss, F.E., Langer, D.H., Moline, K.A. and Maxwell, J.E. (1989) Valproic acid hepatic fatalities. II. US experience since 1984. *Neurology*, **39**, 201–7.

Dulac, O., Figueroa, D., Rey, E. and Arthuis, M. (1983) Monothérapie par le clobazam dans les épilepsies de l'enfant. *La Presse Médicale*, **12**, 1067–9.

Dulac, O., Steru, D., Rey, E., and Arthuis, M. (1986) Sodium valproate monotherapy in childhood epilepsy. *Brain and Development*, **8**, 47–52.

Farwell, J.R., Lee, Y.J., Hirtz, D.G. *et al.* (1990) Phenobarbital for febrile seizures – effects on intelligence and on seizure recurrence. *New England Journal of Medicine*, **322**, 364–9.

Felbamate Study Group in Lennox–Gastaut Syndrome (1993) Efficacy of felbamate in childhood epileptic encephalopathy (Lennox–Gastaut syndrome). *New England Journal of Medicine*, **328**, 29–33.

Feely, M. and Gibson, J. (1984) Intermittent clobazam for catamenial epilepsy. *Journal of Neurology, Neurosurgery and Psychiatry*, **47**, 1279–82.

Gal, P., Tobock, J., Boer, H. *et al.* (1982) Efficacy of phenobarbital monotherapy in treatment of neonatal seizures – relationship to blood levels. *Neurology*, **32**, 1401–4.

Gal, P., Oles, K.S., Gilman, J.T. and Weaver, R. (1988) Valproic acid efficacy, toxicity and pharmacokinetics in neonates with intractable seizures. *Neurology*, **38**, 467–71.

Gram, L., Klosterkov, P. and Dam, M. (1985) γ-vinyl GABA: a double-blind placebo-controlled trial in partial epilepsy. *Annals of Neurology*, **17**, 262–266.

Gram, L., Sabers, A. and Dulac, O. (1992) Treatment of pediatric epilepsies with γ-vinyl GABA (vigabatrin). *Epilepsia*, **33** (suppl 5), 26–29.

Henriksen, O., and Johannessen, S.I. (1982) Clinical and pharmacokinetic observations on sodium valproate – a 5-year follow-up study in 100 children with epilepsy. *Acta Neurologica Scandivavica*, **65**, 504–23.

Herranz, J.L., Armijo, J.A. and Arteaga, R. (1988) Clinical side effects of phenobarbital, primidone, phenytoin, carbamazepine, and valproate during monotherapy in children. *Epilepsia*, **29**, 794–804.

Hrachovy, R.A., Frost, J.D., Kellaway, P. *et al.* (1983) Double-blind study of ACTH vs. prednisone in infantile spasms. *Journal of Pediatrics*, **103**, 641–5.

Iivainen, M. and Himberg, J.J. (1982) Valproate and clonazepam in the treatment of severe progressive myoclonus epilepsy. *Archives of Neurology*, **39**, 236–8.

Ishikawa, A., Sakuma, N., Nagashima, T. *et al.* (1985) Clonazepam monotherapy for epilepsy in childhood. *Brain and Development*, **7**, 610–3.

Jawad, S., Richens, A., Goodwin, G. and Yuen, W.C. (1989) Controlled trial of lamotrigine (Lamictal) for refractory partial seizures. *Epilepsia*, **30**, 35–63.

Jeavons, P.M., Bishop, A. and Harding, G.F.A. (1986) The prognosis of photosensitivity. *Epilepsia*, **27**, 569–75.

Keene, D.L., Whiting, S. and Humphreys, P. (1990) Clobazam as an add-on drug in the treatment of refractory epilepsy of childhood. *Canadian Journal of Neurological Sciences*, **17**, 317–9.

Knudsen, F.U. (1985) Effective short-term diazepam prophylaxis in febrile convulsions. *Journal of Pediatrics*, **106**, 487–90.

Lee, K., Taudorf, K. and Hvorslev, V. (1986) Prophylactic treatment with valproic acid or diazepam in children with febrile convulsions. *Acta Paediatrica Scandinavica*, **75**, 593–7.

Leiderman, D., Garofalo, E. and LaMoreaux, L. (1993) Gabapentin in patients with absence seizures: two double-blind, placebo controlled studies. *Epilepsia*, **34**(suppl. 6), 45.

Livingston, J.H., Beaumont, D., Arzimanoglou, A. and Aicardi, J. (1989) Vigabatrin in the treatment of epilepsy in children. *British Journal of Clinical Pharmacology*, **27**, 109S–12S.

Lombroso, C.T. (1983) A prospective study of infantile spasms: clinical and therapeutic correlations. *Epilepsia*, **24**, 135–58.

Lortie, A., Chiron, C., Mumford, J. and Dulac, O. (1993) The potential for increasing seizure frequency, relapse, and appearance of new seizure types with vigabatrin. *Neurology*, **43**(suppl. 5), S24–7.

Luna, D., Dulac, O., Pajot, N. and Beaumont, D. (1989) Vigabatrin in the treatment of childhood epilepsies: a single-blind placebo-controlled study. *Epilepsia*, **30**, 430–7.

Lundberg, B., Nergardh, A. and Boreus, L.O. (1982) Plasma concentrations of valproate during maintenance therapy in epileptic children. *Journal of Neurology*, **228**, 133–41.

Maheshwari, M.C. and Jeavons, P.M. (1975) The effect of sodium valproate (Epilim) on the EEG. *Electroencephalography and Clinical Neurophysiology*, **39**, 429.

Matsuo, F., Bergen, D., Faught, E. *et al.* (1993) Placebo-controlled study of the efficacy and safety of lamotrigine in patients with partial seizures. *Neurology*, **43**, 2284–91.

Mattson, R.H., Cramer, J.A., Collins, J.F. *et al.* (1985) Comparison of carbamazepine, phenobarbital, phenytoin and primidone in partial and secondarily generalized tonic-clonic seizures. *New England Journal of Medicine*, **313**, 145–51.

Mattson, R.H., Cramer, J.A., Collins, J.F. and the Department of Veterans Affairs Epilepsy Cooperative Study No. 264 Group (1992) A comparison of valproate with carbamazepine for the treatment of complex partial seizures and secondarily generalized tonic-clonic seizures in adults. *New England Journal of Medicine*, **327**, 765–71.

McKinlay, I. and Newton, R. (1989) Intention to treat febrile convulsions with rectal diazepam, valproate, or phenobarbitone. *Developmental Medicine and Child Neurology*, **31**, 617–25.

Mikati, M.A., Trevathan, E., Krishnamoorthy, K.S. and Lombroso, C.T. (1991) Pyridoxine-dependent epilepsy: EEG investigations and long-term follow-up *Electroencephalography and Clinical Neurophysiology*, **78**, 215–21.

Mikkelsen, B., Birket-Smith, E., Brandt, S. *et al.*

(1976) Clonazepam in the treatment of epilepsy. A controlled trial in simple absences, bilateral massive epileptic myoclonus, and atonic seizures. *Archives of Neurology*, **33**, 322–5.

Mireles, R. and Leppik, I.E. (1985) Valproate and clonazepam comedication in patients with intractable epilepsy. *Epilepsia*, **26**, 122–6.

Mitchell, W. and Chavez, J. (1987) Carbamazepine versus phenobarbital for partial onset seizures in children. *Epilepsia*, **28**, 56–60.

Murphy, J.V., Sawaski, F., Marquardt, K.M. and Harris, D.J. (1987) Deaths in young children receiving nitrazepam. *Journal of Pediatrics*, **111**, 145–7.

Obeid, T. and Panayiotopoulos, C.P. (1989) Clonazepam in juvenile myoclonic epilepsy. *Epilepsia*, **30**, 603–6.

Okuno, T., Ito, M., Nakano, S. *et al.* (1989) Carbamazepine therapy and long-term prognosis in epilepsy of childhood. *Epilepsia*, **30**, 57–61.

Oleson, O.V. and Dam, M. (1967) The metabolic conversion of primidone to phenobarbitone in patients under long-term treatment. *Acta Neurologica Scandinavica*, **43**, 348–56.

Oller, L.F.V., Russi, A. and Oller Daurella L. (1991) Lamotrigine in the Lennox–Gastaut syndrome. *Epilepsia*, **32** (suppl. 1), 58.

Oxley, J., Hebdige, S., Laidlaw, J. *et al.* (1980) A comparative study of phenobarbitone and primidone in the treatment of epilepsy, in *Advances in Drug Monitoring* (eds S.I. Johannessen, P.L. Morselli, C.E. Pippenger *et al.*). Raven, New York, pp. 237–45.

Painter, M.J., Pippenger, C., Wasterlain, C. *et al.* (1981) Phenobarbital and phenytoin in neonatal seizures: metabolism and tissue distribution. *Neurology*, **31**, 1107–112.

Pavone, L., Incorpora, G., LaRosa, M. *et al.* (1981) Treatment of infantile spasms with sodium dipropylacetic acid. *Developmental Medicine and Child Neurology*, **23**, 454–61.

Pietz, J., Benninger, C., Schäfer, H. *et al.* (1993) Treatment of infantile spasms with high-dosage vitamin B6. *Epilepsia*, **34**, 757–63.

Powell, C., Painter, M.J. and Pippenger, C.E. (1984) Primidone therapy in refractory neonatal seizures. *Journal of Pediatrics*, **105**, 651–54.

Ramsay, R.E., Wilder, B.J., Murphy, J.V. *et al.* (1992) Efficacy and safety of valproic acid versus phenytoin as sole therapy for newly diagnosed primary generalized tonic-clonic seizures. *Journal of Epilepsy*, **5**, S5–10.

Resor, S.R. and Resor, L.D. (1990) The neuropharmacology of juvenile myoclonic epilepsy. *Clinical Neuropharmacology*, **13**, 465–91.

Richard, M.O., Chiron, C., d'Athis, P. *et al.* (1993) Phenytoin monitoring in status epilepticus in infants and children. *Epilepsia*, **34**, 144–50.

Rimmer, E.M. and Richens, A. (1984) Double-blind study of γ-vinyl GABA in patients with refractory epilepsy. *Lancet*, **i**, 189–90.

Robertson, M.M. (1986) Current status of the 1,4- and 1,5-benzodiazepines in the treatment of epilepsy: the place of clobazam. *Epilepsia*, **27**, S27–41.

Rowan, A.J., Meijer, J.W.A., de Beer-Pawlikowski, N. *et al.* (1983) Valproate–ethosuximide combination therapy for refractory absence seizures. *Archives of Neurology.*, **40**, 797–802.

Sapin, J.I., Riviello, J.J. and Grover, W.D. (1988) Efficacy of primidone for seizure control in neonates and young infants. *Pediatric Neurology*, **4**, 292–5.

Sato, S., Dreifuss, F.E. and Penry, J.K. (1976) Prognostic factors in absence seizures. *Neurology*, **26**, 788–96.

Sato, S., White, B.G., Penry, J.K. *et al.* (1982) Valproic acid versus ethosuximide in the treatment of absence seizures. *Neurology*, **32**, 157–63.

Shaner, M.D., McCurdy, S., Herring, M. and Gabor, A. (1988) Treatment of status epilepticus: a prospective comparison of diazepam and phenytoin versus phenobarbital and optional phenytoin. *Neurology*, **38**, 202–7.

Sher, P.K. (1985) Alternate-day clonazepam treatment of intractable seizures. *Archives of Neurology*, **42**, 787–8.

Singer, W.D., Rabe, E.F. and Haller, J.S. (1980) The effect of ACTH therapy on infantile spasms. *Journal of Pediatrics*, **96**, 485–9.

Smith, D., Baker, G., Davies, G. *et al.* (1993) Outcomes of add-on treatment with lamotrigine in partial epilepsy. *Epilepsia*, **34**, 312–22.

Snead, O.C. (1987) The neuropharmacology of epileptic falling spells. *Clinical Neuropharmacology*, **10**, 205–14.

Snead and Hosey, L.C. (1985) Exacerbation of seizures in children by carbamazepine. *New England Journal of Medicine*, **313**, 916–21.

Snead, O.C. and Hosey, L.C. (1987) Treatment of epileptic falling spells with ethosuximide. *Brain Development*, **9**, 602–4.

Snead, O.C., Benton, J.W., Hosey, L.C. *et al.*, (1989) Treatment of infantile spasms with high-dose ACTH: efficacy and plasma levels of ACTH and cortisol. *Neurology*, **39**, 1027–31.

Spitz, M.C. and Deasy, D.N. (1991) Conversion to valproate monotherapy in nonretarded adults with primary generalized tonic-clonic seizures. *Journal of Epilepsy*, **4**, 33–8.

Takuma, Y., Seki, T. and Hirai, K. (1990) A study of a new treatment for intractable epilepsy with infantile spasms and related disorders using a combination of high-dose pyridoxal phosphate and low-dose ACTH. *Brain Development*, **12**, 641.

Tassinari, C.A., Michelucci, R., Ambrosetto, G. and Salvi, F. (1987) Double-blind study of vigabatrin in the treatment of drug-resistant epilepsy. *Archives of Neurology*, **44**, 907–10.

Timmings, P.L. and Richens, A. (1992) Lamotrigine as add-on drug in the management of Lennox–Gastaut syndrome. *European Neurology*, **32**, 305–7.

UK Gabapentin Study Group (1990) Gabapentin in partial epilepsy. *Lancet*, **335**, 1114–1117.

US Gabapentin Study Group No. 5 (1993) Gabapentin as add-on therapy in refractory partial epilepsy: a double-blind, placebo-controlled, parallel-group study. *Neurology*, **43**, 2292–8.

Vassella, F., Pavlincova, E., Schneider, H.J. *et al.* (1973) Treatment of infantile spasms and Lennox–Gastaut syndrome with clonazepam. *Epilepsia*, **14**, 165–75.

Villareal, H.J., Wilder, B.J., Willmore, L.J. *et al.* (1978) Effect of valproic acid on spike and wave discharges in patients with absence seizures. *Neurology*, **28**, 886–91.

Wallace, S.J. (1990) Add-on trial of lamotrigine in resistant childhood seizures. *Brain and Development*, **12**, 734.

White, P.T., Pott, D. and Norton, J. (1966) Relative anticonvulsant potency of primidone. A double blind comparison. *Archives of Neurology*, **14**, 31–5.

Wolf, S. and Forsythe, A. (1978) Behavior disturbance, phenobarbital and febrile seizures. *Pediatrics*, **61**, 728–31.

Wyllie, E., Wyllie, R., Cruse, R.P. *et al.* (1986) The mechanism of nitrazepam-induced drooling and aspiration. *New England Journal of Medicine*, **314**, 35–8.

Blaise F.D. Bourgeois

Of the various dietary measures that have been tried and advocated in the treatment of epilepsy, the ketogenic diet has the best demonstrated efficacy. The ketogenic diet has been used for several decades and has been shown to be effective against all seizure types. It is usually prescribed after several antiepileptic drugs have failed. Its main indication is in the treatment of young children with the Lennox–Gastaut syndrome and related refractory epilepsies of childhood (Chapter 12). Several variations have been proposed over the years, but they all meet one necessary requirement, which is the production of ketosis and acidosis. They also all share another feature: they are relatively unpalatable. However, newer modifications are more acceptable, and the diet is clearly effective. Complete seizure control is achieved in up to one-half of previously refractory patients, and additional patients derive at least some benefit. The original version tends to increase plasma cholesterol, triglycerides and uric acid, and predisposes to hypo-glycemia. These side-effects appear to be less pronounced with a modified version of the ketogenic diet based on the use of medium chain triglycerides. No matter which version is used, the diet has to be implemented very rigidly in order to be successful.

The original or classic ketogenic diet is generally referred to as the 4:1 ketogenic diet, based on the ratio of fat to non-fat in the diet. It is usually started in the hospital. After initial blood tests that include cholesterol, triglycerides, uric acid, calcium, and phosphate, the first step is a period of fasting of 24–72 hours until the urine is 3–4+ for ketone bodies. If the patient is taking acetazolamide (Diamox), this should be discontinued because of the risk of severe metabolic acidosis. Once started, the diet should contain three or four parts of fat for one part of protein/carbohydrate, enough to maintain ketonuria at 3–4+. The total amount of calories should be 75 cal/kg/day, with 1 g of protein per kg per day. All sugar and sugar-containing medications must be avoided. In addition, the patient should receive supplements of vitamins, including vitamin D 5000 IU per day, and calcium. Hypoglycemia is most likely to occur during the first few days on the diet, and it is asymptomatic in most patients. Ketonuria is monitored for as long as the child is on the diet. If the diet is successful in reducing the seizure frequency, this is usually recognized within the first 2 weeks. Levels of antiepileptic drugs may be altered by the diet. Therefore, drug levels should be monitored and doses should be adjusted as necessary. Noncompliance with the diet will often rapidly lead to break-through seizures or even status epilepticus. If successful, the diet is usually maintained strictly for about 2 years, with a progressive transition to a normal diet.

Kinsman *et al.* (1992) have reviewed the experience at Johns Hopkins with 58 consecutive patients started on the diet between 1980 and 1985. More than half the patients

Epilepsy in Children. Edited by Sheila Wallace. Published in 1996 by Chapman & Hall, London. ISBN 0 412 56860 8

suffered from the Lennox–Gastaut syndrome or had a hypsarrhythmic EEG. The age at the time of initiation of the diet ranged from 12 to 235 months, with an average of 60 months, and the patients had been refractory to an average of 4.9 antiepileptic drugs. A decrease in seizure frequency of at least 50% was achieved in 38% of the patients, and in another 29% seizure control was virtually complete. Thus, a total of 67% of the patients derived a substantial benefit. The median time on the diet was 24 months for those who improved, and 4 months for those who did not. Among those who did improve, 75% remained on the diet for 18 months or more. At least one antiepileptic drug was reduced or discontinued in 64% of those who improved. Improved behavior was reported in 23% and increased alertness in 36% of the patients with reduced seizure frequency. Side-effects included renal stones in three patients, hyperuricemia in two, and acidosis and hypocalcemia in one patient each. One patient refused to eat and another had recurrent infections.

In 1971, Huttenlocher, Wilbourn and Signore introduced a modification of the diet based on the use of medium chain triglycerides (MCT) oil. This oil contains triglycerides of octanoic and decanoic acids, which are more ketogenic than dietary fat, and provides 8.3 calories per gram. The inclusion of MCT achieves a comparable degree of ketosis and acidosis with less restriction of dietary carbohydrates. As proposed, the MCT diet provides 60% of the calories from MCT oil, 11% from other fats, 19% from carbohydrates, and 10% from proteins. The diet starts with a 50-calorie-per-day fast that is maintained until definite ketonuria is achieved. Once the diet begins, MCT oil is served chilled with each meal, blended with at least twice its volume of skimmed milk. The main side-effects of the MCT diet are abdominal cramps, nausea, and occasional vomiting. This can be reduced by having the child take the MCT mixture in small sips throughout the meal. Diarrhea is another side-effect of this diet. Mild asymptomatic hypoglycemia is also observed. The response to the MCT diet in terms of seizure control is at least as good as to the 3:1 ketogenic diet. Results with the MCT diet have been reevaluated in 17 children, aged 12 months to 12 years, who had intractable seizures (Trauner, 1985). Complete seizure control was achieved in five patients, and their antiepileptic drugs could be decreased or even stopped. An additional five patients had some improvement. In three patients, the diet had to be discontinued because of side-effects such as diarrhea, vomiting, or irritability.

Considering the patient population in which it is used, the results achieved with the ketogenic diet are indeed remarkable and are often worth the inconvenience and necessary discipline imposed on the child and on the parents. The mechanism by which the ketogenic diet exerts its antiepileptic effect has not been completely established. Possibilities include: an effect of the ketone bodies themselves; a change in water and electrolyte balance; an alteration in lipid concentration; or a change in acid–base balance resulting in intracellular acidosis and decreased neuronal excitability.

Another diet that has been prescribed in the treatment of epilepsy is the oligoantigenic diet. This was initially introduced for the treatment of children with migraine and hyperactive behavior. However, among those in whom the diet was tested, there was a substantial number who had epileptic seizures, in addition, and whose seizures were noted to decrease in frequency. These 27 patients, together with an additional group of 18 children with refractory seizures and migraine, as well as 18 children with refractory seizures and no migraine, were included in a study of the potential benefit of the oligoantigenic diet in the treatment of epilepsy (Egger *et al.*, 1989). The diet consists of two phases. During the first 4 weeks, the patients receive a strictly oligoantigenic diet that consists of only two meats (lamb and chicken), two carbohydrates (potatoes and rice), two fruits (banana and apple) and vegetables, with calcium and vitamin supplements. Patients who experience a favorable response enter the reintroduction phase, during which one excluded food is reintroduced at weekly intervals. If seizures reoccur, the food is excluded from the diet, otherwise it is reincluded. The following foods were responsible for seizure relapses in more than 20% of the children in the study: cows' milk, cows' cheese, citrus fruits, wheat, and the food additives tartrazine and benzoic acid. In the overall analysis, none of the 18 patients with epilepsy alone benefited from the diet. However, among the 45 patients with migraine and epilepsy, 25 achieved complete seizure control, seven had a more than 50% reduction in their seizure frequency, and four had seizures only during upper respiratory tract infections. All children in whom the seizures were controlled also ceased to have migraine. In conclusion, the oligoantigenic diet is a therapeutic alternative to be considered in children who have both seizures and migraine.

REFERENCES

Egger, J. Carter, C.M., Soothill, J.F. and Wilson, J. (1989) Oligoantigenic diet in the treatment of children with epilepsy and migraine. *Journal of Pediatrics*, **114**, 51–8.

Huttenlocher, P.R., Wilbourn, A.J. and Signore, J.M. (1971) Medium-chain triglycerides as a therapy for intractable childhood epilepsy. *Neurology*, **21**, 1097–103.

Kinsman, S.L., Vining, E.P.G., Quaksey, S.A. *et al.* (1992) Efficacy of the ketogenic diet for intractable seizure disorders; review of 58 cases. *Epilepsia*, **33**, 1132–6.

Trauner, D.A. (1985) Medium-chain triglyceride (MCT) diet in intractable seizure disorder. *Neurology*, **35**, 237–8.

BEHAVIORAL AND SOCIAL THERAPY   23c

Blaise F.D. Bourgeois

Although antiepileptic drugs represent the backbone of epilepsy therapy, behavioral and social issues are essential not only to reduce risk factors, but also to maximize the efficacy of drug therapy. A separate behavioral and social approach to the management of epilepsy is aimed at helping the patient and the family to cope with the diagnosis and the psychosocial consequences of the disease, and this aspect is discussed further in Chapter 25. The present discussion will focus on behavioral and social aspects that will contribute to a reduction in the seizure frequency. There is good general agreement that in any patient with epilepsy external factors can increase the seizure frequency or, in other words, lower the so-called seizure threshold. This lowering of the seizure threshold can be caused by relatively non-specific and common life situations, or it can be related to very specific stimuli or activities. Correspondingly, the seizure frequency can often be effectively reduced by such behavioral and social approaches as improving life hygiene, identification and reduction of stress factors, relaxation techniques and de-sensitization techniques for reflex epilepsies. It is difficult to find objective controlled data that quantify or document the effectiveness of these approaches.

Among patients with refractory epilepsy, it has been estimated that factors known to lower the seizure threshold play an essential role in resistance to therapy in 14% (Aird, 1988). Patients themselves cited intense emotional reactions as the most common precipitating factor, but this was not always corroborated by a more systematic analysis by the physician. There is no question that **psychologic stress** increases the likelihood of true epileptic seizures in patients who have no evidence of experiencing any pseudo-seizures. Inversely, it is common to see a temporary cessation of seizures in patients admitted to hospital for continuous video/EEG monitoring of their seizures. This may well be related to the fact that these patients are in a relatively sheltered environment and get plenty of rest. From a practical point of view, specific stressful situations should be identified and avoided, but the daily challenges of leading a normal life can hardly be eliminated. As a rule, **physical exercise** is not associated with an increase in seizure frequency, unless it is particularly strenuous and leads to exhaustion. Clearly, certain sports predispose to an increase risk of injury if a seizure should occur but, in general, children with epilepsy are too often restricted from participating in sports and games. There is increasing agreement that the potential long-term psychologic damage outweighs the slightly increased risk of injury. Certain sports should clearly be restricted in children with epilepsy, and these include swimming and any activity associated with some form of climbing. Swimming can be allowed in the presence of an adult who:

Epilepsy in Children. Edited by Sheila Wallace. Published in 1996 by Chapman & Hall, London. ISBN 0 412 56860 8

1. Knows that the child has epilepsy, and
2. Constantly watches the child in the water, and
3. Would be able to pull the child out of the water in case of a seizure.

In relation to water safety, it is also important to mention that a child with epilepsy should never take a full bath unless constantly supervised .

Sleep deprivation and disturbances of the circadian sleep cycle are probably the external factors that have been most frequently shown to represent precipitating factors. This seems to apply to patients with generalized epilepsies more than to patients with focal epilepsies. One form of epilepsy that seems to be most exquisitely sensitive to sleep deprivation or sleep disruption is juvenile myoclonic epilepsy (Chapter 14b). Very often, the history given by these patients is that they experienced their first convulsive seizure in the morning following a night of relative sleep deprivation. The seizures are also more likely to occur following provoked awakenings than after spontaneous awakenings (Resor and Resor, 1990). Conversely, patients with juvenile myoclonic epilepsy also seem to experience more sleep disturbances. As a rule, these patients should be advised to adopt a very rigorous sleep hygiene, with limited day-to-day changes in sleeping schedule, and avoidance of caffeinated beverage in the evening.

Opinions regarding the effect of **alcohol** on seizure frequency are somewhat divergent. If alcohol reduces the seizure threshold, this probably occurs during the withdrawal phase rather than at the time of peak alcohol blood level. While some authors advocate complete abstinence from alcohol in patients with epilepsy, others point out that there is no evidence that small to moderate amounts, even on a daily basis, could be demonstrated to be deleterious. One exception is juvenile myoclonic epilepsy (Chapter 14b), which appears to be very sensitive not only to sleep

deprivation, but also to alcohol consumption. It has been suggested that this effect could be mediated indirectly by the disruptive effect on sleep (Resor and Resor, 1990). As a rule, alcohol consumption should be discouraged entirely in patients with juvenile myoclonic epilepsy. There is no evidence that **smoking** has a direct effect on the seizure threshold. However, a significant indirect risk of smoking is the danger of setting a fire associated with a seizure occurring while alone.

There is no good evidence that, besides the ketogenic diet and the oligoantigenic diet discussed earlier, any specific **dietary measures** have a beneficial effect in terms of seizure prevention. Multiple food avoidances or supplements have been advocated without substantiation of the benefit. Two points can be made. Firstly, it is possible that the relative hypoglycemia that could be associated with a missed meal may lower the seizure threshold. For this reason, patients with epilepsy are often advised not to skip meals. Secondly, by preventing sleep, caffeinated beverages could indirectly lower the seizure threshold.

It is well recognized that certain patients with epilepsy are sensitive to certain types of **light stimuli** (Chapter 14d). The seizures that are most commonly precipitated by photic stimuli are absences, and the most powerful stimulus is usually intermittent bright light. These patients will often have been identified by the occurrence of a photoparoxysmal reaction, or the occurrence of a seizure, in response to intermittent photic stimulation during an EEG recording. Practical situations that are likely to trigger seizures in these patients are encountered in a disco, or when the sun is intermittently obscured while the patient rides in a car or in a train, or when the sun is reflected on a water surface, or while watching television. Patients who have been identified as having photosensitive epilepsy should be advised to wear sunglasses when they have to be exposed to known triggering factors. A study of various types of sunglasses has suggested that blue sunglasses are particularly useful in these patients (Takahashi and Tsukahara, 1992)

Finally, **compliance** with the antiepileptic drug regimen is a crucial and often underestimated aspect of the treatment of epilepsy. It is one of the main causes of treatment failure. Significant deviation from the prescribed drug regimen could be shown to occur in up to 50% of patients (Leppik, 1988). Several factors that contribute to lack of compliance have been identified. These include high doses with occurrence of side-effects, frequent daily doses, polytherapy, and insufficient time spent by the physician or the nurse explaining the drug regimen and the possible adverse reactions. Avoidance of these potential risk factors, if feasible, will improve adherence by the patient, or by the parents, to the drug regimen. Additional factors that will improve compliance include regular office visits or telephone contacts, clear explanations regarding the treatment plan and risks of irregular drug intake, and pill boxes containing the medication for a day or for an entire week. Some children may be reluctant to take their medication in school, and it is often possible to change the drug regimen accordingly, with no loss in therapeutic benefit. Patients who are well controlled are also at risk, because they may feel that they no longer need the medication. Blood levels obtained at the time of scheduled office visits are not always reliable indicators of compliance. However, wide fluctuations in levels obtained at the same time of the day on the same dosage regimen should raise suspicions. Finally, the physician's reaction to the lack of compliance by a patient should never have a punitive undertone.

REFERENCES

Aird, R.B. (1988) The importance of seizure-inducing factors in youth. *Brain and Development*, **10**, 73–6.

Leppik, I.E. (1988) Compliance during treatment of epilepsy. *Epilepsia*, **29**(suppl. 2), 79–84.

Resor, S.R. and Resor, L.D. (1990) The neuropharmacology of juvenile myoclonic epilepsy. *Clinical Neuropharmacology*, **13**, 465–91.

Takahashi, T. and Tsukahara, Y. (1992) Usefulness of blue sunglasses in photosensitive epilepsy. *Epilepsia*, **33**, 517–21.

SURGICAL TREATMENT OF EPILEPSY IN CHILDREN

Charles E. Polkey

INTRODUCTION

The surgical treatment of epilepsy has developed via a combination of empiric observations and theoretical proposals. Practised in different ways across the world, the procedures used were often governed by local knowledge and experience. It is possible to place surgical interventions in two groups: resective surgery in which an area of brain is removed, generally because it contains a structural abnormality, and functional surgery in which the procedure is thought to modify brain function so as to improve control of seizures. In the last decade, the explosion in variety and detail of both structural and functional brain imaging techniques has played a significant part in the selection of patients for surgery (Chapter 20). Some procedures combine resective and functional intervention. Examples, at a very simple level, are callosotomy as part of a functional hemispherectomy and multiple subpial transection (MST) combined with a frontal resection. At a more sophisticated level, any resective procedure, such as a standard anterior temporal lobectomy, involves removal of neurons which are ostensibly normal, as well the defined structural abnormality; there is also disconnection of cerebral tissue. It is not possible, or profitable, to dissect the *modus operandi* of resective surgery. For this reason, although the proposals by Lüders and Awad (1991) to separate

and define various deficit and epileptogenic zones are of theoretic interest, they play little part in practical epilepsy surgery beyond the principles of concordance and redundancy as explained later. Epilepsy surgery is a multidisciplinary activity requiring the close cooperation of several specialties. For the pediatric age group a pediatric neurologist or epileptologist with significant pediatric experience is necessary; as are experts in neuropsychologic testing and the interpretation of neurophysiologic and neuroimaging data in childhood. For the purposes of this text only patients aged 15 years or less will be considered.

The practice of epilepsy surgery in children differs from that in adults in three respects. These are firstly, the differing incidence of pathology; secondly the neuropsychologic and neurophysiologic properties of the normal maturing nervous system; and, lastly, the neurophysiologic changes which can occur in the nervous system as a result of chronic, poorly controlled epilepsy and their interaction with the first two factors. With the exception of the structural pathology, the remaining factors are not susceptible to detailed description or analysis, although their influences will be discerned from time to time. Especially with very small children, there are technical problems both in performing the surgery and in postoperative care. Clearly the latter is best carried out by the

Epilepsy in Children. Edited by Sheila Wallace. Published in 1996 by Chapman & Hall, London. ISBN 0 412 56860 8

appropriate pediatric specialist. In addition to these purely technical factors, it must be recalled that the role of the parents, both during the acute phase of management, and in the long term, is important. Therefore suitable accommodation and counseling should be available.

Analysis of current activities on the Maudsley Hospital suggest about 20–30% of epilepsy surgery is performed on children aged 15 years or less. The International League Against Epilepsy (ILAE) survey notes 428 of 1997 (21.4%) operations in this group (H.G. Wieser and H. Silfvenius, 1993, unpublished data). Whether early intervention in children would yield better quality of life and social results remain a matter for debate.

SELECTION BY PHASED MANAGEMENT

In its broad principles the scheme of management for adults, which is summarized in Fig. 23d.1, can be readily adapted to children.

At the Maudsley Hospital, between 1976 and 1993, there were 2340 consultant epi-

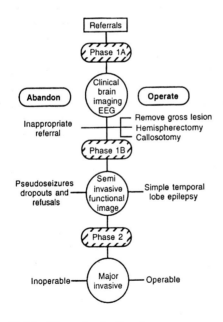

Fig. 23d.1 Phased selection for surgery.

sodes for the surgical management of epilepsy. Of these 598 episodes (24.6%) related to patients of 15 years of age or less. On the whole, the selection for resective surgery and planning of the site and extent of the resection is more susceptible to detail and logical management than that for functional surgery, where most of the selection factors are empiric and based on previous experience. Any scheme of management should aim to reach a positive decision with the least number of tests, thus minimizing patient risk and discomfort; and acknowledging economic aspects. Two principles are involved: concordance and redundancy. Concordance implies that a number of tests or considerations point to a definite decision; redundancy, that if two tests give the same answer then it is only necessary to perform one of them. The application of our adult scheme to children has to accept that some points may be impossible to resolve or may need resolution in a different way. The first phase of this scheme of management consists of collection of clinical data, basic neurophysiologic assessment, basic neuropsychologic or developmental assessment, and structural brain imaging.

PHASE 1A

Every assessment should start with a full clinical history, taking details of both the ictal and the interictal history. The nature of the seizures, including any aura or warning and any peri-ictal or postictal neurologic symptoms or signs, may indicate the area of brain involved. Careful history taking, using the family's expressions for the patient's attacks such as 'turns' or 'do's', may elicit valuable information directly, or indirectly via the parents, down to the age of 5 years or less. Thus, important localizing details such as ipsilateral dystonia, the features of frontal lobe seizures, focal motor seizures, etc., may be obtained. The rate and nature of progression of the seizure, especially when partial, should be determined. Seizures of frontal lobe origin progress more rapidly and lead to unconsciousness more quickly than those of temporal lobe origin. It is particularly important to clarify the meaning of the quasimedical terms, such as 'petit mal', which the patient's relatives may use.

The interictal history is also important in that it reflects the possibility of structural damage or gives evidence of a preexisting lesion, as pointed out by Ounsted, Lindsay and Norman (1966) in their survey of 100 children with temporal lobe epilepsy. Although the mechanism is debatable, there is now no doubt that a prolonged or atypical febrile seizure, characteristically lasting 30 minutes or more, can be associated with later chronic temporal lobe epilepsy and predominantly unilateral scarring of the mesial temporal structures (see Chapter 10). Thus a history of such an episode will be valuable in suggesting a cause for the epilepsy. Likewise histories of cerebral hemorrhage, meningitis, abscess, infarction, etc., may all point to possible causes of the epilepsy.

A general physical examination may identify those children with a neurologic disorder who have an associated structural lesion such as tuberous sclerosis, neurofibromatosis, Sturge–Weber syndrome, etc. In addition, there will be patients with gross neurologic deficits either resulting from previous cerebral insults such as birth injury or, some progressive disease such as Rasmussen's disease (Chapter 15b), or secondary to epilepsy, for example, effective functional hemiplegia as a consequence of epilepsy partialis continuans. Proper and detailed recording of the neurologic state is necessary because it may have a bearing upon the proposed surgery, or may subsequently change so as to modify opinion about what procedure is appropriate. The majority of patients will have no abnormality or a very subtle change.

Basic neurophysiology should be carried out with care so that the examination is technically satisfactory, which is not easy in young or disturbed children. The placement of the electrodes must be appropriate to the question being asked and a sleep recording should be obtained, either by natural sleep, or following sleep deprivation, or by the use of a sedative.

It is important to ascertain cerebral dominance for speech. Basic neuropsychology in older children, or a developmental assessment in younger children, will give an estimate of the overall attainment and demonstrate localized difficulties in those old enough for detailed assessment. When cerebral damage occurs early in life, cerebral reorganization may make the best use of what remains. However, as shown by Rasmussen and Milner (1977), injury to the left brain, even at an early age, leaves some consequences. A bland performance on neuropsychologic testing, especially in patients with temporal lobe epilepsy (TLE) due to mesial temporal sclerosis, does not preclude a focal lesion (Powell, Polkey and McMillan, 1985; McMillan *et al.*, 1987).

The first phase of selection concentrates on structural brain imaging (see Chapter 20). Functional brain imaging is more complex, not always necessary, and easier to interpret when the basic information from phase 1A has been evaluated. Practitioners are obliged to use whatever imaging facilities are available to them. The results obtained depend upon the technique employed and the experience of those interpreting the image. MRI is the 'gold standard' for structural imaging of the brain. Useful results can be obtained from CT provided, for example, the proper views are obtained when examining the temporal lobe (Adams *et al.*, 1987). However, MRI reveals a greater range of tissue change and a greater amount of detail and will show such pathology as cortical dysplasia, which may be missed with CT. It should be emphasized that the examination must be technically satisfactory, even if a general anesthetic is required to obtain the appropriate imaging conditions. Positive lesions such as low-grade tumors, cavernous angiomas, focal cortical dysplasia, and so forth will show up well with proper MRI, which is estimated to detect almost 100% of such lesions. (Kuzniecky *et al.*, 1993a). However the demonstration of the lesion of mesial temporal sclerosis (MTS), found in a large proportion of our resective candidates, is more contentious, possibly because the lesion is known to vary in its laterality and extent. Three techniques are used for examining the temporal lobe for this lesion. These are: simple visual inspection of the standard coronal cuts; volumetric analysis of the hippocampus using a thin slice technique; and tissue changes associated with gliosis, seen as a hyperintense signal on the T_2 image. There are diverse opinions about the sensitivity and specificity of these tests. Good information on the minimal degree of hippocampal sclerosis necessary to act as an epileptogenic focus is lacking. It is thought that an active focus may be associated with as little as 30% cell loss, whereas visual analysis of the MRI alone may only detect 60% cell loss or more. Kuzniecky *et al.* (1993b), describing 44 children, found the MRI abnormalities were concordant with the abnormalities found by other investigations in 84% of patients with a wide distribution and variety of pathology. Similar findings have been reported in adults (Jabbari *et al.*, 1991).

Figure 23d.1 shows the fate of patients at this point. Some will be rejected for surgery for a number of reasons, such as no prospect of a focal lesion or the presence of a nonepileptic attack disorder. Others will be accepted for surgery because the preliminary findings are concordant or there are no further tests which will advance the decision. In yet others it will be necessary to continue with more investigations.

PHASE 1B

The minimally invasive phase involves trying to refine the previous findings in the hope of establishing an electrical focus or an area of dysfunctioning brain.

At this stage, there are a number of tests of brain function which can be used, but many are either research tools or unsuitable, except for older children. Ictal SPECT using HMPAO is a powerful tool for lateralizing temporal lobe attacks in adults, but is less useful in children because of the difficulty in obtaining ictal records and the radiation hazards. Interictal FDG-PET has proved useful both in temporal and extratemporal epilepsies (Chugani *et al.*, 1988; Rintahaka *et al.*, 1993). In the future, MR spectroscopy, especially proton spectroscopy to detect N-aspartate, diminution of which may be representative of tissue loss, could also be contributory.

In teenagers, but not in the younger age group, the traditional carotid amytal test can be used to determine cerebral dominance and memory distribution. In younger children, some workers have used short-acting intravenous anesthesia in the investigation of dominance and memory. Transcranial magnetic stimulation is an alternative means of determining speech dominance. If they are subsequently required for other reasons, subdural grid electrodes can be used for the same purpose. If at all possible, it is important to test the memory function of the temporal lobe in patients scheduled for resective surgery of this region. Details of the variations of the amytal test can be found in a number of reviews (Jack *et al.*, 1988; Rausch *et al.*, 1993). It is of importance that: firstly, early pathology may lead to the location of all memory function in one temporal lobe; and, secondly, that the nature of neuropsychologic testing and subsequent educational and social needs of the child and young adult make deficits of verbal processing and memory more obvious, and more disabling, than nonverbal deficits.

Minimally invasive telemetry should be considered at this point. This term is used advisedly because in some patients the purpose of such recording will be to show the nature of the seizures rather than their origin. For instance frontal seizures, whose description may be misleading, can often be seen to be stereotyped and consistent, although the chance of seeing a focal onset, unless that focus is on the lateral convexity of the frontal lobe, is small. In patients where lateralization to one or other temporal lobe, or differentiation between medial and lateral temporal onset, or between frontal and temporal onset are required, telemetry with sphenoidal or foramen ovale electrodes can be used. The latter have been preferred because they give a true intracranial recording with little increase in risk and can be used in children as young as 5 years. At the end of phase 1B it may be possible to make a decision with regard to surgery. This corresponds to the point of decision on 'noninvasive' criteria as discussed by Sperling *et al.* (1992) and by Rausch on behalf of the UCLA Group (Rausch, 1992)

PHASE 2

If a decision on surgery is not possible at this stage, either the assessment must be abandoned and the patient pronounced inoperable, or major intracranial invasive recording should be commenced. The latter may be indicated for a number of reasons, but, in any particular patient, must be designed to test a specific hypothesis. The type and placement of intracranial electrodes must be chosen with care. We have used complex invasive recording in 15% of 122 children who have undergone surgery for epilepsy. Four children have required a combination of subdural and depth recordings to define a frontal or temporal focus using the method previously described by Van Veelen *et al.* (1990). Fourteen children presented with problems involving the precentral and postcentral cortex. In these, we have been anxious to establish the precise area of cortex involved in the epileptogenic processes and also to

Table 23d.1 Fate of children in the phased selection: Maudsley series

Phase	Stop	Operate	Go to next phase
All 159 children (1976–93)			
1A	18	74	67
1B	15	28	24
2	2	22	—
120 children 1987–93			
1A	17	40	63
1B	18	23	22
2	2	20	

make motor, sensory and speech maps, so as to tailor the surgery to obtain the best combination of maximal eradication of the epileptogenic zone with minimal neurologic or other deficit. For this purpose we have used subdural strips and grids, placed extradurally, as suggested by Goldring and Gregorie (1984). The timing of surgery after the use of grid electrodes is difficult. They should be in place for as short a duration as possible. The patients in whom they are used have frequent seizures and most of our patients have completed the investigations, including stimulation, in the 48 hours after grid insertion. It is preferable to carry out the definitive surgery on the fourth day after their insertion when the grids would normally be removed.

The fate of the patients at the end of phase 2 of the selection process is summarized in Table 23d.1. In all, 159 children had been assessed and operated upon between 1976 and 1993. However, the methods of investigation have changed, so the table also shows the fate of the 120 children seen since 1987 in whom investigations have been taken to the point of offering surgery. This group has had the benefit of consistent and modern methods of selection. During investigation, selection for functional procedures such as callosotomy or MST is also achieved.

Table 23d.2 Pathology in resected specimens in children: Maudsley series

Age (yr)	Pathology (n=75)					
	MTS	Tumor	RD	CD	Other	Non-specific
0–5	0	5	5	4	1	0
6–11	1	6	7	5	4	0
11–15	6	10	4	7	8	2
All	7	21	16	16	13	2
%	9.3	28	21.3	21.3	17.3	2.7

MTS = Mesial temporal sclerosis; RD = Rasmussen's disease; CD = cortical dysplasia.

SURGICAL PATHOLOGY

The extent and nature of the cerebral pathology determines both the possible surgical intervention and the outcome of surgery. Certain pathologies, including nonspecific changes, have been seen regularly in resected specimens from a variety of centers around the world over a number of years. This section deals with these pathologies rather than giving a comprehensive account of pediatric brain pathology, or of the pathology of epilepsy, which is addressed in Chapter 5. The occurrence of these various entities in our series of 75 children is shown in Table 23d.2.

ATROPHIC AND DESTRUCTIVE LESIONS

These range very widely in site and extent as well as etiology. Cerebral infarction due to any cause, the effects of infection, either directly or as a consequence of secondary vascular changes, and the consequences of trauma, whether open or closed head injury, may all lead to such lesions. In general, to be amenable to resective surgery, such changes, whatever their origin, should be circumscribed and unilateral. It can be difficult after a widespread infection or closed head injury, especially in the frontal regions, to be sure that damage is unilateral and that seizure origin is also unilateral. In most of the

patients the solution is local resection, with careful consideration, when it involves eloquent areas. In a few patients with bifrontal damage anterior callosal section may be appropriate.

The range and variety of changes grouped together as mesial temporal sclerosis are dealt with elsewhere. Pathologic evidence suggests that this process is predominantly, rather than exclusively, unilateral. It is possible that in some patients the sclerosis is mainly anterior hippocampal, whereas in others it involves the whole length of the structure. The UCLA Group have shown that surgical outcome can be correlated with the completeness of removal (Babb and Jann-Brown, 1987). Others correlate it with the severity of the neuronal loss (Nakasato, Levesque and Babb, 1992).

VASCULAR LESIONS

Apart from the obvious effects of cerebral hemorrhage from a variety of causes including arteriovenous malformation, which do not require any further special consideration, there are two pathologies which are of importance. Cavernous hemangioma usually comes to light in adult life. On the other hand, Sturge–Weber syndrome is susceptible to surgical treatment at several points in its natural history. Mostly unilateral in extent, and generally having its base in the occipital or frontal regions, not only does its natural history include extension of the lesion itself, but the secondary neurophysiologic consequences arising from processes such as kindling and secondary epileptogenesis may cause diversification of seizure type, increase in seizure severity, and, with these, intellectual deterioration. A number of techniques are available to deal with this problem, varying from local resection to multilobar removals. Hemispherectomy may be the only effective solution if there is a gross hemiplegia. The long-term consequence of this pathology can also be severe. Some centers advise early hemispherectomy, accepting the resulting hemianopia and hemiplegia, which will probably develop anyway, as a reasonable trade-off for freedom from seizures and intellectual deterioration (Hoffman *et al.*, 1979). Erba and Cavazutti (1990) have made a number of suggestions regarding the early management of Sturge–Weber syndrome, but are not supported by others (Moshe and Shinnar, 1993). Brain plasticity and reorganization make the consequences of major intervention at a very young age much less severe than if it is delayed. In a few patients we have used callosotomy to control drop attacks and generalized seizures, where hemispherectomy or multilobar resection would result in too great an increase in the neurologic deficit.

MALFORMATION AND TUMOR-LIKE LESIONS

These are a relatively common but heterogeneous group where the surgeon must rely upon his neuropathologic colleagues for a detailed classification. In practical terms, assuming that it can be seen to be solitary, the location and size of the lesion rather than the precise nature determine outcome. If such lesions can be completely removed when outside of the temporal lobe, or mostly removed as part of a temporal lobe resection, the outcome and long-term prognosis is usually good. Our work, and that of others, has shown that further treatment is seldom necessary, even after the removal is known to be incomplete, either from the surgical account or the pathologic examination (Daumas-Duport *et al.*, 1988; Kirkpatrick *et al.*, 1993). Patients with tuberous sclerosis may develop large areas of focal change and some success in controlling epilepsy has been reported following their removal (Palmini *et al.*, 1992; Vinters *et al.*, 1992). Hypothalamic hamartomata are associated with precocious puberty and gelastic epilepsy. In some patients there may appear to be an associated neurophysiologic target in one temporal lobe. Surgery directed at such a target alone is unrewarding (Cascino *et al.* 1993). If the hamartoma is sufficiently discrete an attempt at direct removal can be made, although this can be a difficult and dangerous task (Machado, Hoffman and Hwang, 1991).

NEURONAL MIGRATION DEFECT (Chapter 4a)

This concept embraces a group of conditions previously described separately under a number of headings, which include hemimegalencephaly, focal and diffuse cortical dysplasia, etc. (Palmini *et al.*, 1991; Janota and Polkey, 1992). The range of changes seen is wide, and when gross, they can be detected by structural and functional brain imaging. When examined in detail these specimens demonstrate both abnormal cells and a gross disruption of cortical lamination and organization with equal disruption and abnormalities of interneuronal connections, features which cannot be detected with current brain imaging methods. This probably accounts for two disappointing aspects of resective surgery in this group: the lesions may be impossible to remove completely; and, even when seizures are controlled, these patients continue to show slow development and poor intellectual progress.

RASMUSSEN'S ENCEPHALITIS OR CHRONIC ENCEPHALITIS WITH EPILEPSY (Chapters 7, 15b)

This rare but definite entity was first described from the Montreal Neurological Institute in 1958, at which time it was labeled encephalitis because this term most accurately described the pathologic findings on light microscopy (Rasmussen, Obozewski and Lloyd-Smith, 1958). In the majority of cases, this a progressive disease in childhood affecting one cerebral hemisphere. However, it is now known that it can occasionally burn out before the hemisphere and its functions are completely destroyed, that cases sometimes have an onset late in life, and, that there are a few well-documented cases of bilateral occurrence. The mechanism is obscure. It has been linked without definite proof to a slow virus infection, in particular to cytomegalovirus (Power *et al.*, 1990). In our series it appears to have a possible autoimmune basis (Coats *et al.*, 1992). Local resection, apart from biopsy, early in the disease, is ineffective, and later it is inappropriate. We have obtained an apparent improvement in seizure control in two cases using MST, but this may have coincided with an arrest of the disease. Otherwise the only effective surgical therapy is hemispherectomy.

MISCELLANEOUS CONDITIONS

Two other conditions deserve mention, namely arachnoid cysts and hydrocephalus. Neither of these will cause focal epilepsy, including partial complex seizures. If such epilepsy, or other localized elements, such as an EEG focus, exist, they must be attributed to some other condition. In arachnoid cyst, the two conditions may be purely coincidental, and in hydrocephalus, there may or may not be a common etiology. We have successfully operated upon the underlying pathology in both instances. Porencephalic cysts are, in effect, enlargement of the ventricular system, usually associated with loss of cerebral substance.

In our series of 75 children the resected material contained no specific pathologic changes in approximately 3% of the specimens. Reports of widespread minor gliotic changes or diffuse microscopic cortical dysplasia cannot be accepted as evidence of focal pathology. In general, but not invariably, such patients do badly from resective surgery.

RESECTIVE TECHNIQUES

The application of resective techniques varies in extent and site. It is best to describe the individual scope of three main groups: extratemporal resections, temporal resections, and major resections. However, a few comments about general techniques, applicable to all groups, are appropriate. With the exception of a few centers the use of local anesthesia to conduct epilepsy surgery is on the wane, and we have consistently found it impossible to conduct such operations below the ages of 15–16 years. However the use of grid electrodes as described above, has resolved many problems. If it is absolutely necessary to explore the central area under local anesthesia, whatever the age of the patient, it is best to conduct craniotomy under general anesthesia on one day and reopen it a few days later under local anesthesia. Anesthetic considerations are much the same as those for general pediatric neurosurgery, except that there is seldom any question of raised intracranial pressure. However, some of the procedures are long and quite major. In young children, metabolic upset and body cooling may make it wise to plan postoperative ventilation in an intensive care unit for 24 hours. Any exposure which goes near the venous sinuses, especially the sagittal sinus, may be accompanied by brisk blood loss, or very rarely air embolism, and in very young children requires an experienced pediatric anesthetist and good cooperation by the surgeon. Particular attention is drawn to the later stages of an anatomic hemispherectomy below the age of 3, when brisk and severe blood loss may occur, if venous hemorrhage is not carefully controlled.

The various areas resected in our pediatric and adult series are shown in Table 29d.3.

EXTRATEMPORAL RESECTIONS

Lesionectomy is a justified technique in extratemporal cases since it produces good results overall (Al Rhodan *et al.*, 1992; Cascino *et al.*, 1992). In general, studies have shown that if the extent of the resection is based upon the extent of the pathology rather

Table 23d.3 Comparison of frequency of resective operations in adults and children: Maudsley series

Operation	Children (no.)	% in children (n = 105)	% in adults (n = 289)
Temporal lobe			
'En bloc'	43	41.0	62.3
Extended	4	0.4	4.1
Selective amygdalohippocampectomy	2	0.2	14.5
Total	49	47.0	81.0
Other resections			
Frontal	18	17.2	7.6
Parietal	7	6.7	4.8
Central	4	4.0	4.8
Occipital	3	2.8	0.3
Total	32	30.5	13.1
Major resection	6	5.7	1.4
Hemispherectomy	18	17.1	4.5
Total	24	22.8	5.9

than electrical abnormalities, it is more likely to be successful. In stereotactic lesionectomy this is determined by the structural appearance of the lesion. Others use frozen sections (Spencer and Ojemann, 1993). Yet others claim that removal of a carefully delineated epileptogenic area using major invasive intracranial recording gives the best results.

Frontal lobe resections are the commonest in this group. A variety of pathologic conditions are found and the overall complete seizure relief rate, for all ages, is around 20% (Van Ness, 1991). Fish *et al.* (1993), describing a pediatric series from the Montreal Neurological Institute, noted excellent results in 13 of 45 children. Morrison *et al.* (1992) report 25 frontal resections: 43% of patients became seizure-free and 79% were improved. In our frontal lobe cases the extent of the resection was determined by the position of the lesion, especially in relation to the precentral cortex or Broca's area, and the extent of changes on the acute electrocorticogram. The ideal situation existed when it was possible to remove the microscopic abnormality plus all the cortex from which spikes were recorded. In our small series of 11 children there was freedom from seizures in four and an overall improvement in eight, leaving three without benefit. Of these eight, all had some positive pathology, tumor in three and cortical dysplasia (CD) in five. Factors associated with a good prognosis were removal of a discrete lesion, even when the EEG had shown widespread changes. A bad prognosis was associated with situations where the disease process may have affected other areas, such as occurs in head injury or infection, or where a lesion was incompletely removed, as was the case in some of those with cortical dysplasia. The acute neurologic complications, provided the central cortex and speech areas were respected, were almost nonexistent. No adverse affect on behavior resulted. Although occasional changes in the neuropsychologic profile were demonstrated, they were not of practical importance.

Resection from the central (parietal) area is rare. When there is a preexisting deficit there is less likelihood of this increasing as a result of operation, and therefore it is more reasonable to attempt surgery (Rasmussen, 1975). Surgical technique is of particular importance, especially care for the deep vessels. These may need to be 'skeletalized', otherwise deficits can result from infarction distant from the site of the resection. Goldring and Gregorie (1984), when first using mat electrodes, found a high proportion of low-grade intrinsic tumours in this region. Especially in children, we have found patches of cortical dysplasia, some of which are visible on brain imaging. In recent years, we have used a combination of MST and resection in these patients.

Occipital resections are also rare. Rasmussen (1975) described experience with 25 cases in almost 40 years, of whom 26% remained seizure free. We have encountered three patients in 105 and all have had a significant reduction in their seizure frequency. The prime consideration in these patients is the introduction or worsening of a visual field defect.

TEMPORAL RESECTIONS

These are the commonest resections in every epilepsy center. Although, in our series, the proportion is lower in the pediatric age group, they nevertheless form almost half of that material. The mechanism of chronic temporal lobe epilepsy probably differs from focal epilepsy in other parts of the brain, which is of importance in assessing the value of various procedures. In temporal lobe epilepsy associated with mesial temporal sclerosis, there is good evidence for the 'amplifier' mechanism proposed by Wieser *et al.* (1993). This asserts that a normal parahippocampal gyrus is part of the neurophysiologic circuit responsible for the persistence of the epilepsy and will need to be removed to obtain a cure. Thus, in many instances, the resection needs to be more extensive than the pathology. In children, preoperative selection must use all the resources available to their particular age group. Some form of temporal resection is indicated if the patient suffers from a chronic epilepsy of a type consistent with a temporal lobe origin. However, especially where younger children are concerned, some latitude may be given with this proscription. If there is a unilateral structural lesion and neurophysiologic evidence of a predominantly unilateral temporal focus, and if the available neuropsychologic data do not contraindicate it, then surgery should be seriously considered. From the surgeon's view there are two points to be considered. The first is that posterior temporal foci tend to migrate forwards with maturation, and the second is that unilateral temporal lobe lesions such as dysembryoplastic neuroepithelial tumors (DNET) may produce relatively widespread unilateral EEG changes or occasionally even bilateral changes.

There is considerable scope for variation in temporal lobe resections. Neocortical removal alone is not very successful and has more or less been abandoned. All other resections involve removal of both superficial and deep structures, and it is the extent of that removal which varies. Certain natural boundaries are imposed upon the surgeon. In the dominant hemisphere the majority of the superior temporal gyrus must be preserved. Figure 23d.2 shows variations which do this, including removal under local anesthesia (Ojemann and Dodrill, 1985), which has been applied to adults, and is included for completeness, since it is hardly practical in children. The insular cortex must remain undisturbed, if the risk of a manipulation hemiplegia is to be avoided (Penfield, Lende and Rasmussen, 1961), but most experienced centers regard persisting postresection spikes there as insignificant. Finally the posterior extent of the resection is governed by the risk of hemianopia. In adults or larger children the limit is around 6.5 cm. In smaller children it is convenient to use the height of the temporal lobe at the mid Sylvian point as a useful guide to the posterior extent of the resection.

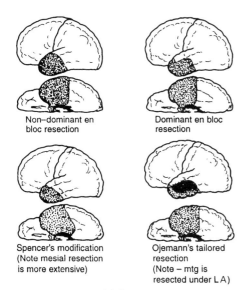

Non–dominant en
bloc resection

Dominant en bloc
resection

Spencer's modification
(Note mesial resection
is more extensive)

Ojemann's tailored
resection
(Note – mtg is
resected under LA)

Fig. 23d.2 Temporal lobe resections – variations. MTG = mesial temporal gyrus; LA = local anesthesia.

A technique for gaining access to the posterior mesial temporal structures without undue neocortical destruction has been described (Spencer *et al.*, 1984).

This approach is very useful in dealing with patients in whom there is a known lesion in the hippocampus close to the trigone. With benign tumours, DNET, hamartomata and similar lesions, complete removal is not absolutely necessary. In our series, these patients did well providing a reasonable 'en bloc' resection was done. These lesions usually respect the arachnoid over the basal cisterns, but may adhere to the trunk of the internal carotid artery, middle cerebral artery, or anterior choroidal artery. Removal can cause hemiplegia if these vessels are damaged. For the same reason, if the tumor is large, it is best to cut through it in order to complete the lobectomy and remove as much of the residual mass as possible, which improves visual access and identification of landmarks. Some surgeons prefer the microscope and the CUSA for the deep parts of a temporal lobe removal.

A further possibility is a restricted removal of the mesial temporal structures, i.e. selective amygdalo-hippocampectomy, using either transylvian techniques (Yasargil *et al.*, 1985) or the transcortical route originally described by Niemeyer (1958). The percentage of children in our own and other published series is not large (Renella, 1989; H.G. Wieser and H. Silfvenius, 1993, unpublished data). Currently the place of this procedure is uncertain. As a technically difficult operation, it should only be used when there is a definite advantage, and is certainly contraindicated in those where the demonstrated pathology cannot be encompassed. In addition, because of the amplifier effect described above, removal of the temporal lobe lesion alone is seldom successful. If such patients' epilepsy is allowed to mature, it is even possible that irreversible changes of secondary epileptogenesis may occur (Morrell, Wada and Engel, 1987).

The seizure outcome following temporal lobe resection is reasonable. For temporal lobe resections overall, i.e. adults and children, the last Palm Desert Symposium described 68% seizure free, 24% improved, and 9% not improved, using the Engel outcome scale (Engel *et al.*, 1993). The ILAE survey gives similar figures of 57% seizure free, 27% improved, and 10% not improved (H.G. Wieser and H. Silfvenius, 1993, unpublished data). Erba *et al.* (1992) described a 96% improvement in seizure control after temporal lobe resections in 46 children studied using noninvasive methods and Fish *et al.* (1993) reported excellent results in 33 children treated at the Montreal Neurological Institute over 40 years. The UCLA group have described a series of 33 children in whom there were positive lesions in 48% (Adelson *et al.*, 1992). In our own series of 41 patients aged 15 years or less, 80% became seizure free, and only one patient (3%) failed to improve. There were adverse effects in five of 50 patients in this age group. Direct operative mortality following temporal lobe resection is rare, and in our series, only occurred in adults. Morbidity in the series as a whole is around 5%, with serious morbidity 1–2%. With correct selection the effects of surgery on intellectual function are equally gratifying; there is little evidence of adverse effect and often considerable improvement. Behavioral problems in children with uncontrolled temporal lobe epilepsy are well documented. Whatever their origin, these will often improve or disappear if seizure control is good. We have not seen schizophreniform psychosis in children. A depressive illness after nondominant temporal lobe resection is extremely rare, although it can occur in the teenage group, and we have once seen it in a younger child who had an unusually large resection. The size of the resection, as well as age, may be critical, since we have not seen depression after selective amygdalo-hippocampectomy.

MULTILOBAR RESECTIONS AND HEMISPHERECTOMY

It is convenient to group these two procedures together because the circumstances under which they are performed and the kind of pathology involved are very similar. In our practice, and that of others, hemispherectomy is commoner than multilobar resection. There are a number of techniques employed for hemispherectomy. The original one described by Krynauw (1950) is in effect a hemi-decortication but is also referred to as an anatomically complete hemispherectomy. This was abandoned in the 1970s by most centres because of the complication of late delayed bleeding (Falconer and Wilson, 1969). Following this, subtotal hemispherectomy was used, but was less effective in the control of seizures. Later, a return to the total hemispherectomy was achieved in the majority of centers by adopting the Montreal technique of a functionally complete hemispherectomy. In this blocks of cortex are left anteriorly and posteriorly but isolated functionally by callosal section (Villemure and Rasmussen, 1990). In addition, a few centers use Adams' modification where, amongst other features, the enormous cavity in contact with the subarachnoid space is converted into an extradural space (Adams, 1983). Multilobar resection involves removal of an epileptogenic area of pathology which does not affect the whole hemisphere. By this means, useful cortex may be salvaged. This technique is used for patients with widespread cortical dysplasia, gross destructive lesions consequent upon trauma or cerebral infarction, or occasionally in patients with Rasmussen's disease.

Hemispherectomy is indicated when there is predominantly unilateral hemisphere disease with seizures uncontrolled by appropriate medication and an effective hemiplegia. As discussed in the section on surgical pathology, some diseases such as Sturge–Weber syndrome (Chapters 16 and 17), may require treatment at an age when the lateralized nature of the seizures and probable hemiplegia are not easy to demonstrate. Hemispherectomy gives a high rate of seizure relief and the incidence of late delayed bleeding is negligible if modern techniques are used (Beardsworth and Adams, 1988; Villemure and Rasmussen, 1993). A number of historic series of hemispherectomy are reported, usually the cases are both adults and children. The overall results were good with 70–80% of patients seizure free. The Palm Desert experience gives 67.4% seizure free with 21.1% improved, and a failure rate of about 11.6% The corresponding figures for multilobar resection are 45.2% seizure free with a failure rate of 19.5% (Engel *et al.*, 1993). In the ILAE survey there were 92 children, of whom 38 underwent functional hemispherectomy and 54 anatomic hemispherectomy. The results for seizure relief from the two procedures used in hemispherectomy are very similar, whereas the results for multilobar resection are slightly worse (H.G. Wieser and H. Silfvenius, 1993, unpublished data). In modern series, hemispherectomy seems less effective than earlier. Differences between functional and anatomic hemispherectomies and differences in the pathology in the patients involved may explain this. Recent series have a higher proportion of patients with Rasmussen's disease (Chapter 15b) or hemimegalencephaly, who are less likely to respond. Other benefits accrue. In many cases the intellectual performance will improve, as will behavior, if the seizures are controlled (Beardsworth and Adams, 1988; Lindsay *et al.*, 1984).

For patients who would otherwise be subjected to hemispherectomy, there have been reports at recent meetings of functional hemispherotomy in which the major fiber tracts are divided without removal of the pathologic brain tissue.

FUNCTIONAL SURGERY

Theoretically functional surgery can work in a number of ways. Possibilities are: abolition of a focus or foci, usually using stereotactic methods; disconnection procedures, traditionally division of part or all of the corpus callosum and more recently, multiple subpial transection; and methods of stimulating the nervous system.

STEREOTACTIC LESIONING

This had considerable vogue 30–40 years ago and is still used sporadically around the world. Long-term follow-up and the methods of patient selection have never been clear. In some series personality disorders, rather than epilepsy, predominate. At best the methods produce a 25–30% improvement in seizure control. When appropriate cases are matched, as in temporal lobe problems, resective surgery is much more efficient. Regrettably modern methods of brain imaging and neurophysiologic investigation have not been applied to this problem (Hood, Siegfried and Wieser, 1983). Recent anecdotal reports describe the use of stereotactically directed radiotherapy for temporal lobe problems, but at present there is no clear information on the efficiency or benefits of this technique.

CALLOSOTOMY

The indications for this operation are disparate. Two or three separate features are required. These are: firstly, unilateral hemisphere disease in which the neurologic deficit would be unacceptably increased by hemispherectomy or major resection; secondly, the most disabling seizure type should be atonic (drop attacks), tonic-clonic and/or bouts of status; and lastly, in patients without unilateral hemisphere disease the routine and sleep scalp EEG should show bilateral synchronous spike and wave discharges. Patients with focal motor or partial complex seizures or frequent myoclonic jerks will not benefit: indeed, if these seizure types are present they may become worse. In patients who are left-handed, or suspected for other reasons to be of mixed speech dominance, a carotid amytal test should be performed, since, if there is a significant amount of speech in both hemispheres, disruption of the transcallosal pathways may have a bad effect (Sass *et al.*, 1988). Modern techniques, including the operating microscope, have made this operation much safer (Wilson, Reeves and Gazzaniga, 1982), but serious complications can still occur. In patients with unilateral hemisphere disease the approach should be from the diseased side. Following the work of Marino (1985), it is our custom to perform the operation with electrocorticographic (ECoG) control, regarding the length of section as adequate when the two sides are desynchronized. Although some have advocated complete callosal section, especially in children, most centers now start with anterior callosal section embracing the trunk and genu. Opinions vary as to whether the section should be completed if it is unsuccessful. The complications of callosal section are acute and long term. The acute complications depend on the extent of the section, being very rare with truncal section and commonest with complete section. Transient paresis, especially of the lower limb, is seen on the side opposite to the maximum retraction. It usually resolves within a few days. Much less common, but more devastating, is a combination of mutism, lower limb paresis and urinary incontinence, probably related to bilateral anterior cerebral artery spasm. In modern series this complication is commendably rare, but may leave permanent damage. Posterior section alone is rare, the one patient we subjected to this procedure had ataxia for 10–14 days afterwards.

There are two long-term complications. The first is the risk, in those of mixed dominance, of speech difficulty which possibly can be avoided by performing the section in stages. The second, associated with posterior section in patients without unilateral hemisphere disease, is the posterior disconnection syndrome in which tasks selected by one hemisphere may not be executed by the other. Some workers believe that the combination of intellectual and personality changes following this operation make the dubious benefits in regard to the seizure control not worthwhile (Ferguson, Rayport and Corrie, 1985). It is certainly true that this surgery seldom provides as complete freedom from seizures as is seen in resective surgery. However, it may relieve certain kinds of seizures in up to 60–70% of patients and therefore can be seen as a useful palliative intervention (Engel *et al.*, 1993; H.G. Wieser and H. Silfvenius, 1993, unpublished data).

MULTIPLE SUBPIAL TRANSECTION

Since the first results were published by Morrell, Whisler and Bleck (1989), many centers have begun to use this ingenious procedure. The operation is based upon the observation that, whereas the essential functions of the cortex are mediated vertically, the interneuronal and other connections, which are likely to affect excitability, and therefore epileptogenicity, are arranged horizontally. Furthermore, if blocks of epileptogenic cortex are reduced in size, their tendency to discharge will be reduced. In essence, therefore, a number of subpial cuts are made, respecting the vessels, and isolating cortical blocks. These are made under ECoG control, so that, when spiking is abolished, the transection is sufficient.

Multiple subpial transection (MST) has been used in a number of different circumstances. Many of the original cases were patients with focal motor epilepsy of unknown etiology; others were patients with known pathology which could not be removed. MST can supplement a resection, where appropriate. In our own series, because of the difficulty of locating the primary motor and sensory cortex anatomically, all our patients have had subdural grids and motor mapping prior to surgery. With patience, this can be achieved even in quite young children. In our experience, this procedure works less well in the presence of specific pathology and we have been unable to reproduce the kind of results reported by Morrell, although some of our patients have undoubtedly benefited. Like Morrell, we have found that when transection is used alone any neurologic deficit is minor and transient. The commonest problem we have seen is a kind of dyscoordination of the upper limb, presumably due to disruption of sensory pathways. Our recommendation would be to use this method in cases of troublesome focal motor or sensory epilepsy of unknown etiology after appropriate invasive studies, and to be less sanguine about its use in association with Rasmussen's disease (Chapter 15b) or focal cortical dysplasia, where it has often proved to be less effective.

A special circumstance in which Morrell and ourselves believe this procedure is useful is that of the Landau–Kleffner syndrome

Table 23d.4   Details of children requiring reoperation: Maudsley series

Patient	Age at first operation (yr)	First operation	Interval between operations	Second operation	Outcome group	Follow-up years
1	9	MST + resection	1.8	R hemisphere	1A	2
2	10	Major resection	0.6	Major resection	3A	1
3	3	Ant call.	3	L occipital	1A	0.5
4	8	L temporal	2	L temporal lobe	4A	1
5	11	MST + resection	1	L hemisphere	1A	3
6	4	L parietal	4.5	L hemisphere	1B	1

Note: outcome scales (Engel, 1987).
1A = completely seizure free; 1B = auras (simple partial seizures only); 3A = seizures reduction > 75%; 4A = no significant change.
MST = multiple subpial transection; Ant call. = anterior callosotomy; L = left.

('acquired aphasia'; Chapter 13d). In brief, this is a disorder in which an epileptic process begins in the dominant hemisphere and subsequently affects the nondominant hemisphere, so that speech is impossible. If it can be shown by appropriate tests that the electrophysiologic situation is as described, MST over the speech area of the dominant hemisphere may give dramatic relief (Morrell, Whisler and Bleck, 1989).

NERVOUS SYSTEM STIMULATION

Deep brain stimulation and cerebellar stimulation for epilepsy have not been used much in children and the results in adults have been disappointing and inconsistent. The idea of altering the level of activity of the nervous system to control the level of seizure activity is a reasonably attractive one. The latest suggestion, which has recently undergone trial in the USA, is vagal nerve stimulation. Used in adults for complex partial seizures, it has produced a mean reduction in seizure frequency of 46%, with a few patients achieving a greater than 50% reduction. This method has not been tried in children and must be seen, at present, as experimental.

REOPERATION

Patients who have already had surgery which has failed may present for further intervention.

In the published series age at surgery is not mentioned, but in general reoperation rates are between 3 and 8% (Polkey *et al.*, 1993). Our experience probably represents the overall situation accurately. We have a reoperation rate of 3.6% overall. There are usually two reasons for reoperation: failure of a previous functional procedure, or inadequate resection of a structural lesion. There were 15 reoperations among approximately 400 operations and six of these patients were children. The details are presented in Table 23d.4.

OUTCOME

It is naïve to document outcome only in terms of seizure control, there are many other factors involved. Information about some of these is difficult to obtain, or more disappointing than one would hope. Although the raw data must be in existence in several centers, follow-up of children into adult life is not very common. Overall, general surveys of large groups, such as that of Guldvog *et al.* (1991), suggest that no overall socioeconomic benefit occurs as a result of epilepsy surgery which has a successful outcome with regard to seizure frequency; but others would argue that this is because such surgery is undertaken too late. Certainly, isolated studies such as those of Ounsted and his colleagues (Lindsay *et al.*, 1984; Ounsted, Lindsay and

Richards, 1987) and Falconer and Davidson (1974) suggest that this may be so. Much of this work assumes that the patient's condition will remain stationary or deteriorate. The surgical treatment of epilepsy, especially resective surgery, is sufficiently successful to make it very difficult to run double-blind trials of this treatment.

It is essential to point out that management in the months and years after surgery for the maturing child and adolescent is important. Readjustment to life without seizures, advice regarding the withdrawal of anticonvulsant medication, and other matters of a like nature are all long-term problems which do not fall within the province of the surgeon. In order to obtain the greatest benefit for the patient from the surgical intervention, it is these aspects which at present, certainly at least in the UK need stricter attention and commitment.

CONCLUSION

In writing this review it is hoped to convince the sceptics that surgical intervention in chronic intractable epilepsy can lead to seizure relief and other benefits, as much or more so, in children as in adults. Amongst all the technical details, it has to be remembered that surgical intervention is usually a unique treatment, rarely repeated or extended. Surgery has to be seen against the background of a maturing nervous system, having to cope with educational and family needs, none of which can be neglected or overlooked. Finally the long-term results of such surgery must be viewed dispassionately against the measure of what might have been, rather than what should have been.

REFERENCES

Adams, C.B.T. (1983) Hemispherectomy – a modification. *Journal of Neurology, Neurosurgery and Psychiatry*, **46**, 617–9.

Adams, C.B.T., Anslow, P., Molyneaux, A. and Oxbury, J. (1987) Radiological detection of surgically treatable pathology, in *Surgical Treatment of the Epilepsies* (ed. J. Engel), Raven, New York, pp. 213–33.

Adelson, P.D., Peacock, W.J., Chugani, H.T. *et al.* (1992) Temporal and extended temporal resections for the treatment of intractable seizures in early childhood. *Pediatric Neurosurgery*, **18**, 169–78.

Al Rodhan, N.R., Kelly, P.J, Cascino, G.D. and Sharbrough, F.W. (1992) Surgical outcome in computer-assisted stereotactic resection of intra-axial cerebral lesions for partial epilepsy. *Stereotactic Functioning in Neurosurgery*, **58**, 172–7.

Babb, T.L. and Jann-Brown, W. (1987) Pathological findings in epilepsy, in *Surgical Treatment of the Epilepsies* (ed. J. Engel), Raven Press, New York, pp. 511–40.

Beardsworth, E.D. and Adams, C.B.T. (1988) Modified hemispherectomy for epilepsy. Early results in 10 cases. *British Journal of Neurosurgery*, **2**, 73–84.

Cascino, G.D., Andermann, F., Berkovic, S.F. *et al.* (1993) Gelastic seizures and hypothalamic hamartomas: evaluation of patients undergoing chronic intracranial EEG monitoring and outcome of surgical treatment. *Neurology*, **43**, 747–50.

Cascino, G.D., Kelly, P.J., Sharbrough, F.W. *et al.* (1992) Long-term follow-up of stereotactic lesionectomy in partial epilepsy: predictive factors and electroencephalographic results. *Epilepsia*, **33**, 639–44.

Chugani, H.T., Shewmon, D.A., Peacock, W.J. *et al.* (1988) Surgical treatment of intractable neonatal-onset seizures: the role of positron emission tomography. *Neurology*, **38**, 1178–88.

Coats, P., Honavar, M., Janota, I. and Polkey, C.E. (1992) Polymerase chain reaction studies in Rasmussen's encephalitis. *Neuropathology and Applied Neurobiology*, **18**, 310.

Daumas-Duport, C., Scheithauer, B.W., Chodkiewicz, J.-P. *et al.* (1988) Dysembryoplastic neuroepithelial tumor: a surgically curable tumor of young patients with intractable partial seizures. Report of thirty-nine cases. *Neurosurgery*, **23**, 545–556.

Engel, J. (ed.) (1987) Outcome with respect to epileptic seizures, in *Surgical Treatment of The Epilepsies*, 1st edn, Raven, New York, pp. 553–71.

Engel, J., Van Ness, P.C., Rasmussen, T. and Ojemann, L.M. (1993) Outcome with respect to epileptic seizures, in *Surgical Treatment of the Epilepsies*, 2nd edn (ed. J. Engel), Raven, New York, pp. 609–22.

Erba, G. and Cavazutti, V. (1990) Sturge–Weber syndrome: natural history and indications for surgery. *Journal of Epilepsy*, **3**, 287–91.

Erba, G., Winston, K.R., Adler, J.R. *et al.* (1992) Temporal lobectomy for complex partial seizures that began in childhood. *Surgical Neurology*, **38**, 424–32.

Falconer, M.A. and Davidson, S. (1974) The rationale of surgical treatment of temporal lobe epilepsy with particular reference to childhood and adolescence, in *Epilepsy. Proceedings of the Hans Berger Centenary Symposium* (eds P. Harris and C. Mawdsley), Churchill Livingstone, Edinburgh, pp. 209–14.

Falconer, M.A. and Wilson, P.J.E. (1969) Complications relating to delayed haemorrhage after hemispherectomy. *Journal of Neurosurgery*, **30**, 413–26.

Ferguson, S.M., Rayport, M. and Corrie, W.S. (1985) Neuropsychiatric observations on behavioral consequences of corpus callosum section for seizure control, in *Epilepsy and the Corpus Callosum* (ed. A.G. Reeves), Plenum, New York, pp. 501–14.

Fish, D.R., Smith, S.J., Quesney, L.F. *et al.* (1993) Surgical treatment of children with medically intractable frontal or temporal lobe epilepsy: results and highlights of 40 years' experience. *Epilepsia*, **34**, 244–7.

Goldring, S. and Gregorie, E.M. (1984) Surgical management of epilepsy using epidural mats to localise the seizure focus. *Journal of Neurosurgery*, **60**, 457–66.

Guldvog, B., Loyning, Y., Hauglie-Hanssen, E. *et al.* (1991) Surgical versus medical treatment for epilepsy. II. Outcome related to social areas. *Epilepsia*, **32**, 477–86.

Hoffman, H.J., Hendrick, E.B., Dennis, M. and Armstrong, D. (1979) Hemispherectomy for Sturge–Weber syndrome. *Child's Brain*, **5**, 223–48.

Hood, T.W., Siegfried, J. and Wieser, H.G. (1983) The role of stereotactic amygdalotomy in the treatment of behavioral disorders associated with temporal lobe epilepsy. *Applied Neurophysiology*, **49**, 19–25.

Jabbari, B., Van Nostrand, D., Gunderson, C.H. *et al.* (1991) EEG and neuroimaging localisation in partial epilepsy. *Electroencephalography and Clinical Neurophysiology*, **79**, 108–13.

Jack, C.R., Nichols, D.A., Sharbrough, F.W. *et al.* (1988) Selective posterior cerebral amytal test for evaluating memory function before surgery for temporal lobe seizure. *Radiology*, **168**, 787–93.

Janota, I. and Polkey, C.E. (1992) Cortical dysplasia in epilepsy – a study of material from surgical resections for intractable epilepsy, in *Recent Advances in Epilepsy No. 5* (eds T.A. Pedley and B.S. Meldrum), Churchill Livingstone, Edinburgh, pp. 37–49.

Kirkpatrick, P.J., Honavar, M., Janota, I. and Polkey, C.E. (1993) Control of temporal lobe epilepsy following en bloc resection of low grade gliomas. *Journal of Neurosurgery*, **78**, 19–25.

Krynauw, R.A. (1950) Infantile hemiplegia treated by removing one cerebral hemisphere. *Journal of Neurology, Neurosurgery and Psychiatry*, **13**, 243–67.

Kuzniecky, R.I., Cascino, G.D., Palmini, A. *et al.* (1993a) Structural neuroimaging, in *Surgical Treatment of the Epilepsies*, 2nd edn (ed. J. Engel), Raven, New York, pp. 197–209.

Kuzniecky, R., Murro, A., King, D. *et al.* (1993b) Magnetic resonance imaging in childhood intractable partial epilepsies: pathologic correlations. *Neurology*, **43**, 681–7.

Lindsay, J., Glaser, G., Richards, P. and Ounsted, C. (1984) Developmental aspects of focal epilepsies of childhood treated by neurosurgery. *Developmental Medicine and Child Neurology*, **26**, 574–87.

Lüders, H. and Awad, I.A. (1991) Conceptual considerations, in *Epilepsy Surgery* (ed. H. Lüders), Raven Press, New York, pp. 51–62.

Machado, H.R., Hoffman, H.J. and Hwang, P.A. (1991) Gelastic seizures treated by resection of a hypothalamic hamartoma. *Childs Nervous System*, **7**, 462–5.

Marino, R. (1985) Surgery for epilepsy. Selective partial microsurgical callosotomy for intractable multiform seizures. Criteria for clinical selection and results. *Applied Neurophysiology*, **48**, 404–7.

McMillan, T., Powell, G.E., Janota, I. and Polkey, C.E. (1987) Relationship between neuropathology and cognitive functioning in temporal lobe patients. *Journal of Neurology, Neurosurgery, and Psychiatry*, **50**, 167–76.

Morrell, F., Wada, J. and Engel, J. (1987) Appendix III: potential relevance of kindling and secondary epileptogenesis to the consideration of surgical treatment for epilepsy, in *Surgical Treatment of the Epilepsies*, ed. J. Engel, Raven, New York, pp.701–7.

Morrell, F., Whisler, W.W. and Bleck, T.P. (1989) Multiple subpial transection. A new approach to the surgical treatment of focal epilepsy. *Journal of Neurosurgery*, **70**, 231–9.

Morrison, G., Duchowny, M., Resnick, T. *et al.* (1992) Epilepsy surgery in childhood. A report of 79 patients. *Pediatric Neurosurgery*, **18**, 291–7.

Moshe, S.L. and Shinnar, S. (1993) Postscript – early intervention, in *Surgical Treatment of the Epilpesies*, 2nd edn (ed. J. Engel), Raven New York, pp.123–32.

Nakasato, N., Levesque, M.F. and Babb, T.L. (1992) Seizure outcome following standard temporal lobectomy: correlation with hippocampal neuron loss and extrahippocampal pathology. *Journal of Neurosurgery*, **77**, 194–200.

Niemeyer, P. (1958) The transventricular amydala-hippocampectomy in temporal lobe epilepsy, in *Temporal Lobe Epilepsy* (eds M. Baldwin, and P. Bailey), Charles C. Thomas, Springfield, pp. 461–82.

Ojemann, G.A. and Dodrill, C.B. (1985) Verbal memory deficits after left temporal lobectomy for epilepsy: mechanism and intraoperative prediction. *Journal of Neurosurgery*, **62**, 101–7.

Ounsted, C., Lindsay, J. and Norman, J. (1966) *Biological Factors in Temporal Lobe Epilepsy*, Heinemann, London.

Ounsted, C., Lindsay, J. and Richards, P. (1987) *Temporal Lobe Epilepsy. A Biographical Study. 1948–1986*, Blackwell Scientific Publications, Oxford, pp. 70–86.

Palmini, A., Andermann, F., Olivier, A. *et al.* (1991) Surgical treatment of patients with intractable seizures due to focal or lateralised neuronal migration disorders. *Epilepsia*, **32** (suppl.1), 93.

Palmini, A., Andermann, F., Tampieri, D. *et al.* (1992) Epilepsy and cortical cytoarchitectonic abnormalities: an attempt at correlating basic mechanisms with anatomoclinical syndromes. *Epilepsy Research Supplement*, **9**, 19–29.

Penfield, W., Lende, R.A. and Rasmussen, T. (1961) Manipulation hemiplegia, an untoward complication in the surgery of focal epilepsy. *Journal of Neurosurgery*, **18**, 769–76.

Polkey, C.E., Awad, I.A., Tanaka, T. and Wyler, A.R. (1993) The place of reoperation, in *Surgical Treatment of the Epilepsies*, 2nd edn (ed. J. Endel), Raven, New York, pp. 663–7.

Powell, G.E., Polkey, C.E. and McMillan, T.M. (1985) The new Maudsley series of temporal lobectomy I: Short term cognitive effects. *British Journal of Clinical Psychology*, **24**, 109–24.

Power, C., Poland, S.D., Blume, W. T. *et al.* (1990) Cytomegalovirus and Rasmussen's encephalitis. *Lancet*, **336**, 1282–4.

Rasmussen, T. (1975) Surgery for epilepsy arising in regions other than the frontal or temporal lobes, in *Advances in Neurology*, vol. 8, *Neurosurgical Treatment of the Epilepsies* (eds D.P. Purpura, J.K. Penry and R.D. Walter), Raven, New York, pp. 207–26.

Rasmussen, T. and Milner, B. (1977) The role of early left brain damage in determining the lateralisation of cerebral speech functions. *Annals of the New York Academy of Sciences*, **299**, 355–69.

Rasmussen, T., Obozewski, J. and Lloyd-Smith, D. (1958) Focal seizures due to chronic localised encephalitis. *Neurology*, **8**, 435–45.

Rausch, R. (1992) Role of the neuropsychological evaluation and the intracarotid sodium amobarbital procedure in the surgical treatment of epilepsy, in *Surgical Treatment of Epilepsy*. (Epilepsy Res. Suppl. 5.), (ed. W.H. Theodore,), Elsevier Science, Amsterdam, pp. 77–86.

Rausch, R., Silfvenius, H., Wieser, H.G. *et al.* (1993) Intraarterial amobarbital procedures, in *Surgical Treatment of the Epilepsies*, 2nd edn (ed. J. Engel), Raven, New York, pp. 341–58.

Renella, R.R. (1989) Outcome of surgery, in *Microsurgery of the Temporal Region*, Springer-Verlag, Wien, pp. 158–64.

Rintahaka, P.J., Chugani, H.T., Messa, C. and Phelps, M.E. (1993) Hemimegalencephaly: evaluation with positron emission tomography. *Pediatric Neurology*, **9**, 21–8.

Sass, K.J., Spencer, S.S., Spencer, D.D. *et al.* (1988) Corpus callosotomy for epilepsy. II Neurologic and neuropsychological outcome. *Neurology*, **38**, 24–8.

Spencer, D.D. and Ojemann, G.A. (1993) Overview of therapeutic procedures, in *Surgical Treatment of the Epilepsies*, 2nd edn (ed. J. Engel), Raven, New York, pp. 455–71.

Spencer, D.D. Spencer, S.S., Mattson, R.H. *et al.* (1984) Access to the posterior medial temporal structures in the surgical treatment of temporal lobe epilepsy. *Neurosurgery*, **15**, 667–71.

Sperling, M.R., O'Connor, M.J., Saykin, A.J. *et al.* (1992) A noninvasive protocol for anterior temporal lobectomy. *Neurology*, **42**, 416–22.

Van Ness, P.C. (1991) Surgical outcome for neocortical (extrahippocampal) focal epilepsy, in

Epilepsy Surgery (ed. H. Lüders), Raven, New York, pp. 613–24.

Van Veelen, C.M.W., Debets, C., Van Huffelen, A.C. *et al.* (1990) Combined use of subdural and intracerebral electrodes in preoperative evaluation of epilepsy. *Neurosurgery*, **26**, 93–101.

Villemure, J.G. and Rasmussen, T. (1990) Functional hemispherectomy – methodology. *Journal of Epilepsy*, **3**, 177–82.

Villemure, J.G. and Rasmussen, T. (1993) Functional hemispherectomy in children. *Neuropediatrics*, **24**, 53–55.

Vinters, H.V., Fisher, R.S., Cornford, M.E. *et al.* (1992) Morphological substrates of infantile spasms: studies based on surgically resected cerebral tissue. *Childs Nervous System*, **8**, 8–17.

Wieser, H.G., Engel, J., Williamson, P.D. *et al.* (1993) Surgically remediable temporal lobe syndromes, in *Surgical Treatment of the Epilepsies*, 2nd edn (ed. J. Engel), Raven, New York, pp. 49–63.

Wilson, D.H., Reeves, A.G. and Gazzaniga, M. (1982) 'Central' commissurotomy for intractable generalised epilepsy: series two. *Neurology*, **32**, 687–97.

Yasargil, M.G. Teddy, P.J. and Roth, P. (1985) Selective amygdalo-hippocampectomy. Operative anatomy and surgical technique, in *Advances and Technical Standards in Neurosurgery*, 12th edn (ed. L. Symon), Springer-Verlag, Wien, pp. 93–123.

COGNITIVE ASPECTS

Dorothée A. Kasteleijn-Nolst Trenité

INTRODUCTION

Epilepsy is a childhood brain disorder; about 60% of all affected patients have an age at onset before 20 years and one-third have their first seizure at junior school.

The appearance of epilepsy in childhood often interferes with normal cognitive development and academic achievement. Several studies show that children with epilepsy perform less well at school than their healthy peers, even during periods without clinical seizures (Stores, 1978; Seidenberg *et al.*, 1986; Aldenkamp *et al.*, 1993). In studies on twins (Lennox and Collins, 1945), differences were found in twins with and without epilepsy and, within twins, if only one had epilepsy. Estimates of prevalence rates of learning problems range from 5 to 50% (Thompson, 1987). Epilepsy in the mentally handicapped is reviewed in Chapter 17, and epilepsies with cognitive symptomatology are discussed in Chapter 13d.

Parents, teachers, and doctors will be confronted with questions concerning the influence of epilepsy on cognitive functioning; for example, how this can be assessed, prevented, or treated. Furthermore, as soon as learning problems arise at school, uncertainty exists concerning the correlation with epilepsy. At the present, it is unclear how and to what extent the different epilepsy factors are involved. Clinicians and researchers have identified several relevant variables, such as age at onset of epileptic seizures, duration of epilepsy, and type and frequency of seizures. Finally, differences in etiology, such as a deteriorating brain disease, localized or generalized brain damage after a trauma or a meningoencephalitis can also give learning problems. The underlying disease or damage generally has a much greater negative effect on the learning problems than the associated epileptic seizures themselves. However, in 75% of children with epilepsy, no etiologic factor can be determined (Hauser, 1978). A genetically determined susceptibility is likely but has not yet been demonstrated for most of the epilepsies. Besides the influence of the epileptic disorder itself on cognitive functioning, side-effects from antiepileptic treatment can affect cognition. Another negative influence relates to the impact of epilepsy on social functioning, which in turn can decrease school performance.

Although the various determinants are interrelated, it is possible to give an impression of the impact of the various factors on cognitive performance and academic achievement. Since the beginning of the twentieth century, and especially in the last 20 years, many studies have been performed.

ASSESSMENT

GENERAL

Around the turn of the century scientists developed methods to determine intellectual behaviour such as the Binet–Simon scales, and Standford Binet and Pintner–Cunningham

Epilepsy in Children. Edited by Sheila Wallace. Published in 1996 by Chapman & Hall, London. ISBN 0 412 56860 8

tests. These tests were applied on a large number of children in order to obtain validation, and subsequently were used in all types of patients, including children with epilepsy.

In 1949 Wechsler developed the Bellevue Intelligence Tests, better known as the Wechsler Intelligence Scales for Children (WISC). Wechsler defined intelligence as 'the aggregate or global capacity of the individual to act purposefully, to think rationally and to deal effectively with his environment'. Intelligence was not considered a mere sum of intellectual ability, but also a function of the way in which the various abilities are combined. Psychologists used the term 'mental products'.

The value of intelligence tests for children was demonstrated soon after their development. The results in school children correlated very highly with scholastic achievement and could therefore be used in proper grading of school children, particularly at the outset of their education. Furthermore, these intelligence tests provided a quantitative measure of the degree of mental deficiency in children. In the first intelligence tests the intelligence quotient (IQ) was calculated by dividing a subject's mental age by his chronologic age. Wechsler (1944) introduced the IQ score as attained or actual score divided by the expected mean score for age. Under normal conditions, an individual's IQ will thus remain the same throughout life (consistency of the IQ scores). The mean IQs are regularly found to be about 100, with deviation of not more than two or three points when repeated from age to age. However, this stability in results is more often found in the Wechsler scale than in the other scales.

Wechsler made a selection of various well-known tests, dividing these subtests into performance or verbal subtests and using subtests which 'hold up' with age for about half of both the verbal and performance items. Division into verbal and performance parts allowed psychologists to guide pupils,

in particular 11 year olds, into appropriate educational programmes: manual workers generally do better on performance, while clerical workers do much better on verbal tests. Large discrepancies between verbal and performance test scores are seen in certain types of mental pathology. Subjects of inferior intelligence do better on performance parts of the examination while subjects of superior intelligence generally do better on the verbal part. Furthermore, patients with organic brain disease perform better on the verbal subtests, whereas congenital mental deficiency is associated with better performance results.

The WISC has also been used in order to examine laterality of seizure foci and differences between verbal and performance IQ. However, the intelligence test was developed for global assessment and not as a means to lateralize. In addition, most of the performance tasks are timed, while those of the verbal tasks are not. Patients with epilepsy, drug intoxication or a combination of these show slowness in cognitive processing, thus performance tests are more affected than verbal ones.

In the 1970s behavioral neurologists started to select neurobehavioral tasks primarily in terms of their face validity. Clinical experience helped in selecting specific items sensitive to neurobehavioral impairment (Luria, 1973). Standardized neuropsychologic tests and test batteries were subsequently designed for assessment of brain-damaged patients. Neuropsychologic assessment, especially in children, includes issues such as functional brain organization, information processing, cerebral hemispheric lateralization, and plasticity (Cohen *et al.*, 1992). While the intelligence tests are primarily developed in children and later modified for adults, the neuropsychologic test batteries most commonly employed, the Luria–Nebraska Childrens' Revision and the Halstead–Reitan, are modifications of adult tests (Cohen *et al.*,

1992). These tests include simple tasks such as finger tapping, as well as more complex tasks such as digit symbol, visual retention, and visual and performance memory tests.

Due to lack of function-specific tests, discrimination of localized brain functions is, however, difficult. Although the various tests can be divided into categories such as tactile-perceptual, visual-perceptual, problem-solving, etc., a considerable overlap exists between them. Isolation of functions in test material is minimal in tests of reaction, however. Memory tasks, for example, always include verbal or visual functions as well.

Recent development of computerized, neuropsychologic tests has improved precision in timing of test parameters such as stimulus and response-time and item frequency, which is of importance in studies of speed and attention. Furthermore, computerized testing should be favored in multicenter studies because tester bias and variability of test application is avoided (Alpherts and Aldenkamp, 1990).

However, children who are moderately or severely physically and/or mentally handicapped are unable to cope with computers, or are unable to understand test instructions (Johnson, 1991). Aman (1991) investigated the use of computerized testing with the Standford Binet Intelligence Scale in 30 children whose ages ranged from 5 to 13 years, with below average IQs, and who were hyperactive or had conduct disorders. These children could successfully meet the test requirements if their IQs were at least 50. In 70 subjects with a mean age of 11 years (range 6–15 years), the use of microcomputer-generated short-term memory tasks for routine clinical testing of children with epilepsy was evaluated (Kasteleijn-Nolst Trenité *et al.*, 1990). Two self-pacing microcomputer tests were presented in the form of a video-game consisting of nonverbal and visual spatial material, similar to Corsi's block test (Aarts *et al.*, 1984). Only nine of the 70 children were unable to perform verbal tasks appropriately.

The visual spatial task could be performed by all children.

INTELLIGENCE TESTS

One of the most commonly used tests in children with epilepsy is the Intelligence Test. As early as 1935, Sullivan and Gahagan investigated 103 children with epilepsy with a Binet–Simon intelligence test; the average IQ of these children was 92.4, whilst that of a normal control group was 105. The IQ was relatively higher in children whose epilepsy appeared after the age of 6 years and in children with only 'minor seizures'. These findings have been confirmed by other studies (Ledeboer, 1941; Tarter, 1972; Bourgeois *et al.*, 1983; Farwell, Dodrill and Batzel, 1985), and it is generally agreed that the IQ score of those with epilepsy is lower than that of normal children, and depends on type, frequency and severity of epileptic seizures as well as on etiology. Rutter, Graham and Yule (1970) found the distribution of intelligence in children with epilepsy closely resembling the normal distribution values. However, the children with epilepsy who were investigated all attended normal schools and were those with the least severe epilepsy.

It was also recognized in the early forties that different intelligence tests such as the Pintner–Cunningham and Binet–Simon tests, could give different results in the same children with epilepsy (Ledeboer, 1941). If the Pintner–Cunningham test was used, the overall results were better than if the Binet–Simon test was used. This difference in results in the same children appeared to be mainly due to the time factor in the latter, and it was therefore concluded that children with epilepsy seemed to suffer more from psychomotor slowing (slowness) than normal children.

Since the 1950s and especially since the 1970s, the WISC IQ test, more accurately WISC-R (the revised WISC) (Wechsler Intelligence Test for Children – Revised) has been used most often. The various studies in which these IQ tests were used, confirm that IQ levels of children with epilepsy tend to be below mean intelligence. A relatively high test–retest variability can be found in repeated IQ testing of these children (Bourgeois *et al.*, 1983; Rodin, Schmaltz and Twitty, 1986). During a follow-up period of an average of 10 years, these authors found a positive or negative fluctuation as high as 10 points in patients performing verbal or performance subtests at any IQ level. Although in both studies a steady rise in IQ was observed in children in remission rather than in those with continued epileptic seizures, no significant relationships were found between age, sex, presence or absence of etiologic factors by history, EEG results, seizure type, frequency or duration of epilepsy and verbal performance or total IQ. Only higher initial verbal IQ and epilepsy starting at an earlier age were correlated with much lower performance IQ at follow-up. In another study of 45 children referred to the Epilepsy Centre, Heemstede (Aldenkamp *et al.*, 1990), no significant test–retest differences were found between test results at the mean ages of 9, 10, and 13 years. In the latter study, however, all the children had a high seizure frequency, starting several years before the first assessment and continuing during the follow-up period. Furthermore, in comparison to the studies of Rodin and Bourgeois, fewer children were treated with phenobarbitone and phenytoin and lower dosages of all antiepileptic drugs (AEDs) were prescribed. Subtest score analysis revealed, in both studies, below average scores in vocabulary (fluency, verbal language skill), coding or digit-symbol (attention, sensory-motor coordination), and information (verbal language skill).

Ellenberg, Hirtz and Nelson (1986) examined the IQ before and after the onset of seizures in 62 children. These children had their first seizure between the age of 4 and 7 years. Comparison of IQ could be made between 7-year-old children with and without epileptic seizures. No differences were found in IQ if children with seizures were compared with those matched for the same initial IQ at 4 years of age, sex, race, and socioeconomic status. Neurologic and developmental status before the initial seizure appeared to be a major determinant of outcome. The epileptic seizures themselves did not cause intellectual deterioration. Wallace and Cull (1979) investigated the long-term outcome for children whose first seizure occurred with fever. In contrast to the previous study, the age range was much more extended: 2 months to 7 years. All children were investigated after the age of 8 or 9 years of age. The IQs of the group as a whole showed normal means and distribution. However, some subgroups performed less well: a lower social class and persisting neurologic abnormality were related with lower psychologic functioning in boys and girls. Remarkably, however, girls appeared to be much more affected than boys when they had a history of recurrent seizures. Furthermore, girls, especially those with right-sided seizures, carried a poor prognosis if the attacks occurred early in life (between 13 and 18 months).

Apart from factors such as age of onset and duration of epilepsy, differences can be found in performance depending on seizure type. Generalized tonic-clonic seizures have a greater impact than short-lasting partial seizures. Psychologic investigations should not be performed within a few days after generalized tonic-clonic convulsions. Fedio and Mirsky (1969), comparing children with generalized tonic-clonic seizures to patients with partial seizures, found the former group to have specific disorders of attention and constructional apraxia. This finding was confirmed by Giordani *et al.* (1985), who discovered that patients with a partial epilepsy showed better results on the subtests of the WISC-R (picture arrangement, coding, block design, and object assembly) than those with generalized epilepsy. These performance subtests require visiospatial problem solving and sequencing and also attention and concentration. One would expect that children with an epileptic focus in the left or right temporal lobe would show hemisphere-specific dysfunction. The left side of the brain is generally specialized in verbal information processing and the right in visual spatial information processing. Some studies (Fedio and Mirsky, 1969; Lavadas, Umilta and Provinciali, 1979) have indeed demonstrated hemisphere-specific dysfunctions in patients with epileptic foci in the left versus right temporal lobe (Camfield *et al.*, 1984). This is however difficult to investigate: first one has to select children exclusively with seizures that start and are confined to the region of the epileptic focus. Most children will not only show partial seizures but also secondarily generalized seizures. Furthermore, most children will show seizures from both the right and left temporal region or from other regions as well. In order to select children with 'pure' localization-related seizures, detailed seizure histories in combination with simultaneous EEG recordings are necessary. A second problem, especially in children, is that the area of the epileptic focus cannot necessarily be inferred from neuropsychologic functioning. Finally, due to adaptation, a functional reorganization (plasticity) might occur if some parts of the brain are not functioning well. This is likely in children who develop epilepsy at an early age. Some mentally retarded children, for example, who have severe neuronal loss in one hemisphere, show epileptic seizures arising in the relatively good functioning side of their brains, whilst the other side functions less well and is nonepileptogenic. Thus, even children who show a consistent epileptic focus in their EEGs are not necessarily a homogeneous group.

Furthermore, the commonly used Wechsler Intelligence Test does not provide a consistent and reliable index of lateralization. The visual perceptual and constructional tests (e.g. picture completion, picture arrangement, block design, object assembly) of the Wechsler test are timed. Apart from having a lower intelligence, epilepsy, drug intoxication, or a combination of these, influence performance on these nonverbal subtests in a negative manner. These confounding factors must thus be taken into consideration. In addition, unnoticed seizures or subclinical EEG discharges during intelligence testing have a more negative influence on outcome of some subtests than others, which will be relatively unaffected (Siebelink *et al.*, 1988). Siebelink *et al.* (1988) investigated 21 school children with or without seizures attending outpatient clinics for epilepsy or an academic hospital. Those with epilepsy were recruited among patients with known subclinical epileptiform EEG discharges in the waking state, regardless of whether they had social-emotional or educational problems. The children were tested with the Revised Amsterdam Child Intelligence Test (Revised Amsterdam Kinder Intelligentie Test, RAKIT) with simultaneous continuous EEG and video monitoring. The mean IQ of the 21 children was 87.4, which is significantly lower than the standard normal value for this test battery (mean, 100; standard deviation, 15). The test profile proved to be significantly abnormal due chiefly to poor performance on a paired-associates task (learning names). The child is asked to reproduce the proper names for animal pictures, which demands short-term verbal learning. The subsequent abnormal test profile was accounted for almost entirely by poor performance on the paired-associates task in those children who exhibited epileptiform discharges during the testing; this demonstrates that differences in results between various studies, and test–retest discrepancies within the same patients, can be due to subclinical epileptiform discharges, apart from other contributing factors.

NEUROPSYCHOLOGIC TESTS

Attention and concentration deficits are often recognized as a special problem in children with epilepsy (Holdsworth and Whitmore, 1974; Stores, 1978). Holdsworth and Whitmore found that teachers described 36 of the 85 affected children as lethargic, dull, and apathetic. In only five children could this be attributed to possible short-lasting seizures (absences). Reaction time as measured by simple and choice reaction time tests was found to be markedly increased and psychomotor speed decreased in patients with epilepsy (Bruhn, 1970). However, the extent to which intellectual functioning contributes to this effect is not clear, since IQ and disease are often confounded.

Speed of information processing is found to be lower in children with epilepsy than in controls, as demonstrated by Alpherts and Aldenkamp (1990) using a computerized visual-search task (CVST).

Although clinically the relationship between memory disturbances and epilepsy was made as early as the beginning of the twentieth century (Gowers, 1885), not much research has been done concerning memory and epilepsy. In the studies performed, it has been shown that memory impairment is especially correlated with partial complex seizures of temporal lobe origin: verbal memory impairment in patients with left-sided temporal foci and nonverbal memory impairment in patients with right-sided foci (Fedio and Mirsky, 1969; Lavadas, Umilta and Provinciali, 1979). Memory impairment has also been found during the occurrence of epileptiform EEG discharges using short-term memory tasks (Kasteleijn-Nolst Trenité *et al.*, 1990). Antiepileptic drugs such as phenytoin can also negatively influence memory (Thompson, Huppert and Trimble, 1981).

ACADEMIC ACHIEVEMENT

Children with epilepsy perform less well at school than their healthy peers, even during periods without clinical seizures (Stores, 1978; Seidenberg *et al.*, 1986). Seidenberg *et al.*, demonstrated in 122 children with a full-scale IQ of at least 70 (WISC-R) that the children made less academic progress than expected for their IQ level and age. These deficiencies were most pronounced for arithmetic and spelling, followed by reading comprehension and word recognition. Older children were further behind in their achievement levels in all areas when compared with younger children. Earlier age of seizure onset, longer duration of epilepsy and the presence of generalized seizures, were associated with poor arithmetic achievement scores. Other factors such as the number of AEDs did not influence the results.

READING AND ARITHMETIC

Rutter, Graham and Yule (1970), Stores and Hart (1976), and Long and Moore (1979) have focused on reading. Rutter, Graham and Yule (1970) found that 18% of children with epilepsy were 2 or more years below grade level in reading comprehension, although their IQ scores were normal or above average. Boys, even more than girls, show reading impairment. This sex difference in reading ability is not found in arithmetic skills (Seidenberg *et al.*, 1986). Children with mainly left-sided epileptiform discharges show lower reading performance than children with right-sided epileptiform discharges (Stores and Hart, 1976; Kasteleijn-Nolst Trenité *et al.*, 1990). Again, this difference is not found with regard to arithmetic (Kasteleijn-2olst Trenité *et al.*, 1990). However, a consistent relationship between a left-sided focus and reading disabilities has not always been found (Camfield *et al.*, 1984; Seidenberg *et al.*, 1986). Seidenberg's patients with right focal epileptiform discharges performed less well in reading comprehension, but preserved reading rate. A possible explanation could be that memorizing of the spatial component of reading is impaired. Camfield *et al.* (1984) found lower scores on mental arithmetic in children with left temporal foci. With the exception of that of Kasteleijn-Nolst Trenité *et al.* (1990), none of the above-mentioned studies simultaneously correlated epileptiform discharges in the EEG with test performance, but relied only on findings during a routine diagnostic EEG. Furthermore the findings of Stores and Hart (1976) and Kasteleijn–Nolst Trenité *et al.* (1990) are consistent with the accepted data, that reading is generally supported in the left hemisphere (Bakker and Vinke, 1985), while arithmetic is a function involving both hemispheres (Levin and Spiers, 1985). Arithmetic underachievement is also a common finding in nonepileptic learning and mentally disabled children (Strang and Rourke, 1985).

Not only children, but also adolescents, with epilepsy showed poorer comprehension of reading material than their controls matched for age, sex, and general ability (Clement and Wallace, 1990). The lowest overall reading scores were found in patients with myoclonic seizures, partial seizures with secondary generalization, or generalized tonic-clonic seizures. This is more or less in agreement with Seidenberg *et al.* (1986), who found that children with both generalized tonic-clonic and absence seizures did less well than others.

SPELLING

Jennekens-Schinkel *et al.* (1987) investigated the writing-to-dictation results in mildly epileptic children of at least average intelligence who were attending ordinary elementary schools, and compared them to normal controls. Boys with epilepsy, followed by girls with epilepsy and control boys, made the highest number of errors per hundred dictated words. Significantly more letter perseveration errors were made by children with epilepsy, who also made more corrections and left more errors uncorrected (performance errors). Skill-related errors were not seen more often.

No relation with other variables, such as type of epilepsy, etc., could be made.

Few studies have included EEG data other than that necessary for diagnosis and classification. Baird *et al.* (1980) investigated the EEG more systematically using quantitative assessment. They evaluated whether children who are school underachievers exhibit more EEG and evoked potential abnormalities than those who perform at grade level. In addition comparisons were made with healthy non-epileptic achievers and underachievers. All children with epilepsy were well controlled with medication. Underachievers with epilepsy showed more beta bursts and excessive theta and delta rhythms in the resting EEG, and greater hyperreactivity of evoked responses to visual and auditory stimuli in the frontal and frontopolar regions. In those with epilepsy, both achievers and underachievers showed widespread sharp waves. Healthy underachievers showed more abnormal spectral bands, greater asymmetry and a higher incidence of sharp waves when compared with healthy achievers. The finding that children with learning disability, whether associated with epilepsy or not, showed a high incidence of sharp waves indicates that these subclinical epileptiform discharges cause cognitive impairment.

SUBCLINICAL EPILEPTIFORM EEG DISCHARGES AND COGNITION

Shortly after the discovery of the EEG, Berger noticed that absence seizures were accompanied by 3 Hz generalized spike-waves (Berger, 1933). However, Gibbs, Lennox and Gibbs (1936) observed that not all short-lasting generalized spike-waves gave clinical manifestations. Some patients continued singing and counting during the discharges. Discharges of about 10 seconds or less duration are generally not noticed by clinical observation of the patient, and are referred to as subclinical EEG discharges. They can however disturb cognition, as was first demonstrated by Schwab (1939). Patients were asked to respond to a visual stimulus (150-watt lamp) by squeezing a rubber ball that was connected to a marker on the EEG. Schwab noticed individual differences. Some patients had a normal or even shorter reaction time during the generalized discharge. Others did not respond at all, and in yet others, the reaction time was twice or three times as long as normal. Since then, many authors have reported cognitive impairment during epileptiform discharges using simple motor reaction tasks, such as tapping or writing on the EEG record itself, and more complex tasks, such as forwards or backwards subtraction, simple or choice-reaction-time-tests, and short-term memory tests. (For a review see Aarts *et al.* (1984).) Most tests were performed during evoked epileptiform discharges using hyperventilation or photic stimulation as provocative methods.

To summarize, the likelihood of demonstrating cognitive impairment by generalized spike-wave discharges depends on the complexity of the task: choice reaction-time tests and short-term memory tests are more sensitive than simple motor tasks. Although cognitive impairment can be demonstrated during discharges of half a second duration, the likelihood of impairment increases greatly if the discharges last more than 3 seconds.

Various authors have tried to determine maximal impairment related to time of occurrence of discharges during the trials: Grisell *et al.* (1964) and Goode *et al.* (1970) found maximal impairment when the discharges occurred in the middle of the stimulus. Tizard and Margerison (1963) and Browne *et al.* (1974) demonstrated maximal impairment shortly before or at the beginning of the stimulus, and Mirsky and Van Buren (1965), from 5 seconds before until 5 seconds after. Interaction between performance of the task and occurrence of epileptiform discharges had already been described by Schwab (1939).

In general, cognitive activity reduces the frequency and duration of spontaneous epileptiform discharges (Guey *et al.*, 1956; Vidart and Geier, 1967). Hutt, Newton and Fairweather (1977) reported, futhermore, that the frequency of epileptiform discharges was lowest when patients performed psychologic tasks at their own levels of performance, when compared with tasks of greater or lesser difficulty. Apart from scientific purposes, the study of cognitive impairment during subclinical discharges is of practical importance. Such cognitive impairment may cause educational problems, or even danger (falling down stairs or hazardous behavior in traffic situations). Therefore, a routine test for detection of transitory cognitive impairment (TCI) fulfilling various criteria was developed by Aarts *et al.* (1984). In order not to suppress epileptiform activity and make assessment impossible, the test was made self-pacing: patients could perform at their own submaximal level. The test is continuous and is presented in the form of a video game, attractive enough to make performance possible over a sufficiently long period of time (at least half an hour) in order to 'catch' enough discharges. This self-pacing, microcomputer-generated short-term memory test is similar to Corsi's blocks test (Milner, 1971). Both a nonverbal (maximum seven coloured rectangles) and verbal version (maximum seven-letter words for common animals) were developed. The stimuli are presented randomly with changing colours and the presentations and responses are all automatically annotated on the EEG. Thus, after visual identification of the type and location of epileptiform discharges, temporal relationships between discharges and the phase of the trial could be made. The number of correct or incorrect answers per patient per session are compared with occurrence or absence of epileptiform discharges. Results are analyzed using the Fisher Exact Probability Test and patients who make significantly more errors during the discharge periods are considered to suffer from transitory cognitive impairment. This

Table 24.1 Waveform and distribution of EEG discharges as function of number of test sessions*

	Type of discharge							
	Generalized bilateral synchronized		Right-sided		Left-sided		Total	
	No.	%	No.	%	No.	%	No.	%
Isolated or irregular (poly) spike-waves	29		10		8		47	65
Spikes, sharp waves	7		2		—		9	13
Sharp delta/theta waves	11		2		3		16	22
Total	47	65	14	20	11	15	72	100

*72 pooled visual-spatial and verbal test sessions.

design, in which the patient serves as his or her own control, eliminates possible confounding influences of different types of epilepsy or medication. Evaluation of 91 patients of various ages by Binnie *et al.* (1987), showed that cognitive impairment occurred in approximately half the patients during subclinical generalized and also isolated focal EEG discharges. Right-sided discharges were associated with impaired performance in the spatial memory task, whilst left-sided discharges were associated with errors in the verbal tasks. Further research using the modified Corsi blocks test was done to determine the temporal relationship of the discharges to the various phases of the trial (stimulus presentation, stimulus-response interval, response and intertrial interval). The increase in error rate appeared to be most marked if the epileptiform activity was present during the stimulus. Secondly most disruptive, was the occurrence of epileptiform activity within 2 seconds before the stimulus, and in the period between stimulus and response. The least increase in error rate was found when epileptiform activity occurred during the response phase.

The use of this microcomputer-generated short-term memory task for routine clinical testing of children with epilepsy has been evaluated. A total of 70 children (34 boys, 36 girls) at a mean age of 11 years (range 6–15 years) was tested in 101 sessions. They were

Table 24.2 Test sessions showing significant ($P<0.05$) transient cognitive impairment (numerator) versus total of test sessions evaluated (denominator) as function of test tasks

Type of discharge	Visual-spatial (n=69)		Verbal (n=61)		Either or both (n=72)	
	No.	%	No.	%	No.	%
Generalized	10/46	22	8/37	22	15*/47	32
Right-sided	7/13	54	0/13		7/14	50
Left-sided	1/10	10	4/11	36	4/11	36
All types	18/69	26	12/61	20	26/72	36

*One patient was left-handed.

selected from those referred for routine EEGs who were found to have frequent subclinical epileptiform discharges in the 'waking-eyes-open' state. At least one discharge every 5 minutes, and at most a discharge every 5 seconds, was necessary to compare periods of discharges with periods without discharges, in the same patient. Of the total number of children, nine were unable to perform the verbal task. Consequently, the results of 69 visual spatial tests and 61 verbal tests could be evaluated for 53 children. These are shown in Tables 24.1 and 24.2.

Thirty-six per cent of the children showed transitory cognitive impairment in either or both tasks, corresponding to 47% of all children tested. Right-sided discharges impaired performance in 50% of test sessions and had a more profound influence on the visual spatial task. Left-sided discharges appeared to exert greater influence on the verbal task. Thus, short-lasting and even isolated subclinical epileptiform discharges, generalized or focal, can influence cognitive functioning in children.

The consequences of these transitory cognitive impairments for academic achievement in children were unknown. Therefore, further studies were performed to determine the face validity of the test. Twenty children with subclinical epileptiform discharges were asked to perform reading, arithmetic and writing tests with continuous EEG and video monitoring (Kasteleijn-Nolst Trenité *et al.*, 1988). The following hypotheses were tested:

1. Do children with frequent subclinical discharges show poorer performance than children with infrequent epileptiform discharges?
2. Does the type of cognitive activity (domain) and its degree of difficulty (level) affect the incidence of epileptiform discharges?
3. Is reading performance impaired during the discharges and what is the relation between the duration of the discharge and reading performance?

Four domains of activity were studied: reading, mental arithmetic, a motor dexterity task, and rest. After determination of the current levels of attainment of reading and arithmetic, the reading and arithmetic tasks were presented at three levels of difficulty corresponding to the child's current level. Each of these activities lasted for 10 minutes. Both reading and arithmetic were performed out loud to permit continuous monitoring; the reading and writing task, as well as the arithmetic tasks, were sampled from primary school books. The EEG record was scored for nature, time-of-onset, and duration of every single epileptiform discharge, and subsequently a copy of the test material was annotated with information concerning time, duration and period of discharge, as well as

information concerning performance (videotape). Reading errors comprised repetitions, corrections, hesitations, omissions, additions, and words read wrongly. Reading and arithmetic quotients were established on the basis of the child's current attainments as measured with the Brus 2 min Reading and Maths Tests (school level tests), i.e. the current level minus expected level divided by the expected level. A positive quotient means better achievement than expected according to age and education. Both the mean reading and arithmetic quotients were respectively 0.7 and 0.73 compared to 1.0 in normal control populations. High discharge rates were associated with low scholastic performance, particularly arithmetic, but the differences were not significant.

Surprisingly, the discharge rate was found to be lower at rest than during the three task domains. The highest discharge rate for both reading and arithmetic was at the children's own level. In addressing effects of individual discharges on performance, only measures of reading performance could be employed. Reading efficiency was significantly reduced during discharges, in comparison with nondischarge periods in the same child. More reading errors were also made when the discharge length was longer than 3 seconds. The reading impairment was also detected in the predischarge period, although less marked than during the discharges. The results are thus in accordance with those obtained with the short-term memory test of Corsi.

In order to investigate, in addition, the relationship between lateralization of the subclinical epileptiform discharges and the scholastic tasks, the children were placed in three groups according to the results obtained in the simultaneous EEG recording. Group I had generalized or multifocal epileptiform discharges involving both hemispheres (five girls, four boys). Group II had localized or clearly lateralized right-sided epileptiform discharges, with or without secondary, bilateral synchrony (four girls, four boys), and group III had localized or clearly lateralized left-sided discharges without secondary bilateral synchrony (three girls, one boy). The children from the left-sided discharge group performed significantly less well on reading tasks than children with right-sided discharges, i.e. the left-sided discharge group performed at a level of about 2 years below expected school level, and children with right-sided discharges at a level of 1 year below expected school level. These differences between the groups were not found in arithmetic quotients: all three groups performed on levels about 1 year below the school level. These findings agree with those of Stores and Hart (1976), but not with those of Camfield *et al.* (1984). However, neither of these former studies correlate simultaneous EEG discharges with test performance.

Similar studies were performed correlating subtests scores of the RAKIT with subclinical EEG discharges. Twenty-one children were investigated (13 boys and eight girls), with an average age of 9 years and 3 months. Fifteen children exhibited subclinical EEG discharges while six had no or only two or three discharges during the whole testing period. The discharge group showed a significantly abnormal test profile, due chiefly to poor performance on a subtest concerned with short-term verbal memory. Item performance of all subtests was impaired during epileptiform discharges, with the exception of the subtest that involved recall of material learnt previously (long-term memory). Thus, examiners of cognitive tests should indeed be aware of the negative effect of discharges on performance. The high test – retest variability found in many studies can (partly) be due to the effect of the discharges occurring during testing itself, or even during the explanation phase.

However, the ultimate evidence that transitory cognitive impairment is due to subclinical EEG discharges is improvement of performance after suppression of the EEG discharges. Aarts *et al.* (1984) demonstrated this in an individual case. A 13-year-old boy complained of difficulty with his schoolwork. In his EEG repeated runs of generalized sharp waves or irregular spike-wave activity were seen and transitory cognitive impairment was demonstrated using the Corsi test. Due to repeated errors he never advanced beyond a series length of two blocks or two words. After intravenous injection of diazepam, epileptiform activity was completely suppressed. After 15 minutes, performance testing was repeated and he gave correct answers to a series of three blocks. An hour later, while his epileptiform activity was still absent but he felt less drowsy, he managed to respond correctly to a series of four blocks.

In 1989, having demonstrated that children are impaired in their schoolwork by EEG discharges, we started a double-blind controlled trial in children with subclinical EEG discharges with well-controlled or no clinical seizures, to investigate the effects on school performance of treatment with valproic acid monotherapy or as add-on therapy. Following a period of 6 weeks on placebo the patients were randomized into a 6-week period of valproic acid (VPA), followed by 6 weeks on placebo, or vice versa. At the start and at the end of each period the patients were assessed with a battery of tests, including scholastic achievements tests, under continuous EEG and video monitoring. A standard dosage of 600 mg valproic acid was chosen in order to maintain 'blindness'. In four of the six children, the suppression of the clinical EEG discharges was complete or nearly complete. Changes were seen in all but one patient. Cognitive performance increased significantly in two of the four patients who had a good suppression of EEG discharges. The other two had either no change in, or even lowering of, school performance, but they suffered from VPA-induced behavior disturbance, thus influencing the performance negatively. In summary, about half of the children who were treated with VPA with subsequent suppression of clinical EEG discharges, showed an increase in cognitive performance, indicating also that not all children with subclinical EEG discharges will benefit from drug therapy.

The same type of study was performed by Marston *et al.* (1993) in 12 children. With the exception of two patients, all were treated with relatively high dosages of VPA (1000–2000 mg) as add-on therapy. Two children were already on VPA and were treated in the double-blind phase with 20 mg clobazam. Two patients dropped out because of behavioral side-effects (one on clobazam and one on valproic acid); eight of the 10 children showed an improvement in performance on the Neale reading test, digit-span, and Bender time. However, only one child was seizure free throughout the trial; the others showed a clear reduction in seizure rate due to additional treatment with VPA. Therefore, the results obtained could be ascribed to lowering of seizure frequency itself.

The percentages of normal children or those with epilepsy who have subclinical epileptiform discharges while awake are not known. Petersén and Eeg-Olofsson (1971) found that about 10% of children with a history of seizures show epileptiform activity in their EEG. However, EEG data are normally obtained via routine EEG recordings, i.e. lying on a bed with the eyes closed for about 15 minutes. No data are available on the frequency of epileptiform discharges during the daytime, comparing, for example, periods of rest, learning and exercise. The impact of having EEG discharges during the night is another unknown factor. There are reports of children who exclusively have continuous spikes and slow waves during sleep and have learning problems (see Chapter 13d). Individual differences are found throughout. In summary, there are many questions which still have to be answered. However, it is important to realize that, in individual cases, suppression of epileptiform discharges

can be beneficial. In the evaluation of the effect of treatment, it is necesary to standardize EEG and cognitive performance measures, before and after treatment. Otherwise, parents, teachers and physicians will not know whether or not suppression of the EEG discharges is beneficial. A complicating factor is the effect of the antiepileptic drugs on cognition itself.

ANTIEPILEPTIC DRUGS

Antiepileptic drugs prevent a child from having further seizures, without curing the underlying cause. After a first unprovoked seizure, further seizures occurred in 52% of untreated children (Camfield *et al.*, 1985). Currently no consensus exists as to whether children should be treated immediately after the first seizure, in order to prevent epilepsy becoming more active (Reynolds, Elwes and Shorvon, 1983), or whether it is better to wait until the second seizure so that children are not treated unnecessarily. Should antiepileptic drugs only have very minor side-effects, this dilemma would not arise. However, antiepileptic drugs are psychoactive and can affect cognition.

After the introduction of phenobarbitone in the 1920s and, again, after the introduction of phenytoin in the 1930s, these drugs were thought to make the patients less drowsy in comparison with respectively, bromide and phenobarbitone. Although the effects are less severe than with bromide, phenobarbitone and phenytoin are considered to impair cognitive function (Trimble, 1987).

Up to the 1970s children with epilepsy were generally treated with standard dosages of phenobarbitone, phenytoin or a combination of these. The fear of subsequent seizures prevailed over the well-being of the child. Therefore, many children were treated with high dosages of antiepileptic drugs leading to sleepiness and drowsiness with consequent psychomotor impairment. The impact on cognition was even greater, since epilepsy was considered a life-long disorder that required continuous medication, whether or not further seizures occurred. Moreover, treatment often started in the early years of life when the nervous system is still developing. With the later introduction of nonsedative antiepileptic drugs, such as VPA and carbamazepine, and the individualization of treatment, therapy changed accordingly (Hekster *et al.*, 1993). This individualization of treatment was enhanced by the introduction of routine determinations of antiepileptic drug-blood levels and the development of so-called therapeutic ranges (Meijer, 1991; Kasteleijn-Nolst Trenité, 1993). One of the major advantages of the newer drugs, VPA and carbamazepine, appeared to be that the children became more active. Carbamazepine even was supposed to have psychotropic effects (Trimble and Thompson, 1983). Since then, many studies in adults have been performed to investigate cognitive changes associated with the various antiepileptic drugs (Sommerbeck *et al.*, 1977; Dodrill, 1975; Thompson and Trimble, 1982, 1983; Andrewes *et al.*, 1986; Smith, 1987). In order to systematically assess the cognitive side-effects of the antiepileptic drugs phenytoin, carbamazepine, sodium valproate, and clobazam, Trimble and Thompson (1983) performed double-blind placebo controlled studies in healthy volunteers. The latter group took the drugs for a period of 2 weeks and functions such as tension, short-term memory speed, and decision-making were measured. Even within the therapeutic ranges, all drugs showed a negative influence on performance. Phenytoin had a negative effect on all tests, while the other drugs did not impair memory function. However, only short-term effects of the drugs could be investigated in healthy volunteers. Other studies have mainly involved adult patients. Combination of the results led to the general agreement that toxic dosages of antiepileptic drugs, as well as, and especially, polytherapy, can impair concentration, motor-speed and memory function. Moreover, phenytoin and phenobarbitone especially, can negatively influence cognition more than carbamazepine and valproate. A complicating factor, however, is that therapy-resistant children with severe epilepsy will, in particular, be treated both with polytherapy (including phenobarbitone and phenytoin) and high dosages of drugs.

In a matched control study in 622 newly diagnosed patients of 18 years and older, comparison of the influence of four antiepileptic drugs (carbamazepine, phenytoin, phenobarbitone or primidone) was carried out with regard to behavioral and cognitive effects. Smith (1987) found that interrelations existed between age, education, and IQ. If the data were controlled for these factors, no dramatic differences were found in performance between the four drug groups. The carbamazepine group showed significantly fewer cognitive effects than the others. If age, education, and IQ seem to be important confounding factors in adult studies, these certainly must be of great importance in studies in children (Smith, 1987). Ideally the effects of drugs should be investigated in children who serve as their own controls. Vining *et al.* (1987), therefore, investigated 21 children of normal intelligence and with relatively mild seizure disorders in a double-blind cross-over study to measure the effects of phenobarbitone and VPA on cognitive functioning. The children had different types of seizures (tonic-clonic seizures or partial complex seizures); the EEGs prior to the study entry were either normal in five patients, slightly abnormal in nine, or markedly abnormal in seven of the cases. Ten boys and 11 girls underwent a complete neuropsychologic battery including the WISC-R before entry into the trial: the mean full-scale IQ was 94.0 (standard deviation 14.4). The majority of the children were already receiving medication prior to the study, either phenobarbitone, phenytoin, primidone, or carbamazepine. Although the study consisted of two, 6-month double-blind periods, patients were assessed every month to achieve either seizure reduction or blood levels within the therapeutic range. Both continuous performance reaction tests, as measures of vigilance and concentration, as well as complete neuropsychologic testing, were repeatedly carried out. The children served as their own controls. There was statistical difference between the VPA and phenobarbitone periods in control of seizures, but children receiving phenobarbitone performed less well ($P < 0.01$) on four tests of neuropsychologic functioning, i.e. block-design (timed constructional praxis), performance IQ, full-scale IQ, and Berkeley paired-association learning tasks (attention and short-term learning). Thus, VPA produced significantly less cognitive impairment in children when compared with phenobarbitone. This study proved that different drugs can have different effects on higher cortical functions, even at lower or average dosages. Recently, a number of studies have been performed using the discontinuation of antiepileptic drugs in children, usually when they have been seizure free for at least 2 years. Aldenkamp *et al.* (1993) reported the Multicenter Holmfrid Study in which 100 children between 7 and 18 years with various forms of epilepsy were tested with a computerized test battery during and after treatment with monotherapy, carbamazepine, VPA, or phenytoin. The majority of children received carbamazepine prior to withdrawal. Reassessment was performed 6 months after the start of the 3-month withdrawal period. Children matched for age, sex and school level were used as controls. Many tests showed an improvement for the patients with epilepsy after withdrawal. However, these changes were not significantly different from those observed in their matched controls. Thus, improvement could be attributed to both retest effects, in combination with maturation, and was not exclusively a function of drug withdrawal. Only one test was

performed significantly better in the epilepsy group after drug withdrawal than in matched controls: finger-tapping for the dominant hand, i.e. psychomotor speed. Furthermore, patients who took phenytoin had a different cognitive profile when compared with children on carbamazepine. However, these differences continued after withdrawal of the drug. It seems unlikely that a drug effect can last for more than 3 months, and a possible explanation is therapy bias, i.e. children with more severe seizures are predominantly treated with phenytoin, whilst those with mild seizures received carbamazepine.

Aman *et al.* (1987) investigated 46 children with well-controlled seizures receiving sodium valproate monotherapy. Cognitive and motor tests were administered in three sessions, usually at weekly intervals. During the last two sessions, the morning medication was administered either about two and a half hours before testing, or was delayed until after testing. Half of the subjects were randomly assigned to receive delayed medication first, and the others delayed medication second. The subjects were thus tested both at trough levels and at peak levels. Data were analysed for effect of the type of epilepsy (partial versus generalized epilepsy), high or low dose, i.e. below 20 mg per kg per day, and time of medication (peak and trough levels). The children with generalized epilepsy and those with the lower doses performed best. In contrast with results found in the same type of study comparing patients with phenytoin and carbamazepine monotherapy (Aman, Paxon and Werry, 1983), no effect was found in relation to time of medication. During high concentrations of both phenytoin and carbamazepine, psychomotor deterioration was observed. However, both the pharmacokinetics and the dynamics of VPA and phenytoin and carbamazepine are different, which may explain these differences in results. Differences in the effect of the most commonly used antiepileptic drugs were confirmed in patients on monotherapy within the therapeutic ranges, using EEG spectral analysis (Drake *et al.*, 1990). Sixty-three age-matched patients with generalized tonic-clonic seizures and no neurologic abnormalities were investigated. Pheno-barbitone (at normal range and toxic levels) and to a lesser extent phenytoin (only at high levels) slowed the EEG. Carbamazepine did not give this effect, while valproate mainly had a suppressive effect on the alpha rhythm. An effect on the EEG of the introduction of valproate in children was found by Benniger, Mattis and Scheffner (1985). Although benzodiazepines such as diazepam, clonazepam and more recently clobazam are frequently used in antiepileptic treatment in children, little research has been done on the cognitive effects of these drugs. The benzodiazepines have been thoroughly invest-igated in animal models, healthy volunteers (e.g. in driving tests) (Mortimer and Howat, 1986), and psychiatric patients, but not in patients with epilepsy. Benzodiazepines can cause sedation with resultant impairment of various cognitive functions, especially shortly after introduction of the drug.

In clinical practice this sedating effect of benzodiazepines is well known, and epi-leptologists prefer using these drugs only for IV or rectal use in status epilepticus. In patients with severe therapy-resistant epi-lepsy their use, however, is sometimes unavoidable.

A number of new antiepileptic drugs such as vigabatrin, lamotrigine and gabapentin are now available in many countries. In the phase II and III controlled studies with these drugs, no important cognitive side-effects were reported, though vigabatrin has been associated with psychosis in adults. A study has been undertaken to determine the effect of vigabatrin on cognitive functions and mood (McGuire, Duncan and Trimble, 1992). Thirty adults with intractable epilepsy were compared with 15 controls matched for age, sex and IQ; assessments took place before the start of vigabatrin as add-on medication and 4 weeks later when the patients were on 2 g/day. No negative effect of vigabatrin was found using a diversity of neuropsychologic tests, including mood. Some positive effects were even seen, e.g. on reaction time, atten-tion and visuospatial ability.

The effect on cognitive function will become an issue in future searches for and competition between new antiepileptic drugs. Rating scales as tools for quantitative assess-ment of adverse drug events, in combination with neuropsychologic tests, will help to discriminate these differences (Mattson and Cramer, 1993)

SUMMARY

It is recognized by many clinicians and scientists that children with epilepsy have a higher risk of deficits in cognitive function-ing. However, many different factors contrib-ute to cognitive impairment and most of these are interrelated. Epilepsy is a sign or symptom and cannot be considered a disease entity. This explains why the various avail-able studies are difficult to compare. At one end of the scale, children with severe brain damage and neurologic dysfunction, includ-ing epileptic seizures, are found; at the other end, normal intelligent children, without any detectable brain dysfunction besides epileptic seizures, are seen.

Underlying brain 'damage' will have a continuous negative influence on cognitive functioning. Epileptic seizures and sub-clinical EEG discharges influence cognitive functioning intermittently. After a seizure the child can catch up with his/her previous level of functioning. However, if the number, in combination with the degree of severity, of seizures, and/or number of subclinical EEG discharges is high, the influence can be considered very substantial. Etiology and severity of epileptic seizures and EEG dis-charges are normally related to each other. Antiepileptic drug treatment generally de-creases the number of seizures and subclinical EEG discharges and thus exhibits a positive influence on cognitive functioning. However, the antiepileptic drugs, being psychoactive in nature, have a suppressive effect on cognitive function itself. The negative effect of antiepileptic drugs is basically continuous in nature, although fluctuations in drug levels during the day can also give differences in impairment. Currently, it is not known how pharmacodynamic effects are related to pharmacokinetics of the various antiepileptic drugs. The effects on cognitive functioning of interactions between the various antiepileptic drugs are even less well known. In addition, there are relationships between etiology of epilepsy, severity of epilepsy, choice of antiepileptic drug, dosage and number of drugs prescribed. Finally, psychosocial factors also have their impacts on cognitive functioning, and will be dependent on severity of seizures; although children who have to compete with normal children at school can be relatively more handicapped by having epilepsy than those living in an institution for the handicapped.

These factors explain why the literature on cognitive aspects of children with epilepsy is often contradictory and confusing. Ideally, studies should be performed in homogeneous groups. Another possibility is to use a design in which the children are their own controls; differences in etiology, seizure type, and medication are then no longer important variables. Furthermore, children should be investigated in association with continuous EEG and video monitoring, in order to discriminate between continuous disturbing factors such as underlying brain function disorders and medication and transitory cognitive impairment due to epileptiform discharges or seizures.

In clinical assessment, it is of utmost importance to carry out psychologic investigations when the children are medically stable, i.e. no changes in seizure frequency or type and not during drug withdrawal or shortly after changes in dosage or type of drug. The neuropsychologist, too, should be aware of the type of epilepsy, the frequency and severity of seizures, including the last occurring seizure, as well as the type of medication. All these factors should be taken into account for evaluation of the results. The tests should be able to measure global function disorders, such as attention and psychomotor speed, as well as more specific areas, namely long-term and short-term memory. Academic achievement tests (reading and arithmetic) must be part of the tests employed. Eventually, a combination of historic data on the child, including seizure and medication history, will give a complete picture of intellectual ability and functioning. It must always be remembered that not all children with epilepsy have impairment in cognitive functions, and not all problems arising at school can be assigned to epilepsy or medication.

ACKNOWLEDGMENTS

The research on subclinical EEG discharges was supported by a grant from the CLEO (Commissie Landelijk Epilepsie Onderzoek). I would like to thank B.M. Siebelink for his critical comments and A. Tierlier-Long for her help in preparing the text.

REFERENCES

Aarts, J.H.P., Binnie, C.D., Smit, A.M. and Wilkins, A.J. (1984) Selective cognitive impairment during focal and generalized epileptiform EEG activity. *Brain*, **107**, 293–308.

Aldenkamp, A.P., Alpherts, W.C.J., Dekker, M.J.A. and Overweg, J. (1990) Neuropsychological aspects of learning disabilities in epilepsy. *Epilepsia*, **31**(suppl.4), S9–20.

Aldenkamp, A.P., Alpherts, W.C.J., Blennow, G. *et al.* (1993) Withdrawal of antiepileptic medication in children – effect on cognitive function: the multicenter Holmfrid study. *Neurology*, **43**, 41–50.

Alpherts, W.C.J. and Aldenkamp, A.P. (1990) Computerized neuropsychological assessment in children with epilepsy, in Epilepsy and

Education; Cognitive Factors in Learning Behavior (eds A.P. Aldenkamp and W.E. Dodson). *Epilepsia* (suppl.4), S35–40.

Aman, M.G. (1991) Applications of computerized cognitive-motor measures to the assessment of psychoactive drugs, in *The Assessment of Cognitive Function in Epilepsy* (eds W.E. Dodson, M. Kinsbourne and B. Hiltbrunner), Demos Publications, New York, pp. 69–96.

Aman, M.G., Paxon, J.W. and Werry, J.S. (1983) Fluctuations in steady-state phenytoin concentrations as measured in saliva in children. *Pediatric Pharmacology*, **3**, 87–94.

Aman, M.G., Werry, J.S., Paxton, J.W. and Turbott, J.W. (1987) Effect of sodium valproate on psychomotor performance in children as a function of dose, fluctuations in concentration and diagnosis. *Epilepsia*, **28**, 115–24.

Andrewes, D.G., Bullen, J.G., Tomlinson, L. *et al.* (1986) A comparative study of the cognitive effects of phenytoin and carbamazepine in new referrals with epilepsy. *Epilepsia*, **27**, 128–34.

Bakker, D.J. and Vinke, J. (1985) Effects of hemispheric-specific stimulation on brain activity and reading in dyslectics. *Clinical and Experimental Neuropsychology*, **7**, 505–25.

Baird, H.W., John, E.R., Ahn, H. and Maisel, E. (1980) Neurometric evaluation of epileptic children who do well and poorly in school. *Electroencephalography and Clinical Neurophysiology*, **48**, 683–93.

Benninger, C., Mattis, P. and Scheffner, D. (1985) Spectral analysis of the EEG in children during the introduction of anti-epileptic therapy with valproic acid. *Neuropsychobiology*, **13**, 93–6.

Berger, H. (1933) Ueber das Elektrenkephalogramm des Menschen: siebente Mitteilung. *Archive für Psychiatrie und Nervenkranckheiten*, **100**, 301–20.

Binnie, C.D., Kasteleijn-Nolst Trenité, D.G.A., Smit, A.M. and Wilkins, A.J. (1987) Interactions of epileptiform EEG discharges and cognition. *Epilepsy Research*, **1**, 239–45.

Bourgeois, B.F.D., Prensky, A.L., Palkes, H.S. *et al.* (1983) Intelligence in epilepsy: a prospective study in children. *Annals of Neurology*, **14**, 438–44.

Browne, T.R., Penry, J.K., Porter, R.J. and Dreifuss, F.E. (1974) Responsiveness before, during and after spike-wave paroxysms. *Neurology (Minneapolis)*, **24**, 659–65.

Bruhn, P. (1970) Disturbances of vigilance in subcortical epilepsy. *Acta Neurologica Scandinavica*, **46**, 442–54.

Camfield, P.R., Gates, R., Ronen, G. *et al.* (1984) Comparison of cognitive ability, personality profile and school success in epileptic children with pure right versus left temporal lobe EEG foci. *Annals of Neurology*, **15**, 122–6.

Camfield, P.R., Camfield, C.S., Dooley, J.M. *et al.* (1985) Epilepsy after a first unprovoked seizure in childhood. *Neurology*, **35**, 1657–60.

Clement, M.J. and Wallace, S.J. (1990) A survey of adolescents with epilepsy. *Developmental Medicine and Child Neurology*, **32**, 849–57.

Cohen, M.J., Branch, W.B., Grant Willis, W. *et al.* (1992) Childhood, in *Handbook of Neuropsychological Assessment: A Biopsychosocial Perspective*, (eds A.E. Puente and R.J. McCaffrey), Plenum, New York, pp. 49–79.

Dodrill, C.B. (1975) Diphenylhydantoin serum levels, toxicity and neuropsychological performance in patients with epilepsy. *Epilepsia*, **16**, 593–600.

Drake, M.E. Jr, Huber, S.J., Pakalnis, A. and Denio, L. (1990) Electroencephalographic effects of antiepileptic drug therapy. *Journal of Epilepsy*, **3**, 75–9.

Ellenberg, J.H., Hirtz, D.G. and Nelson, K.B. (1986) Do seizures in children cause intellectual deterioration? *New England Journal of Medicine*, **314**, 1085–8.

Farwell, J.R., Dodrill, C.B. and Batzel, L.W. (1985) Neuropsychological abilities of children with epilepsy. *Epilepsia*, **26**, 395–400.

Fedio, P. and Mirsky, A.F. (1969) Selective intellectual deficits in children with temporal lobe or centrencephalic epilepsy. *Neuropsychologia*, **7**, 287–300.

Gibbs, F.A., Lennox, W.G. and Gibbs, E.L. (1936) The electroencephalogram in diagnosis and in localization of epileptic seizures. *Archives of Neurology and Psychiatry*, **36**, 1225–35.

Giordani, B., Berent, S., Sackellares, J.C. *et al.* Intelligence test performance of patients with partial and generalized seizures. *Epilepsia*, **26**, 37–42.

Goode, D.J., Penry, J.K. and Dreifuss, F.E. (1970) Effects of paroxysmal spike wave and continuous visual-motor performance. *Epilepsia*, **11**, 241–54.

Gowers, W.R. (1885) *Epilepsy and Other Chronic Convulsive Diseases: Their Causes, Symptoms and Treatment*. Reprint of the work first published by William Wood, New York, American Academy of Neurology, reprint series, vol.1.

Grisell, J.L., Levin, S.M., Cohen, B.D. and Rodin, E.A. (1964) Effects of subclinical seizure activity on overt behavior. *Neurology*, **14**, 133–5.

Guey, J., Tassinari, C.A., Charles, C. and Coquery, C. (1956) Variations du niveau déficience en relation avec des décharges épileptiques paroxystiques. *Revue Neurologique*, **112**, 311–7.

Hauser, W.A. (1978) Epidemiology of epilepsy, *Advances in Neurology*, vol.19 (ed. B. C. Schoenberg), Raven, New York, pp.313–39.

Hekster, Y.A., Wijsman, D.J.P., Wuis, E.W. *et al.* (1993) Individualization of antiepileptic drug therapy, in *Quantitative Assessment in Epilepsy Care* (eds H. Meinardi, J.A. Cramer, G.A. Baker and A. Martins da Silva), Plenum, New York, pp. 109–16

Holdsworth, L. and Whitmore, K. (1974) A study of children with epilepsy attending ordinary schools. I: Their seizure patterns, progress and behaviour in school. *Developmental Medicine and Child Neurology*, **16**, 746–58.

Hutt, S.J., Newton, S. and Fairweather, H. (1977) Choice reaction time and EEG activity in children with epilepsy. *Neuropsychologia*, **15**, 257–67.

Jennekens-Schinkel, A., Linschooten-Duikersloot, E.M.E.M., Bouma, P.A.D., *et al.* (1987) Spelling errors made by children with mild epilepsy: writing-to-dictation. *Epilepsia*, **28**, 555–63.

Johnson, T. (1991) Statistical issues in the computerized assessment of cognitive function, in *The Assessment of Cognitive Function in Epilepsy*, (eds W.E. Dodson, M. Kinsbourne and B. Hiltbrunner), Demos Publications, New York, pp. 137–53

Kasteleijn-Nolst Trenité, D.G.A. (1993) Drug choice and replacement, in *Quantitative Assessment in Epilepsy Care* (eds H. Meinardi, J.A. Cramer, G.A. Baker and A. Martins da Silva), Plenum, New York, pp. 103–7.

Kasteleijn-Nolst Trenité, D.G.A., Bakker, D.J., Binnie, C.D. *et al.* (1988) Psychological effects of subclinical epileptiform EEG discharges. I. Scholastic skills. *Epilepsy Research*, **2**, 111–6.

Kasteleijn-Nolst Trenité, D.G.A., Smit, A.M., Velis, D.N. *et al.* (1990) On-line detection of transient neuropsychological disturbances during EEG discharges in children with epilepsy. *Developmental Medicine and Child Neurology*, **32**, 46–50.

Làvadas, E., Umilta, C. and Provinciali, L. (1979) Hemisphere-dependent cognitive performances in epileptic patients. *Epilepsia*, **20**, 493–502.

Ledeboer, B.Ch. (1941) Over epilepsieën by kinderen; een klinische studie van het epilepsievraagstuk. Thesis.

Lennox, W.G. and Collins, A.L. (1945) Intelligence of normal and epileptic twins. *American Journal of Psychiatry*, **99**, 174–80.

Levin, H.S. and Spiers, P.A. (1985) Acalculia, in *Clinical Neuropsychology* (eds K.M. Heilman and E. Valenstein), Oxford University Press, New York, pp. 97–115.

Long, C.G. and Moore, J.R. (1979) Parental expectations for their epileptic children. *Journal of Child Psychology and Psychiatry*, **20**, 313–24

Luria, A.R. (1973) *The working brain*, New York, Basic Books.

Marston, D., Besag, F., Binnie, C.D. and Fowler, M. (1993) Effects of transitory cognitive impairment on psychosocial functioning of children with epilepsy: a therapeutic trial. *Developmental Medicine and Child Neurology*, **35**, 574–81.

Mattson, R.H. and Cramer, J.A. (1993) Quantitative assessment of adverse drug effects, in *Quantitative Assessment in Epilepsy Care* (eds H. Meinardi, J.A. Cramer, G.A. Baker and A. Martins da Silva), Plenum, New York, pp. 123–35.

McGuire, A.M., Duncan, J.S. and Trimble, M.R. (1992) Effects of vigabatrin on cognitive function and mood when used as add-on therapy in patients with intractable epilepsy. *Epilepsia*, **33**, 128–34.

Meijer, J.W.A. (1991) Knowledge, attitude and practice in antiepileptic drug monitoring. *Acta Neurologica Scandinavica*, **83**, 134.

Milner, B. (1971) Interhemispheric differences in the localization of psychological processes in man. *British Medical Bulletin*, **27**, 272–7.

Mirsky, A.F. and Van Buren, J.M. (1965) On the nature of the 'absence' in centrencephalic epilepsy: a study of some behavioural, electroencephalographic and autonomic factors. *Electroencephalography and Clinical Neurophysiology*, **18**, 334–48.

Mortimer, R.G. and Howat, P.A. (1986) Effects of alcohol and diazepam, singly and in combination, on some aspects of driving performance, in *Drugs and Driving* (eds J.F. O'Hanlon and J.J. de Gier), Taylor & Francis, London, pp. 163–78.

Petersén, I. and Eeg-Olofsson, O. (1971) The development of the electroencephalogram in normal children from the age of 1 through 15 years. Non-paroxysmal activity. *Neuropädiatrie*, **2**, 247–304.

Reynolds, E.H., Elwes, R.D. and Shorvon, S.D. (1983) Why does epilepsy become intractable? Prevention of chronic epilepsy. *Lancet*, **ii**, 952–4.

Rodin, E.A., Schmaltz, S. and Twitty, G. (1986) Intellectual functions of patients with childhood epilepsy. *Developmental Medicine and Child Neurology*, **28**, 25–33.

Rutter, M., Graham, P. and Yule, W. (1970) *A Neuropsychiatric Study in Childhood*, Lippincott, Philadelphia.

Schwab, R.S. (1939) A method of measuring consciousness in petit mal epilepsy. *Journal of Nervous and Mental Disease*, **89**, 690–1.

Seidenberg, M., Beck, N., Geisser, M. *et al.* (1986) Academic achievement of children with epilepsy. *Epilepsia*, **27**, 753–9.

Siebelink, B.M., Bakker, D.J., Binnie, C.D. and Kasteleijn-Nolst Trenité, D.G.A. (1988) Psychological effects of subclinical epileptiform EEG discharges in children. II. General intelligence tests. *Epilepsy Research*, **2**, 117–21.

Sommerbeck, K.W., Theilgaard, A., Rasmussen, K.E. *et al.* (1977) Valproate sodium: evaluation of so-called psychotropic effect. A controlled study. *Epilepsia*, **18**, 159–67.

Smith, D.B. (1987) Anticonvulsants, seizures and performance: the veteran's administration experience, in *Epilepsy, Behaviour and Cognitive Function* (eds M.R. Trimble and E.H. Reynolds), John Wiley, Chichester, pp. 67–78.

Stores, G. (1978) School children with epilepsy at risk of learning and behaviour problems. *Developmental Medicine and Child Neurology*, **20**, 502–8.

Stores, G. and Hart, J. (1976) Reading skills of children with generalized or focal epilepsy attending ordinary school. *Developmental Medicine and Child Neurology*, **18**, 705–15.

Strang, J. and Rourke, B.P. (1985) Adaptive behavior of children who exhibit specific arithmetic disabilities and associated neuropsychological abilities and deficits, in *Neuropsychology of Learning Disabilities. Essentials of Subtype Analysis* (ed. B.P. Rourke), Guildford, New York, pp. 302–31.

Sullivan, E.B. and Gahagan, L. (1935) On intelligence of epileptic children. *Genetic Psychology Monographs*, **17**, 309–75.

Tarter, R.E. (1972) Intellectual and adaptive functioning in children with epilepsy. *Diseases of the Nervous System*, **33**, 763–770.

Thompson, P.J. (1987) Educational attainment in children and young people with epilepsy, in *Epilepsy and Education* (eds J. Oxley and G. Stores), The Medical Tribune Group, London pp. 15–24.

Thompson, P.J. and Trimble, M.R. (1982) Anticonvulsant drugs and cognitive functions. *Epilepsia*, **33**, 531–4.

Thompson, P.J. and Trimble, M.R. (1983) Anticonvulsant serum levels: relationship to impairments of cognitive functions. *Journal of Neurology, Neurosurgery and Psychiatry*, **46**, 227–33.

Thompson, P., Huppert, F.A. and Trimble, M. (1981) Phenytoin and cognitive function: effects on normal volunteers and implications for epilepsy. *British Journal of Clinical Psychology*, **20**, 155–62.

Tizard, B. and Margerison, J.H. (1963) Psychological functions during wave-spike discharge. *British Journal of Social and Clinical Psychology*, **3**, 6–15.

Trimble, M.R. (1987) Anticonvulsant drugs: mood and cognitive function, in *Epilepsy, Behaviour and Cognitive Function* (eds M.R. Trimble and E.H. Reynolds), John Wiley, Chichester, pp. 135–43.

Trimble, M.R. and Thompson, P.J. (1983) Anticonvulsant drugs, cognitive function, and behavior. *Epilepsia*, **24**(suppl.1), S555–63.

Vidart, L. and Geier, S. (1967) Enregistrements télé-encephalographiques chez des sujets épileptiques pendant le travail. *Revue Neurologique*, **117**, 475–80.

Vining, E.P.G., Mellits, E.D., Dorsen, M.M. *et al.* (1987) Psychologic and behavioural effects of antiepileptic drugs in children: a double-blind comparison between phenobarbital and valproic acid. *Pediatrics*, **80**, 165–74.

Wallace, S.J. and Cull, A.M. (1979) Long-term psychological outlook for children whose first fit occurs with fever. *Developmental Medicine and Child Neurology*, **21**, 28–40.

Wechsler, D. (1944) *The Measurement of Adult Intelligence*, Williams & Wilkins, Baltimore.

David C. Taylor

I am not God's little lamb
I am God's sick tiger

Stevie Smith

INTRODUCTION

Caring for the sick always requires an element of psychologic concern. Because of the trivial or transient nature of the engagement, in many medical encounters that concern can be set aside at modest risk. Because most people are psychologically robust they will, mostly, even when seriously sick, tolerate our failure to meet all their needs. But in the seriously ill, chronically sick, brain-affected child the risk factors for psychologic distress and psychiatric illness are summed to a point where they cannot be overlooked. This was confirmed in Graham and Rutter's classic study (1968) which spelled out the increasing association between sickness and behavioral problems as cerebral dysfunction was more and more closely specified. Hippocrates had concluded: '. . . so long as the brain is still, a man is in his right mind' (Hippocrates, 1947). What stands in the way of the general acceptance of this, recently confirmed, 2000-year-old proposition?

The child in the epilepsy clinic has, by definition (well, almost by definition), epilepsy. He/she does not necessarily have any particular form of associated disorder. The relationships between epilepsy and associated psychologic problems are experienced either as sporadic clinical issues or come from reading research studies. These studies depended upon labels, categories, and samples of patients that may be dissimilar to our own experience.

Perhaps the psychiatry of epilepsy should be thought of as 'formal' or 'informal'. The informal, I argue, characterizes everyday clinical practice where live problems are seen to be highly idiosyncratic, contingent, personal and familial problems which do not seem to meet, or be contained within, the categories used by psychiatrists. The formal approach to psychiatry, as I see it, has developed from a need to codify its entities by previously agreed tight definitions so that researchers into etiology and outcome can share this information.

The severe and obvious, clear-cut, mental illnesses which would be easiest to codify, though increased in frequency, are still relatively rare and form only a small part of the psychiatric aspects of managing children with epilepsy. It matters little to the pediatrician if the child described to them as disturbingly overactive does not appear to meet the criteria of a consensus definition if it is the way in which a serious management problem manifests itself to the family.

Finally, both clinical experience and research studies also depend upon the constraints put upon the definitions used for the category 'epilepsy', for example the age range of the sample, the time since the last seizure. The same is true of the category 'psychiatric disorder'. These will profoundly affect the nature of the associations seen, or held to

Epilepsy in Children. Edited by Sheila Wallace. Published in 1996 by Chapman & Hall, London. ISBN 0 412 56860 8

exist, when these categories are brought into conjunction. Such sample characteristics underlie much of the discordance of views which are recorded in good reviews about the subject, such as that of Kim (1991).

In this chapter, following some discussion about the categorization of those people who present as 'sick', a largely informal approach will be taken to the psychiatric aspects of childhood epilepsy. First, they can be viewed simply as an example of the associations between psychiatric illness and any chronic sickness, though a particular set of associations is additionally seen with epilepsy. Then, issues such as the effect upon parents of the loss of a perfect child and the threats imposed upon parenting by a chronically sick child will be considered. Attention will be drawn to psychologic mechanisms coming into play in sufferers, parents, witnesses, and doctors and other carers.

DISEASE, ILLNESS, AND PREDICAMENT

I have argued for a tight definition of these terms (Taylor, 1979, 1982a). They can be used to distinguish disorder of structure (things: diseases) from function (processes: illness) from the specific background situation against which the issues are played out (predicament). Consider carefully what 'epilepsy' is. Several definitions will be given elsewhere in this book and yet others implied. I suggest that epilepsy is an increased propensity to exhibit certain behaviors at some future time as a consequence of unwanted neuronal discharges. Exhibiting them 'now' is called a seizure; having 'epilepsy' is thus an abstraction to do with the chances of doing it again, and again. If the attacks stop with treatment it is only the propensity which has been treated. If they do not stop it is hard to know what has been treated. Similarly, psychiatric illness is a disposition towards exhibiting a particular set of behaviors without a necessary presumption that they are manifest at any given moment. To say 'this little boy with

epilepsy is overactive' is a truth for only particular moments in time. On the other hand, to speak of his tuberous sclerosis, though it suggests many possible things about him, rashes, heart problems, learning difficulties, actually only implies certain tangible tissue changes. However, these persist in time even in the absence of any unwanted behaviors or seizures at any given time. So the disease diagnosis is a truth for all time but may be of no measurable consequence. A person presents as sick because their 'disease', or their 'illness', or an interaction between them, has come to affect their life by producing a change in their situation, the predicament in which they find themselves. For instance, a child may have lived comfortably with their epilepsy and the disease underlying it until the moment of a humiliating seizure in front of peers at school. The remedy for their distress could come:

1. From removing the diseased tissue.
2. Altering the propensity to the illness in other ways, through medicines.
3. Altering the vulnerable (depressed say) mental state of the child.
4. Changing the probability of experiencing humiliation by work on the group of peers.

These operations might be viewed as more or less real doctoring, more or less marginal, more or less in the moral domain ('now children be kind to Sandra'). Certain considerations that can be applied to the three components of sickness are outlined in Table 25.1. Doctors vary in their degree of preparation and their preferences and skills for work in their different worlds of sickness (Taylor, 1982b). Yet almost any sickness account can be shown to require a capacity to cope with each of them as it unfolds.

An attractive and intelligent adolescent of good and stable family has suffered classic complex partial seizures following some years after her infantile febrile status epilepticus. It is established that she has unequivocal right-sided mesial temporal sclerosis and surgical treatment has been proposed. But the girl declines operation and prefers to live within the limits created by her seizures. Exploring this apparently irrational [non-compliant] decision reveals a sibling who, it now emerges, has serious learning difficulties. Having knowledge of an even darker side of handicap, she seems to have accepted, or have a rational fear, that her plight could be worse.

Time and maturity might alter the balance of her decision. In the meantime her doctors can only keep faith with her by continuing their care, hoping to influence her beliefs which presently oppose what they see as the rational approach. Having had the experience of doubt will affect her views on the outcome of surgery even if she should change her mind.

HISTORY TAKING

In recognizing the need to diagnose the disease, the illness, and the predicament, the sort of history which needs to be taken in a difficult case of chronic epilepsy becomes clearer. The natural lead from patients or parents is to offer an account of the illness. This can sometimes be so robust as to 'stand for' the disease (pathognomonic), as in the example of mesial temporal sclerosis above. Or with guidance it will be seen to correspond with one of the epilepsy syndromes

Table 25.1 Considerations which may be applied to a sickness

Diseases	Illnesses	Predicaments
Discernible as physical reality Not necessarily organ specific	The declaration of the disease in its specific forms. More probably organ specific	The complex of psychosocial ramification with immediate bearing on the individual
Specific changes in structure or functional organization of tissue	Essentially a social manifestation, a limitation, a commentary, a role, a behavior pattern	Diffuse, multifactorial, personal but not necessarily unique
May be trivial	May change for better or worse without reclassifying 'the disease'. Capable of being recast as a role	Very unstable structure
Valid without 'illness'. Does not depend upon its implications	Valid without discoverable disease	Valid without disease or illness
Amoral	Probably judged 'morally'. Psychosocial processes modify	Highly charged with moral implication Dependent upon social mores
Diagnosis is discovery-specifying structural-functional change	Diagnosis is description and semantic reattribution	Diagnosis is discernment
Space, place, and time irrelevant	Space, place, and time relevant. Developmental process modifies. Significance contracts and expands	Space, place, and time paramount
Knowledge grows with investigation	Knowledge grows with classification	Knowledge grows with 'understanding'
Scope for specific therapy, scope for reconciliation	Scope for palliation, scope for personal change	Scope for social and political remedies

Reproduced with permission from Taylor (1982b).

expounded elsewhere in this book. The disease will be confirmed by evidence from investigation revealing or implying altered structure. Tying disease to illness is an exhibition of the specialist's rational expertise. It is intensely satisfying; but it is not enough. The predicament, from which this is emerging (a very much overvalued late adoption to a childless couple for example), or which is created by the illness (extreme pressure on a previously working mother), will be highly germane to the success of proposed management. Its understanding depends upon the discernment of the pediatrician and the quality of the account which is evoked between doctor and patient.

The centrepiece of this is the account of the 'coming into being' of the family and in particular the child in question within the context of that family. Many pediatricians use a thumbnail family tree in their notes; it is a question of expanding upon this excellent device. Setting a child in this context can, of course, elicit painful and difficult, even embarrassing, issues. It is easier to take the mother aside to some quiet and comfortable place to listen to her. Learn about her pregnancies, a brief history of each, their fathers, the dates of the births, the survivors' fates, and the modes of death or loss of others. (The preciousness of certain children becomes apparent and may help explain the impassable attachment disorder.) Dates of birth not only remain valid in the notes forever, whereas ages are soon wrong, they also highlight possible shifts in family dynamics (absent father; new father). They can focus on the special position given to the child in question (long expected first born; unlooked for afterthought). Raising these issues allows for an assessment of the quality of the family group within which the long-term care of a chronically sick child will be undertaken. The impact of the sickness is revealed. Naming the siblings brings them alive, allows them to be discussed freely then and later. Their birth accounts may help explain current dynamics.

Jean was 4 when her first sibling arrived. Sister Sharon was dramatically delivered by spontaneous labour at 32 weeks and required intensive care which claimed much parental involvement. A mild infantile hemiplegia gradually resolved and her subsequent development was normal. Aged 10, Sharon experienced some mild complex partial seizures which were easy to treat. Jean was at that time coping with her puberty and emergent sexuality in a very enmeshed puritanical family. At a public event Jean swooned repeatedly. An EEG was made which revealed that some spike and wave forms were indeed present. A diagnosis of epilepsy was awarded partly on the grounds of familial association. That was at least dynamically accurate.

For certain families the chronically sick child will prove a salve and a focus for good; for others it will prove to be the 'last straw'. The health and sickness careers of the family are important; not least for Meadow's syndrome (Meadow, 1977), which most frequently manifests through phenomena that look like epilepsy often against a background of excessive maternal health-care seeking. More often it is useful to know how parents are placed when a burden of treatment is going to be placed upon them. Hoare and Kerley (1992) showed, firstly, that half their clinic sample of children with epilepsy had high psychosocial morbidity but also, secondly, that few of the parents who came seeking 'treatment' expressed interest in an intervention program and, thirdly, almost none completed it. The study revealed elegantly the gap between care seeking on behalf of the sick and the apparent capacity to respond to that care. Presumably some unmeasured needs had been met. To achieve the sort of care that the doctor deems appropriate may require much work on behalf of the child by a team of carers.

CHRONIC SICKNESS AND PSYCHOPATHOLOGY

The nature, extent, and the management of behavioral problems arising among the chronic sick vary substantially with the way in which the child is received, perceived, and handled within their family. It is important to be acquainted with the stresses which the family will experience as a consequence of the sickness. These are rarely systematically reviewed.

I argue that the perception of 'epilepsy' held within a social group must be a product of its corporate experiences of seizures and their outcome and its oral traditions about these. At its simplest level, for example, 50% of mothers systematically questioned about their reaction to witnessing their child's first febrile seizure said they feared it was dying (Baumer *et al.*, 1981). While the fear of death is to some extent irrational (Verity, Ross and Golding, 1993), it is also true that a group of children, identified as suffering from epilepsy in early childhood, show substantially increased mortality. Sillanpää and Helenius (1993) in their superb community study revealed a death rate of 37 of their original sample of 245 at a mean of 27 years' follow-up. In Harrison and Taylor's (1976) 25-year follow-up, 10% were dead from a sample which had included all children with fits associated with fever as well as all other epilepsies. The cohort study of all the births in the first week of March 1946 (Britten *et al.*, 1986) showed that 92 of 130 patients who had developed epilepsy by the age of 36 had an onset of epilepsy under 14 years of age. Of these, 20% had died by the 36-year follow-up. In Sweden 11 of 194 had died by the 12-year follow up, 'only' 11% of the test group still had seizures (Brorson and Wranne, 1987). In a State-wide study of deaths in children aged 1–14 years in Victoria, 8.5% were associated with epilepsy. Twenty-two per cent of these deaths were attributed directly to epilepsy. Over 90% of the epilepsies were

classed as 'secondary' (Harvey, Nolan and Carlin, 1993). When the broad swathe of neurologic, cognitive, and behavioral morbidity is added, it is scarcely surprising that childhood epilepsy excites deep concern and negative feelings in the community. These feelings become the basis of prejudice, irrationality, and distortions of relationships which can themselves become self-fulfilling prophesies. An article entitled 'Low morbidity and mortality of status epilepticus in children', nicely reveals medical bias in the interpretation of outcome. From an excellent center of care the local people would perceive that seven of 193 children died within 3 months and that 'neurological sequelae' followed for 29% of children under 1 year old and 11% of 1–3 year olds (Maytal *et al.*, 1989).

Part of the increased mortality comes from a risk of sudden death 'out of the blue', a risk associated with relatively few other chronic illnesses. Ten per cent of the deaths in the Harvey *et al.* study occurred in that way. Each seizure provides a reminder of this possibility.

Following upon a series of seizures, called initially febrile convulsions, but of escalating duration and severity the parents of the child, both of whom were medically qualified, took it in turns to co-sleep with the child and deliver rectal diazepam. This practice continued over several years.

The persistent concern which is experienced between attacks of a recurrent sickness is dread. This specific anxiety is intermittently (i.e. very powerfully) reinforced by reality. It can survive prolonged intervals of well-being, even of 'recovery'. Dread motivates preoccupation with seizure control as the primary goal of treatment, sometimes to the detriment of general well-being. Dread distinguishes the parents' from the doctors' perspective on how well treatment is going. Treatment failures also reinforce dread.

The anguish of parents is added to by the impairment of brain functioning which becomes gradually apparent in so many children with epilepsy. The best evidence that 'being prone to seizures recurrently' does impair cerebral functioning comes in the improvement seen after successful surgical treatment (Ounsted, Lindsay and Richards, 1987). There is also adequate evidence that subclinical epileptic events create impairment (Marston *et al.*, 1993; see also Chapters 13d, 24). It is important that children known to have conditions that reduce learning ability even in the absence of seizures do not have their impairment attributed solely to that cause when epilepsy is also present. Improving the seizure management can make crucial improvement to learning ability. Some of the learning problems arise from limitations upon sensory input. Children with epilepsy are liable to be deprived of: (1) experiences; such as cycling, swimming, risk taking; (2) information; ordinarily gathered from wandering about exploring their surroundings, 'following their noses'; (3) relationships; because callers are fewer, the traffic of friendships is likely to be uneven because of limitations imposed on the sick child, and because the limitations and manifest concerns for safety are liable to create anxious attachments and reduced expectations of the child (Long and Moore, 1979).

Epilepsy is a stigma. The seizures are powerfully aversive and frightening to onlookers. Voiding may occur. There may be dysmorphisms, scars of old injuries, peculiarities of gait. Protective clothing also stigmatizes, it declares minority group membership.

There are certain problems in personality traits and structure. There are more problems for the more obviously affected children (Britten, Woolsworth and Fenwick, 1984).

These traits arise from 'organic psychosyndromes' which impose limitations from deficits of function, observed as lack of social skills for example. More psychologically, the life lived as a sick person can become the only conceivable life and rehabilitation after loss of seizures becomes very difficult. The image of the 'self' as the controlling agent in the life being lived is contradicted by the evidence of the support, sustenance, medications, ingestions, insertions, intrusions that are a commonplace aspect of medical care. Sick people, moreover, are expected to be 'compliant' with all that!

Sociologists have provided a view about the rules governing being sick (Mechanic, 1968). Certain proscriptions apply (driving) as an immediate consequence of 'class membership'. 'Epileptics' as a class of person, irrespective of any personal considerations or characteristics, qualify for certain proscriptions. The chronic sick from whatever cause are also liable to negative connotation. 'Get well soon', expressed as a wish, seems more like an admonition. The sick become liable to various forms of exploitation and also to set up defences against such exploitation.

Carers for the sick are also liable to exploitation by uninvolved members of society who prefer to remain uninvolved. The burden of care can be computed as a financial cost as well as a profound burden. The sorrow and grief of those caring for others who can never realize the ordinary ambitions that were had for them is measurable only as rates of depression, sickness rates in care units, and 'care provider burn out'. Most exits are blocked to parents who are carers.

The impact of a sickness will depend on the scale of the organic deterioration, but also upon the resources of development which are available. Very early onset disorders preclude any significant 'premorbid' life and no life tasks have been achieved. As will be seen elsewhere (Chapters 22–24), the treatments can themselves be harmful at their best; at worst they can be degrading, noxious and ineffective, but endlessly administered, however useless they prove. Doctors appear to feel legally obligated to provide 'antiepileptics' for 'epileptics' lest some ictal catastrophe should occur which, it is imagined, the medication might have prevented.

The logic and statistics to support this are hard to imagine – most sudden deaths in epilepsy occur to people on drugs.

PSYCHOLOGIC DEFENSES

All these potential portents and impacts from chronic epilepsy evoke responses from the ordinary psychologic defenses. Just as the skin and immune system work against intrusions and just as, at times, the work of these defenses becomes painfully apparent, so painful work will be done by psychologic defenses. The chronically sick child is not the child that was hoped for, and the possibility of that child must be grieved. (I assume that parents would not, a priori, hope to have a child with serious health problems.)

Parents and child will be discovered at some point in the grieving process which, like the grief of a death, follows from shock, to denial, to anger, to depression, to coming to terms. Usually these are only partially sequential. Passing through these states may be made quite uneven by variations in the cause of the illness, sudden crises, variable remissions. These normal reactions are painful states of being. 'Sorrow' is the word which conveys my meaning best.

Denial is the most common defense against intolerable pain. It stands in the way of clear communication when news is being given, future plans discussed, or treatment outlined. It accounts for post hoc trivialization of expert advice, often including disparaging the capability, sensitivity, and manners of the newsgiver. It accounts for the surprising revelation, after years of discussion about the child, that the parents had never previously been told, or understood, the impact of some vital piece of information.

The mother of a child with hemiplegia following on a very long convulsion in early childhood with subsequent brain swelling and atrophy explained the absence of her husband from consultations at the epilepsy clinic. In the early hours of the morning of the original prolonged seizure he had got up to help his daughter go to the bathroom. On returning to bed he remarked to his wife that their son appeared unwell. She found him convulsing, profoundly unconscious, anoxic, and soaked in sweat. Father's beliefs were fatalistic and avoidant not just of the acute episode but to all subsequent care. It would be wrong to think that this mother was supported just because a family structure appeared to exist.

Repression is less active, more simple, 'Its no use, I just can't bear to think about it'. In this state people agree to decisions which they may later regret. Taking a decision gives rise to an action which triggers a reaction. This is one basis of not following through an agreed treatment strategy. **Projection** means ascribing to others feelings and actions in oneself that are not owned up to. These unowned feelings are likely to be negative, wishing to be rid of the burden of care, wondering whether the quality of the life at issue is worth the distress to all concerned, etc. The doctor may be aware of hostility directed at them despite their best efforts. (In effect they are the only apparent owners of negative feelings in the dyad since the parent is denying them.) Or doctors may be manipulated into giving heroic and extreme treatments. A negative outcome of these will give rise to righteous indignation or a lawsuit. **Reaction formation** allows extreme degrees of self-denial and blind and exhausting committment to what parents see as the best interests of the child. Some parents can never entrust their child to others to allow themselves respite or recreation. The understandable sense of the child as a burden is buried under total devotion. Altering the dynamics is fraught with danger: there may be sudden rejection, more often anger and criticism of the resources offered. **Displacement** is a diversion of distress from its proper object, the grief at the loss of a perfect child, on to professionals who are seen as standing in the way of restoring the child. Caring professionals are used to being made to feel impotent despite their best efforts. They are just next in line to prove to be a disappointment.

Rationalization makes certain thoughts and courses of action seem reasonable when they are not. It is a justification for therapies which are noxious or tiresome. Professionals should be warned when fixed beliefs are made evident as part of the therapeutic encounter. To demur from meeting the demands is likely to lead to termination of treatment. **Sublimation** is a substitute activity for what is 'forbidden'. It deflects the energies of grief and pain and aggression into creative outlets. Some of the most helpful organizations which represent the interests of various 'disease' sufferers stem from sublimated energies.

Through these various defenses the prolonged pain, distress, and grief are made tolerable. The best way of altering the painful dynamics in the distressed family of a child with epilepsy is to alter the basis of the distress. Cure is often expected of doctors. It is mostly not available for epilepsy. Often the seizure disorder is only the most pressing but not the only or even the worst dysfunction. This truth is revealed whenever unwanted effects of treatment throw the other components of the sickness into high relief. The example below touches on many of the issues outlined above.

A lovely looking boy, now aged 8, still displays a range of difficult behaviors 1 year after a temporal lobectomy relieved him of all his seizures. These behaviors are mostly aspects of the organic psychosyndrome which followed from the cataclysmic febrile seizures, two of which lasted several hours, in early childhood. The parents have no grasp on the massive degree of the child's cognitive difficulties, they have no grasp of psychogenesis or of the effects upon the child of his anxious attachment to his mother. The parents brush aside any gains which may come from relief of seizures; their focus is entirely upon the unremitting behavior dis-

order. It is readily apparent that the massive seizures and dire threat to this infant wrecked attachment, left mother profoundly depressed for most of the child's life, and utterly destroyed the resources the parents needed to help remedial management. Yet they have insisted upon removing him from a place of care and raising him themselves.

PSYCHIATRIC DISORDERS AND EPILEPSY

The Introduction referred to 'informal' and 'formal' psychiatry. Hitherto the issues discussed have been 'psychosocial' in the strict sense, referring to the interaction of behavioral and social factors, and the influence of social factors upon the individual mind or behavior. Psychiatric disorders are the more formal constructs of psychiatry, representing the current state of its capacity to define the characteristics of certain illnesses. The terms should not be abused; protocols are available (DSM III R (IV), see American Psychiatric Association (1987); ICD 9, (10), see World Health Organization (1977)).

On the other hand, the variety of behavioral dysfunction in neurologically dysfunctional children is considerably wider than the categories available and matching the strict protocols is problematic. This may partly account for how little fresh research is done in the field. Descriptive diagnoses for clinical purposes can be less demanding than those applied for research.

PSYCHOSES

Autism

Autism was viewed as 'psychosis' because it did not seem possible to share reality with the child. Epilepsy, or a past history of epilepsy, is common in children with autism and the spectrum of 'autistic-like' disorders. These are children who, while failing to meet with strict diagnostic criteria needed for a formal diagnosis of autism, nevertheless show a number of features in common with children labeled 'autistic'. These range from language and communication problems, to a lack of real warmth in relationships and a poor understanding of the feelings of others, to play lacking in imagination, and to rather fixed and limited interests. The closest associations are through infantile spasms and myoclonic epilepsies of the types seen in the Lennox–Gastaut syndrome (Gillberg and Coleman, 1992). The epilepsy most frequently arises in the first year of life, either from previous developmental normality or minor abnormality, and the autistic syndrome appears to be a sequel.

Wong (1993) confirmed early findings by Schain and Yannet (1960) and Kolvin, Roth and Ounsted (1971). Of 145 'autistic' children in Wong's study (sex ratio 4.5 : 1, male to female), 7.6% had developed epilepsy, as had 5% of 101 children with 'autistic features' (1.5 : 1, male to female). The study did not reveal a secondary peak of epilepsy onsets (Olsson, Steffenberg and Gillberg, 1988). My own experience is that autistic children without previous epilepsy may develop seizures for the first time towards puberty. This is usually a mild epilepsy with complex partial seizures. In earlier studies (Schain and Yannet, 1960; Rutter and Lockyer, 1969), up to 40% eventually had suffered from epilepsy. Mostly the autism follows the early onset seizures ineluctably despite successful treatment, but there are some reports that the autistic features can remit when the seizures remit (Gillberg and Coleman, 1992; I. Jambaqué *et al.*, 1994, personal communication). The various natures of the association between 'autistic disorders' and 'epilepsies' suggest that the appearance of causality between them is spurious and that both are aspects of an underlying neurodevelopmental disorder within the limbic system (Deonna *et al.*, 1993). Diseases such as tuberous sclerosis can be regarded as having both illnesses in its symptomatic repertoire.

Asperger's syndrome

The recent acknowledgement of Asperger's syndrome as an important developmental deviation stems from the work of Wing (1981) and of Gillberg (Gillberg and Coleman, 1992). The rise in interest among neuropediatricians has led to overdiagnosis. Diagnostic criteria require:

1. Severe impairment in reciprocal social interaction.
2. All-absorbing narrow interests.
3. The imposition of these routines and interests upon others.
4. Speech and language problems (pedantic; odd prosody).
5. Nonverbal communication problems (gauche; inappropriate gaze).
6. Motor clumsiness.

There are genetic links with infantile autism in some families.

The relevance of these traits to people with epilepsy is in course of classification. Personal experience within specialist centers has been that young people with these traits are seen regularly. The traits also come within the massive adjectival vocabulary of the so-called 'epileptic personality'. That concept proved too compendious to be useful (Tizard, 1962). Imaging studies reviewed by Gillberg and Coleman (1992) reveal some abnormalities, notably neuronal migration defects, which are less in degree but continuous with those seen associated with seizures. The syndrome may denote no more than a certain form of oddity of personality. Those who come to psychiatric attention may have a poor prognosis even without epilepsy. It is helpful for the traits to be recognized and explanations offered for them outside the moral frame in which they are otherwise construed.

Schizophrenia

Schizophrenia in childhood is rare. It is less commonly associated with epilepsy than are the autistic disorders. For schizophrenia to be diagnosed, delusions, hallucinations, loose associations and incoherence, catatonia, and inappropriate or flattened affect must be present (Volkmar, 1991). There is often notable and increasing social maladaptation with withdrawal from normal pursuits. Pediatricians will also be concerned, however, with the long-term psychiatric prognosis of childhood epilepsies.

The association between epilepsy and schizophrenia was formalized in the classic papers of Slater, Beard and Glitheroe (1963). In that study of 63 subjects, six males and nine females started their epilepsy under the age of 10, and one male and four females became schizophrenic before the age of 20. Twelve females, compared with two males, had onset of both epilepsy and psychosis under the age of 20. Flor-Henry (1969) and Taylor (1975) found a bias towards left-sided foci among those developing schizophrenia. In Ounsted's study (Ounsted, Lindsay and Richards, 1987), the bias was towards males developing schizophrenia (as diagnosed and treated by persons other than the authors), though the left-sided emphasis, on EEG foci, was confirmed. Ten per cent of their original 100 sample had been diagnosed by 1977 (i.e. there may have been others later). The notion of 'interval' or 'delay' as having some causal relevance became prominent, but it was discounted by Slater and Moran (1969) and shown to be artefactual by Taylor (1971). In 10% of Slater's series both conditions were either diagnosed synchronously, or within 1 year. There is some evidence (Taylor and Marsh, 1977; Bruton, 1988) that some types of lesion, notably gangliogliomata, bear a higher risk of association with later psychosis. It is not certain that early operation will eliminate the risk because a notable case of Falconer's operated on the aged two and a half became schizophrenic at age 17, despite being seizure free (Falconer, 1973). However Caplan *et al.* (1993) have shown in a pilot study that thought disorder and illogical thinking in children with TLE is improved by successful lobectomy. The precise nature of the link between schizophrenia and epilepsy remains to be found, but evidence suggests that the link is through an aspect of 'brain damage' (Bruton, Stevens and Frith, 1994).

AFFECTIVE DISORDERS

Strictly, mood disorders constitute unipolar depressive disorder and bipolar disorders. There is no reason to suppose they would be less frequent in children with epilepsy. At issue is understanding the mechanism of association via the location, lateralization, and type of lesion; potential interactions between such disorders and the treatment of epilepsy; and increases of risk of a non-specific nature through the vicissitudes of chronic illness. There is a marked increase in the diagnosis of these disorders around puberty. For some years psychiatrists were reluctant to diagnose depression in children. Theoretically they were not considered susceptible until the super ego was developed. There is recognizable development of the experience and recognition of sadness (Garber and Kashani, 1991), but clinically relevant affective disorder may not be continuous with either normal or marked sadness. Hermann *et al.* (1989) showed in a study of 6–11 year olds that 'depression' as a function of responses to a behavioral checklist was related to the items 'inadequate seizure control' and 'parental divorce or separation'. These two items were also the most important predictors of all the behavioral problems and of social competence in their study.

Much of the research with children is fashioned around checklists and questionnaires given to parents. My view is that these have strong potential as projective tests. Given the sorts of issues discussed earlier in this chapter, the vocabulary provided by the questionnaire may provide as much evidence of the mental state of the parent as of the child. But child behavior is essentially interactive with the immediate environment of persons, and the behavior and attitudes of those persons will be germane to the child's behavior.

There are contradicting reports concerning the lateralization of focal abnormalities and depression. No data exists directly concerning children. Taylor (1989) reviewed the topic. Firstly, certain characteristics of depression in people with epilepsy differed from those in nonepileptic depressives (Mendez, Cummings and Benson, 1986). These were similar to traits in the 'Organic Personality Syndrome'. Only adults were studied, but pediatricians should be aware that certain traits, chronic enough to seem characterologic, may be depressive and modifiable by treatment. Secondly, Taylor argued that the reason why bipolar disorder is rarely recorded before puberty is that the hypomanic dimension may be interpreted as hyperkinesis as there are overlapping characteristics to these diagnoses. Thirdly, he gave examples, and referred to others, where hypomanic symptoms had been associated with deep right temporal/perithalamic lesions.

Differences in behavioral outcome dependent upon the hemisphere affected are in a limbo of their own. Lateralization of language centers is clearly established. If there is parallel lateralization of other specializations to the right brain, it is less certain what those specializations are. It would not be surprising if they were skills that were independent of language and hence symptoms of dysfunction would not be easy to express in language. Voeller (1986) coined a 'Right Hemisphere Deficit Syndrome' in children, with marked deficits in performance skills. These children had problems picking up affective clues in social interactions, and 14 of the 15 subjects were 'hyperactive'.

More research is needed, but it seems plain that what appears as 'personality' will be subtly but powerfully shaped by particular sorts of deficits and overactivities within the dysfunctional brain.

SUICIDE

Suicide statistics in adults with epilepsy show various levels of increase dependent on the nature of the sample (Barraclough, 1981), with temporal lobe epilepsy showing markedly increased risks. This is some further incentive towards surgical treatment. Suicide rates in children are low but a marked increase occurs around puberty. Suicide attempts have been shown to be disproportionately increased in adolescents with epilepsy (Hawton, Fagg and Marsuck, 1980; Brent, 1986). Since the mortality of young people with epilepsy is markedly increased, and since they have a variety of means of ending their lives without recourse to obvious self-killing, it is clear that much consideration should be given to the mental state of young people with epilepsy (Lund and Gormsen, 1985).

HYPERKINETIC SYNDROME (ADHD, CONDUCT DISORDER)

All pediatricians are aware of the fulminant hyperkinetic syndrome precipitated in certain children with epilepsy when treated by some anticonvulsant drugs. The original study of Kramer and Pollnow (1932) and the astonishing account by Ounsted (1955) describe children in behavioral chaos. Probably anticonvulsants were in part responsible. But some children who are not on drugs, especially those with lower IQs and some with autistic syndromes, produce ranges of overactivity, dangerous tricks, tempers, demandingness which far exceed normal standards. Eric Taylor (1986), summarizing years of study, draws clear distinctions between overactivity, hyperactivity, and hyperkinesis. Entering a study of the Maudsley Child Psychiatry clinic through a definition of hyperkinesis, James and Taylor (1990) found that 25 of the 79 hyperkinetic children (discovered in 6525 clinic attenders) suffered epilepsy. Though males were overrepresented in the sample of 79 (3.38 :1), proportionately more females with hyperkinesis suffered from epilepsy. Children must be monitored and parents advised about hyperkinesis. Too many are left, for months between appointments, with intolerable behavior. Drug variation, and adjunctive therapy with methylphenidate or dexamphetamine might be needed.

CONDUCT DISORDER

Conduct disorder may be associated with attention deficit and hyperactivity. The child with epilepsy whose behavioral problems are complained of in the clinic usually has more diffuse behavioral deviations. The profile of these abnormalities will vary substantially with etiology, intelligence, seizure type, family background, but also upon the research techniques and 'instruments' used. Research produces strikingly anomalous results. Aman, Werry and Turbott (1992) used a sample of 112 children aged 6–12 years with well-controlled seizures and average or more IQ. (This design is often seen as providing evidence about the effect of 'epilepsy' alone; I have remarked elsewhere that this is an elusive concept.) On Conner's scale, **teachers** of these children regarded them as the equals or superiors of their matched controls. But their **parents** rated their children with epilepsy as significantly worse on all six scales. Boys were generally rated worse than girls. (It would be pointless to discuss who was **right** as that would imply that children's behavior could be described in anything **but** some other persons standards.) In our own study (Hackney and Taylor, 1976) comparing children with and without epilepsy admitted to a Child Pyschiatry Hospital, we found comparable, high rates on the 'Neurotic' and 'Antisocial' components of Rutter's Questionnaire as filled in by teachers. Boys were more antisocial than girls. Children with epilepsy in the community compared to their controls showed much lower rates of disorder. But all epileptic children were rated on more items than controls. These items, which did not contribute to the

Antisocial and Neurotic scales produced a picture of a child with epilepsy, not much liked by other children, squirmy and fidgety, solitary, irritable, with tics and mannerisms, unresponsive, and resentful when corrected. This profile seems to link, via 'organicity', to the picture described in adults. There was some evidence that teachers (and parents?) suddenly lose patience with difficult children and then use the questionaires to express their problem.

TICS AND OBSESSIVE COMPULSIVE DISORDER

A florid, somewhat grotesque, obsessionality was described once as 'organic' obsessionality. An adolescent patient of Murray Falconer's had retained all her sanitary towels in cases in her room together with any garment which had become 'touched' by her mother, washed but wet in plastic bags. She never changed her bed linen. The association of elements of Tourette's, Asperger's, and compulsive disorder has been seen by me several times in people with epilepsy. Treatment may require behavioral psychotherapy (Marks, 1986), but the obsessive symptoms might be responsive to anticonvulsants (Kroll and Drummond, 1993).

NEUROSES

The category 'neurosis' is falling from use, though 'neurotic' traits persists. Attention is given to anxiety, panic disorder, phobias, and to somatoform disorder (similar to 'hysterical'). The level of fears, worries, miseries, is generally raised in chronically sick children (Taylor and Eminson, 1994), but the specific illnesses and their relationship to epilepsy is too little studied.

HYSTERICAL EPILEPSY, PSEUDO-SEIZURES, NONEPILEPTIC SEIZURES

There are two serious problems relating to these labels. The first is that neither 'epilepsy' nor 'seizures' are appropriate descriptions of the untoward behavior. The second is our problem in naming what we think is going on in some sort of medical terms without giving offense, seeming presumptuous, or being wrong. We give offence by implying that the behavior is 'deliberate', as it firmly suggests a moral fault in the patient and foolishness in those who have been duped. The concept of unconscious behavior has been thought a useful camouflage and is manifest in the literature as 'not trying to deceive' and such like. It is presumptuous to imply that we can perceive unconscious motivation for a behavior which, by definition, would be inaccessible. We are wrong to misconstrue the behavior in any way, and to confuse medical and psychiatric labels with moral judgements such as malingering. (If malingering could be substantiated it would be a form of fraud or theft and, by definition, not a medical event.) It is probably wrong to give a child to understand that a behavior is unconscious when only the child knows whether it is or not. Treatment is variably effective (Saccomani, Cirrincione and Savoini, 1993).

NONEPILEPTIC ATTACK DISORDER

Betts (Betts, 1990; Betts and Boden, 1991) coined this label which is the best description of the unwanted behavior. It covers alternative medical conditions as well as what he calls 'emotional' attacks. These he subcategorizes as swoons, tantrums, abreactions, and pseudostatus (epilepticus). His work however has been principally with adults.

For children Meadow's syndrome is a major consideration (see also Chapter 2). Seizures are imposed upon young children in various ways. Outlandish factitious illness (Taylor, 1991) describes a condition of older children who are inveigled into enactments of illnesses which conform to parental beliefs. Some of these were among the cases I called 'The Falling Sickness' (Taylor, 1986a) as being

the least prejudicial, most ancient, and most eloquent of labels for the untoward behavior.

The ideas that give rise to the untoward behavior may originate:

1. Within the illness of epilepsy just as, at times, symptom exaggeration with various degrees of personal awareness marks many chronic illnesses.
2. Or opportunistically, snatched from a dramatic moment in the biography to meet dynamic needs (see 'Elaine' in Taylor, 1986a).
3. Or it may be a stage in the development of hysteria, Briquet's syndrome, persistent, polysymptomatic and very problematic.
4. Or the needs of the situation may only be met by flagrant and prolonged exhibition of the behaviour into 'status', thus precipitating serious medical intervention.

Betts sees his categories as various forms of communication from persons who have limits on their ordinary communication; the impaired, the mentally ill, the sexually abused. 'The body speaks what the tongue cannot utter' (Taylor, 1986b). Betts' concepts open the possibility of various types of psychologic treatment.

The need is considerable, since most estimates provide that at least one case in ten has a nonepileptic attack disorder.

CONCLUSION

The pediatrician who wants to be responsive to the psychologic needs of children and recognize the possibility of psychiatric disorder will need certain strategies.

Firstly, a recognition of the threat component of epilepsy. This is a feared condition because of its morbidity and mortality.

Secondly, a tactic in the clinic for identifying those cases who have (or who will) become chronic. All chronic sickness creates special problems.

Thirdly, a realization that brain dysfunction and cerebroactive medications are likely to disrupt behavior and learning in the short term. Psychiatric disorder may arise concurrently or supervene at any time.

Fourthly, a system of personal audit should be considered so that 'chronic' cases, which have exhausted initial enthusiasm, should be regularly, personally, reconsidered. Might anything better be done? Might the cost, in suffering and in loss of facility, deserve another opinion?

Awareness can be increased by ensuring that management of chronic illness is undertaken with a clear picture of the real family and the available support system, carefully given in detail to the pediatrician in person and kept up to date.

Many of the behavioral problems do not constitute 'formal' psychiatric disorder but are compounded of organic, toxic, cognitive, situational, and management elements. Listening with understanding, agreeing mutual aims, and taking a flexible approach to therapy will be helpful. An awareness of helpful and unhelpful defenses among everyone concerned will prevent pediatricians from feeling too bruised, which is bad for them, or moralizing, which is bad for everybody concerned.

REFERENCES

Aman, M., Werry, J. and Turbott, S. (1992) Behaviour of children with seizures. Comparison with norms and effect of seizure type. *Journal of Nervous and Mental Diseases*, **180**, 124–9.

American Psychiatric Association (1987) *Diagnostic and Statistical Manual of Mental Disorders*, revised 3rd edn, Americal Psychiatric Association Washington DC.

Barraclough, B. (1981) Suicide and epilepsy, in *Epilepsy and Psychiatry* (eds E. Reynolds and M. Trimble), Churchill Livingstone, Edinburgh.

Baumer, J.H., David, T.J., Valentine, S. *et al.* (1981) Many parents think their child is dying when having a first febrile convulsion. *Developmental Medicine and Child Neurology*, **23**, 462–4.

Betts, T. (1990) Pseudoseizures: seizures that are not epilepsy. *Lancet*, **336**, 163–4.

Betts, T. and Boden, S. (1991) Pseudoseizures (non-epileptic attack disorder), *Women and Epilepsy* (ed. M. Trimble), John Wiley, Chichester, pp. 243–58.

Brent, D.A. (1986) Overrepresentation of epileptics in a consecutive series of suicide attempters seen at a children's hospital 1978–1983. *Journal of the American Academy of Child and Adolescent Psychiatry*, **25**, 242–6.

Britten, N., Wadsworth, M. and Fenwick, P. (1984) Stigma in patients with early epilepsy: a national longitudinal study. *Journal of Epidemiology and Community Health*, **38**, 291–5.

Britten, N., Morgan, K., Fenwick, P. and Britten, H. (1986) Epilepsy and handicap from birth to age 36. *Developmental Medicine and Child Neurology*, **28**, 719–28.

Brorson, L. and Wranne, L. (1987) Long term prognosis in childhood epilepsy: survival and seizure prognosis. *Epilepsia*, **28**, 324–30.

Bruton, C. (1988) *The Neuropathology of Temporal Lobe Epilepsy*, Oxford University Press, Oxford.

Bruton, C., Stevens, J. and Frith, C.D. (1994) Epilepsy, psychosis, and schizophrenia: clinical and neuropathologic correlations. *Neurology*, **44**, 34–42.

Caplan, R., Guthrie, D., Shields, D. *et al.* (1993) *Journal of American Academy of Child and Adolescent Psychiatry*, **32**, 604–71.

Deonna, T., Ziegler, A.L., Mourra-Serra, J. and Innocenti, G. (1993) Autistic regression in relation to limbic pathology and epilepsy: report of two cases. *Developmental Medicine and Child Neurology*, **35**, 158–76.

Falconer, M.A. (1973) Reversibility by temporal-lobe resection of the behavioral abnormalities of temporal lobe epilepsy. *New England Journal of Medicine*, **289**, 451–5.

Flor-Henry, P. (1969) Psychosis and temporal lobe epilepsy. *Epilepsia*, **10**, 363–95.

Garber, J. and Kashani, J.H. (1991) Development of the symptom of depression, in *Child and Adolescent Psychiatry* (ed. M. Lewis), Williams and Wilkins, Baltimore, pp. 293–309.

Gillberg, C. and Coleman, M. (1992) *The Biology of Autistic Syndromes*, 2nd edn, MacKeith Press, Blackwell, Oxford, chap. 6.

Graham, P. and Rutter, M. (1968) Organic brain dysfunction and child psychiatric disorder. *British Medical Journal*, **3**, 695–700.

Hackney, A. and Taylor, D.C. (1976) A teachers' questionnaire description of epileptic children. *Epilepsia*, **17**, 275–81.

Harrison, R.M. and Taylor, D.C. (1976) Childhood

seizures: a 25 year follow up. Social and medical prognosis. *Lancet*, **5**, 948–51.

Harvey, A.S., Nolan, T. and Carlin, J.B. (1993) Mortality in children with epilepsy. *Epilepsia*, **34**, 597–603.

Hawton, K., Fagg, J. and Mrazek, P. (1980) Association between epilepsy and attempted suicide. *Journal of Neurology, Neurosurgery and Psychiatry*, **43**, 168–70.

Hermann, B., Whitman, S. and Dell, J. (1989) Correlates of behaviour problems and school performance of children with epilepsy aged 6–11, in *Childhood Epilepsies: Neuropsychological, Psychosocial and Intervention Aspects* (eds. B.P. Hermann and M. Seidenberg), pp. 143–58.

Hippocrates (1947) The Sacred Disease, in *The Medical Works of Hippocrates* (trans J. Chadwick and W. Mann), Blackwell, Oxford.

Hoare, P. and Kerley, S. (1992) Helping parents and children with epilepsy cope successfully: the outcome of a group programme for parents. *Journal of Psychosomatic Research*, **36**, 759–67.

James, A. and Taylor, E. (1990) Sex differences in the hyperkinetic syndrome of childhood. *Journal of Child Psychology and Psychiatry*, **31**, 437–46.

Kim, W.J. (1991) Psychiatric aspects of epileptic children and adolescents. *Journal of the American Academy of Child and Adolescent Psychiatry*, **30**, 874–86.

Kolvin, I., Roth, M. and Ounsted, C. (1971) Studies in the childhood psychoses V: cerebral dysfunction and childhood psychoses. *British Journal of Psychiatry*, **118**, 407–14.

Kramer, F. and Pollnow, H. (1932) Uber eine hyperkinetische Erkrankung im Kindesalter. *Monatsschrift für Psychiatrie und Neurologie, Berlin*, 82.

Kroll, L. and Drummond, L. (1993) Temporal lobe epilepsy and obsessive compulsive symptoms. *Journal of Nervous and Mental Disease*, **181**, 457–8.

Long, C.G. and Moore, J.R. (1979) Parental expectations for their epileptic children. *Journal of Child Psychology and Psychiatry*, **20**, 299–312.

Lund, A. and Gormsen, H. (1985) The role of antiepileptics in sudden death in epilepsy. *Acta Neurologica Scandinavica*, **72**, 444–6.

Marks, I. (1986) Behavioural and drug treatments of phobic and obsessive-compulsive disorders. *Psychotherapy and Psychosomatics*, **46**, 35–44.

Marston, D., Besag, F., Binnie, C. and Fowler, M. (1993) Effects of transitory cognitive impairment on psychosocial functioning of children with

epilepsy: a therapeutic trial. *Developmental Medicine and Child Neurology*, **35**, 574–81.

Maytal, J., Shinnar, S., Moshe, S.L. and Alvarez, L.A. (1989) Low morbidity and mortality of status epilepticus in children. *Pediatrics*, **3**, 323–31.

Meadow, R. (1977) Munchausen syndrome by proxy – the hinterland of child abuse. *Lancet*, **ii**, 391–407.

Mechanic, D. (1968) *Medical Sociology: A Selective View*, Free Press, New York.

Mendez, M., Cummings, J. and Benson, D.F. (1986) Depression in epilepsy. *Archives of Neurology*, **43**, 766–70.

Olsson, I., Steffenberg, S. and Gillberg, C. (1988) Epilepsy in autism and autistic-like conditions: a population based study. *Archives of Neurology*, **45**, 666–8.

Ounsted, C. (1955) The hyperkinetic syndrome in epileptic children. *Lancet*, **ii**, 303–11.

Ounsted, C., Lindsay, J. and Richards, P. (1987) *Temporal Lobe Epilepsy: A Biographical Study 1948–1986*, MacKeith Press, Blackwell, Oxford.

Rutter, M. and Lockyer, L. (1969) A five to fifteen year follow-up study of infantile psychosis 1. Description of sample. *British Journal of Psychiatry*, **113**, 1169–82.

Saccomani, L., Cirrincione, M. and Savoini, M. (1993) Pseudo-epileptic seizures in children and adolescents. *Developmental Medicine and Child Neurology*, **35**, 359–61.

Schain, R. and Yannet, H. (1960) Infantile autism: an analysis of 50 cases and a consideration of certain relevant neuropsychological concepts. *Journal of Pediatrics*, **57**, 560–7.

Sillanpää, M. and Helenius, H. (1993) Social competence of people with epilepsy: a new methological approach. *Acta Neurologica Scandinavica*, **87**, 335–41.

Slater, E. and Moran, P. (1969) The schizophrenia-like psychoses of epilepsy: relation between ages of onset. *British Journal of Psychiatry*, **115**, 599–600.

Slater, E., Beard, A.W. and Glithero, E. (1963) The schizophrenia-like psychoses of epilepsy. *British Journal of Psychiatry*, **109**, 95–150.

Taylor, D.C. (1971) Ontogenesis of epileptic psychosis: a reanalysis. *Psychological Medicine*, **1**, 247–53.

Taylor, D.C. (1975) Factors influencing the occurrence of schizophrenia-like psychosis in patients with temporal lobe epilepsy. *Psychological Medicine*, **5**, 249–54.

Taylor, D.C. (1979) The components of sickness: diseases, illnesses and predicaments. *Lancet*, **ii**, 1008–10.

Taylor, D.C. (1982a) The components of sickness: diseases, illnesses and predicaments, In: *One Child* (eds J. Apley and C. Ounsted) Spastics International I, Heineman, London.

Taylor, D.C. (1982b) Epilepsy: a model of sickness, *Psychopharmacology of Anticonvulsants* (ed. M. Sandler), Oxford University Press, Oxford.

Taylor, D. (1986a) The falling sickness: a reorientation to hysterical epilepsy, In *Neurologically Handicapped Children*, vol I (eds N. Gordon and I. McKinlay), Blackwell, Oxford, pp. 286–96.

Taylor, D.C. (1986b) Hysteria, play-acting and courage. *British Journal of Psychiatry*, **149**, 37–41.

Taylor, D.C. (1989) Affective disorders in epilepsies: a neuropsychiatric review. *Behavioural Neurology*, **2**, 49–68.

Taylor, D. (1991) Outlandish factitious illness, in *Recent Advances in Paediatrics* (eds T.J. David), Churchill Livingstone, Edinburgh, pp. 63–76.

Taylor, D.C. and Eminson, M. (1994) Psychological aspects of chronic physical sickness, in *Child and Adolescent Psychiatry* (eds M. Rutter, L. Hersov and E. Taylor), Blackwell, Oxford.

Taylor, D.C. and Marsh, S. M. (1977) Neuropathology and social pathology: the effects of small lesions in the temporal lobe, in *Tegretol in Epilepsy: Proceedings of an International Meeting*, Geigy, Macclesfield.

Taylor, E. (1986) 'Overactivity, hyperactivity and hyperkinesis', in *The Overactive Child* (ed. E. Taylor), Spastics International Medical Publication, Blackwell, Oxford, chap. 1.

Tizard, B. (1962) The personality of epileptics: a discussion of the evidence. *Psychological Bulletin*, **59**, 196–210.

Verity, C.M., Ross, E.M. and Golding, J. (1993) Outcome of status epilepticus and lengthy febrile convulsions: findings of national cohort study. *British Medical Journal*, **307**, 225–8.

Voeller, K. (1986) Right-hemisphere deficit syndrome in children. *American Journal of Psychiatry*, **143**, 1004–9.

Volkmar, F. (1991) Childhood schizophrenia, in *Child and Adolescent Psychiatry* (ed. M. Lewis), Williams and Wilkins, Baltimore.

Wing, L. (1981) Asperger's syndrome: a clinical account. *Psychological Medicine*, **11**, 115–29.

Wong, V. (1993) Epilepsy in children with autistic spectrum disorder. *Journal of Child Neurology*, **8**, 316–22.

World Health Organization (1977) *Manual of the International Statistical Classification of Diseases, Injuries and Causes of Death*, WHO, Geneva.

SPECIAL CENTERS FOR CHILDHOOD EPILEPSY

26

Frank M.C. Besag

INTRODUCTION

The concept of segregating people simply on the basis of suffering from a disease or disorder is no longer either accepted or acceptable. At various times in the past, the leper colony, the mental asylum and the tuberculosis sanatorium were considered to be not only acceptable but desirable. The purpose of these institutions was sometimes not so much to offer a service to those with the condition as to segregate them from society, sparing the general public the inconvenience or perceived risk of having such people in the community. Attitudes have changed in a major way. The emphasis now is on ensuring that the child with epilepsy leads as normal a life as possible. This necessarily implies that there should be no hint of institutionalization in his or her management. Against this background, why should a chapter on special centers be included in a modern book on childhood epilepsy? The answer lies in viewing the needs of the child with epilepsy in context. Most children with epilepsy have well-controlled seizures, attend regular mainstream schools and do not require much attention from the specialist services. However, a significant proportion will need additional help and a few will require a short- or longer-term placement in a special center if their needs are to be fulfilled adequately.

HISTORY OF THE SPECIAL CENTERS

Grant (1981) and Laidlaw and Laidlaw (1982) have summarized the history of the epilepsy centers. Although Hippocrates tried to dispel the attitude that epilepsy was the result of possession by evil spirits, the feeling that epilepsy might be a bad influence on others, or might even be infectious, continued. One of the earliest recorded establishments with a more caring attitude was founded at the end of the fifteenth century, when the monks at the Priory of St Valentine at Rufach in Alsace provided a 'hospice for epileptics'. The Bishop of Wurzburg started a home for people with epilepsy in 1773. Esquirol in 1815 was said to have suggested that special provision be made for people with epilepsy because he thought that the sight of an epileptic attack might make a healthy person develop epilepsy. The National Hospital for the Paralysed and Epileptic was opened in Queen Square, London, in 1860. In 1867, one of the most influential centers was established in a farmhouse near the town of Bielefeld, Germany. This was taken over, in 1872, by Pastor Friedrich von Bodelschwing and has become the famous Bethel Centre. Subsequently the colony at Meer en Bosch in Heemsteede, Holland and the Filadelfia colony at Dianalund in Denmark were founded. Based on the Bethel experience, several centers opened in the UK, including the Chalfont Centre

Epilepsy in Children. Edited by Sheila Wallace. Published in 1996 by Chapman & Hall, London. ISBN 0 412 56860 8

in Buckinghamshire in 1894; the center at Lingfield, now known as St Piers Lingfield, in 1898; and, the David Lewis Centre in Cheshire in 1904. These three centers remain, and, together with the Park Hospital in Oxford, form the nucleus for intensive work with people who have difficult epilepsy. There are other adult assessment units in the UK, e.g. Bootham Park Hospital, York. Most of those started in the USA did not survive. The National Centre for Epilepsy in Sandvika in Norway continues to provide a base for research and assessment. This list illustrates some of the developments which have taken place over the centuries, but is by no means comprehensive. Of particular importance, however, is the change in attitude. The epilepsy center is no longer viewed as being a place in which people can be segregated from society. Instead, it enables those who attend to fulfil a greater role within society by offering specialist assessment, treatment, education, and rehabilitation. This philosophy has successively grown out of a number of reports including, in the UK, the 1944 Education Act, the Reid Report ('People with Epilepsy', 1969), the Winterton report (1986), the 1978 Warnock Report and the subsequent 1981 Education Act. Several other reports have also been influential in this area. Particular attention should be drawn to the Warnock Report (1978), which emphasized the importance of educating children in mainstream schooling, wherever this is feasible, while acknowledging the important role of special schools in providing for children whose needs could not adequately be fulfilled by mainstream schooling, even with additional help.

EPILEPSY AND EDUCATIONAL DIFFICULTIES
(see also Chapters 13d, 17, 24, 25)

Difficulties in the management of the child with epilepsy almost inevitably impinge on education. In a recent review (Besag, 1995), it has been emphasized that the contrasting assumptions that epilepsy always has a major effect on education or that epilepsy seldom affects school performance are equally wrong. A number of studies have made it clear that, although many children with epilepsy have no educational problems, a large proportion encounter some difficulty. Not all of these papers are based on true epidemiologic studies, but the emerging pattern is nevertheless consistent. Earlier publications by Pond and Bidwell (1960) and Ounsted, Lindsay and Norman (1966) revealed educational difficulties in a high proportion of children with epilepsy. The Isle of Wight Study (Rutter, Graham and Yule, 1970) found an excess of reading retardation in children with epilepsy around 10 years of age. Studies by Green and Hartlage (1971) and Holdsworth and Whitmore (1974) also confirmed a high proportion of children were performing poorly in school. Other studies include those of Pazzaglia and Frank-Pazzaglia (1971) in Cesena, Italy, Stores (1971, 1978, 1981) and Stores and co-workers (Stores and Hart, 1976; Stores, Hart and Piran, 1978). The best epidemiologic investigation in the UK was the National Child Development Study, based on a cohort of 17 733 children born in the week 3–9 March 1958 in England, Scotland, and Wales. This has led to a number of publications, including Ross *et al.* (1980), Verity and Ross (1985), and Kurtz, Tookey and Ross (1987). Amongst their findings it was noted that 34% of the children with epilepsy were in special education by age 16. In the USA, Ellenberg, Hirtz and Nelson (1985) based their publication on results from a national collaborative perinatal project of the National Institute of Neurological and Communicative Disorders and Stroke, which followed the outcome of 54 000 pregnancies in 1959. Although their results suggested that there was no difference in IQ between the children with epilepsy and sibling controls, the IQ scores of the former were less than those of the general population.

Outstanding epidemiologic studies have been carried out by Sillanpää in Finland. In a recent publication (Sillanpää, 1992), data on 143 children with epilepsy from a population of 21 104 children aged 4–15 years was examined. The most frequent impairments were mental retardation (31.4%), speech disorders (27.5%), and specific learning disorders (23.1%). In earlier reviews (Sillanpää, 1990, 1983) it was concluded that 27.5% of children with epilepsy did not complete their basic education or required schooling in establishments for learning disability. Taking these studies overall, it would appear that about half of the population of children with epilepsy will experience some educational difficulty and a smaller proportion, perhaps about one-third, will not remain in mainstream schooling. A much smaller proportion, in the UK less than 1% of children with epilepsy, attend the epilepsy special centers or schools.

The results of these studies raise some interesting questions both with regard to additional input for children attending mainstream schooling and in relation to the provision in the special centers. In particular, they suggest that a larger proportion of children might benefit from specialist reassessment of the effect of epilepsy on learning, although the type and extent of such a reassessment in each case deserves further consideration. The reasons for referral to an epilepsy specialist centre and the ways in which the center might be of value are discussed in the following sections.

REASONS FOR REFERRAL

The possible reasons for referral to a residential epilepsy special school have been discussed elsewhere (Besag, 1986, 1988a, 1988b, 1995). They are summarized in Tables 26.1 and 26.2.

A distinction must be made between a **residential** center for children with epilepsy, offering the possibility of intensive, medium-term or long-term multidisciplinary intervention, and **outpatient** services, which are sometimes also referred to as centers. An example of the latter would be the 'Epilepsy Center' recently formed by drawing together a number of experienced people in the field from the Maudsley and King's College Hospitals, London and St Piers Lingfield. Although the range of expertise assembled in this 'center' is impressive, the service is currently mainly based at two London teaching hospitals. The close cooperation between the various members of the team is considered to be of great value. The way in which this 'center' will use residential facilities remains to be determined.

Most of the following comments will refer to the four residential centres for childhood epilepsy in the UK, listed in Table 26.3.

There are certain factors which distinguish these residential special schools for epilepsy from other facilities. As would be expected, the emphasis is on allowing the child to take a full part in educational and social activities,

Table 26.1 Problems leading to referral

Difficult epilepsy
Other medical
Cognitive
Behavioral
Peer group
Family and social
Psychiatric
Multiple

Table 26.2 Difficult epilepsy

Frequent seizures
Injury in seizures
Risk of status epilepticus
Variable seizure frequency
Postictal disturbances
Antiepileptic drug problems
Inadequate control
Difficult to recognize epilepsy

Table 26.3 Residential centres for epilepsy in the UK

The Park Hospital, Oxford
Outpatient services, short- and medium-term
  intensive inpatient assessment

The David Lewis Centre, Cheshire
Medium-term intensive assessment in a
  designated assessment centre and long-term
  placements

St Elizabeth's School, Much Hadham,
  Hertfordshire
Most placements are long term

St Piers, Lingfield, Surrey
Medium-term and long-term placements. Children
  accepted for intensive assessment

---

together with a suitable peer group. A strong emphasis is also placed on relationships with the community, both locally and further afield. Although this does not differ, in principle, from what should happen in any other school, the training and experience of the staff, together with the specialist medical back-up, in the special center, allow access to a broader curriculum and a much wider range of activities to children with severe or problematic epilepsy.

A further important distinction should be drawn in relation to antiepileptic drug reviews carried out in such a center. The concept of admitting a child to hospital for 2 or 3 weeks to 'sort out their antiepileptic drugs' often has little basis in reality. A common situation is that the child enters hospital and, because of the changed environment, the seizures improve. The professionals are then puzzled about how to proceed. The child is discharged 2 or 3 weeks later and the seizures recommence. The exercise has been counterproductive by raising the expectations of the family, only to dash them again, and by disrupting the child's routine by admitting him to hospital. The residential center, in contrast, has the opportunity of observing the child in a number of different situations over a period of some weeks before instituting any changes. In general, assessment of changes in antiepileptic drug cannot be hurried. Although some children will respond immediately to a drug change, others may take several weeks. Sometimes drugs may take 2 months or more before they are effective. On occasions a child may continue with severe epilepsy for several weeks and then suddenly respond, even becoming seizure-free. A hasty judgment about the efficacy of the drug in such circumstances could lead to conclusions which were quite wrong and the child might be denied the opportunity of improving. In theory, it might be possible to admit a child to a hospital ward for several months to carry out such changes. However, it is difficult to provide a sufficiently 'normal' environment for the child, offering the full range of facilities he or she requires, in the hospital setting. These facilities should include education, recreation, leisure, a peer group, and much opportunity for interaction with the world outside.

Any epilepsy center, whether residential or not, should offer an interdisciplinary approach capable of assessing the whole child. The epilepsy often forms only part of the problem. To ignore the other aspects is to give poor service to the child and the family. Again, these matters have been discussed well elsewhere (Taylor, 1979; Chapter 25).

The epilepsy center can also fulfil a role in the presurgical assessment and the post-surgical rehabilitation of children undergoing epilepsy neurosurgery. Abolition of seizures may imply a major change in life-role. Some children and teenagers find it very difficult to come to terms with this and require much support. If the child has been in a dependent role for many years and is suddenly expected to take responsibility, the outcome may be traumatic unless the appropriate support is provided.

In the future it is anticipated that the childhood epilepsy centers might be used much more for short-term assessment and intervention, including the preparation for and aftercare of epilepsy surgery. The tendency has been to consider recommending that a child should attend an epilepsy center only if the epilepsy has been severe for many years and if there has been a major failure to progress, either in terms of response to treatment or in educational and social development. There is a place for a different model of referral, in which the child is referred early when the epilepsy **begins** to interfere in a major way with quality of life and as soon as it is clear that the problem is unlikely to be solved rapidly using local services. It is anticipated that such a child might stay in a center for approximately 6–12 months, during which a major antiepileptic drug review could be undertaken. Even if the review were not complete at the end of that period, there would be a good chance that it would be so advanced that the plan could be continued in the community. Towards the end of the assessment period a multi-disciplinary case review is recommended. This gives all concerned the opportunity to document the child's special needs, taking into account the effect of any interventions which have taken place at the epilepsy center, and to plan for the future. In difficult cases, in which the epilepsy has proved highly resistant to intervention or when there are other major problems, longer-term placement might be considered to be appropriate. This model of medium-term assessment is already available in some of the childhood epilepsy centers in the UK.

The centers also have a major role to play in research. For example, research on new antiepileptic drugs can be conducted much more safely when children are observed 24 hours a day in an establishment which has an on-site doctor, with full EEG and nursing facilities. The epilepsy centers have provided the basis for important research into drug treatment, cognitive changes and behavioral disturbance in children with epilepsy, leading to a number of key publications over recent years.

A further important role of the epilepsy centers is to provide teaching for other professionals. The recent trend in the UK has been for the centers to join with the epilepsy associations in holding courses for teachers, general practitioners, hospital doctors, and other staff who have responsibility for the management of children with epilepsy. It is important that the specialist knowledge gained at these centers is shared.

OUTCOME

The major changes in the pattern of referral of children and young people with epilepsy to the epilepsy centers make it difficult to make global statements about outcome. In previous years a much larger proportion of children with epilepsy were referred to such centers. Employment rates in the general population were also higher. Consequently the outcome was relatively good, against the background of relatively poor outcome for people with epilepsy in general (e.g. Harrison and Taylor, 1976). In recent years, the tendency has been to refer only children and young people with particularly difficult epilepsy. These young people often had other special needs which prevented most of them entering open employment, for example, additional brain abnormalities, learning disability or other medical conditions. The current suggestion is that the epilepsy center should be used more for short-term assessments and rehabilitation, including those related to epilepsy surgery. If this becomes accepted, with the result that children are referred earlier and stay for relatively short periods, the outcome should be particularly good. There is relatively little chance of a good outcome if a child is referred after years of neurologic, educational and social damage from recurrent bouts of inadequately treated, prolonged status epilepticus, as has been the case all too often in the past.

CONCLUSIONS

Most children with epilepsy should attend a mainstream school and do not need the services of a special center. However, it is important to recognize that a large proportion of children with epilepsy, approximately half of the total number, will have some educational difficulty and professionals should be prepared to offer the additional support that such children require within the community. A relatively small proportion will require the specialist services of an epilepsy center. Past trends of waiting until the child and family had suffered many years of severe epilepsy, fragmented education and grossly restricted quality of life should certainly be discouraged. Early recognition of problematic epilepsy, coupled with early referral, intensive assessment and appropriate specialist management, should allow the child a much better chance of returning to the local community and re-establishing a satisfactory quality of life.

REFERENCES

Besag, F.M.C. (1986) The role of the special centres for children with epilepsy, in *Symposium on Epilepsy and Education, Royal College of Physicians*, (eds J. Oxley and G. Stores), Education in Practice, Medical Tribune Group, pp. 65–71.

Besag, F.M.C. (1988a) Schooling the child with epilepsy. *The Royal College of General Practitioners Members' Reference Book*, Royal College of General Practitioners, London, pp. 370–2.

Besag, F.M.C. (1988b) Which school for the child with epilepsy? *MED*, 2(2), 16–17.

Besag, F.M.C. (1994) Epilepsy, education and the role of mental handicap, in *Epilepsy* (eds E. Ross and R. Wood), Ballière's Clinical Paediatrics, Ballière Tindall, London pp.561–84.

Ellenberg, J.H., Hirtz, D.G. and Nelson, K.B. (1985) Do seizures in children cause intellectual deterioration? *Annals of Neurology*, 18, 389.

Grant, R.H. (1981) Special centres, in *Epilepsy and Psychiatry* (eds E.H. Reynolds and M.R. Trimble), Churchill-Livingstone, Edinburgh pp. 347–61.

Green, J.B. and Hartlage, L.C. (1971) Comparative performance of epileptic and non-epileptic children and adolescents. *Diseases of the Nervous System*, 32, 418–21.

Harrison, R. and Taylor, D. (1976) Childhood seizures: a 25-year follow-up. Social and medical prognosis. *Lancet*, i, 948–51.

Holdsworth, L. and Whitmore, K. (1974) A study of children with epilepsy attending ordinary schools. I: Their seizure patterns, progress and behaviour in school. *Developmental Medicine and Child Neurology*, 16, 759–65.

Kurtz, Z., Tookey, P. and Ross, E. (1987) The epidemiology of epilepsy in childhood, in *Epilepsy in Young People* (eds E. Ross, D. Chadwick and R. Crawford), John Wiley, Chichester, pp. 13–21.

Laidlaw, J. and Laidlaw, M.V. (1982) in *A Textbook of Epilepsy*, 2nd edn (eds J. Laidlaw and A. Richens), Churchill Livingstone, Edinburgh, pp. 513–44.

Ounsted, C., Lindsay, J. and Norman, R. (1966) Biological factors in temporal lobe epilepsy, in *Clinics in Developmental Medicine*, no. 22, Spastics Society/Heinemann Medical, London.

Pazzaglia, P. and Frank-Pazzaglia, L. (1976) Record in grade school of pupils with epilepsy: an epidemiological study. *Epilepsia*, 17, 361–6.

Pond, D. and Bidwell, B. (1960) A survey of epilepsy in fourteen general practices. II Social and psychological aspects. *Epilepsia*, 1, 285–99.

Reid, J.J.A. (Chairman) (1969) Central Health Services Council, Advisory Committee on the Health and Welfare of Handicapped Persons, in *People with Epilepsy. Report of a Joint Sub-Committee of the Standing Medical Advisory Committee and the Advisory Committee on the Health and Welfare of Handicapped Persons*, HMSO, London.

Ross, E.M., Peckham, C.S., West, P.B. and Butler, N.R. (1980), Epilepsy in childhood: findings from the National Child Development Study. *British Medical Journal*, 1, 207–10.

Rutter, M., Graham, P. and Yule, W. (1970) A neuropsychiatric study in childhood, in *Clinics in Developmental Medicine*, Nos 35/36 SIMP, Heinemann Medical, London.

Sillanpää, M. (1983) Social functioning and seizure status of young adults with onset of epilepsy in childhood. An epidemiological 20-year follow-up study. *Acta Neurologica Scandinavica*, 68(96), 1–81.

Sillanpää, M. (1990) Prognosis of children with epilepsy, in *Paediatric Epilepsy* (eds M. Sillanpää, S.I. Johanessen, G. Blennow and M. Dam), Wrightson Biomedical, Petersfield, pp. 341–68.

Sillanpää, M. (1992) Epilepsy in children: pre-valence, disability and handicap, *Epilepsia*, **33**, 444–9.

Stores, G. (1971) Cognitive function in children with epilepsy. *Developmental Medicine and Child Neurology*, **13**, 390–3.

Stores, G. (1977) Behaviour disturbance and type of epilepsy in children attending ordinary school, in *Epilepsy: Proceedings of the Eighth International Symposium* (ed. J.K. Penry), Raven, New York, pp. 245–9.

Stores, G. (1978) School-children with epilepsy at risk for learning and behaviour problems. *Developmental Medicine and Child Neurology*, **20**, 502–8.

Stores, G. (1981) Problems of learning and behaviour in children with epilepsy, in *Epilepsy and Psychiatry*, Churchill Livingstone, London, pp. 33–48.

Stores, G. and Hart, J. (1976) Reading skills of children with generalised or focal epilepsy attending ordinary school. *Developmental Medicine and Child Neurology*, **18**, 705–16.

Stores, G., Hart, J.A. and Piran, N. (1978), Inattentiveness in school children with epilepsy. *Epilepsia*, **19**, 169–75.

Taylor, D.C. (1979) The components of sickness: diseases, illnesses and predicaments. *Lancet*, **ii**, 1008–10.

Verity, C.M. and Ross E.M. (1985), Longitudinal studies of children's epilepsy, in *Paediatric Perspectives on Epilepsy* (eds E.M. Ross and E.H. Reynolds), John Wiley, Chichester, pp. 133–40.

Warnock Report (1978) Special educational needs, in *Report of the Committee of Enquiry into the Education of Handicapped Children and Young People*, HMSO, London.

Winterton, P.M.C. (Chairman) (1986) *Report of the Working Group on Services for People with Epilepsy. A Report to the Department of Health and Social Security, The Department of Education and Science and the Welsh Office*. HMSO, London.

EPILEPSY CONTINUING INTO ADULTHOOD

27

David Chadwick

INTRODUCTION

The prevalence of epilepsy during adolescence is greater than during childhood (Hauser and Hesdorfer, 1990), and the success or otherwise of treatment during the second decade of life is likely to have a formidable impact on the consequences of epilepsy through the rest of life. Thus the literature on epilepsy in adolescence and its psychosocial consequences is surprisingly limited when compared with the quantities of information available on epilepsy in childhood and in adult life.

The poverty of literature is mirrored by a lack of provision of specialized services for adolescents. At a time in their lives when their own needs and ambitions are changing rapidly, adolescents with epilepsy often find themselves transferred from a highly integrated pediatric service with direct links with community and educational services, to an adult service which is less well integrated and has less time to address their specific needs.

This chapter briefly reviews those epilepsies that continue into adult life and the problems that are particularly relevant to adolescents, and makes some suggestions for the management of these difficulties.

EPILEPSY SYNDROMES CONTINUING INTO ADULT LIFE

A systematic classification of epilepsy syndromes has been proposed (Commission on Classification and Terminology of the International Leauge Against Epilepsy, 1989). Most epilepsy syndromes are age related and occur for the first time in childhood, whilst the majority of the epilepsies with onset in adult life are symptomatic partial epilepsies. For this reason the classification of epilepsy syndromes has less relevance to adults in whom accurate localization of the onset of partial seizures and determination of their etiology is of greater importance. Those specific epilepsy syndromes where seizures tend to continue into adult life, are of major importance to the current discussion.

IDIOPATHIC GENERALIZED EPILEPSIES

Childhood absence epilepsy (see also Chapter 13a)

This syndrome accounts for about 8% of epilepsy in school age children (Cavazzuti, 1980). Between 33% (Oller-Daurella and Sanchez, 1981) and 80% (Dalby, 1969) of those with childhood absence epilepsy (CAE) achieve long-term remission. Figures at the lower range of these estimates include patients followed up for longer periods. Approximately 6% of patients with CAE have absences which persist into adult life (Oller-Daurella and Sanchez, 1981). Tonic-clonic seizures, however, commonly de-

Epilepsy in Children. Edited by Sheila Wallace. Published in 1996 by Chapman & Hall, London. ISBN 0 412 56860 8

velop, usually between 5 and 10 years after the onset of absences (Loiseau *et al.*, 1983). Varying lengths of follow-up make it difficult to determine the exact proportion developing tonic-clonic seizures, but between 40% (Loiseau *et al.*, 1983) and 60% of patients (Oller-Daurella and Sanchez, 1981) can be affected. There is some evidence that tonic-clonic seizures are more likely to develop in subjects whose absences initially respond poorly to appropriate antiepileptic drug therapy (Oller-Daurella and Sanchez, 1981).

When tonic-clonic seizures occur in subjects with CAE persisting to adulthood, they occur without an aura and usually present within 1–2 hours of wakening. Sodium valproate is undoubtedly the drug of choice for the treatment of persisting seizures in adults with this syndrome (Loiseau, 1985).

The idiopathic epilepsies of adolescence

Three specific age-related syndromes share many similarities and may potentially be regarded as different phenotypic presentations of what may be a single genetic disorder. They are juvenile myoclonic epilepsy, juvenile absence epilepsy, and epilepsy with tonic-clonic seizures on awakening (Chapter 14a, b, c). All tend to commence after puberty but rarely commence after the age of 20–25, are strongly associated with spike-wave activity (4–6 Hz) and are characterized by seizures most prominent on wakening and often precipitated by sleep deprivation.

Juvenile absence epilepsy

Juvenile absence epilepsy (JAE) is much less common than CAE. Absence seizures begin in the second decade of life but tend to be much less frequent than those of CAE. A greater proportion (80%) also have tonic-clonic seizures, of which 75% occur on awakening (Janz and Christian, 1957; Janz, 1969). Myoclonic seizures can also be present in this syndrome (Wolf and Inoue, 1984).

Valproate is again the drug of choice, with remission in 85% of patients (Wolf and Inoue, 1984). The small proportion of patients with only absence seizures will almost certainly remit with appropriate therapy.

Juvenile myoclonic epilepsy

Juvenile myoclonic epilepsy (JME) accounts for approximately 6% of the epilepsies. Seizures can begin between the ages of 8 and 26, but 80% commence between the ages of 12 and 18 (Janz, 1969). Myoclonic jerks are usually symmetric and mostly affect the upper limbs. Myoclonus can on occasion be associated with absences, or typical absence seizures can occur independently. Seizures most commonly occur after wakening, but there may also be a second peak in seizure susceptibility during the evening. Sleep deprivation appears to be a potent provocative factor for seizures.

Ninety per cent of patients have generalized tonic-clonic seizures; 10% of patients may have absence seizures. However, usually, the tonic-clonic seizures precipitate medical referral; patients may not recognize the important association with jerks which may have preceded the first tonic-clonic seizure by some time. It is important in identifying this syndrome to ask specifically for a history of myoclonus, particularly soon after awakening.

The EEG typically shows polyspike and spike-wave activity at a more rapid rate than the classic 3 cycle/second spike-wave (Janz, 1969). Photosensitivity is common and usually identified in about 30% of patients, though this phenomenon may frequently be blocked by treatment with valproate (Goosses, 1984). Valproate is the drug of choice in JME. Indeed, remission may be uncommon if patients are treated with other antiepileptic drugs (Delgado-Escueta and Enrile-Bascal, 1984). Remissions of JME are drug dependent: 90% of patients with it will relapse if drugs are withdrawn (Janz *et al.*, 1983).

Tonic-clonic seizures on awakening

Tonic-clonic (or clonic-tonic-clonic) seizures predominate in this syndrome, though the presence of occasional myoclonus or absence does not preclude the diagnosis. Janz (1962) examined the timing of tonic-clonic seizures in 2825 patients; 33% had tonic-clonic seizures on awakening compared to 44% occurring during sleep and 23% occurring at random. There was a strong association between tonic-clonic seizures occurring on wakening and generalized spike-wave activity in the EEG.

Precipitating factors seem particularly important. Sleep deprivation and alcohol intake are relevant precipitants, but sudden arousal from sleep and catamenial seizures are also prominent factors.

Avoidance of precipitating factors is important in management, and valproate is probably the drug of choice for this syndrome. The occurrence of seizures on wakening seems to increase the risk of relapse if drugs are withdrawn after a period of remission (Janz *et al.*, 1983; MRC Antiepileptic Drug Withdrawal Study Group, 1991).

SYMPTOMATIC GENERALIZED EPILEPSIES

These childhood epilepsies are frequently malignant and are associated with a significant mortality. However, many children with such epilepsies will survive into the adult age range. They are frequently mentally handicapped and may also have motor disability (cerebral palsy). In adult life there is often a change in the nature of seizures with myoclonic, tonic, atonic, and complex absence seizures becoming less frequent, whereas more typical simple partial and complex partial seizures become evident. These seizures characteristically appear multifocal from a clinical and electroencephalographic point of view. Although such patients may continue to have severe epilepsy during adult life, seizure frequency tends to be less than in childhood.

PARTIAL (LOCALIZATION-RELATED) EPILEPSIES

The idiopathic age-related syndromes (eg. Rolandic epilepsy) are not seen in adult life as they have an early age of onset in childhood and a uniformly excellent prognosis. In contrast, many of the most difficult epilepsies of adult life are those partial (often symptomatic) epilepsies which have their onset in childhood but do not enter significant remission. The international classification divides symptomatic epilepsies into frontal, temporal, parietal, and occipital lobe epilepsies, on the grounds of the site of origin of the seizures. This adds little further help or information to classifying a patient's seizures.

ADOLESCENTS WITH EPILEPSY

Epilepsy is the most common neurologic problem in adolescence (Cooper, 1965; Castle and Fishman, 1973), and during this critical period of development, its effect may include behavioral problems, noncompliance with medication and psychosocial difficulties (McKinlay, 1987). Young people with epilepsy may be particularly susceptible to the psychosocial effects of epilepsy and its impact is not necessarily related to the frequency or severity of the seizure disorder (Thornton, 1987). A number of studies of adolescents with epilepsy have demonstrated several problem areas, including: absence of friendships; difficulties within the family; difficulties with peer relationships; poor self-confidence, self-esteem and social adjustment, and depressive feelings (Richardson and Freidman, 1974; Freeman *et al.*, 1984; Dorenbaum *et al.*, 1985; Viberg, Blennow and Polski, 1987).

Adolescence is a period of development where the young adult seeks to become more autonomous, more independent from the family, to develop more intimate relationships, and strives to establish roles in work and society. The constraints for adolescents with epilepsy are numerous and include restrictions on driving, leisure activities, career options, and opportunities for engaging in social relationships. The impact of epilepsy can thus severely impede the natural process of entering adulthood (Pellock, 1991). If the burden of epilepsy is heavily felt, then adolescence may represent a critical period of confusion, rather than of normal development.

Taylor (1969) has argued that the need to conform and identify with one's peer groups is essential during adolescence. Being different may have significant consequences in terms of social isolation, self-esteem, and self-awareness. Comparison with a peer group is an important source of evaluating self-worth and self-image. Having epilepsy during adolescence can only serve to remind the individual of differences and subsequently impede the natural process of 'growing up'. Unfortunately, normal adolescent behavior that includes drinking and irregular patterns of sleeping may precipitate seizures. The restrictions of such activities may result in the adolescent being more isolated from his or her peer group and subsequently lead to anxiety and depression.

The implications of being perceived to be treated differently or actually being treated differently have been well documented (Scambler, 1989), but the relationship between stigma and psychosocial functioning requires further investigation. One recent study which investigated the relationship between stigma and self-esteem in adolescents (Westbrook, Bauman and Shirinar, 1992) using a multivariate approach showed that the belief that epilepsy is stigmatizing predicted low self-esteem.

Coming to terms with epilepsy is a problem for people with epilepsy of all ages, but has different significance for the adolescent who also faces the challenge of leaving school, finding and starting work, and striving for independence. It is not surprising, therefore, that some adolescents will have difficulty in coping with these demands. Denial of the disorder is one of the strategies adolescents may adopt; dissociating themselves from the management of their epilepsy is another. Noncompliance with medication is a recognized problem in this age group, as is the increased incidence of psychosomatic complaints and psychiatric disorders (Goodyer, Kolvin and Gatzanis, 1985).

Sexual development and sexual identity are of considerable concern for the adolescent with epilepsy (Betts, 1992). Knowledge of sexual development and sexual behavior is often lacking among adolescents with poorly controlled epilepsy and this may, in part, be the consequence of parental overprotection (Thompson and Oxley, 1992). The need for education about sexual development is important in adolescence, independent of whether the individual has epilepsy or not. There is some evidence that adolescents with epilepsy may have heightened concerns about sexual performance (Strang, 1987). Betts (1992) suggests that the most frequent concerns for people with epilepsy are lack of practise due to social isolation and fear of having a seizure during intercourse: behavioral programming and counseling appear to be effective in the treatment of these concerns.

Viberg, Blennow and Polski (1987) compared personality and development in adolescents with epilepsy to that of normal control subjects, and found significant differences in a number of areas. The authors used interviews to investigate self-esteem and personality traits in 16 patients with epilepsy and 16 controls. The patients with epilepsy were found to have a greater discrepancy between their actual and ideal self-images than the controls. They also reported poor self and body images and had less stable sexual identities. Most described their seizures as frightening and said that their relatives were also frightened. They also found it difficult to discuss their epilepsy with other adolescents for fear of a negative reaction. The authors conclude that adolescents with epilepsy, regardless of the frequency or severity of their seizures, are often disturbed in their basic trust of their bodies and themselves. Hodgman *et al.* (1979) found low self-esteem and poor expectation for the future in adolescents with epilepsy, particularly in those without associated neurologic deficits.

When onset of epilepsy occurs in adolescence, schooling is often interrupted and the stress experienced during intensive study periods or examinations may provoke seizures. Adolescence is an important time for embarking on a career path, and epilepsy can delay or diminish career opportunities. A recent study by Elwes *et al.* (1991) found that people with epilepsy were less likely to leave school with formal qualifications or to undergo subsequent training apprenticeships.

While there exist clear limitations on employment opportunities for people with epilepsy, legislation does provide for special employment services. In the UK the Manpower Services Commission provides a full range of services for disabled people to which adolescents with epilepsy have full entitlement (Edwards, Espir and Oxley, 1986). In addition, the 1981 Education Act ensures that early recognition of educational needs are identified and specialist services are provided to maximize employment prospects. The efficacy of this legislation in securing or improving employment prospects for adolescents with epilepsy remains uncertain.

In conclusion there is a considerable evidence of emotional disturbance among adolescents with epilepsy. The way in which adolescents adjust to epilepsy will depend on a number of complex factors. As yet little is understood of this process, or of how some adolescents are successfully able to minimize the impact.

ADDRESSING THE NEEDS OF THE ADOLESCENT WITH EPILEPSY

The changing needs of the adolescent with epilepsy demand as integrated an approach to the clinical, psychological and social problems created by epilepsy as that in childhood. Unfortunately, these needs are rarely met, and the adolescent is transferred from a holistic pediatric system of care to one that is orientated towards more strictly clinical care of adults, often with the acceptance and expectation that epilepsy will be lifelong and associated with psychosocial deprivation. In spite of the fundamental importance for this period of life in determining long-term success or failure in employment and social relationships, the special needs of the adolescent are rarely addressed.

OPTIMIZING SEIZURE CONTROL

Whilst in childhood many pediatricians feel able to accept less than optimal control of seizures in order to avoid any untoward effects of antiepileptic drugs on learning and behavior, in adolescents a much greater emphasis needs to be put on the best possible control of seizures. An adolescent epilepsy service therefore needs to reassess the management of an individual's epilepsy. It is essential to review the diagnosis of epilepsy and ensure that both seizures and epilepsy syndromes are satisfactorily classified, and that the most appropriate drug therapy is being used. It is the author's experience that, largely due to the restricted number of pediatric neurologists practising in the UK, many adolescents have been misdiagnosed, or not given adequate trials of those antiepileptic drugs likely to be most effective. While families often have very fixed ideas about adverse effects of some antiepileptic drugs used previously during childhood, the same drug in adolescence may have a radically different outcome.

Another area in which reappraisal of the diagnosis may be important is that of pseudo-seizures (see Chapters 2, 25). Such non-epileptic attacks most commonly develop in the late teenage years. On occasions, children with a history of epilepsy may develop pseudo-seizures at this time as a means of negotiating their way through the changing demands and expectations from their family and peers.

The issue of compliance must also be discussed with the adolescent and his or her family. The individual needs to be encouraged to take responsibility for his or her own management. In particular, the importance of taking antiepileptic drugs on a regular basis and the problems that are likely to develop if good compliance is not maintained must be understood.

The final method of management to be considered in the adolescent is surgical treatment where there is clear evidence of intractability (see Chapter 23d). The outcomes for temporal lobe surgery, in particular, are now so satisfactory, with most centers achieving 70–80% cure rates, that any young person with intractable partial epilepsy should have the opportunity of a full presurgical evaluation at this time in their life. The literature on psychosocial outcome of surgical treatment emphasizes that very few mature adults undergoing surgical treatment of epilepsy find employment for the first time or make up any acquired deficit in social skills, even if their seizures are completely controlled. To have maximum impact surgical treatment of epilepsy needs to be targeted very clearly at the adolescent age group, or earlier.

ADDRESSING THE INFORMATIONAL NEEDS OF ADOLESCENTS

The chief concern of most adolescents shifts from schooling to the possibility of future employment and a career. It is vital that adolescents receive sensible, realistic, but supportive advice on such matters from the careers services, disablement resettlement officers, and their doctors. Certain occupa-

tions and professions may be closed to people with epilepsy. These would include vocational driving, the police and armed services. However, many other careers can be pursued with success as long as inappropriate restrictions are avoided and a sensible method of disclosure is used (Thompson and Oxley, 1992). Too often, young people with epilepsy encounter ill-informed opinions about epilepsy from those running employment training schemes and from employers. It is important that young people with epilepsy have a clear-cut goal that is appropriate to their own skills and talents and compatible with a realistic estimate of seizure control. The definition of such a goal requires sensitive and sensible input and discussion, and most particularly good advice about filling in application forms.

It is the author's practice to advise people not to complete any medical section of a first application form for employment. This is best left blank. However, it must be emphasized that if a firm job offer is made, epilepsy must be disclosed, along with a reassurance that a medical reference is available from someone with genuine expertise in the area of epilepsy. An optimal code of practice for assessing medical aspects of fitness to work has been adopted in the British Civil Service and should be more widely applied (Espir, Semmence and Floyd, 1987).

Providing information about driving regulations is very important. For the young person with a relatively mild or well-controlled epilepsy, obtaining a driving licence may be a major goal and one which can be beneficial for both employment prospects and the individual's own self-esteem. There are often areas of confusion in the regulations related to epilepsy during sleep, and, whether antiepileptic drugs have to be discontinued before driving can commence, which need to be discussed.

For young women with epilepsy the effects of their epilepsy and its drug treatment on contraception and pregnancy need a full discussion. The interaction between enzyme-inducing antiepileptic drugs such as carbamazepine and phenytoin and oral contraceptives must be emphasized, as should the small risks of teratogenicity associated with antiepileptic drugs. The desire for future drug-free pregnancies may be one important reason for discussing the possibility of discontinuation of antiepileptic drugs after any significant period of remission of epilepsy. Equally, young women need to have the offer of preconceptual counseling so as to optimize any essential drug therapy prior to pregnancy and to ensure that preconceptual folate is administered to reduce the small risk of neural tube defects.

Overall, adolescents and their families need considerable help and support in allowing young people to develop independence and personality. Inevitably, there are always parental concerns about demands for increasing freedom. However, the ability to pursue independent activity is so important at this age that a sensible approach to risk-taking in everyday life has many benefits.

In order to address the needs of adolescents with epilepsy, we have, in Liverpool, developed an adolescent epilepsy clinic which is run jointly by an adult neurologist and pediatric neurologist. Most patients are referred between the ages of 14 and 16 and continue to attend the clinic up to the age of 18 before their care is taken over by the adult clinic. This system allows a more satisfactory continuity of care throughout this difficult period and a more effective communication between the clinicians involved concerning the past problems of childhood and the future challenges of adult life. There is invaluable support from an epilepsy nurse specialist whose skills are particularly important in addressing the complex informational needs of the adolescent with epilepsy. While the effectiveness of this system has not been formally tested, we believe that it has been successful in offering an improved quality of care for adolescents with epilepsy, and that it is a model that could be adopted more widely.

REFERENCES

Betts, T.A. (1992) Neuropsychiatry, in *A Textbook of Epilepsy*, 3rd edn (eds J. Laidlaw, A. Richens and D. Chadwick), Churchill Livingstone, Edinburgh, pp. 397–457.

Castle, G.F. and Fishman, L.S. (1973) Seizures in adolescent medicine. *Pediatric Clinics of North America*, **20**, 819–35.

Cavazzuti, G.B. (1980) Epidemiology of different types of epilepsy in school-age children of Modena, Italy. *Epilepsia*, **21**, 57–62.

Commission on Classification and Terminology of the International League Against Epilepsy (1989) Proposal for revised classification of epilepsies and epileptic syndromes. *Epilepsia*, **30**, 389–99.

Cooper, J.E. (1965) Epilepsy in a longitudinal survey of 5000 children. *British Medical Journal*, **1**, 1020–2.

Dalby, M.A. (1969) Epilepsy and 3 per second spike and wave rhythms. A clinical, electroencephalographic and prognostic analysis of 346 patients. *Acta Neurologica Scandinavica*, **45**(suppl.), 40.

Delgado-Escueta, A.V. and Enrile-Bascal, F. (1984) Juvenile myoclonic epilepsy of Janz. *Neurology*, **34**, 285–94.

Dorenbaum, D., Cappelli, M.C., Keene, D. and McGrath, P.J. (1985) Use of a child behaviour checklist in the psychosocial assessment of children with epilepsy. *Clinical Pediatrics*, **24**, 634–7.

Edwards, F., Espir, M. and Oxley, J. (1986) *Epilepsy and Employment: A Medical Symposium on Current Problems and Best Practices*, Royal Society of Medicine Services, London.

Elwes, R.D.C., Marshall, J., Beattie, A. and Newman, P.K. (1991) Epilepsy and unemployment: a community based survey in an area of high unemployment. *Journal of Neurology, Neurosurgery and Psychiatry*, **54**, 200–3.

Espir, M., Semmence, A. and Floyd, M. (1987) The recruitment to the Civil Service of people with epilepsy. *Journal of the Society of Occupational Medicine*, **37**, 16–8.

Freeman, J.M., Jacob, S.H., Vining, E. and Rabin,

C.E. (1984) Epilepsy and inner city schools: a school-based program that makes a difference. *Epilepsia*, **25**, 438–42.

Goodyer, I.M., Kolvin, I. and Gatzanis, S. (1985) Recent undesirable life events and psychiatric disorder in childhood and adolescence. *British Journal of Psychiatry*, **147**, 517–23.

Goosses, R. (1984) *Die Beziehung der Fotosensibilitat zu den verschiedenen epileptischen Syndromen.* University of West Berlin. Thesis.

Hauser, W.A. and Hesdorfer, D.H. (1990) *Epilepsy: Frequency, Causes and Consequences*, Demos, New York.

Hodgman, C.H., McAnarney, E.R., Myers, G. *et al.* (1979) Emotional complications of adolescent grand mal epilepsy. *Journal of Pediatrics*, **95**, 309–12.

Janz, D. (1962) The grand-mal epilepsies and the sleeping-waking cycle. *Epilepsia*, **3**, 69–109.

Janz, D. (1969) *Die Epilepsien*, Thieme, Stuttgart.

Janz, D. and Christian, W. (1957) Inpulsiv-petit mal. *Journal of Neurology*, **176**, 346–86.

Janz, D. Kern, A. Mossinger, H.J. and Puhlmann, U. (1993) Rückfall-prognose nach Reduktion der Medikamente bei Epilsiebehandlung. *Nervenarzt*, **54**, 525–9.

Loiseau, P. (1985) Childhood absence epilepsy, in *Epileptic Syndromes in Infancy, Childhood and Adolescence* (eds J. Roger, C. Dravet, M. Bureau *et al.*), John Libbey, London, p.106–20.

Loiseau, P., Pestre, M., Dartigues, J.F., *et al.* (1983) Long-term prognosis in two forms of childhood epilepsy; typical absence seizures and epilepsy with rolandic (centrotemporal) EEG foci. *Annals of Neurology*, **13**, 642–8.

McKinlay, I. (1987) Epilepsy care: the problem of the child to adult, in *Epilepsy in Young People* (eds. E. Ross, D. Chadwick and C. Crawford), John Wiley, Chichester.

MRC Antiepileptic Drug Withdrawal Study Group (1991) Randomized study of antiepileptic drug withdrawal in patients in remission. *Lancet*, **337**, 1175–80.

Oller-Daurella, L. and Sanchez, M.E. (1981) Evolucion de las ausencias tipicas. *Revue Neurologique (Barcelona)*, **9**, 81–102.

Pellock, J. (1991) The adolescent female with epilepsy, in *Women and Epilepsy* (ed. M.R. Trimble), John Wiley, Chichester, pp. 87–106.

Richardson, D.W. and Freidman, S.B. (1974) Psychosocial problems and the adolescent patient with epilepsy. *Clinical Paediatrics*, **13**, 121–6.

Scambler, G. (1989) *Epilepsy*, Tavistock, London.

Strang, J. (1987) Medical aspects of learning problems in children with epilepsy, In *Epilepsy and Education* (eds J. Oxley and G. Stores), Medical Tribune Group, London, pp. 25–30.

Taylor, D. (1969) Aggression and epilepsy. *Journal of Psychosomatic Research*, **13**, 229–36.

Thompson, P. and Oxley, J. (1992) Social aspects of epilepsy, in *A Textbook of Epilepsy*, 4th edn (eds J. Laidlaw, A. Richens and D. Chadwick), Churchill Livingstone, Edinburgh, pp. 667–704.

Thornton, L. (1987) Personal relationships, in *Epilepsy in Young People* (eds E. Ross, D. Chadwick and C. Crawford), John Wiley, Chichester.

Viberg, M., Blennow, G. and Polski, B. (1987) Epilepsy in adolescence: implications for the development of personality. *Epilepsia*, **28**, 542–6.

Westbrook, L.E., Bauman, L.J., and Shinnar, S. (1992) Applying stigma theory to epilepsy: a test of a conceptual model. *Journal of Pediatric Psychology*, **17**, 133–49.

Wolf, P. and Inoue, Y. (1984) Therapeutic response of absence seizures in patients of an epilepsy clinic for adolescents and adults. *Journal of Neurology*, **231**, 225–9.

Index

Note: abbreviations used are as explained on pages xix–xxii.